MW01105199

ORTHOTADS
The Clinical Guide and Atlas

What the EXPERTS *are saying about OrthoTADs...*

ORTHODONTICS

I have been in the writing and publishing field for a lifetime, but this volume is truly a once-in-a lifetime experience and it will have a significant impact on the profession. Kudos to Dr. Cope and his team!

—Tom Graber, Editor-in-Chief,
World Journal of Orthodontics

The practicing clinician has sorely needed a text that provides a step-by-step approach for TAD implementation. I can't imagine any orthodontist not having and using this text on a frequent basis.

—Larry White, past Editor
Journal of Clinical Orthodontics

This excellent collection of basic information, accompanied by a generous dose of clinical cases, is arriving at precisely the right time. Congratulations to Dr. Cope for being in front of the curve.

—Robert J. Isaacson, Editor
The Angle Orthodontist

This book will soon become a necessity for every orthodontist in search of the broad-based experience reflected so well by the experts who have contributed to this textbook.

—David L. Turpin, Editor-in-Chief
American Journal of Orthodontics & Dentofacial Orthopedics

This text is a 'must have' for practitioners of modern orthodontics. It will, without doubt, be a signature reference for Temporary Anchorage Devices in Orthodontics.

—P. Lionel Sadowsky, Editor
Seminars in Orthodontics

It is gratifying to witness all the current interest in implant-anchored orthodontics. I am pleased that Dr. Cope has organized the current text to review many of the temporary anchorage devices currently available.

—W. Eugene Roberts

This book is urgently needed by orthodontists and surgeons. It provides an excellent review of the different anchorage systems in use today, and the reader will benefit by learning from the experienced clinicians in this field who will, without doubt, shed light on a body of knowledge that is new to most of us.

—Anoop Sondhi

Anchorage has not changed, the method has. From tip-back bends to miniscrew implants, we have come a long way; and this book illustrates exactly how to harness the power of this exciting new technique.

—R.G. Wick Alexander

Dr. Cope's book will be the landmark text pertaining to contemporary TADs in orthodontics. It is pertinent, practical, and well written. It belongs in every orthodontist's professional library.

—Jack Sheridan

This text aptly demonstrates how to place and use all of the major TAD systems available, as well as illustrates a myriad of clinical applications for the various cases we treat clinically.

-—Richard P. McLaughlin

OrthoTADS: The Clinical Guide and Atlas is a must read and study for all of us who are serious about providing successful orthodontic treatment for our patients.

—Jack Dale

PERIODONTICS

This state of the art book addresses the emerging and essential aspect of modern orthodontic therapy—temporary anchorage devices…a must read.

—Thomas G. Wilson, Jr, Editor
Quintessence International

ORAL SURGERY

Dr. Cope has compiled a most impressive and comprehensive treatise of TADs. This treatment adjunct may circumvent the need for orthognathic surgery in some patients, while providing a significant improvement in presurgical orthodontic set-ups to further enhance surgical results in other patients.

—Larry Wolford

The provision of osseous anchorage takes the handcuffs off the orthodontist and permits tooth movements that were heretofore not feasible and in much shorter time than thought possible. This book presents what will prove to be the greatest advance in orthodontic mechanics since headgears, facemasks, and chin-cups.

—Edward Ellis, III

ORTHOTADS
The Clinical Guide and Atlas

JASON B. COPE, DDS, PhD
Diplomate, America Board of Orthodontics
Adjunct Clinical Assistant Professor, Department of Orthodontics,
Adjunct Assistant Professor, Department of Oral & Maxillofacial Surgery and Pharmacology,
Texas A&M University System—Health Science Center, Baylor College of Dentistry
Private Practice of Orthodontics, Dallas, Texas

With more than 2350 illustrations and tables

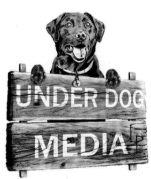

Under Dog Media, LP
Dallas, Texas, 2007

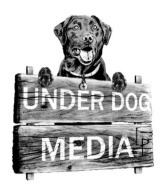

Editor: Jason B. Cope
Copy editor: Warren Perkins
Book layout: Susan LBFF Pittman and Jason B. Cope
Cover design: Jason B. Cope
Illustration editor: Carmen DoDah Banks
Photograph editors: Jason B. Cope and Alexander Cherkashin
Printer: Taylor Publishing Company

NOTICE

Medical/dental knowledge is constantly changing. Standard safety precautions must be followed, but as new research and clinical experience broaden our knowledge, changes in treatment and drug therapy may become necessary or appropriate. Readers are advised to check the most current product information provided by the manufacturer of each drug to be administered to verify the recommended dose, the method and duration of administration, and contraindications. It is the responsibility of the practitioner, relying on experience and knowledge of the patient, to determine dosages and the best treatment for each individual patient. The publisher, the editor, and the authors do not assume any liability for any injury and/or damage to persons or property arising from this publication.

The purpose of this manual is not to reprint all of the information that is otherwise available to the dental/medical practitioner but instead to complement, amplify, or supplement other texts. The reader is urged to read all the available material, learn as much as possible about temporary anchorage devices, and tailor the information to your individual needs. Every effort has been made to make this manual as complete and accurate as possible. However, there may be mistakes, both typographic and in content. Therefore, this text should be used only as a general guide and not as the ultimate or definitive source of temporary anchorage device information. Furthermore, this manual contains information on temporary anchorage devices that is current only up to the printing date. If you do not wish to be bound by the above, you may return this book to the publisher for a full refund within 10 days of purchase. A dated receipt is required.

Under Dog Media, LP
7015 Snider Plaza, Suite 200
Dallas, Texas 75205
www.orthotads.com

Printed in the United States of America

International Standard Book Number 10: 0-9776301-0-2
13: 978-0-9776301-0-3

Library of Congress Control Number 2005909955

    Cope, Jason B.
        OrthoTADs: the clinical guide and atlas / Jason B. Cope.
        p. cm.
        Includes bibliographical references and index.
        LCCN 2005909955
        ISBN 10: 0-9776301-0-2
            13: 978-0-9776301-0-3

        1. Dental implants. 2. Dental implants—Atlases.
    I. Title.

RK667.I45C67 2007   617.6'93
                  QBI05-600197

CONTRIBUTORS

George Anka, DDS, MS
Adjunct Clinical Assistant Professor,
Department of Orthodontics
Nihon University
Private Practice in Orthodontics
Tokyo, Japan

Claudio Arcuri, MD, DDS
Associate Professor, Department of Oral Pathology
University of Rome "Tor Vergata"
Fatebenefratelli Hospital—Isola Tiberina
Rome, Italy
Private Practice of Oral Surgery
Rome, Italy

John R. Bednar, DMD
Assistant Clinical Professor,
Department of Orthodontics
Boston University School of Dental Medicine
Private Practice of Orthodontics
Nashua, New Hampshire, USA

Siegrid Brix, DDS
Private Practice of Orthodontics
Gotha, Thuringia, Germany

Axel Bumann, DDS, PhD
Clinical Assistant Professor,
Department of Craniofacial Sciences and Therapy
University of Southern California
Private Practice of Orthodontics and
Craniomandibular Disorders
Berlin, Germany

Aldo Carano, DDS, MS (Deceased)
Adjunct Professor, Department of Orthodontics
St. Louis University, St. Louis, Missouri, USA
Adjunct Professor, Department of Orthodontics
University of Ferrara, Ferrara, Italy

Kyu-Rhim Chung, DMD, PhD
Chairman,
The Korean Society of Speedy Orthodontics
Private Practice of Orthodontics
Seoul, Korea

Jason B. Cope, DDS, PhD
Adjunct Clinical Assistant Professor,
Department of Orthodontics
Adjunct Assistant Professor,
Department of Oral & Maxillofacial Surgery
TAMUSHSC—Baylor College of Dentistry
Private Practice of Orthodontics
Dallas, Texas, USA

Antonio Costa, DDS, MS
Clinical Professor, Department of Orthodontics
University of Siena
Private Practice of Orthodontics
Parma, Italy

Michel Dalstra, PhD
Associate Professor, Department of Orthodontics
School of Dentistry, University of Aarhus
Aarhus, Denmark

Thomas S. Drechsler, DDS
Private Practice of Orthodontics and
Craniomandibular Disorders
Wiesbaden, Germany

Pedro F. Franco, DDS
Adjunct Clinical Assistant Professor,
Department of Oral & Maxillofacial Surgery
TAMUSHSC—Baylor College of Dentistry
Private Practice of Oral and Maxillofacial Surgery
Dallas, Texas, USA

Minayo Funatsu, DDS, PhD
Clinical Assistant Professor,
Department of Orthodontics
Tohoku University Dental Hospital
Sendai, Japan

Tomas Gedrange, DDS, PhD
Professor and Director,
Department of Orthodontics, Preventive, and
Pediatric Dentistry
Ernst-Moritz-Arndt University
Greifswald, Germany

Aldo Giancotti, DDS, MS
Assistant Professor, Department of Orthodontics
University of Rome "Tor Vergata"
Fatebenefratelli Hospital—Isola Tiberina
Rome, Italy
Private Practice of Orthodontics
Rome, Italy

Peter Goellner, DDS, MS
Private Practice of Orthodontics
Bern, Switzerland

John W. Graham, DDS, MD
Private Practice of Orthodontics
Litchfield Park, Arizona, USA

Richard P. Harper, DDS, PhD, FRCD(C)
Private Practice of Oral & Maxillofacial Surgery
Corsicana, Texas, USA

Shiori Hashimoto, DDS, PhD
Clinical Assistant Professor,
Department of Orthodontics
Tohoku University Dental Hospital
Sendai, Japan

Robert J. Herman, DDS, MS
Assistant Professor of Research,
Department of Orthodontics
University of Oklahoma College of Dentistry
Lieutenant, Dental Corps, U.S. Navy
Okinawa, Japan

Ryoon-Ki Hong, DDS, PhD
Chairman, Department of Orthodontics
Chong-A Dental Hospital
Clinical Professor, Department of Orthodontics
College of Dentistry, Seoul National University
Clinical Professor, Department of Orthodontics
College of Dentistry, Dankook University
Clinical Professor, Department of Dentistry
University of Ulsan
Seoul, Korea

Sarandeep S. Huja, DDS, PhD
Assistant Professor,
Section of Orthodontics and Oral Biology
College of Dentistry, The Ohio State University
Columbus, Ohio, USA

Masayoshi Kawakami, DDS, PhD
Assistant Professor,
Department of Oral and Maxillofacial Surgery
Nara Medical University Kashihara
Nara, Japan

Hiroshi Kawamura, DDS, PhD
Professor and Chair,
Division of Maxillofacial Surgery
Graduate School of Dentistry, Tohoku University
Sendai, Japan

Seong-Hun Kim, DMD, MSD
Instructor, Department of Orthodontics
The Catholic University of Korea,
Uijeongbu St. Mary's Hospital
Uijeongbu, Gyeonggido, Korea

Yoon-Ah Kook, DDS, PhD
Associate Professor, Department of Orthodontics
The Catholic University of Korea,
Gangnam St. Mary's Hospital
Seoul, Korea

Isao Koyama, DDS, PhD
Visiting Professor,
Fourth Military Medical University
Part-Time Lecturer, Osaka Dental University
Private Practice of Orthodontics
Osaka, Japan

Hee-Moon Kyung, DDS, MSD, PhD
Professor, Department of Orthodontics
School of Dentistry,
Kyungpook National University
Daegu, Korea

Johnny J.L. Liao, DDS
Adjunct Clinical Director,
Department of Orthodontics
National Taiwan University Hospital
Private Practice of Orthodontics
Taipei, Taiwan

Joong-Ki Lim, DDS, MS
Clinical Assistant Professor,
Department of Orthodontics
College of Dentistry, Yonsei University
Clinical Assistant Professor,
Department of Orthodontics
School of Medicine, Sungkyunkwan University
Private Practice of Orthodontics
Seoul, Korea

James C.Y. Lin, DDS
Consultant Orthodontist, Department of
Orthodontics and Craniofacial Dentistry
Chang Gung Memorial Hospital
Visiting Lecturer,
Graduate Institute of Craniofacial Medicine
Chang Gung University
Private Practice of Orthodontics
Taipei, Taiwan

Eric J.W. Liou, DDS, MS
Director and Assistant Professor,
Department of Orthodontics and Craniofacial
Dentistry
Chang Gung Memorial Hospital
Chang Gung University,
Institute of Craniofacial Medicine
Taipei, Taiwan

James Mah, DDS, BSc, MSc, DMSc
Clinical Assistant Professor,
Department of Craniofacial Sciences and Therapy
University of Southern California
Los Angeles, California, USA

B. Giuliano Maino, MD, DDS
Visiting Professor,
Department of Oral & Maxillofacial Surgery
Parma University
Private Practice of Orthodontics
Vicenza, Italy

Birte Melsen, DDS
Professor, Dr.Odont.,
Department of Orthodontics
School of Dentistry, University of Aarhus
Aarhus, Denmark

Kuniaki Miyajima, DDS, MS, PhD
Adjunct Professor,
Center for Advanced Dental Education
St. Louis University
St. Louis, Missouri, USA
Private Practice of Orthodontics
Tokyo, Japan

Paola Mura, DMD
Private Practice of Orthodontics
Vicenza, Italy

Hiroshi Nagasaka, DDS, PhD
Director,
Department of Oral and Maxillofacial Surgery
Miyagi Children's Hospital
Sendai, Japan

Makoto Nishimura, DDS, PhD
Clinical Assistant Professor,
Department of Orthodontics
Tohoku University Dental Hospital
Sendai, Japan

Shannon E. Owens, DDS, MS
Private Practice of Orthodontics
Jackson, Wyoming, USA

Cheol-Ho Paik, DDS, PhD
Clinical Assistant Professor,
Department of Orthodontics
Seoul National University Dental College
Private Practice, SAI Orthodontic Center
Seoul, Korea

Hyo-Sang Park, DDS, MSD, PhD
Associate Professor, Department of Orthodontics
School of Dentistry,
Kyungpook National University
Daegu, Korea

Shuichi Saeki, DDS, PhD
Instructor, Division of Orthodontics and
Dentofacial Orthopedics
Graduate School of Dentistry, Tohoku University
Sendai, Japan

Shigeru Saito, DDS, PhD
Mayumi Orthodontic Office
Private Practice of Orthodontics
Kawasaki, Japan

Masaru Sakai, DDS
Director, Sakai Orthodontic Office
Private Practice of Orthodontics
Nagoya, Japan

Takamasa Sannohe, DDS
Graduate Student,
Division of Orthodontics and Dentofacial
Orthopedics
Graduate School of Dentistry, Tohoku University
Sendai, Japan

Renya Sato, DDS, PhD
Clinical Assistant Professor,
Department of Orthodontics
Tohoku University Dental Hospital
Sendai, Japan

Junji Sugawara, DDS, PhD
Associate Professor, Division of Orthodontics and
Dentofacial Orthopedics
Graduate School of Dentistry, Tohoku University
Sendai, Japan

Ichiro Takahashi, DDS, PhD
Lecturer,
Division of Orthodontics and Dentofacial
Orthopedics
Graduate School of Dentistry, Tohoku University
Sendai, Japan

Paul M. Thomas, DMD, MS
Senior Research Fellow
Eastman Dental Institute for Oral Healthcare Sciences
London, England
Adjunct Professor, Department of Orthodontics
University of North Carolina at Chapel Hill
Chapel Hill, North Carolina, USA

Mikako Umemori, DDS, PhD
Clinical Associate Professor, Division of
Orthodontics and Dentofacial Orthopedics
Graduate School of Dentistry, Tohoku University
Sendai, Japan

Stefano Velo, MD, MS
Adjunct Professor, Department of Orthodontics
University of Ferrara
Ferrara, Italy

Thomas G. Wilson, Jr., DDS
Clinical Associate Professor,
Department of Periodontics
TAMUSHSC—Baylor College of Dentistry
Private Practice of Periodontics and Dental
Implants
Dallas, Texas, USA

Satoshi Yamada, DDS, PhD
Instructor,
Division of Orthodontics and Dentofacial
Orthopedics
Graduate School of Dentistry, Tohoku University
Sendai, Japan

Tadashi Yamada, DDS
Graduate Student,
Division of Orthodontics and Dentofacial
Orthopedics
Graduate School of Dentistry, Tohoku University
Sendai, Japan

ABOUT THE EDITOR

Jason B. Cope was born in Dallas, Texas, and raised in Bossier City, Louisiana. Upon receiving his dental degree from Baylor College of Dentistry in 1995, he was the first student at Baylor to undertake a dual program in both orthodontics and craniofacial biology. After completion of his orthodontic certificate in 1997, he joined the orthodontic department as an adjunct clinical assistant professor. At the same time, he continued his postdoctoral program in craniofacial biology as a National Research Service Award Fellow for an additional 2 years, and began practicing orthodontics. In 1999, after only 4 years of combined training, Jason defended his dissertation *Bilateral Mandibular Lengthening by Osteodistraction: Biologic and Biomechanical Parameters* and earned a PhD.

During his young career, Dr. Cope has published 22 refereed journal articles, 35 book chapters, and a research handbook and has co-edited a multimedia CD-ROM and a 600-page textbook on distraction osteogenesis. In addition, he has given more than 100 lectures nationally and internationally. He also has been recognized with 6 national awards for his distraction research including the Thomas M. Graber Award of Special Merit awarded by the American Association of Orthodontists. He has been an investigator on 21 funded research grants. Dr. Cope is an ad hoc reviewer for the *American Journal of Orthodontics and Dentofacial Orthopedics,* the *Angle Orthodontist,* the *Journal of Clinical Orthodontics,* the *World Journal of Orthodontics, Archives of Oral Biology,* and the *Journal of Dental Research;* is a past associate editor for *Quintessence International;* and was the guest editor for the March 2005 issue Temporary Anchorage Devices in Orthodontics in *Seminars in Orthodontics.* His private practice is located in Dallas, Texas, where he treats patients 4 days a week and continues both clinical and basic science research on OrthoTADs.

In the span of one month in March 2002, he presented cases to the Texas Tweed Group, the Southwest Component of the Edward H. Angle Society, and the American Board of Orthodontics, passing all three exams and becoming board certified. In July 2004, he presented his scientific paper to become a full member of the SW component of the Edward H. Angle Society of Orthodontists. In January 2005, he was awarded the Baylor College of Dentistry Alumni Association Outstanding Young Alumnus Award for his contributions to the dental profession.

His complete curriculum vitae is available at *http://www.orthotads.com/editor.*

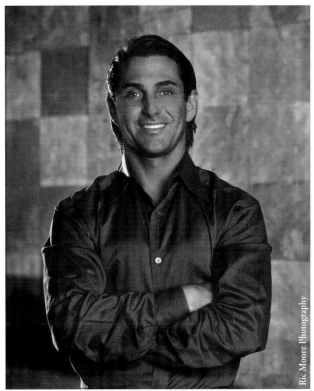

Ric Moore Photography

DEDICATION

I have often been asked why I work so much. I am not so sure that there is a simple answer. Perhaps it is because, as the firstborn son of an orthodontist, I saw firsthand the dedication of my father to his craft ... his sitting around the swimming pool on those hot summer days reading the *American Journal of Orthodontics* as my brothers, Matt and Cameron, and I played, or perhaps it was the evening meetings he had with H.O. (Blackwood) to discuss difficult cases. Maybe, it was that impression of seeing my Dad's passion and work ethic for orthodontics that pushed me down this road.

Or maybe it was the fact that I was quite average physically, athletically, and academically and decided that I wanted to be more than average. And in order for me to compete with and beat those who were more talented, I had to work harder, stay up later, and get up earlier. On top of that, my Mom, who would sacrifice anything for her kids, somehow convinced me that I could do anything I conceived, believed, and was willing to pay the price to achieve.

Perhaps it was enlightenment from the Scriptures. Luke 12:48 reads, "From everyone who is given much, much will be demanded; and from the one who is entrusted with much, much more will be asked." In my first 37 years, I have been extremely blessed, first by my Dad's and then by my own involvement in dentistry. I have been given the opportunity to attend the best universities, to travel the world, to have been befriended by orthodontic legends, and to have had the opportunity to discuss orthodontic mechanics with the most brilliant minds in the field. These are things that 95% of the world's population will never have the chance to experience.

What I do know is that I have been given much more than my share of blessings. My hope and prayer is that in the next 37 years, I can be more of a benefactor than a beneficiary of both the dental profession and my family. The short answer: I guess I work so much because, at the end of this journey we call life, my hope is that I can say I have at least given as much as I have received, although I'm quite sure that is impossible.

Sir Isaac Newton once said, "If I see further than others, it is only because I stand on the shoulders of giants." We all have giants in our lives, those people who lift us up and empower us to be more than we are capable of becoming on our own. The two most prominent giants in my life have been my Mom and Dad, whom I can never possibly repay for their encouragement, support, acceptance, and love of someone who has not always been that lovable. Thank you. I am proud to be your son. If the true measure of parents is the success of their children, both in life and in spirit, you have succeeded three times over. This book is dedicated to my parents, and to my Lord and Savior, Jesus Christ, who makes it all possible.

Jason B. Cope, DDS, PhD
Dallas, December 2006

I would rather be ashes than dust! I would rather that my spark should burn out in a brilliant blaze than it should be stifled by dryrot. I would rather be a superb meteor; every atom of me in magnificent glow, than a sleepy and permanent planet. The proper function of man is to live, not to exist. I shall not waste my days in trying to prolong them. I shall use my time ...

—Jack London

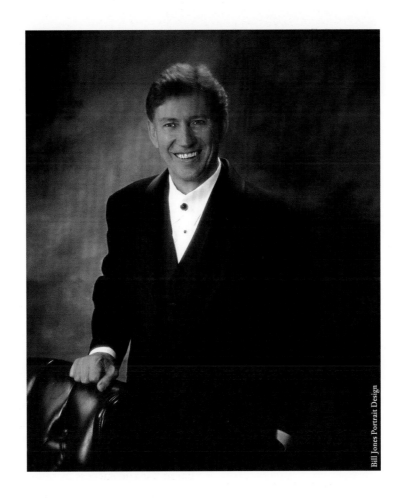

Donald D. Cope, DDS, MSD

February 16, 1944 - June 11, 2006

IN LOVING MEMORY...

...THE GREATEST MAN I HAVE EVER KNOWN

FOREWORD

It is a real privilege to write the foreword for this avant-garde book on orthodontic temporary anchorage devices (OrthoTADs). It is truly the first comprehensive magnum opus in this area and is long overdue. And the contributing authors read like a list from "Who's Who" in this rapidly developing field.

For too long, orthodontists have struggled to establish anchorage for a myriad of tooth movements of individual teeth and segments and as a stable base for growth guidance. Complex wire geometries, brackets, and auxiliary appliances have been used but have been only partially successful at best. The iatrogenic response to our clinical manipulations has been encountered frequently, with anchorage loss, root resorption, crestal bone loss, gingival recession, and even disfiguration of the enamel surfaces from prolonged mechanotherapy. The term *stationary anchorage* has been a misnomer, as slippage and untoward responses are encountered all too frequently. Orthognathic surgery has been one answer to this gnawing problem, with its own set of problems—all of these building up a risk management problem for

orthodontists and a good financial resource for trial lawyers.

Dr. Jason B. Cope, who has been a leader in distraction osteogenesis, has turned his attention to this Achilles heel problem of anchorage. What a welcome contribution!

Section 1 addresses the historical development and evolution of temporary anchorage devices—a short but fascinating discourse.

Section 2 presents the biologic basis of bone adaptation to miniscrew implants by world-class researchers and clinicians in the field.

Section 3 develops the clinical basis of TAD applications by Jason B. Cope and associates, with treatment planning, biomechanics, hard and soft tissue dimensions, and potential complications.

Section 4 is devoted to miniscrew implants by the developers themselves, people such as Kyu-Rhim Chung, Axel Bumann, Birte Melsen, Eric Lou, Jason B. Cope, and Paul Thomas, just to mention a few.

The miniscrew implant clinical case reports alone (20 of them in Section 5!) make this book a major contribution to our compendium of knowledge, again by leading clinicians from around the world. The examples cover many problem cases (i.e., anterior decrowding, en masse retraction, molar distalization, extraction treatment, lingual orthodontics, Class II correction, space closure, missing teeth, use in surgical cases, and occlusal plane canting). Clinicians will avidly read and reread this section as an essential, indispensable chairside adjunct.

Sections 6 and 7 are on palatal implants, again by world leaders and developers such as Tomas Gedrange, Jason B. Cope, Aldo Giancotti, Giuliano Maino, and Peter Goellner.

Sections 8 and 9 present miniplate implants, such as the C-plate® and C-tube® and the Skeletal Anchorage System, by the groups of Dr. Chung and Dr. Sugawara, respectively. Again, this is a veritable gold mine for handling intrusion, traction of impacted teeth, protraction of molars in both arches, distalization of molars, and Class III correction.

Indeed, the whole gamut of skeletal and dental malocclusions is covered, and teamwork with surgical orthodontic treatment, together with miniplate anchorage, is described.

Truly, superlatives still do not do justice to this clinical guide and implant atlas. I have been in the writing and publishing field for a lifetime, but this volume is truly a once-in-a lifetime experience, and it will have a significant impact on the profession itself for those fortunate enough to read it. Kudos to Dr. Cope and his team!

Tom Graber
T.M. Graber, DMD, MSD, PhD,
Odont Dr, ScD, DSc, MD, FRCS
Professor, Department of Orthodontics,
University of Illinois
Editor-in-Chief,
World Journal of Orthodontics

ACKNOWLEDGEMENTS

I am extremely proud of the text contained within. From its inception a year and a half ago until now, I have dedicated the majority of my professional and personal life to seeing it come to fruition. This book, however, is the product of more than 50 clinicians and researchers from around the world, all of whom have spent countless hours dedicated to the highest-quality patient care and clinical/experimental research.

My colleague and dear friend Dr. Pedro Felipe Franco has worked with me to develop and test concepts and ideas both clinically and in the laboratory. Brainstorming sessions with him and other devoted colleagues from around the world are the stimulus that keeps me passionate about our profession.

The eminent leader in orthodontics, Dr. Tom Graber, who has become a friend, a colleague, and a mentor, rolled out the proverbial red carpet for me, giving me opportunities to speak, write, and publish in venues that were so far above my reach that it would have taken me years to knock down the door and gain entry. Tom graciously agreed to write the foreword to this, my second textbook, and in so doing has validated it as a worthwhile endeavor and worthy of his respected name. Tom, I thank you for your trust and friendship.

For the contributors who spent their valuable time compiling their clinical and experimental research and experience into logical, thought-provoking chapters, I sincerely thank you. Your hard work, scientific knowledge, and clinical experience has helped make this text live up to its potential. I also understand the sacrifices you made over the past year—time taken away from your practices, families, and friends. It is my sincere hope that your sacrifices will be repaid many times over in the form of professional accolades, clinical success, and in a greater appreciation of the true value of family and friends.

I would like to thank the people who said I could and should pursue this independent publishing venture when it was nothing more than a thought; Dr. Jim and Charlene McNamara, Dr. Lionel Sadowsky, and Dr. Ron Bulard, I cannot possibly express my appreciation for your confidence and insight. And although perhaps counterintuitive, I would also like to thank those who, with all sincerity and concern for my best interests, said it could not be done. Disbelief fans the flames of my passion and drive more so than any other single factor. If we do not push ourselves past the point of what we *know* we can accomplish, we will never understand the true potential and strength within.

Thanks also to those freelancers in the publishing industry who offered their advice, services, and moral support. I gave you a challenge to equal or surpass the quality of the major medical/dental publishers, and you came through with flying colors. I cannot begin to express how appreciative I am for your hard work and patience in dealing with my relentless, perfectionist ideals of what the final product could and should be. I am extremely pleased with the quality of the book and hope that you are equally as satisfied.

Finally, I would like to acknowledge the many patients around the world who have agreed to undergo OrthoTAD placement in conjunction with orthodontic treatment. In our unending search for the ideal treatment to overcome orthodontic anchorage limitations, you have agreed to be our student, our colleague, and our teacher—with the implicit trust that we will do no harm. As we march on into this wonderful future of OrthoTAD therapy, we thank you and all of those who will come after you. We will always strive to do our best!

Jason B. Cope, DDS, PhD
Dallas, December 2006

PREFACE

Most innovative new concepts or products, no matter how significant, usually cannot avoid the frustrating evolution from harebrained idea to possible widespread acceptance. In their infancy, they are initially rejected by almost all potential users who claim that it cannot be done or it is too complicated. Shortly thereafter, it is accepted by a few; the vast majority, however, contends that it is just not there yet or might be applicable later. After a period of time, most people adopt the new technique and begin to question why their colleagues are not using it. Finally, after years of clinical and experimental documentation, it becomes the standard of care—the technique by which all others are compared.

So it was with the conversion from banding every tooth in the mouth to gluing those tiny little brackets on the teeth, as well as with using titanium miniplates and screws for maxillomandibular fixation instead of using intermaxillary wire fixation. Let us not forget that crazy Russian surgeon who thought it possible to actually grow bone with a mechanical device that pushed cut bone segments apart. It is interesting, though, that Ilizarov and his distraction osteogenesis technique has grown more bone with what started out as used bicycle spokes and wheel rims than all of the world's most brilliant scientists combined.

Oh the times, they are a changing indeed! The practice of orthodontics is different from what it was 10 years ago, not to mention how it was practiced 100 years ago. It goes without saying that anchorage control, or the ability to control the movement of teeth during orthodontic mechanotherapy, currently looks nothing like what the Angles and Bonwills of the 1800s envisioned it would look like. Even today, with all of our technological advances, it is not uncommon that we first treatment plan a case via camouflage therapy instead of going through the exercise of establishing an ideal treatment plan using all 28 teeth (omitting the third molars, of course), and then working backward if, and only if, costs, time, or risk factors are more important to the patient. Unfortunately, we have become so accustomed to our lack of control over tooth movement that we assume that *we can't* before we envision that *we can*.

Ah, but we can! We are in the second stage of the evolution of *Orthodontic Temporary Anchorage Devices (OrthoTADs)*, implantlike devices that are placed temporarily in or on bone for the purpose of moving teeth and that are removed and discarded later. Our Asian orthodontic colleagues are placing OrthoTADs routinely, but clinicians of North and South America look upon the placement of a miniscrew implant (MSI) for orthodontic anchorage as if it were witchcraft, hypocrisy, or insanity. Perhaps it is due to our litigious society, or the lack of understanding of what exactly is clinically possible with OrthoTADs, or the costs associated with having a surgeon place them, or fear of the possible complications—or downright resistance to change. Regardless of the reason, OrthoTADs are here to stay; they are a reality, and they will change the way orthodontics is practiced from this point forward.

Over the past 10 to 15 years, several different attempts at skeletally based anchorage have been attempted clinically: fixation wires, bone plates, fixation screws, miniaturized dental implants in the palate and retromolar areas, and palatal onplants. From this point forward, though, the single most important of these will be the MSI (see Chapter 1 for the classification of these) for several reasons. First, the American Association of Orthodontists has amended the liability insurance policy to cover "the placement of micro implants that do not involve the reflection of a surgical flap." Although this technically also covers some palatal implants, most orthodontists will not place palatal implants because they are usually placed under intravenous sedation. Miniscrew implants, however, are customarily placed without a flap or after a punch incision under topical anesthetic or local infiltration only. For this reason, as well as the added costs for placement by surgeons, many orthodontists may begin to place MSIs. Almost certainly, many clinicians who have not given an injection in years may be uncomfortable with this scenario; but to be sure, most young orthodontists will be comfortable with this. Many recent graduates placed or were involved in the placement of dental implants during their dental school training. So, even though *who* places MSIs may be a current topic of discussion, 10 to 20 years from now, this will most likely not even be a consideration.

It is important, however, to realize that the potential complications are relatively insignificant relative to major orthognathic surgical procedures; however, oroantral fistulae, tooth root damage, bony and soft tissue infection, and implant failure are possible. Although this relatively new clinically methodology of temporary anchorage offers tremendous benefits, those clinicians venturing into the "surgical" placement of OrthoTADs would be well-advised to review, in a more formal fashion, all of the anatomic and drug interactions associated with the surgical placement of implants before moving forward. This is no different from the field of distraction osteogenesis. Dr. G.A. Ilizarov, the noted Russian pioneer, once remarked, "What seems at first a simple procedure, can lead to a catastrophic outcome if the fixator is applied with insufficient knowledge of the basic principles and techniques."

The ability of orthodontists to overcome previously insurmountable anchorage limitations appears to be truly within our grasp. This textbook first introduces OrthoTADs from a historic point of view to give a clear definition and current classification system. The next section contains chapters that outline the basic biologic factors associated with OrthoTAD use. The third section covers placement locations for OrthoTADs in the oral cavity, treatment planning, biomechanics, and potential complications. The three subsequent clinical sections cover the three most common TADs in use today: miniscrew implants, palatal implants, and miniplate implants. These chapters were designed to serve as a "how to" guide, relying on text and photographs to explain the design and use of the system, but without complete clinical cases. This was to show the reader the information necessary to implement the particular system. After each of these clinical sections are a series of case reports, which were designed with minimal text covering only the basics of the case and relying heavily on the use of photographs for documentation and illustration of the case. This was done to give the reader the many different ways that OrthoTADs could be applied and used clinically.

It is my greatest hope that *OrthoTADs: The Clinical Guide and Atlas* will provide the profession with a comprehensive, scientifically based, yet clinically relevant resource that will benefit our patients with better treatment results than could have been obtained otherwise with traditional orthodontic anchorage.

Jason B. Cope, DDS, PhD
Dallas, December 2006

CONTENTS

SECTION 1

HISTORICAL DEVELOPMENT

CHAPTER

1

Historical Development and Evolution of Temporary Anchorage Devices

Jason B. Cope, Shannon E. Owens

INTRODUCTION TO ORTHODONTIC ANCHORAGE

Traditionally, orthodontists have used teeth, intraoral appliances, and extraoral appliances to control anchorage, thus minimizing the movement of certain teeth while carrying out the desired movement of other teeth. However, because of Newton's third law—that is, for every action there is an equal and opposite reaction—the ability to completely control all aspects of tooth movement is limited. For example, orthodontists often have inadequate mechanical systems with which to control anchorage, which leads to a loss of anchorage in the reactive unit and thus incomplete correction of intraarch and interarch alignment problems. Moreover, in an attempt to overcome these limitations, clinicians often incorporate bulky acrylic appliances or extraoral appliances, which when combined with the ever challenging problem of uncooperative patients, are often a futile attempt at best.

Although definitive research on palatal implants was published in the 1990s,[1-3] the orthodontic literature has only recently seen a flurry of published case reports documenting the possibility of using a number of different types of orthodontic temporary anchorage devices (OrthoTADs) in approximation to bone with the intent of enhancing or overcoming the limitations of traditional anchorage.[4-9] Case reports, although important in describing what is possible clinically, are inadequate for documenting the basic biologic and biomechanical parameters necessary for the implementation of a new

clinical modality on a broad scale. The literature is just beginning to see the publication of clinical trials[10-14] and basic science experiments,[15-21] which should begin to definitively answer some of the most essential questions. To this end, the purpose of this chapter is to clearly define these devices, introduce their historical development, organize them into a simple but adaptable classification system, and outline several pertinent terms and definitions associated with their use.

Orthodontic Anchorage

Although the principle of orthodontic anchorage has been implicitly understood since the seventeenth century, it does not appear to have been clearly articulated until 1923 when Louis Ottofy[22] defined it as "the base against which orthodontic force or reaction of orthodontic force is applied." Most recently, Daskalogiannakis[23] defined anchorage as "resistance to unwanted tooth movement." Orthodontic anchorage can also be defined as the amount of allowed movement of the reactive unit. This, however, requires a definition of the reactive unit (tooth/teeth acting as anchorage during movement of the active unit) and the active unit (tooth/teeth undergoing movement) (Fig. 1-1).

Ottofy[22] also summarized the anchorage categories previously outlined by Edward H. Angle and others as simple, stationary, reciprocal, intraoral, intermaxillary, or extraoral. Since that time, several noted authors have modified or developed their own classification. For

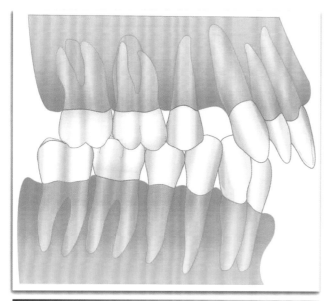

Fig. 1-1

Class II dental malocclusion with upper premolar extraction to facilitate maxillary anterior retraction. The active unit is the tooth or teeth undergoing movement (*anterior teeth*). The reactive unit is the tooth or teeth acting as anchorage during movement of the active unit (*posterior teeth*).

example, Moyers[24] expanded Ottofy's classification system by clearly outlining the different categories of extraoral anchorage and subcategorizing simple anchorage into single, compound, and reinforced subcategories. Later, others developed their own classification terminology. Gianelly and Goldman[25] suggested the terms *maximum*, *moderate*, and *minimum* to indicate the extent to which the teeth of the active and reactive units should move when a force is applied. Marcotte[26] and Burstone[27] classified anchorage in three categories—*A*, *B*, and *C*—depending on how much of the anchorage unit contributes to space closure. Tweed[28] went further to define anchorage preparation, or the uprighting and even the distal tipping of posterior teeth in order to use the mechanical advantage of the tent peg concept before retracting anterior teeth.

Considering the foregoing classification systems, it becomes apparent that a lack of consensus exists on the terminology for describing anchorage. Moreover, these systems are outdated and currently do not provide clear guidelines with which the orthodontist can communicate clearly and concisely. For example, these classification systems only account for anteroposterior dental relationships and do not really account for vertical or transverse relationships. They also only account for the anteroposterior extent of the dental

bases and do not account for distalizing the dentition to create a Class I dental relationship without the need for extractions or surgery. Moreover, they only account for groups of teeth; they do not account for individual teeth, nor do they account for the entire occlusal plane as would be required for occlusal cant correction via differential intrusion and extrusion. The reason for the latter is most likely due to the fact that at that time these classification systems were developed, the possibility of, for example, intruding posterior teeth to correct a skeletal anterior open bite without surgery was unimaginable. Given the recent advances in biology, materials, and clinical treatment, this type of tooth movement is not only a possibility but also a reality.[11,29-31] Thus it becomes apparent that a new anchorage classification system is needed to fully characterize the nature and extent of the problem and treatment.

Temporary Anchorage Devices

A temporary anchorage device (TAD) is a *device that is temporarily fixed to bone for the purpose of enhancing orthodontic anchorage by supporting the teeth of the reactive unit or by obviating the need for the reactive unit altogether and which is subsequently removed after use.* Temporary anchorage devices can be located transosteally, subperiosteally, or endosteally; and they can be fixed to bone mechanically (cortically stabilized) or biochemically (osseointegrated). It should also be pointed out that dental implants placed for the ultimate purpose of supporting a prosthesis, regardless of the fact that they may be used for orthodontic anchorage, are not considered TADs because they are not removed after orthodontic treatment. An important note, however, is that the initial incorporation of dental implants into orthodontic treatment made possible *infinite anchorage*, which has been defined in terms of implants as showing no movement (zero anchorage loss) as a consequence of reaction forces.[23]

HISTORICAL DEVELOPMENT OF TEMPORARY ANCHORAGE DEVICES

The evolution of OrthoTADs was based on the development and improvement of traditional orthodontic anchorage, dental implants, and orthognathic fixation methods. Later, modifications of these techniques were unified with basic biologic and biomechanical principles of osseointegration into orthodontic mechanics that were finally improved based on experiences with interdisciplinary dentistry.

Orthodontic Anchorage

Very early in their history, orthodontists realized the limitations of using teeth as anchorage to move other teeth. As early as 1728, Fauchard described the use of the expansion arch, which by ligating the teeth to an ideally shaped *rigid* metal plate, broadened the crowded dentition to a more normal form. A few decades later, Bourdet improved the technique by using a slightly flexible plate (Fig. 1-2).[32,33] About 100 years later, Gunnell claimed to have used occipital anchorage in 1822 but did not describe its use until 1841. At the same time, Schange perfected the "crib" of Delabarre and used it for attaching the palatal plate as anchorage, which allowed the use of a labial arch and ligatures of silk or gold wires to accomplish various tooth movements. Desirabode in 1843 is reported to have used teeth with longer and stronger roots as anchorage to move other teeth. Of course, no discussion of orthodontic anchorage would be complete without the contributions of Edward H. Angle, who introduced the idea of stationary anchorage in 1887 and occlusal anchorage in 1891.[33]

Dental Implants

Although Brånemark[34,35] pioneered the original experimental work that established the principle of osseointegration, he followed by about 50 years those who originally imagined the possibility of using biocompatible materials to replace missing teeth. This has been overlooked, however, because much of the background information is not available in the clinical literature but primarily in patent documents. In addition, the lack of online accessibility of the original dated journals limits their use to those who are willing to venture into the library.

Greenfield, in a patent of 1909 titled *Mounting for Artificial Teeth,*[36] envisioned a replacement for teeth, the basis of which was a metal frame that would be inserted into a cavity drilled into the jaw bone (Fig. 1-3). This predecessor of the hollow basket implant concept would allow bone to grow into the cage followed by cementation of a crown onto the frame. However, according to Strock,[37] the iridioplatinum meshwork of Greenfield was not strong enough to withstand the forces placed on it. Moreover, the cage frequently was placed in the molar and canine region with a gold bridge suspended between the two cages. Strock implied that the bridge was placed and loaded without sufficient time for osseointegration.

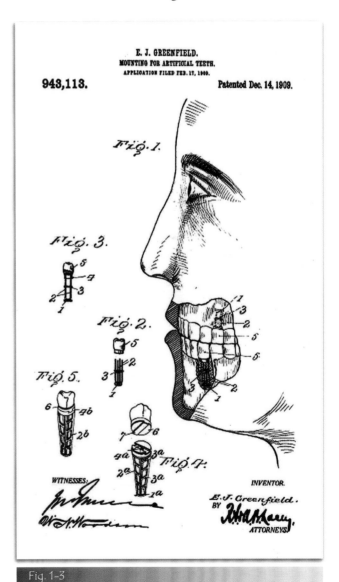

Fig. 1-3

Greenfield's implant patent. (Reprinted from Greenfield EJ, inventor. Mounting for Artificial Teeth. US patent 943,113, 1-3. December 14, 1909.)

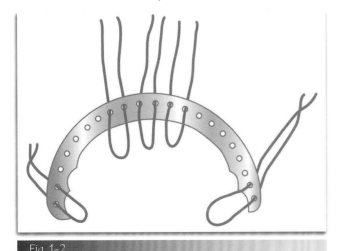

Fig. 1-2

Bourdet's type of expansion arch.

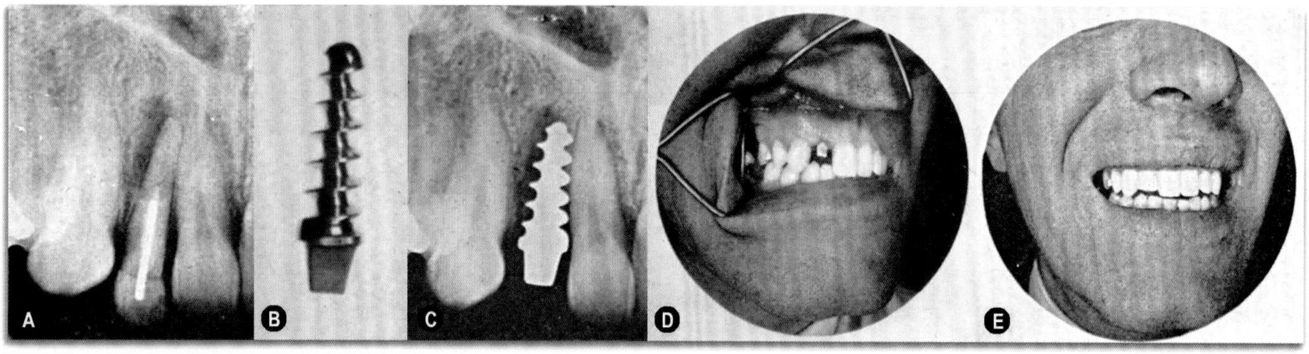

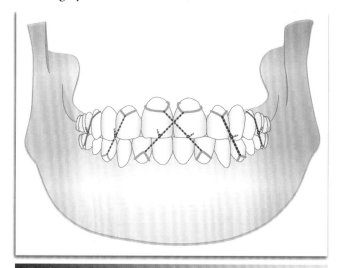

Fig. 1-4

Strock's replacement of missing incisors. **A,** Radiograph of failed endodontic treatment. **B,** Photograph of Vitallium screw implant. **C,** Radiograph of Vitallium screw implant. **D,** Photograph of Vitallium screw implant in place. **E,** Photograph of celluloid crown on implant. (Reprinted from Strock AE. Experimental work on a method for the replacement of missing teeth by direct implantation of a metal support into the alveolus. *Am J Orthod.* 25:467-472, 1939, with permission from the American Association of Orthodontists.)

Alvin Strock, a dentist from Boston, began to search for his own methods of tooth replacement.[37] At that point in the 1940s, implants were frequently made of lead and iron, which eroded intraorally and also caused bone resorption. Because Greenfield's cage was not suitable, Strock began to use the screw principle of fixation combined with a recently developed alloy called Vitallium, which Venable and Stuck[38] had determined to be completely inert in bone. Strock used a $5/8$-inch Vitallium Venable screw for immediate replacement of incisors lost as a result of trauma or endodontic failure (Fig. 1-4). Of interest is the fact that in the 1940s Strock discussed several salient points that remain critical even today: immediate placement is feasible if enough bone remains for the implant to be secure from the start, and the occlusion must be favorable to prevent occlusal trauma to the implant. For example, he routinely left the celluloid (temporary) crown out of occlusion for 4 to 6 months until it was replaced by a porcelain jacket crown.

Not until the late 1950s did Per Ingvar Brånemark come onto the scene. It was then that this young researcher was using specially designed optical titanium chambers to study the intravascular dynamics of bone marrow circulation by transillumination in vivo.[35] At this point in time the titanium chambers were custom-made and extremely expensive; therefore they were to be removed and reused. However, bone grew into the thin spaces in the titanium, and the chambers could not be easily removed. This finding prompted the detailed experimentation on osseointegration that ensued. Based on these and other findings by Brånemark's group,[34,35,39] for osseointegration to be successful, a healing time of 4 to 6 months was advocated prior to functional loading. Loading prior

to this point was thought to allow micromotion, which permitted fibrous tissue growth and subsequent failure.

Orthognathic Fixation

Although current fixation techniques for orthognathic surgery are performed primarily using bone plates and screws, most fractures before the 1800s were treated with splints, bandages, and combinations of intraoral and extraoral appliances. Gordon Buck[40] is credited with being the first to place an interosseous wire in a mandibular fracture in 1847. However, Milton Adams[41] popularized the practice. In the late 1800s, Thomas Gilmer[42] was the first American to use the dentition to secure maxillomandibular fixation (wires) in the treatment of jaw fractures (Fig. 1-5).

Christiansen[43] originally introduced bone plates to oral surgery in 1945. However, not until the late 1960s

Fig. 1-5

Gilmer's method of maxillomandibular fixation using interdental wires.

was enough experimental data and the biomechanical understanding of long bone fracture healing applied to the mandible.[44] Hans Luhr[45] is credited with introducing the compression plate to maxillofacial surgery in the late 1960s. His Vitallium compression plate used the gliding screw principle to achieve compression across the fractured segments, thereby allowing the possibility of fracture healing without the need for maxillomandibular fixation (Fig. 1-6).

Screw fixation using the lag screw technique was first introduced to maxillofacial surgery in 1970 by Brons and Boering,[46] who demonstrated the possibility of fracture reduction with screws of only 2.7 mm in diameter. Finally, in 1973, Michelet and colleagues[47] began a small revolution by reporting on the treatment of mandibular fractures using miniaturized plates and monocortical screws placed intraorally. Champy and colleagues[48-50] substantiated that the technique was scientifically sound (Fig. 1-7). Miniaturized bone screws, as the sole source of fixation, were first reported by Jeter and colleagues[51] in 1984 (Fig. 1-8). Their group placed three 2.0-mm diameter bicortical bone screws bilaterally through a transoral approach to successfully fixate the mandible after osteotomy.

Initial Temporary Anchorage Device Experiences

Although the concept of temporary implant anchorage has only recently been described, it was envisioned as early as 1945. Gainsforth and Higley,[52] understanding that "the teeth selected for the anchorage often move simultaneously with those in which movement is desired," sought "a method of basal bone anchorage." Using a 2.4-mm pilot hole, a 3.4-mm diameter by 13-mm long Vitallium screw was placed in the ascending ramus of six dogs (Fig 1-9). A rubber band delivering between 140 to 200 g of force was attached from the screw head to a 0.040-inch wire

that slid through a tube on the upper molar band and was soldered to the upper canine band. The system was designed to distally tip and retract the canine by immediately loading the screws with the rubber bands. Unfortunately, all of the screws were lost within 16 to 31 days. The authors did not describe frank infection; however, the failures may have been due to the lack of well-developed antibiotics at the time and to the *dynamic* loading of the screws.

The first clinical report in the literature of the use of a TAD appeared in 1983 when Creekmore and Eklund[53] used a Vitallium bone screw to treat a patient with a deep impinging overbite. The screw was inserted in the anterior nasal spine to intrude and root correct

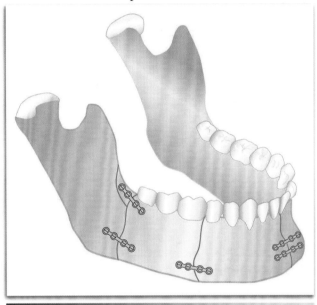

Fig. 1-7

Champy's method of mandibular fixation using bone plates.

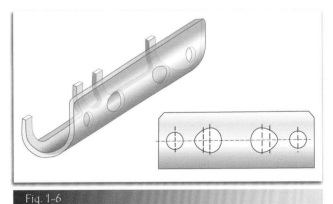

Fig. 1-6

Luhr's mandibular compression plate using the gliding screw principle.

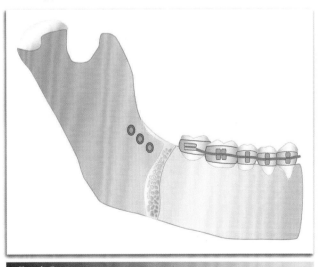

Fig. 1-8

Miniscrew fixation of a mandibular sagittal split advancement.

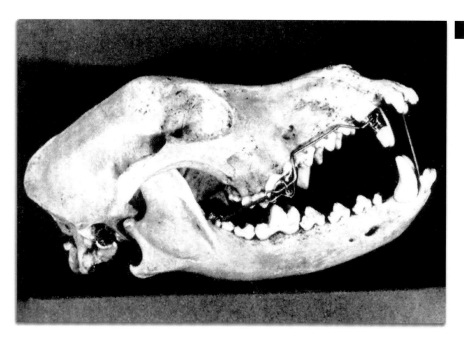

Fig. 1-9

Gainsforth's Vitallium screw for orthodontic anchorage. Note the miniscrew is placed in the ascending ramus and attached via a rubber band to a wire connected to the maxillary canine. (Reprinted from Gainsforth BL, Higley LB. A study of orthodontic anchorage possibilities in basal bone. *Am J Orthod Oral Surg.* 31:406-416, 1945, with permission from the American Association of Orthodontists.

the upper incisors using an elastic from the screw to the incisors 10 days after the screw was placed (Fig. 1-10).

Even though this first clinical procedure documented the successful application of a TAD, the technique did not gain immediate acceptance. This was most likely due to the lack of the widespread acceptance of surgical procedures, the still as of yet unaccepted field of implant dentistry, the lack of scientific data on the use of implantable materials, and the fear of complications. Instead, traditional anchorage mechanics remained the principal treatment modality for managing orthodontic problems.

Interdisciplinary Dentistry

The first report concerning the use of osseointegrated implants for both restorative and orthodontic purposes appeared in 1969 when Linkow[54] used a blade implant in the mandibular first molar region as a partial abutment for a bridge that was restored before orthodontics. Class II elastics were worn from the implant-supported bridge to the upper arch to facilitate tooth movement (Fig. 1-11). Since this initial application, the use of osseointegrated dental implants for orthodontic anchorage has been well documented. Kokich[55] and Smalley[56,57] have developed protocols for determining how to place dental implants accurately in the final desired location for restorative procedures before orthodontic therapy such that the implants can be used for both orthodontic anchorage and the subsequent restorative therapy.

EVOLUTION OF CURRENT TEMPORARY ANCHORAGE DEVICES AND TECHNIQUES

Temporary Anchorage Device Types

In an attempt to overcome the limitations with tooth-based anchorage and compliance-based intraoral and extraoral appliances, several authors have developed so-called compliance-free appliances.[58-61] However, these appliances usually have resulted in less than ideal treatment outcomes[61] and could not fulfill the requirements of infinite anchorage. It has been suggested that only ankylosed teeth and skeletal anchorage can deliver infinite anchorage and thus not be mobilized by orthodontic forces.[62] These bone-based devices have commonly been referred to as OrthoTADs.[63-66] The following section gives a historical perspective of the various OrthoTADs in use based on their chronological appearance in the literature.

Ankylosed Tooth Roots

Although infinite anchorage is usually thought of in terms of biochemically inert foreign objects introduced into the body, this is not necessarily the case. Biologic materials can also be used for infinite anchorage. For example, the use of ankylosed teeth as anchorage was described first in a study carried out on rhesus monkeys in 1980 where Guyman and colleagues[67] ankylosed lateral incisors using the method described by Parker and colleagues.[68] The teeth to be ankylosed were extracted and kept outside the socket for approximately 75 minutes before being reimplanted. During that period, the pulp was extirpated and the roots were allowed to

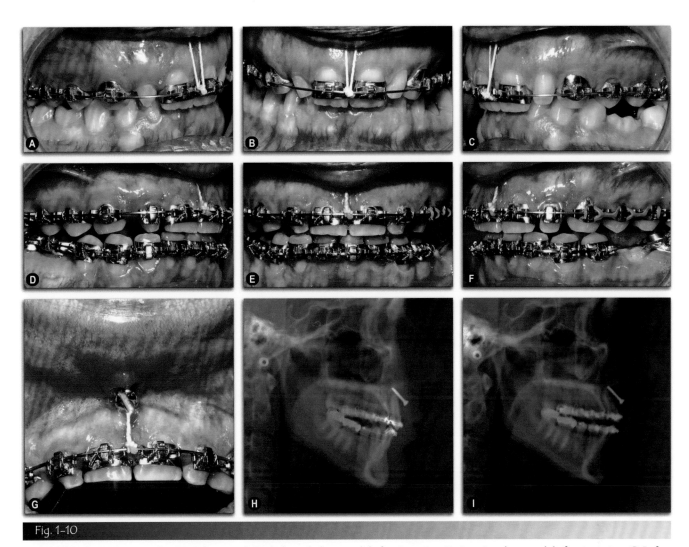

Fig. 1-10

Creekmore's miniscrew anchorage technique. **A,** Right buccal photograph before intrusion. **B,** Anterior photograph before intrusion. **C,** Left buccal photograph before intrusion. **D,** Right buccal photograph after intrusion. **E,** Anterior photograph after intrusion. **F,** Left buccal photograph after intrusion. **G,** Photograph showing screw emergence through soft tissues and elastic force. **H,** Lateral cephalometric radiograph before intrusion. **I,** Lateral cephalometric radiograph after intrusion. (Courtesy the Dr. Tom Creekmore family.)

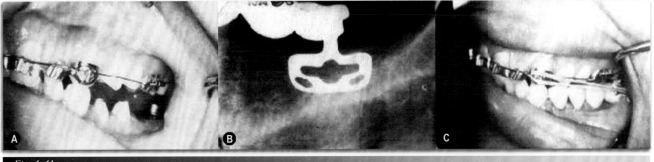

Fig. 1-11

Linkow's blade implant for orthodontic anchorage. **A,** Buccal photograph before placement of four-unit bridge. **B,** Radiograph of blade implant incorporated into four-unit bridge. **C,** Implant-supported bridge used to wear Class II elastics. (Reprinted with permission from Linkow LI. Implanto-Orthodontics. *J Clin Orthod.* 4:685-705, 1970, www.jco-online.com.)

desiccate. Eight weeks later, the teeth demonstrated signs of ankylosis and were loaded. Posttreatment histologic examination confirmed the teeth had undergone

replacement resorption on the root surfaces.

Kokich and colleagues[69] and Omnell and Sheller[70] later used a similar approach clinically on deciduous canines for maxillary protraction in children (Fig. 1-12). Use of ankylosed deciduous teeth has proved efficient and effective; however, the technique is limited for the most part to patients with deciduous teeth. Theoretically, this technique also can be used in cases for protraction of posterior teeth, retraction of anterior teeth, or distalization of the entire arch. Another concern with this type of treatment is that in older adolescent patients, the therapeutically ankylosed teeth could interfere with the eruption of the permanent teeth. In spite of these limitations, this technique is an option in select cases.[71,72]

Miniscrew Implants

Although the first clinical report of miniscrew use appeared in 1983 by Creekmore and Eklund,[53] relatively little interest was generated at that time. Not until the late 1990s were several reports published to introduce the use of miniscrews for orthodontic anchorage. In 1997, Kanomi[73] introduced a mini-implant specifically for orthodontic use (Fig. 1-13). The surgical protocol, however, was extensive and involved local anesthesia, a flap, pilot hole, implant placement, a healing period for osseointegration, and a second flap for orthodontic mechanics attachment. A year later Costa and colleagues[74] introduced another miniscrew with a much simplified placement procedure that involved only local anesthesia, placement of a drill-free screw, and immediate loading (see Chapter 12). Two years afterward, Gray and Smith[75] introduced the use of transitional dental implants, originally designed for supporting a temporary fixed prosthesis, as a tool for orthodontic tooth movement. The transitional implants were placed distal to the upper premolars in edentulous areas to successfully retract the anterior teeth.

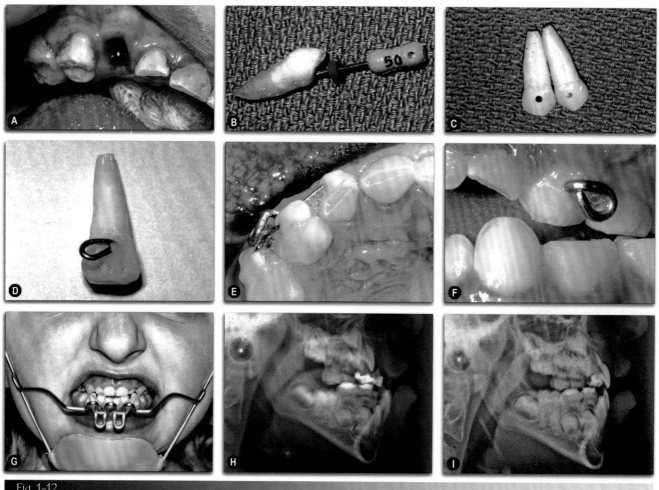

Fig. 1-12

Ankylosed tooth roots for orthodontic-orthopedic anchorage. **A,** Extraction of deciduous canine. **B,** Root canal therapy on extracted canine. **C,** Holes are drilled through the crowns of the canines. **D,** A stainless steel wire is passed through the holes and bonded to the canines. **E,** The canines are temporarily bonded to the adjacent teeth for stabilization until ankylosis occurs. **F,** The bonding material is removed after ankylosis. **G,** The ankylosed canines are attached directly to a protraction face mask via elastics. **H,** Lateral cephalometric radiograph before protraction. **I,** Lateral cephalometric radiograph after protraction. (Courtesy Dr. Lena Omnell.)

Unlike many other TADs, miniscrews are ideally suited for orthodontic anchorage. First, they are not site specific; they can be placed just about anywhere in the oral cavity where ample bone stock is available (usually about 3.5 mm in diameter). Second, the surgical protocol is minimal; no flap is necessary, and many can be placed without a pilot hole. Third, they are designed to achieve primary stability by cortical stabilization. Therefore, they can be loaded immediately without a healing period.

Miniplate Implants

Although Sugawara's group[11,12,76-79] has popularized the use of miniplates for orthodontic anchorage recently, the first report in the literature appeared in 1985. Interestingly, after a mandibular advancement in which the mandibular segments were stabilized by fixation wires, Jenner and Fitzpatrick[80] placed a four-hole bone plate lateral to the ascending ramus to distalize a lower first molar for crowding resolution in the premolar region (Fig. 1-14).

In 1992, Sugawara[81] first applied the precursor of the Skeletal Anchorage System® (SAS) to correct a severe anterior crossbite without using mandibular molars for anchorage. Because of the missing lower molars and extensive horizontal bone loss in the posterior mandible, conventional implants were not an option for anchorage. So Sugawara used a bone screw on one ramus and a modified bone plate on the other to retract the mandibular arch en masse. Essentially, the Skeletal Anchorage System (Dentsply-Sankin, Tokyo, Japan; see Chapter 21) is a modification of rigid fixation using miniplates and bone screws with a portion of the miniplate exposed in the oral cavity for attachment. The primary use of this system has been in the ramus and infrazygomatic regions. However, this limits its use in that when placed in the region of the dentition, it must be placed apical to the roots of the teeth. More recently, Chung and colleagues[82] have introduced the C-plate® and C-tube® (KLS Martin LP, Jacksonville, Florida; see Chapters 19 and 20) for use in the palate and buccal alveolar process, respectively.

Miniplates are probably the second most applicable TAD. They are somewhat site specific in that their different configurations are larger than miniscrews, so they can be placed only in certain locations. However, miniplates are malleable, so they can be cut, bent, and shaped to different bony anatomy. The surgical procedure is also more involved; an incision and flap is necessary, so postoperative discomfort is somewhat higher. The surgical protocol may also increase the risk of infection slightly. Similar to miniscrews, miniplates can also be loaded immediately, so there is no delay in treatment.

Retromolar Implants

Roberts and colleagues[83] reported on the development of a miniaturized dental implant for placement in

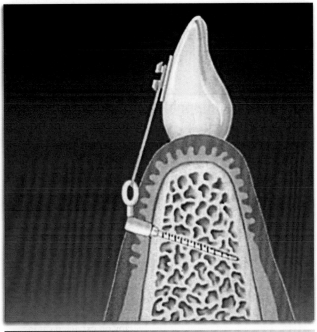

Fig. 1-13

Kanomi's miniscrew implant technique. (Reprinted with permission from Kanomi R. Mini-implant for orthodontic anchorage. *J Clin Orthod.* 31:763-767, 1997, www.jco-online.com.)

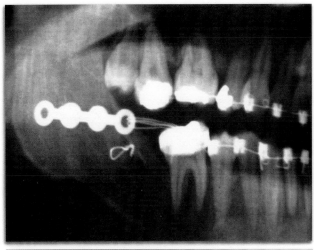

Fig. 1-14

Miniplate implant for orthodontic anchorage. (Reprinted with permission from Jenner JD, Fitzpatrick BN. Skeletal anchorage utilising bone plates. *Aust Orthod J.* 9:231-233, 1985; courtesy of the Australian Orthodontic Journal.)

the retromolar region. The patient, who completed treatment in 1986, was treated with a retromolar implant to intrude and protract the left lower second and third molars to eliminate the edentulous area left by a missing first molar and to avoid the need for dental implant placement and restoration (Fig. 1-15). Roberts and colleagues have also substantiated the technique and use of miniaturized dental implants for orthodontic anchorage experimentally[84-88] and clinically.[89,90] More recently, Higuchi and Slack[91] have also reported the use of retromolar implants. Interestingly, their technique was different from that of Roberts. The former used the implant as direct anchorage to push the molars forward; the latter used the implant as indirect anchorage to stabilize the canine, which was used to pull the molars forward. The main disadvantage of retromolar implants, besides being larger than miniscrew implants, is that they are site specific and so do not lend themselves to many different cases. Moreover, a healing period is required to allow for osseointegration before loading.

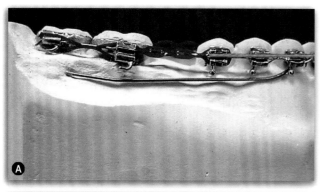

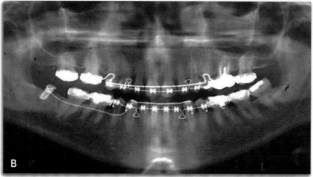

Fig. 1-15

Retromolar implant for orthodontic anchorage. **A,** The standard set-up includes a titanium-molybdenum alloy (TMA) arch wire extending from the retromolar implant anteriorly to the canine, which then is used indirectly to protract the molars. **B,** Panoramic radiograph after molar protraction into a missing premolar space. (Courtesy Dr. Bill Hohlt.)

Palatal Implants

The first reported use of the palate for placement of a screw-type implant appeared in 1988, when Fontenelle[92] demonstrated the clinical use of an osteosynthesis screw for orthodontic purposes. The screw was placed in the palate and connected via a cast bar to the upper posterior segments as indirect anchorage for retracting the anterior teeth. Several years later Triaca and colleagues[1] used the anterior hard palate for placement of a palatal implant for orthodontic anchorage. Perhaps it was these first few reports that spurred Wehrbein and colleagues[2,3,93-98] to report extensively on the basic biology and clinical use of palatal implants (see Chapter 18), small dental implants placed specifically in the palate for maxillary anchorage. The benefit of palatal implants is that they can be placed most anywhere in the hard palate with minimal concern for dental anatomic structures such as tooth roots. As with retromolar implants, their limitation lies in their site-specific nature and required healing period (Fig. 1-16).

Fixation Wire Implants

Screws, plates, and miniaturized implants are not the only possibilities for enhancing orthodontic anchorage. Another orthognathic fixation technique has also been advocated for orthodontic purposes. In 1998, Melsen and colleagues[99] introduced the use of fixation wires through the zygomatic arch (see Chapter 12) for retraction and intrusion of flared and overerupted upper anterior teeth in patients with insufficient posterior anchorage. Although the report was published in 1998, the first case was treated about 10 years earlier. The procedure was fairly successful and allowed immediate loading; however, the ligatures were site specific and were only useful for about 3 to 6 months, after which they often pulled through the bone. The authors felt that this failure was due to inadequate cortical purchase upon initial wire insertion. More recently, Sfondrini and colleagues[100] used a similar technique in the ascending ramus to deimpact a mesioangularly impacted lower second molar.

Palatal Onplants

Similar to palatal implants, palatal onplants, developed by Block and Hoffman[101,102] in the early 1990s, were designed specifically for placement in the hard palate. Unlike implants, however, the onplant was not designed to be placed within the cortical and medullary bone but rather to sit on top of the cortical bone. The physical characteristics were a thin disk (2 mm tall by

10 mm in diameter). The surgical procedure involved elevation of a soft tissue flap, subperiosteal tunneling, placement of the onplant in intimate bony contact,

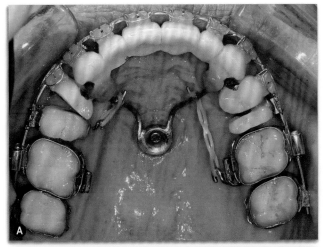
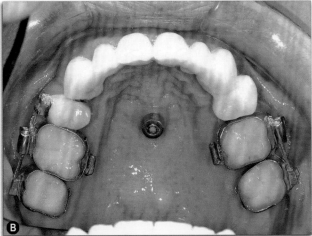
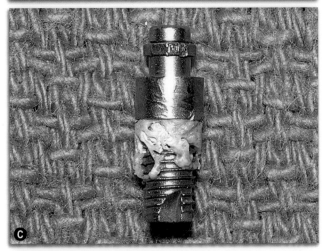

Fig. 1-16

Palatal implant used to protract upper buccal segments and eliminate premolar pontics. **A,** Occlusal photograph at initial loading. **B,** Occlusal photograph after protraction. **C,** Palatal implant upon removal. Note extensive bone ingrowth around implant.

followed by soft tissue closure. In a second procedure approximately 4 months later, after osseointegration, the abutment of the onplant was uncovered for orthodontic attachment.

Although effective for orthodontic anchorage as demonstrated by several clinical reports,[103-105] the surgical procedure is more complex, time consuming, and invasive than other TAD placement procedures. Moreover, a considerable amount of laboratory and chair time is needed to deliver the attachment mechanisms, increasing the orthodontic cost (Fig. 1-17).

Dilacerated Tooth Roots

Ankylosed teeth are not the only type of biologic material that can be used for absolute anchorage. Another option is the use of severely dilacerated tooth roots, which apparently have been overlooked heretofore (Fig. 1-18). The patient presented with DiGeorges syndrome or congenital absence of the thymus and parathyroid glands. The syndrome is usually characterized by kidney, heart, and ear involvement. However, the patient did not have heart involvement, but rather dental involvement, which mimicked amelogenesis imperfecta with primary failure of eruption. At the time of initial presentation, the 16-year-old girl had already undergone three surgeries to uncover the unerupted teeth. Understanding that if the 90-degree dilacerated lower second premolars did move, they would move at such a slow rate to be effectively ankylosed relative to the adjacent teeth, the treatment plan was to sacrifice them for orthodontic treatment. Crowns were waxed, cast, and cemented to the final desired occlusal plane. The orthodontic mechanics were then designed to extrude the adjacent teeth, followed by extraction of the lower second premolars with eventual replacement via dental implants and restoration. Although this is a relatively rare situation, it demonstrates that teeth can be used as TADs, whether by ankylosis or severe dilaceration.

Classification

Characteristics of an ideal anchorage device include: simple to use, inexpensive, small dimensions, immediately loadable, able to withstand orthodontic forces, immobile, does not require compliance, biocompatible, and provides clinically equivalent or superior results compared with traditional anchorage systems. At a minimum, when initially placed, TADs must have primary stability and must be able to withstand orthodontic force levels. For integrated implants the maximum load is proportional to the quantity of osseointegration, whereas for nonintegrated implants the maximum load is proportional to the surface area contact of the bone to the implant.

The currently available TADs can be classified as biocompatible or biologic (Fig 1-19).[64,65] Both groups can be subclassified based on the manner in which they are attached to bone: biochemical (osseointegrated) or mechanical (cortical stabilization). For instance, an ankylosed tooth temporarily used for orthodontic anchorage and subsequently replaced would be considered a biologic TAD that is biochemically fixed to bone. Likewise, a significantly dilacerated tooth can be used as

a biologic TAD that is mechanically fixed to bone.

The biocompatible TADs are a modification of (1) a dental implant or (2) a surgical fixation method. For example, a palatal implant is a miniaturized dental implant placed in the palate with the intention of osseointegration and subsequent use for orthodontic anchorage. However, a miniscrew implant is a fixation device placed in many locations for anchorage control without the intention of osseointegration but only for mechanical stability. Recently, a hybrid device was developed.[9] Interestingly, the 1.8-mm C-Implant® (Cimplant Co., Seoul, Korea) is a miniscrew but also

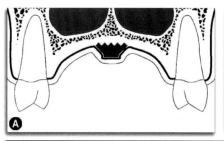 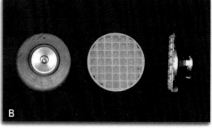 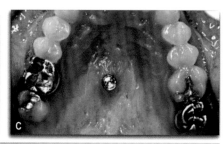

Fig. 1-17

Palatal onplant used for maxillary anchorage. **A,** Diagram illustrating subperiosteal position. **B,** Photograph of the onplant showing superior, inferior, and lateral views. **C,** Occlusal photograph of onplant in place. (Courtesy Dr. Bill Hohlt.)

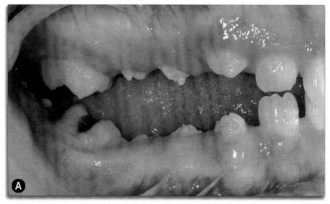 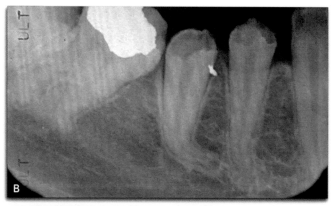

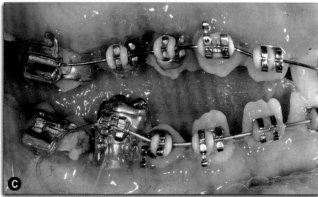 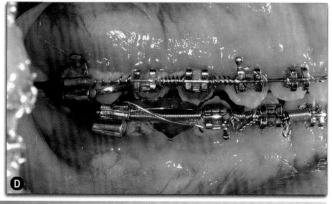

Fig. 1-18

Dilacerated tooth roots used to extrude posterior teeth. **A,** Initial buccal photograph. **B,** Initial periapical radiograph. **C,** Progress buccal photograph at initial crown cementation and loading. **D,** Progress buccal photograph after posterior extrusion and dilacerated tooth extraction.

has a treated surface to enhance the possibility of osseointegration (see Chapter 17). The authors suggest that it can be used in heavier loading conditions than with traditional miniscrew implants.

The ability of orthodontists to communicate with each other clearly and concisely is important. Previously, several different terms have been used to refer to the same entity. To explain, what heretofore has been referred to as a miniscrew implant has been referred to in the literature as a microimplant,[106] microscrew implant,[107] mini-implant,[108] mini dental implant,[109] miniscrew,[20] and screw-type implant.[7] *Mini* is simply the shortened form of miniature, which traditional dictionaries refer to as "something small compared to other things of its type" or "small in relation to others of the same kind." *Micro*, however, is the shortened form of the word *microscopic*, which traditional dictionaries refer to as "requiring magnification" or "revealed by or having the structure discernible only by microscopic examination." By definition then, it follows that something microscopic conceivably has no viable use in orthodontic mechanics at present; therefore, the term *mini* is more correct and is preferable.

The difference between a screw and an implant also can be debated. Both can be defined based on function or design. For instance, the original historical function of a screw was to use the mechanical advantage of the inclined plane wrapped around a central body to lift objects. The screw was later used to join two objects together. Screw designs are defined by length, diameter, thread depth, thread pitch, and head/end configuration. The original historical function of the implant was to replace or augment a body part. Many of the original dental implants were designed with a screw shape for initial mechanical stability[37] because the initial basket and other shapes did not offer immediate mechanical stability.[36,37] Implant designs also are defined by length, diameter, thread depth, thread pitch, and head/end configuration.

According to the United States Food and Drug Administration,[110] an endosseous dental implant is a "device made of titanium or titanium alloy that is surgically placed in bone of upper or lower jaw." The governmental regulatory agency goes on to characterize a root-form endosseous dental implant by four geometrically distinct types: basket, screw, solid

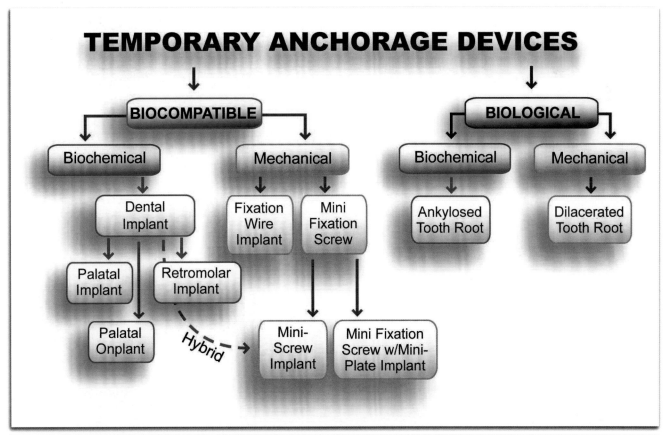

Fig. 1-19

Temporary anchorage device classification.

cylinder, and hollow cylinder. To be fair, the European Economic Community, which awards the CE mark and is the regulatory body in Europe closely analogous to the Food and Drug Administration, defines an implantable device as one "intended to remain in place after the procedure for at least 30 days."[111]

Using this available information, it appears that all biocompatible TADs should be considered implants. Further, for the entity described as a small or miniaturized screw-shaped implant, the term *miniscrew implant* (MSI) is most appropriate and will be used herein. Furthermore, *miniscrew implant* will be defined as having a diameter of between 1.0 and 2.5 mm. Following is a list of simple yet distinct acronyms for all of the currently available TADs.[64,65] For example, shorthand terminology for a palatal implant would be TAD-PI.

OrthoTAD	Orthodontic Temporary Anchorage Device
ATR	Ankylosed Tooth Root
DTR	Dilacerated Tooth Root
FWI	Fixation Wire Implant
MPI	Miniplate Implant
MSI	Miniscrew Implant
PO	Palatal Onplant
RMI	Retromolar Implant
PI	Palatal Implant

Considering the surgical protocol and armamentarium, the future of OrthoTADs will most probably be reserved primarily for MSIs. They are easier to place than other TADs, they do not require pilot holes or flaps, they are more cost-effective, they now can be placed frequently with topical anesthetic only (see Chapter 9), and they are much easier for orthodontists to place. Recently, the American Association of Orthodontists has amended its liability policy to include coverage of MSI placement so long as no soft tissue flap is raised.[112]

TERMS AND DEFINITIONS

In using OrthoTADs, however, the inexperienced clinician is sure to be bombarded and overwhelmed with new and unfamiliar terms. What follows is a brief explanation of the more commonly used terms associated with OrthoTADs.

Delayed, Early, and Immediate Loading

Delayed loading is the term used to describe an extended healing period after surgical implant placement prior to functional loading. This period has traditionally ranged from 6 weeks[113] to 6 months.[34,35,39,86] Two terms have been used to describe loading of an implant earlier than traditional delayed loading. *Immediate loading* has been defined as functional implant loading within 48 hours of surgical implant placement. *Early loading* has been defined as functional implant loading at least 48 hours after implant placement, but shorter in time frame than conventional healing, which is usually 6 or more weeks.[114]

Originally, based on Brånemark's work,[34,35,39] it was thought that all implants should undergo a 4- to 6-month healing period prior to functional loading. This was because the authors, based on clinical and experimental evidence, felt that premature loading caused micromotion of the implants, which allowed the invasion of fibrous tissue and implant failure. This was supported by the findings of Roberts and colleagues,[86] using a rabbit model to study static orthodontic-type implant loading of 100 g after 6, 8, or 12 weeks of healing. Based on these findings, Roberts and colleagues felt that 6 weeks (in rabbits) was the earliest an implant should be loaded after placement. Because sigma, or the duration of remodeling, in human beings is about 3 times longer than in rabbits, he felt that the same duration equaled 18 weeks in human beings.

In the early 1990s, several groups began to publish their findings of immediately loading dental implants after initial surgical placement. Lum and colleagues,[115] comparing hydroxylapatite-coated to uncoated blade-type implants in rhesus monkeys, found that immediately loaded implants were comparable clinically and histologically to delayed-loaded implants; that is, both were stable and had direct bone contact without fibrous tissue invasion. Importantly, all implants were stabilized by a fixed prosthesis, thereby minimizing micromotion of the implant.

Several years later, Tarnow and colleagues[116] reported similar findings in human patients. Their study used a minimum of 10 mandibular implants, 5 of which were loaded immediately via a multiimplant retained single-unit prosthesis and the other 5 of which remained buried/unloaded in case any of the immediately loaded implants failed. Only 2 out of 69 immediately loaded implants failed, both of which were placed into an immediate extraction site. These findings suggested that immediate loading of implants also may be possible clinically as long as the implants are splinted together, thereby minimizing local micromotion.

Dynamic and Static Loading

Dynamic loading is the term used to describe implant loading under intermittent loads of variable force levels, much as would be seen during mastication. These types of loads have been referred to as jiggling forces and are reported to cause implant failure.[117] *Static loading* is the term used to describe constant loads of uniform force levels, similar to what is seen with orthodontic forces; usually loaded in one direction only, with a relatively uniform force over an extended period.

Duyck's group[118] recently evaluated the differences in load type on osseointegrated implants. After 10-mm long Brånemark implants were allowed to heal for 6 weeks, the implants were loaded for 14 days statically (constant loads of uniform force levels) or dynamically (cyclic loads of variable force levels) or were left unloaded. Interestingly, similar bone-to-implant contact was seen for all implants, but a difference was seen in the marginal bone around the implant. The statically loaded and unloaded controls showed a more dense cortical lamellar bone at the neck and apex of the implants, whereas the dynamically loaded implants revealed bony craters and Howship's lacunae around the implants necks, indicating a higher level of bony resorption. Gotfredsen and colleagues[119] found similar results in laterally loaded experimental implants: higher bone density and bone-to-implant contact for the statically loaded implant compared with unloaded controls.

Based on some of the more relevant studies, it appears that implants can be loaded earlier than previously thought as long as the implants are splinted together (i.e., micromotion is minimized). The same has also been found with MSIs designed for immediate loading under static loading conditions.[74,120] According to Szmukler-Moncler and colleagues,[117] micromotion should be less than about 100 μm. Furthermore, statically loaded implants have more dense cortical lamellar bone and higher bone-to-implant contact on the loaded surface than dynamically loaded or unloaded control implants.

Self-Tapping, Drill-Free, and Non–Drill-Free Screws

A distinction should be made regarding screw-shaped implant nomenclature. Often misused terms include *self-tapping*, self-drilling (also referred to as *drill-free*), and *non–self-drilling*. *Self-tapping* simply refers to the ability of a screw to advance when turned while creating its own thread. There are two types of self-tapping screws: *thread-forming* and *thread-cutting*. Both screw types have sharp threads for forming the internal bony threads during screw advancement. In addition, a thread-cutting screw has a notch cut parallel to the long axis and located at the apex of the implant, such that as the screw is advanced into the bone, the notched surface of the implant actually cuts or taps and removes bone out of the way of the advancing threads.[59] The notch also aids in removal of *swarf*, or bone debris, created during screw placement. Importantly, the notch feature may tend to weaken smaller screw-shaped implants, possibly necessitating a pilot hole. Moreover, when the screws are left in place for long periods, bone may have grown into the notch, thereby making screw removal difficult.[121,122]

A self-drilling or *drill-free implant* is one in which its apex is sharp and tapered to allow for placement without a predrilled pilot hole. For example, the Ortho Implant (IMTEC Corp, Ardmore, Oklahoma; see Chapter 9) is drill-free and self-tapping (thread-forming). Recent evidence suggests that drill-free screws have better bone-to-implant adaptation than non–drill-free screws.[16] Finally, a *non–drill-free implant* requires the placement of a pilot hole before implant insertion because the apex is not sharp enough to perforate the outer bony layer or because the implant is too small in diameter to allow placement into bone without the possibility of fracture.

Direct and Indirect Anchorage

Two different terms have been developed to differentiate how the orthodontic mechanics attach to TADs. Direct anchorage is the term used when the TAD is attached directly to the teeth of the active segment for tooth movement. Indirect anchorage is the term used when the TAD is attached to and reinforces the teeth of the reactive segment, which is directly used to move the teeth of the active segment. Unlike the previously mentioned terms, direct and indirect attachment mechanisms are not determined based on scientific data but rather on a case-by-case basis for the specific mechanics requirements.

SUMMARY

The use of OrthoTADs is a relatively new application of more established clinical methodologies. Although the clinician can look to the literature for many answers, much is unknown and will be answered only by well-designed prospective basic scientific experiments and clinical trials. The future development of TADs for orthodontic anchorage will establish a more complete understanding of the biology and biomechanics associated with integrated and nonintegrated TADs.

REFERENCES

1.   Triaca A, Antonin M, Wintermantel E. Ein neues titan-flaschrauben implantat zur orthodontischen verankerung am anterion gaumen. *Int Orthod Keiferorthop.* 24:251-257, 1992.

2.   Wehrbein H, Glatzmaier J, Mundwiller U, Diedrich P. The Orthosystem: a new implant system for orthodontic anchorage in the palate. *J Orofac Orthop.* 57:142-153, 1996.

3.   Wehrbein H, Mertz B, Diedrich P, Glatzmaier J. The use of palatal implants for orthodontic anchorage: design and clinical application of the orthosystem. *Clin Oral Implants Res.* 7:410-417, 1996.

4.   Park HS, Bae SM, Kyung HM, Sung JH. Simultaneous incisor retraction and distal molar movement with microimplant anchorage. *World J Orthod.* 5:164-171, 2004.

5.   Bae SM, Park HS, Kyung HM, Sung JH. Ultimate anchorage control. *Tex Dent J.* 119:580-591, 2002.

6.   Giancotti A, Muzzi F, Santini F, Arcuri C. Mini-screw treatment of ectopic mandibular molars. *J Clin Orthod.* 37:380-383, 2004.

7.   Kawakami M, Miyakawa S, Noguchi H, Kirita T. Screw type implants used as anchorage for lingual orthodontic mechanics: a case of bimaxillary protrusion with second premolar extraction. *Angle Orthod.* 74:715-719, 2004.

8.   Kyung SH, Hong SG, Park YC. Distalization of maxillary molars with a midpalatal miniscrew. *J Clin Orthod.* 37:22-26, 2003.

9.   Chung K-R, Kim S-H, Kook Y-A. The C-Orthodontic micro-implant. *J Clin Orthod.* 38:478-486, 2004.

10. Liou EJ, Pai BCJ, Lin JC. Do miniscrews remain stationary under orthodontic forces? *Am J Orthod Dentofacial Orthop.* 126:42-47, 2004.

11. Sugawara J, Baik U, Umemori M, et al. Treatment and posttreatment dentoalveolar changes following intrusion of mandibular molars with application of a skeletal anchorage system (SAS) for open bite correction. *Int J Adult Orthodon Orthognath Surg.* 17:243-253, 2002.

12. Sugawara J, Daimaruya T, Umemori M, et al. Distal movement of mandibular molars in adult patients with the skeletal anchorage system. *Am J Orthod Dentofacial Orthop.* 125:130-138, 2004.

13. Miyakawa S, Koyama I, Inoue M, et al. Factors associated with the stability of titanium screws placed in the posterior region for orthodontic anchorage. *Am J Orthod Dentofacial Orthop.* 124:373-378, 2003.

14. Cheng SJ, Tseng IY, Lee JJ, Kok S-H. A prospective study of the risk factors associated with failure of mini-implants used for orthodontic anchorage. *Int J Oral Maxillofac Implants.* 19:100-106, 2004.

15. Melsen B, Costa A. Immediate loading of implants used for orthodontic anchorage. *Clin Orthod Res.* 3:23-28, 2000.

16. Kim J, Ahn S, Chang Y. Histomorphometric and mechanical analyses of the drill-free screw as orthodontic anchorage. *Am J Orthod Dentofacial Orthop.* 128:190-194, 2005.

17. Owens S, Buschang PH, Cope JB, et al. Experimental evaluation of mini-screw-implant stability and tooth movement in the beagle dog. *Am J Orthod Dentofacial Orthop.* In press.

18. Deguchi T, Takano-Yamamoto T, Kanomi R, et al. The use of small titanium screws for orthodontic anchorage. *J Dent Res.* 82:377-381, 2003.

19. Ohmae M, Saito S, Morohashi T, et al. A clinical and histological evaluation of titanium mini-implants as anchors for orthodontic intrusion in the beagle dog. *Am J Orthod Dentofacial Orthop.* 119:489-497, 2001.

20. Dalstra M, Cattaneo PM, Melsen B. Load transfer of miniscrews for orthodontic anchorage. *Orthodontics.* 1:53-62, 2004.

21. Huja S, Litsky A, Beck FM, et al. Pull-out strength of monocortical screws placed in the maxillae and mandibles of dogs. *Am J Orthod Dentofacial Orthop.* 127:307-313, 2005.

22. Ottofy L. *Standard Dental Dictionary.* Chicago, Ill: Laird & Lee Inc, 1923.

23. Daskalogiannakis J. *Glossary of Orthodontic Terms.* Leipzig, Germany: Quintessence Publishing Co, 2000.

24. Moyers R. Handbook of *Orthodontics for the Student and General Practitioner.* Chicago, Ill: Year Book Medical Publishers Inc, 1973.

25. Gianelly A, Goldman H. *Biologic Basis of Orthodontics.* Philadelphia, Pa: Lea & Febiger, 1971.

26. Marcotte M. *Biomechanics in Orthodontics.* Toronto, Canada: BD Decker, 1990.

27. Burstone CJ. En masse space closure. In: Burstone CJ, ed. *Modern Edgewise Mechanics and the Segmented Arch Technique.* Glendora, Calif: Ormco Corp, 1995:50-60.

28. Tweed C. *Clinical Orthodontics.* St Louis, Mo: CV Mosby Co, 1966.

29. Sherwood KH, Burch JG, Thompson WJ. Closing anterior open bites by intruding molars with titanium miniplate anchorage. *Am J Orthod Dentofacial Orthop.* 122:593-600, 2002.

30. Paik CH, Woo YJ, Boyd RL. Treatment of an adult patient with vertical maxillary excess using miniscrew fixation. *J Clin Orthod.* 37:423-428, 2003.

31. Park HS, Kwon T-G, Kwon OW. Treatment of open bite with microscrew implant anchorage. *Am J Orthod Dentofacial Orthop.* 126:627-636, 2004.

32. Weinberger BW. The history of orthodontia, VI. *Int J Orthod.* 2:103-117, 1916.

33. Weinberger BW. *Orthodontics: An Historical Review of Its Origin and Evolution.* St Louis, Mo: CV Mosby Co, 1926.

34. Brånemark PI, Breine U, Adell R, et al. Intra-osseous anchorage of dental prostheses, I: experimental studies. *Scand J Plast Rencontr Surg.* 3:81-100, 1969.

35. Brånemark PI. Osseointegration and its experimental background. *J Prosthet Dent.* 50:399-410, 1983.

36. Greenfield EJ, inventor. Mounting for Artificial Teeth. US patent 943 113, 1-3. December 14, 1909.

37. Strock AE. Experimental work on a method for the replacement of missing teeth by direct implantation of a metal support into the alveolus. *Am J Orthod.* 25:467-472, 1939.

38. Venable S, Stuck W. *The Internal Fixation of Fractures: An Historical Review of Its Origin and Evolution.* Springfield, Ill: Charles C Thomas, 1947.

39. Adell R, Lekholm U, Rockler B, Brånemark PI. A 15-year study of osseointegrated implants in the treatment of the edentulous jaw. *Int J Oral Surg.* 10:387-416, 1981.

40. Hamilton F. *A Practical Treatise on Fractures and Dislocations.* Philadelphia, Pa: Blanchard & Lea, 1860.

41. Adams W. Internal wiring fixation of facial fractures. *Surgery.* 12:523-530, 1932.

42. Gilmer T. A case of fracture of the lower jaw with remarks on treatment. *Arch Dent.* 4:388-392, 1887.

43. Christiansen G. Open operation and tantalum plate insertion for fracture of the mandible. *J Oral Surg.* 3:194-204, 1945.

44. Ellis E III. The internal fixation of fractures: historical perspectives. In: Tucker MR, Terry BC, White RP Jr, Van Sickels JE, eds. *Rigid Fixation for Maxillofacial Surgery.* Philadelphia, Pa: JB Lippincott Co, 1991:3-29.

45. Luhr H. Zur stabilen osteosynthese bei unterkieferfrakturen. *Dtsch Zahnarztl Z.* 23:754-759, 1968.

46. Brons R, Boering G. Fractures of the mandibular body treated by stable internal fixation: a preliminary report. *J Oral Maxillofac Surg.* 28:407-415, 1970.

47. Michelet F, Deymes J, Dessus B. Osteosynthesis with miniaturized screwed plates in maxillofacial surgery. *J Oral Maxillofac Surg.* 1:79-84, 1973.

48. Champy M, Wilk A, Schnebelen J. Die behandlung der mandibularfrakturen mittels osteosynthese ohne intermaxillare ruhigstellung nach der technik von Michelet. *Dtsch Zahn Mund Kieferheilkd.* 63:339-346, 1975.

49. Champy M, Lodde J, Jaeger J. Osteosyntheses mandibulaires selon la technique de Michelet, I: bases biomechaniques. *Rev Stomatol Chir Maxillofac.* 77:569-575, 1976.

50. Champy M, Lodde J, Jaeger J. Osteosyntheses mandibulaires selon la technique de Michelet, II: presentation d'un nouveau materiel resultats. *Rev Stomatol Chir Maxillofac.* 77:577-582, 1976.

51. Jeter T, Van Sickels J, Dolwick M. Modified techniques for internal fixation of sagittal ramus osteotomies. *J Oral Maxillofac Surg.* 42:270-272, 1984.

52. Gainsforth BL, Higley LB. A study of orthodontic anchorage possibilities in basal bone. *Am J Orthod Oral Surg.* 31:406-416, 1945.

53. Creekmore TD, Eklund MK. The possibility of skeletal anchorage. *J Clin Orthod.* 17:266-269, 1983.

54. Linkow LI. The endosseous blade implant and its use in orthodontics. *Int J Orthod.* 7:149-154, 1969.

55. Kokich VG. Managing complex orthodontic problems: the use of implants for anchorage. *Semin Orthod.* 2:153-160, 1996.

56. Smalley WM. Implants for tooth movement: determining implant location and orientation. *J Esthet Dent.* 7:62-72, 1995.

57. Smalley WM, Blanco A. Implants for tooth movement: a fabrication and placement technique for provisional restorations. *J Esthet Dent.* 7:150-154, 1995.

58. Ghosh J, Nanda R. Evaluation of an intraoral maxillary molar distalization technique. *Am J Orthod Dentofacial Orthop.* 110:639-646, 1996.

59. Keles A, Sayinsu K. A new approach in maxillary molar distalization: intraoral bodily molar distalizer. *Am J Orthod Dentofacial Orthop.* 117:39-48, 2000.

60. Ngantung V, Nanda R, Bowman S. Posttreatment evaluation of the distal jet appliance. *Am J Orthod Dentofacial Orthop.* 120:178-185, 2001.

61. Bolla E, Mruatore F, Carano A, Bowman S. Evaluation of maxillary molar distalization with the distal jet: a comparison with other contemporary methods. *Angle Orthod.* 72:481-494, 2002.

62. Rozencweig G, Rozencweiz S. Use of implants and ankylosed teeth in orthodontics: a review of the literature. *J Paradontol.* 8:179-184, 1989.

63. Cope JB. Introduction. *Semin Orthod.* 11:1-2, 2005.

64. Cope JB. Temporary anchorage devices in orthodontics: a paradigm shift. *Semin Orthod.* 11:3-9, 2005.

65. Cope J. Temporary anchorage devices in orthodontics. Available at: www.OrthoTADs.com. Accessed March 1, 2005.

66. Mah J, Bergstrand F. Temporary anchorage devices: a status report. *J Clin Orthod.* 39:1-5, 2005.

67. Guyman G, Kokich VG, Oswald R. Ankylosed teeth as abutments for palatal expansion in the rhesus monkey. *Am J Orthod.* 77:486-499, 1980.

68. Parker W, Frische H, Grant T. The experimental production of dental ankylosis. *Angle Orthod.* 34:103-107, 1964.

69. Kokich VG, Shapiro PA, Oswald R, et al. Ankylosed teeth as abutments for maxillary protraction: a case report. *Am J Orthod Dentofacial Orthop.* 88:303-307, 1985.

70. Omnell M, Sheller B. Maxillary protraction to intentionally ankylosed deciduous canines in a patient with cleft palate. *Am J Orthod Dentofacial Orthop.* 106:201-205, 1994.

71. Sheller B, Omnell M. Therapeutic ankylosis of primary teeth. *J Clin Orthod.* 25:499-502, 1991.

72. Silva Filho OG, Ozawa TO, Okada CH, et al. Intentional ankylosis of deciduous canines to reinforce maxillary protraction. *J Clin Orthod.* 37:315-320, 2003.

73. Kanomi R. Mini-implant for orthodontic anchorage. *J Clin Orthod.* 31:763-767, 1997.

74. Costa A, Raffaini M, Melsen B. Miniscrews as orthodontic anchorage: a preliminary report. *Int J Adult Orthodon Orthognath Surg.* 13:201-209, 1998.

75. Gray JB, Smith R. Transitional implants for orthodontic anchorage. *J Clin Orthod.* 34:659-666, 2000.

76. Sugawara J, Nishimura M. Mini bone plates: the skeletal anchorage system. *Semin Orthod.* 11:47-56, 2005.

77. Umemori M, Sugawara J, Mitani H, et al. Skeletal anchorage system for openbite correction. *Am J Orthod Dentofacial Orthop.* 115:166-174, 1999.

78. Daimaruya T, Nagasaka H, Umemori M, et al. The influence of first molar intrusion on the inferior alveolar neurovascular bundle and root using the skeletal anchorage system in dogs. *Angle Orthod.* 71:60-70, 2001.

79. Daimaruya T, Takahashi I, Nagasaka H, et al. Effects of maxillary molar intrusion on the nasal floor and tooth root using the skeletal anchorage system in dogs. *Angle Orthod.* 73:158-166, 2003.

80. Jenner JD, Fitzpatrick BN. Skeletal anchorage utilising bone plates. *Aust Orthod J.* 9:231-233, 1985.

81. White L, Sugawara J. Dr. Junji Sugawara on the skeletal anchorage system. *J Clin Orthod.* 33:689-696, 1999.

82. Chung K, Kim Y, Linton JL, Lee Y. The miniplate with tube for skeletal anchorage. *J Clin Orthod.* 36:407-412, 2002.

83. Roberts WE, Marshall KJ, Mozsary PG. Rigid endosseous implant utilized as anchorage to protract molars and close an atrophic extraction site. *Angle Orthod.* 60:135-151, 1990.

84. Roberts WE, Helm FR, Marshall KJ, et al. Rigid endosseous implants for orthodontic and orthopedic anchorage. *Angle Orthod.* 59:247-256, 1989.

85. Roberts WE, Poon LC, Smith RK. Interface histology of rigid endosseous implants. *Angle Orthod.* 12:406-416, 1986.

86. Roberts WE, Smith RK, Zilberman Y, et al. Osseous adaptation to continuous loading of rigid endosseous implants. *Am J Orthod Dentofacial Orthop.* 86:95-111, 1984.

87. Chen J, Chen K, Garetto LP, Roberts WE. Mechanical response to functional and therapeutic loading of a retromolar endosseous implant used for orthodontic anchorage to mesially translate mandibular molars. *Implant Dent.* 4:246-258, 1995.

88. Chen J, Esterle M, Roberts WE. Mechanical response to functional loading around the threads of retromolar endosseous implants utilized for orthodontic anchorage: coordinated histomorphometric and finite element analysis. *Int J Oral Maxillofac Implants.* 14:282-289, 1999.

89. Roberts WE, Arbuckle GR, Analoui M. Rate of mesial translation of mandibular molars using implant anchored mechanics. *Angle Orthod.* 66:331-338, 1996.

90. Roberts WE, Nelson CL, Goodacre CJ. Rigid implant anchorage to close a mandiublar first molar extraction site. *J Clin Orthod.* 28:693-703, 1994.

91. Higuchi KW, Slack JM. The use of titanium fixtures for intraoral anchorage to facilitate orthodontic tooth movement. *Int J Oral Maxillofac Implants.* 6:338-344, 1991.

92. Fontenelle A. Esthetics in orthodontics: lingual appliances. *Actual Odontostomatol.* 42:743-766, 1988.

93. Glatzmaier J, Wehrbein H, Diedrich P. Biodegradable implants for orthodontic anchorage: a preliminary biomechanical study. *Eur J Orthod.* 18:465-469, 1996.

94. Wehrbein H, Merz BR. Aspects of the use of endosseous palatal implants in orthodontic therapy. *J Esthet Dent.* 10:315-324, 1998.

95. Wehrbein H, Glatzmaier J, Yildirim M. Orthodontic anchorage capacity of short titanium screw implants in the maxilla: an experimental study in the dog. *Clin Oral Implants Res.* 8:131-141, 1997.

96. Wehrbein H, Yildirim M, Diedrich P. Osteodynamics around orthodontically loaded short maxillary implants: an experimental study. *J Orofac Orthop.* 60:409-415, 1999.

97. Wehrbein H, Merz BR, Diedrich P. Palatal bone support for orthodontic implant anchorage: a clinical and radiological study. *Eur J Orthod.* 21:65-70, 1999.

98. Wehrbein H, Feifel H, Diedrich P. Palatal implant anchorage reinforcement of posterior teeth: a prospective study. *Am J Orthod Dentofacial Orthop.* 116:678-686, 1999.

99. Melsen B, Petersen JK, Costa A. Zygoma ligatures: an alternative form of maxillary anchorage. *J Clin Orthod.* 32:154-158, 1998.

100. Sfondrini MF, Cacciafesta V, Sfondrini D. The uprighting of mesially tipped and impacted mandibular second molars: the use of the mandibular ramus as orthodontic anchorage. *Orthodontics.* 1:3-12, 2004.

101. Block MS, Hoffman DR. A new device for absolute anchorage for orthodontics. *Am J Orthod Dentofacial Orthop.* 107:251-258, 1995.

102. Armbruster PC, Block MS. Onplant supported orthodontic anchorage. *Atlas Oral Maxillofac Surg Clin North Am.* 9:53-74, 2001.

103. Hohlt WF. Using the palatal onplant for absolute anchorage. In: McNamara JA Jr, ed. *Implants, Microimplants, Onplants, and Transplants: New Answers to Old Questions in Orthodontics,* Ann Arbor: Center for Human Growth and Development, University of Michigan, 2005:145-158.

104. Bondemark L, Feldmann I, Feldmann H. Distal molar movement with an intra-arch device provided with the onplant system for absolute anchorage. *World J Orthod.* 3:117-124, 2002.

105. Janssens F, Swennen G, Dujardin T, et al. Use of an onplant as orthodontic anchorage. *Am J Orthod Dentofacial Orthop.* 122:566-570, 2002.

106. Chung K, Kim S-H, Kook Y. C-Orthodontic microimplant for distalization of mandibular dentition in Class III correction. *Angle Orthod.* 75:119-128, 2004.

107. Park HS, Kwon T-G. Sliding mechanics with microscrew implant anchorage. *Angle Orthod.* 74:703-710, 2004.

108. Hong R-K, Heo J-M, Ha Y-K. Lever-arm and mini-implant system for anterior torque control during retraction in lingual orthodontic treatment. *Angle Orthod.* 75:129-141, 2004.

109. Herman R, Cope J. Miniscrew implants: IMTEC mini ortho implants. *Semin Orthod.* 11:32-39, 2005.

110. US Food and Drug Administration, Department of Health and Human Services. Code of Federal Regulations. Title 21 Food and Drugs, Vol 8, Chap I, Subch H, Medical Devices. 4-1-2004. 21 CFR 872.3640.

111. The Council of the European Communities. Council directive 93/42/EEC of 14 June 1993 concerning medical devices. *Official Journal L.* 169, 12/7/1993, 0001-0043. 12-7-1993, 31993L0042.

112. American Association of Orthodontists Insurance Company. Orthodontist Professional Liability Insurance Policy. Montpelier, Vt: American Association of Orthodontists Insurance Company, 2004:1-16.

113. Barewal RM, Oates TW, Meredith N, Cochran DL. Resonance frequency measurement of implant stability in vivo on implants with a sandblasted and acid-etched surface. *Int J Oral Maxillofac Implants.* 18:641-651, 2003.

114. Ganeles J, Wismeijer D: Early and immediately restored and loaded dental implants for single-tooth and partial-arch applications. *Int J Oral Maxillofac Implants.* 19:92-102, 2004.

115. Lum LB, Beirne R, Curtis DA. Histologic evaluation of hydroxylapatite-coated versus uncoated titanium blade implants in delayed and immediately loaded applications. *Int J Oral Maxillofac Implants.* 6:456-462, 1991.

116. Tarnow DP, Emitaz S, Classi A. Immediate loading of threaded implants at stage 1 surgery in edentulous arches: ten consecutive case reports with 1- to 5-year data. *Int J Oral Maxillofac Implants.* 12:319-324, 1997.

117. Szmukler-Moncler S, Salama H, Reingewirtz Y, Dubruille JH. Timing of loading and effect of micromotion on bone-dental implant interface: review of experimental literature. *J Biomed Mater Res.* 43:192-203, 1998.

118. Duyck J, Ronold HJ, Van Oosterwyck H, et al. The influence of static and dynamic loading on marginal bone reactions around osseointegrated implants: an animal experimental study. *Clin Oral Implants Res.* 12:207-218, 2001.

119. Gotfredsen K, Berglundh T, Lindhe J. Bone reactions adjacent to titanium implants subjected to static load. *Clin Oral Implants Res.* 12:1-8, 2001.

120. Freudenthaler JW, Haas R, Bantleon HP. Bicortical titanium screws for critical orthodontic anchorage in the mandible: a preliminary report on clinical applications. *Clin Oral Implants Res.* 12:358-363, 2001.

121. Ansell R, Scales J. A study of some factors which affect the strength of screws and their insertion and holding power in bone. *J Biomech.* 1:279-302, 1968.

122. Bechtol C. Internal fixation with plates and screws. In: Bechtol C, Ferguson A, Laing P, eds. *Metals and Engineering in Bone and Joint Surgery.* Baltimore, Md: William & Wilkins, 1959:152-171.

SECTION 2

BIOLOGIC BASIS

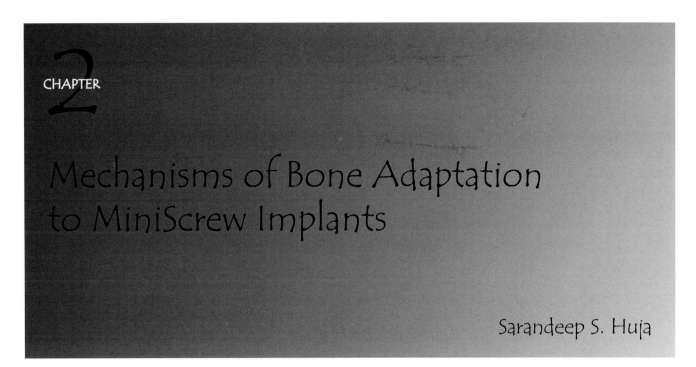

Mechanisms of Bone Adaptation to MiniScrew Implants

Sarandeep S. Huja

Recently, temporary anchorage devices have been used increasingly in orthodontics. These devices are basically surgical screws that have been modified to allow for orthodontic force application to the screw head. These surgical screws (also referred to as miniscrews, mini-implants, or miniscrew implants) provide anchorage for orthodontic tooth movement.[1,2] Both animal and human studies have provided the basis for their clinical use.[3-5] Creekmore and Eklund[6] were probably the first to suggest that screws could be used for orthodontic applications clinically. The primary advantages of miniscrews are their low cost, the ease with which they are placed and removed, and the ability to place them in interradicular locations. However, their anchorage value is lower relative to that of endosseous implants. One problem associated with miniscrews is loosening, which is usually a result of torsional forces; therefore, a higher failure rate is currently seen with miniscrews than with endosseous implants.[7] Screw design (e.g., pitch, thread form, and thread depth) also plays a role in the success rate. Nevertheless, either endosseous implants or miniscrews can be used by orthodontists for treatment of patients with mutilated and/or compensated dentitions depending on anchorage requirements. Due to space requirements, however, endosseous implants will probably be precluded from traditional orthodontic anchorage applications henceforth.

A large body of information is available on the biologic adaptation of titanium and titanium alloy devices to bone and soft tissue. Titanium endosseous implants are routinely used in dentistry and have high success rates.[8,9] In order for these implants to be suitable for clinical use, a prerequisite is osseointegration. Most temporary anchorage devices, however, and miniscrews in particular, are not required to osseointegrate, thereby facilitating removal without the need for a trephine. In order to understand the difference between endosseous implants and miniscrews, the biologic factors that govern the success of these devices must be thoroughly understood.

BONE ADAPTATION PHYSIOLOGY OF ENDOSSEOUS IMPLANTS AND MINISCREWS

Because endosseous implants and miniscrews have a great deal in common in adaptation physiology, the commonalities of bony adaptation responses is discussed initially. The physiology of bone adaptation to endosseous implants has been well described in the literature[10,11] and comes primarily from animal experiments. However, some data also have been obtained from human biopsy or retrieval specimens of failed implants. Regardless of the source, most of the available data provide an understanding of *short-term adaptation* of bone to an implant (approximately 6 to 12 months). This is due in large part to the costs and ethical considerations of long-term animal studies.

Although implants are known to be predictably successful on average for more than 10 years, the goal of treatment is that the endosseous implant remains integrated for the life span of the patient, which may be 50 to 60 years after implant placement. The success of endosseous implants in this *long-term period* is not entirely understood. This is especially important because the medical status and oral health of the patient will most likely change as the person ages. For example, the effect of long-term bisphosphonate therapy (a drug often used to treat osteoporosis or cancer) on implants is not entirely understood. This is important because it is likely that long-term drug therapy may significantly alter bone remodeling around an implant. Because of the similarities in material composition and anatomic design, the large body of information available on short-term bone adaptation around a dental implant can be applied to miniscrews.

The foregoing observations were made by placing endosseous implants in either edentulous sites in the maxilla or mandible, or in dog femoral sites. The canine femur was chosen because of its uniform cortical thickness. The bone healing events following surgical placement of an endosseous implant are similar to those involved in fracture healing.[12] The formation and consolidation of a periosteal and endosteal callus, interfacial bone repair and remodeling events, maturation of the interfacial bone, and eventual resorption of the callus are typical events associated with short-term implant healing.[11,13] A basic understanding of these events and their biologic implications is a prerequisite to understand the concepts presented in this chapter. In addition, the reader should have a clear understanding of the distinctions between modeling and remodeling events in bone.[14] Briefly, bone modeling is a larger change in bone volume or shape seen primarily in response to mechanical loads, whereas bone remodeling is a relatively steady state of bone turnover as a result of the coupled activity of osteoclasts and osteoblasts. Another histologic observation in implant healing is the elevated remodeling in the bone adjacent to the implant.[15] This initial increase in remodeling is likely a healing response to bone injury.[16] However, the persistence of this elevated remodeling is suggested to be a unique mechanism of long-term bone adaptation to an implant (Fig. 2-1).

Mechanism and Sequence of Bone Adaptation to Implants

At the bone-implant interface, a mismatch exists in the elastic modulus of the two materials on the magnitude of approximately sixfold to tenfold. For example, although there is a wide range for the elastic modulus of cortical bone (10 to 17 GPa), the mean modulus is estimated to be 13.4 GPa, whereas titanium has a modulus of 104 GPa.[17-19] Because of this modulus of elasticity mismatch, stresses concentrate in the bone. Ordinarily, these stresses would result in fracture of the bone around an implant. Evidence suggests that in order to avoid this problem, elevated bony remodeling occurs at the bone-implant interface. This elevated remodeling serves to remove the devitalized bone at the interface and increases the compliance (decreases the stiffness) of the bone adjacent to the implant.[15,20] Without this compliant layer of bone, the stress concentration at the bone-implant interface would result in fracture and microcracking of the bone (Fig. 2-2).

The process of implant site preparation (osteotomy) and placement creates stresses in the bone resulting in microcrack formation.[16,21,22] These microcracks are removed by bony remodeling during the initial healing process.[23] If remodeling remains elevated over a longer duration, then it is possible that similar stresses within the interfacial bone (at the bone-implant interface) would not result in microcracks or microdamage in the implant-supporting bone immediately adjacent to the implant. In support of this, research in the author's laboratory suggests that over the short term (12 weeks), bone within 1 mm of the implant interface has a lower elastic modulus and hardness.[2] This is a result of the regional elevated bone turnover that prevents secondary mineralization and maturation of the osteonal bone. Unfortunately, direct measurements of remodeling rates and elastic properties of bone adjacent to implants in place for longer time periods (3 to 15 years, for example) are not available even though clinical data suggest that implants are successful for 1 to 2 decades or more.

Based on limited data, the assumption can be made that high remodeling rates (100% to 200% per year) occur in the implant-supporting bone well beyond the initial healing period of 6 to 12 months. This increased remodeling is considered unusual for cortical bone, which typically only turns over at a rate of 2% to 10% per year. The hypothesis being advanced is as follows: At time points well beyond the healing period typically required for bone (6 to 12 months), an elevated remodeling rate exists in implant-supporting bone (i.e., within 1 to 2 mm of the bone-implant interface). This elevated bone remodeling is considered a *localized* bone adaptation response. This localized response exists because the bone in the immediate vicinity of the implant is mechanically loaded and stressed.[24] Bone further away (e.g., 3 to 4 mm away from the implant interface), however, does not experience altered

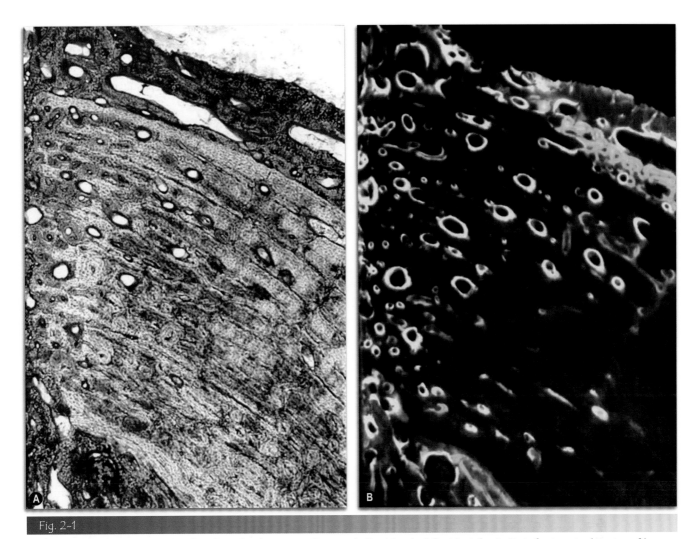

Fig. 2-1

Characteristic photomicrographs of implant placed in canine femur and allowed to heal for 12 weeks. **A,** Basic fuscin-stained section of bone adjacent to implant. **B,** Same image viewed under epifluoroscence. Note the periosteal callus and high rate of remodeling as indicated by the large number of bone labels in the bone adjacent to the implant. Implant is not seen but the interface is at the left edge of images. Endocortical callus is seen at the bottom left corner of images. (Reprinted from Huja S, Roberts EW. Mechanism of osseointegration: characterization of supporting bone with indentation testing and backscattered imaging. *Semin Orthod.* 10:162-173, 2004, with permission from Elsevier.)

mechanical stresses and strains and does not demonstrate the same adaptation response.

Placement of an implant in bone creates a tissue level discontinuity (a hole), which alters the localized stress environment. As a result, an adaptation response is seen in the immediate vicinity of the implant. A more *generalized* remodeling response that affects a larger area of bone is commonly seen with orthopedic hip implants inserted into the femoral cavity. This more generalized response presumably occurs because of increased loading by walking or running and is probably not necessary for maxillary/mandibular bone under the forces of mastication. The reader is referred to a recent chapter to understand the differences in a localized vs. a generalized adaptation response.[25]

Microdamage Physiology and Bone Adaptation to Implants

It was previously thought that local bony microdamage stimulated bone turnover or remodeling in the implant-supporting bone.[25] However, an alternate hypothesis is that after the initial 4- to 6-month healing period, a compliant layer of bone surrounding and supporting the implant (implant-supporting bone) actually prevents microdamage from occurring.[22] Based on a series of experiments,[20,22,26,27] it appears that after the initial implant healing takes place, increased microdamage is seen in the implant-supporting bone even if physiologic fatigue-type loads are applied to the implant and its supporting bone. If any such microdamage does accumulate, it is at a level that can be removed by remodeling invoked in the surrounding bone (Fig. 2-3, *A*). However, if hyperphysiologic forces were applied, it is likely that linear microcracks would been seen in bone further away (e.g., greater than 1 mm) from the implant (Fig. 2-3, *B*).

Understanding microdamage physiology of bone adaptation to implants is important conceptually. This is even more important because drugs such as bisphosphonates or parafunctional habits may increase

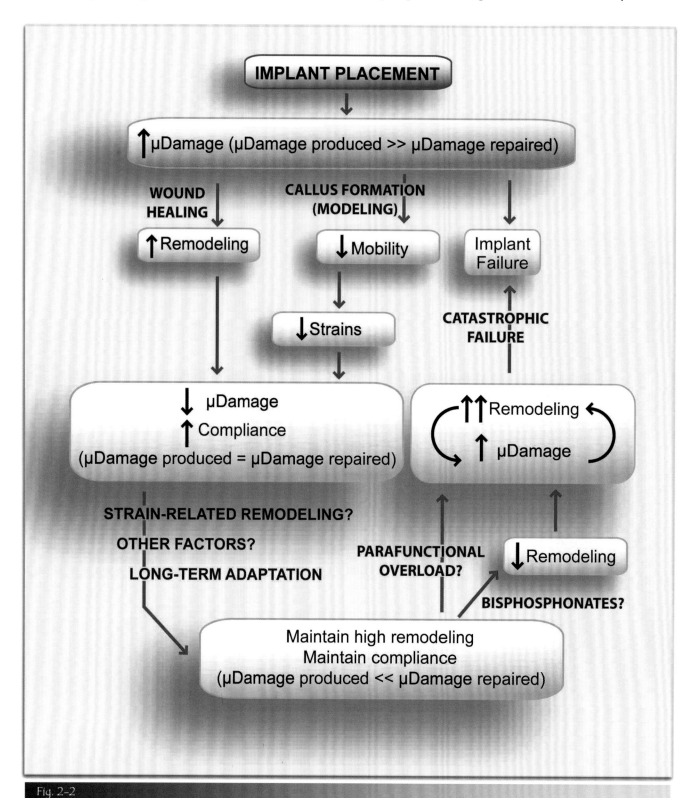

Fig. 2-2

Schematic of events associated with implant adaptation based on microdamage (μdamage) physiology.

the microdamage burden of the implant-supporting bone. This microdamage burden, if excessive, may lead to a cycle of remodeling that may increase bone porosity and decrease the strength of implant-supporting bone.[28] This could possibly lead to the ultimate failure of the implant. Because the design of experiments to test these long-term adaptation events is expensive, the aforementioned sequence of events is more hypothetical than proven. In light of this, the development of a registry for retrieved failed implants might provide cumulative data for better understanding the long-term bone-implant adaptation events.

Histologic Events in Bone Adaptation to Miniscrews

The following observations are derived from insertion of miniscrews into maxillary and mandibular alveolar cortical bone. The primary difference between these alveolar sites and the previously tested sites for dental implant healing is the increased anatomic variation and the potentially decreased cortical bone thickness in the alveolar bone. Alveolar cortical bone thickness ranges from approximately 0.7 to 2.6 mm, which may lead to variable adaptation responses. For example, a screw placed into a 2.0-mm cortex would exhibit more primary stability than a screw placed into a 1.0-mm cortex, all other factors being equal. This may lead to a better prognosis for the screw in thicker cortical bone because primary stability (discussed in detail later) is an important factor that determines the amount of micromotion exhibited by an implant.

Importantly, the forces delivered during mastication bend the jaw bone, creating measurable strains at bone surfaces.[29-31] Thus the bony discontinuity, or hole, in

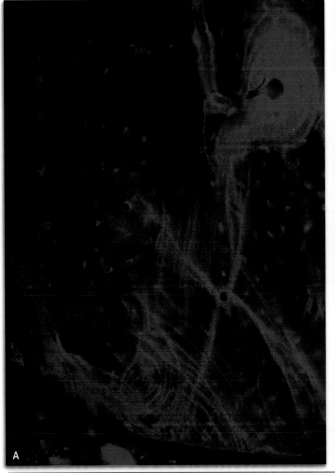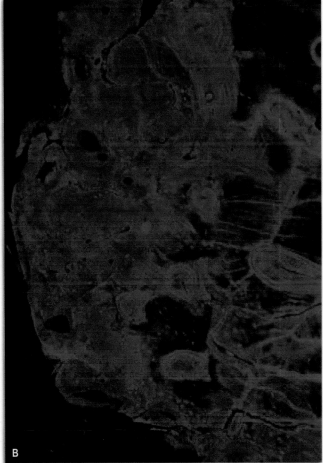

Fig. 2-3

Photomicrograph of microdamage detected by using epifluorescent methods in basic fuscin stained sections. **A,** Linear microcracks are apparent after fatigue loading of bone on the day of implant placement. Implant not seen, but bone-implant interface is to the bottom of image. Some of the damage may be due to implant placement. Linear cracks are removed in bone by invoking remodeling. Details of the experiment are described in Huja and colleagues.[22] **B,** Appearance of bone around the implant at 12 weeks postimplantation. Nonphysiologic (approximately 400 N in cantilever bending) fatigue loads were inadvertently applied to the implant, resulting in extensive fracturing of bone. Close to the implant is new bone which is compliant and does not readily demonstrate linear cracks. However, more mineralized bone, approximately 0.8 μm from the implant interface demonstrates linear microdamage. Implant seen on the left hand side is black).

which the miniscrew was placed, plus the superimposed masticatory forces, result in even greater strains about the miniscrew. Moreover, the masticatory forces themselves presumably vary depending on the location in the jaws.[32,33] For example, greater changes in compressive strains in the posterior maxilla would be expected relative to the posterior mandible after screw insertion, primarily based on cortex thickness.

Bone responds to increased strain by modeling, or depositing bone, thereby increasing bone volume, which decreases the strain at the bone surfaces and within the bone. If the new modeled bone surface of woven bone is needed for a long period of time, the woven bone in the callus is replaced by composite and load-bearing bone over time. In essence, the weaker woven bone volume is replaced by stronger compact bone with a smaller volume. As this occurs, the bone strains reach a more steady state and the bone volume is maintained at that level. This type of adaptation response (modeling, increase in bone volume, and lamellar compaction) is observed in the thin maxillary bone at 6 weeks after miniscrew placement (Fig. 2-4).

A different type of adaptation response is seen in the mandible. This is likely due to the mandibular alveolar cortical bone being thicker. This thicker bone provides greater primary stability. The strains in the mandible dissipate more readily because of the increased bone volume present; hence, there is no biologic urgency to invoke a robust modeling response. In mandibular bone, especially at thick cortical sites, a remodeling response is seen at the implant interfacial bone at 6 weeks after miniscrew placement (Fig. 2-5). A fracture callus is not readily observed.

We speculate that remodeling, as opposed to modeling, is seen in mandibular bone for the following reasons: (1) Osteonal arrangements in the mandible are clearly identifiable. In the maxilla, such osteonal arrangements may not be in the plane of section and thus not easily quantifiable. (2) In the maxilla the initial modeling response is required to decrease the strains in the immediate vicinity of the implant. Once the localized adaptation modeling phase is complete, then the remodeling response is invoked. Currently, not enough information is available to indicate the extent of the long-term adaptation events around miniscrew implants. Based on preliminary data, placement of a surgical screw into thin (0.7 to 1.2 mm) cortical bone results in a modeling response. Placement of the screw in thicker

(1.5 to 2 mm) bone with greater primary stability results in an observable remodeling response, with limited or no observable modeling.

BIOLOGIC PARAMETERS THAT DETERMINE MINISCREW SUCCESS

The following section attempts to provide the biologic basis for determining the success of miniscrews used for orthodontic anchorage.[34] Primary stability, immediate loading, orthodontic force magnitude, and attached vs. mobile mucosa are discussed in light of miniscrew implant success.

Primary Stability

Because primary stability, or the lack of micromotion, upon initial placement has been shown to be an important factor for dental implant healing, it is logical to think that primary stability would also be important for miniscrews.[35,36] Pluripotential cells in bone are well known to differentiate into fibrous tissue, cartilage, and bone.[37] Bone formation can result from a cartilaginous intermediate, but fibrous tissue cannot be converted to bone. The reason primary stability is important is that micromotion at the implant interface can result in the formation of fibrous tissue, which has been seen with blade-type implants.[38-42] However, with endosseous implants, a larger amount of cortical surface area is present at the bone-implant interface. As a result, micromotion is decreased, and direct occlusal loading is kept to a minimum during the initial 3- to 4-month unloaded healing period.

More recently, immediate and early implant loading has been advocated.[38,43] This is usually accomplished by increasing the number of implants that are connected to each other (i.e., splinting to decrease micromotion), and is in contrast to Brånemark's original two-stage procedure. Although implant technology has changed, bone biology has not. It has been suggested that early loading may actually enhance bone formation. However, this early loading increases bone strain within weeks of implantation and most likely results in a modeling response, which is responsible for the increased bony dimension because of its increased mechanical use.[44] Roberts[11] estimates that the repair of devitalized interfacial bone typically takes about 12 to 18 weeks in human beings. Moreover, this interfacial bone does not likely respond to the initial or early load bearing.

The primary stability of screws used to enhance orthodontic anchorage is largely obtained from the cortical plate. Most screws use monocortical anchorage,

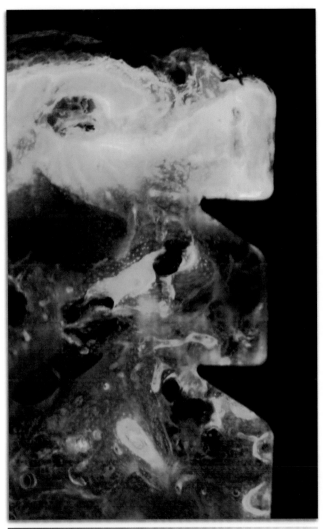

Fig. 2-4

Epifluorescent radiomicrograph (×40) of surgical screw at 6 weeks after placement in maxillary posterior region. The cortical bone into which the implant was placed is thin and essentially is contained between the first two screws threads at the top of the image. Bone below these two threads also is labeled and formed after implant placement. Contrast this with Fig. 2-5.

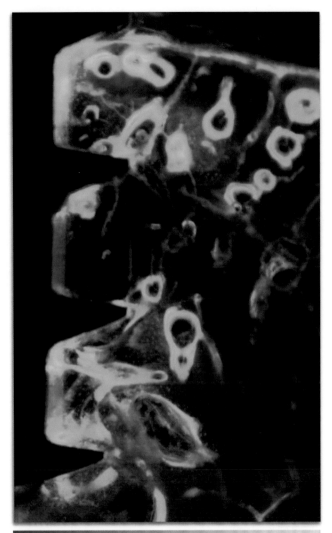

Fig. 2-5

Epifluorescent radiomicrograph (×40) of surgical screw at 6 weeks after placement in mandibular posterior region. Bone remodeling and calcein green (fluorescent bone label) is clearly seen. Note about four screw threads traverse the cortical bone thickness (approximately 1.7 mm thick). Importantly, no periosteal or endosteal callus is visible.

though bicortical anchorage is possible in partially edentulous areas and in extraalveolar sites. An approximately twofold difference exists in the thickness of the buccal cortical plates in the jaws (maxilla versus mandible) of dogs. Likewise, significant differences exist in pullout strengths of monocortical screws in the mandibular posterior region relative to the mandibular anterior region. Pullout strengths are an indication of the holding power of these screws. One pullout strength study suggests that the screw used would adequately withstand orthodontic loads from a purely physical standpoint.[45] However, the pullout tests were conducted in tension and not in cantilever bending.

Unlike endosseous implants, which receive vertical and off-axis loads, screws used in orthodontics receive primarily bending and torsional loads (Fig. 2-3). The strain distribution to these cantilever loads in the bone (moments generated at the bone surface) and the strains generated during occlusal loading are different, and it might also be anticipated that the adaptation responses would also be different.[26] However, whether this strain affects the primary stability of a miniscrew or whether a lack of primary stability increases the modeling responses at the periosteal and endosteal bone surfaces is unclear.

Immediate Loading

The issues of immediate loading and primary stability are inseparable. Immediate or early loading of screws to move a single tooth is possible clinically without subsequent failure of the screw. However, a short healing period of 1 week before loading (similar to the latency period in distraction) may be advisable. Specific information on this subject does not exist in the scientific literature, but the rationale for such an approach would be to allow the healing responses to commence before the application of relatively light (3 to 5 N) loads. This should not cause a problem in terms of timing because orthodontists plan their treatment well in advance, and the planning sequence could include time for the insertion of a screw or screws and healing time.

Evidence suggests that loading of endosseous implants increases bone mass in the vicinity of the implant.[46] For screws, there is no clear evidence to suggest that an undisturbed screw would have less bone support than a screw to which a 2- to 5-N load was applied 1 week after placement. Because these screws are used for a short time, for example, 1 to 2 years, the success of these screws is assessed only over this short period. This is in contrast to endosseous implants, the service of which is judged over a 30- to 40-year period or the patient's life span.

In the literature, it is well established that when an inert object (implant or screw) is placed in the jaw bone, there is a stress concentration at the interface because of the elastic modulus mismatch between a titanium implant and bone.[47,48] Additionally, even though no force is placed on the implant, the implant is still under indirect load. This indirect load is due to the bending of the jaws during physiologic functions (e.g., mastication, speech, and deglutition). Tensile and compressive strains have been recorded on the bone surfaces during various functional activities.[49,50] These deformations are even greater at the interface because of the discontinuity created by the implant. Some researchers believe that the bone adaptation response around an implant may be related, in part, to these physiologic forces in addition to the loads received from direct occlusal loading. These indirect loads should be taken into consideration when a screw is placed into bone. Judicious immediate or early loading should not be a concern for a screw that has good primary stability.

Orthodontic Force Magnitude

Orthodontic load applications are typically on the order of 1 to 3 N for tooth movement. Bite forces and loads on implants are typically in the range of 200 to 300 N.[32,51] Even if multiple teeth are moved en masse against an orthodontic anchor, the forces on the anchor will probably not exceed 20 to 30 N. With an endosseous

implant as an anchor, it may be possible to use the 10-2 anchorage strategy, that is, two anchors to move 10 teeth simultaneously, to decrease treatment time. However, such a strategy with a single screw may be close to the maximum force that could be applied to such an anchor. The clinician must apply force judiciously depending on the location of the screw and its anchorage potential. For example, using a monocortical screw in the mandibular anterior region to protract molars and premolars simultaneously may not be advisable. In this situation, a retromolar implant may serve as a better indirect anchor. With retromolar implant anchorage, it is routine to move teeth through relatively atrophic areas. Tooth movement into these atrophic areas is accompanied by the tooth bringing its supporting alveolar and periodontal tissues. This regenerative response has been referred to as "tissue engineering" of atrophic areas.

Attached Mucosa vs. Mobile Mucosa

Various techniques exist for placement of miniscrews. If a screw is to be placed at the level of the attached mucosa, then a self-drilling screw can be inserted directly through the mucosa without a prior incision. At most locations, however, the interradicular space is insufficient for placement of a 1.5-mm screw at the level of the attached mucosa without damage to the adjacent roots.[52] Placing these screws at an angle and pointing them apically and away from the crowns has been advocated to prevent root damage, but the alveolar bone is thinner at its most coronal locations and thicker at its base. The other option is to place the screws further apically in the movable mucosa. When screws are placed through movable mucosa without a prior incision, the tendency is for the mucosa to "wind" around the screw. This situation can be avoided by making a small incision. The soft tissue is reflected to the bone and the screw is inserted directly into the bone while the soft tissue is retracted away from the threads of the screw.

It is important that the head of the screw have a mechanism to which a ligature or orthodontic wire can be attached. This attachment needs to be exposed to the oral cavity. The orthodontist attaches the force-generating mechanism (e.g., coil spring or elastics) to this point of purchase. The point of emergence into the oral cavity is where soft tissue irritation can be a concern. Sometimes, irritation may result in an inflammatory response that could possibly cover the entire screw. In addition, the proinflammatory cytokines could result in failure of the screw by a process similar to that described for endosseous implants. The patient must maintain meticulous oral hygiene in the direct vicinity of the screw.

OSSEOINTEGRATION

Osseointegration is defined as some form of direct contact of load-bearing living bone with an inert object.[53] Unfortunately, there are multiple interpretations of this concept. For example, removal torque is used as an outcome measurement for the level of osseointegration.[54] However, it is difficult to define at what removal torque value osseointegration has occurred. Another variable that has been used to measure the level of osseointegration is amount of bone contact.[55] Again, there is no clear consensus regarding the minimal amount of bone contact required for an implant to be considered osseointegrated. Theoretically, an implant can be integrated if there are three distinct and permanent points of contact between the implant and the adjacent bone. However, bone remodeling at the implant interface is a dynamic process.[15] Bone in contact at the initial phase of implant healing may be resorbed subsequently, and new areas of bone contact to the implant surface may occur.

In any respect, based on the clinical observation that miniscrews placed intraorally for the short-term purpose of enhancing orthodontic anchorage can be easily removed, they are not osseointegrated. Because bone contact and thread mechanical interlock are well known to increase by etching titanium surfaces or by applying a surface coating, such as plasma spraying,[55,56] one reason for easy removal is that miniscrews have smooth polished surfaces and a low tensile bond strength of titanium to bone.

One study compared initial bone contact for two screw types.[57] Self-drilling screws had greater bone contact than screws (implants) that were placed using the conventional pilot drilling process followed by tapping of the implant. It should be remembered that the cortical plates are thin, so there is minimal area to support screws used for anchorage. If the diameter of a screw is approximately 2 mm, the circumference at a particular cross section of the screw will be 6.24 mm. If this screw were placed in bone with 1-mm thickness, the area of the bone in contact with the tooth would be 6.24 mm². This obviously does not include increases in surface area caused by the threads. Additionally, because of the bone response (modeling), the area in contact with the screw increases, and this adaptation response may help the screw to bear loads. This area could increase twofold because of a modeling adaptation response. The amount of bone contact around craniofacial screws is not well described in the literature.

If 50% bone contact exists with current screws, it might be tempting to suggest that the surface of the screws could be roughed to increase contact. However, this might make removal of the screw difficult, and trephining of the screw with surrounding bone may be required for removal.

SUMMARY

A large body of evidence suggests that screws are an effective way of enhancing anchorage in select cases. However, it is important to note that even experienced clinicians have initial failures. Understanding bone biology and the biomechanics of bone and screws is imperative to decreasing miniscrew failure rate in clinical practice.

ACKNOWLEDGMENTS

I am indebted to my mentors Drs. Eugene Roberts, Thomas Katona, David Burr, and Lawrence Garetto from Indiana University Schools of Dentistry and Medicine. Many of the ideas discussed in this chapter originate from long discussions with these supportive mentors. Funding was made possible from the American Academy Implant Dentistry, Synthes USA, the College of Dentistry Start Up Funds, and The Ohio State University for the miniscrew research.

REFERENCES

1. Costa A, Raffaini M, Melsen B. Miniscrews as orthodontic anchorage: a preliminary report. *Int J Adult Orthod Orthognath Surg.* 13:201-209, 1998.
2. Kanomi R. Mini-implant for orthodontic anchorage. *J Clin Orthod.* 31:763-767, 1997.
3. Ohmae M, Saito S, Morohashi T, et al. A clinical and histological evaluation of titanium mini-implants as anchors for orthodontic intrusion in the beagle dog. *Am J Orthod Dentofacial Orthop.* 119:489-497, 2001.
4. Paik CH, Woo YJ, Boyd RD. Treatment of an adult patient with vertical maxillary excess using miniscrew fixation. *J Clin Orthod.* 37:423-428, 2003.
5. Park YC, Lee SY, Kim DH, Jee SH. Intrusion of posterior teeth using mini-screw implants. *Am J Orthod Dentofacial Orthop.* 123:690-694, 2003.
6. Creekmore TD, Eklund MK. The possibility of skeletal anchorage. *J Clin Orthod.* 17:266-269, 1983.
7. Melsen B, Verna C. A rational approach to orthodontic anchorage. *Prog Orthod.* 1:10-22, 1999.
8. Albrektsson T, Zarb G, Worthington P, Eriksson AR. The long-term efficacy of currently used dental implants: a review and proposed criteria of success. *Int J Oral Maxillofac Implants.* 1:11-25, 1986.
9. Smith DE, Zarb GA. Criteria for success of osseointegrated endosseous implants. *J Prosthet Dent.* 62:567-572, 1989.
10. Brunski JB, Puleo DA, Nanci A. Biomaterials and biomechanics of oral and maxillofacial implants: current status and future developments. *Int J Oral Maxillofac Implants.* 15:15-46, 2000.
11. Roberts WE. Bone tissue interface. *J Dent Educ.* 52:804-809, 1988.
12. Schenk RK, Hunziker EB. Histologic and ultrastructural features of fracture healing. In: CT Brighton, GE Friedlaender, JM Lane, eds. *Bone Formation and Repair.* Rosemont, Ill: American Academy of Orthopaedic Surgeons, 1994:117-146.

13. Roberts WE, Poon LC, Smith RK. Interface histology of rigid endosseous implants. *J Oral Implantol.* 12:406-416, 1986.

14. Roberts WE, Roberts JA, Huja SS. Fundamental principles of bone modeling applied to orthodontics. *Semin Orthod.* 10:123-161, 2004.

15. Garetto LP, Chen J, Parr JA, Roberts WE. Remodeling dynamics of bone supporting rigidly fixed titanium implants: a histomorphometric comparison in four species including humans. *Implant Dent.* 4:235-243, 1995.

16. Hoshaw SJ, Watson JT, Schaffler MB, Fyhrie DP. Microdamage at bone-implant interfaces affects bone remodeling activity. *Trans Orthop Res Soc.* 20:188, 1995.

17. Ashman RB, Rho JY. Elastic modulus of trabecular bone material. *J Biomech.* 21:177-181, 1988.

18. Currey JD. Mechanical properties of bone tissues with greatly differing functions. *J Biomech.* 12:313-319, 1979.

19. Reilly DT, Burstein AH, Frankel VH. The elastic modulus for bone. *J Biomech.* 7:271-275, 1974.

20. Huja SS, Katona TR, Moore BK, Roberts WE. Microhardness and anisotropy of the vital osseous interface and endosseous implant supporting bone. *J Orthop Res.* 16:54-60, 1998.

21. Hoshaw SJ, Fyhrie DP, Schaffler MB. The effect of implant insertion and design on bone microdamage. In: Davidovitch Z, ed. *The Biological Mechanisms of Tooth Eruption, Resorption and Replacement by Implants.* Boston, Mass: Harvard Society for the Advancement of Orthodontics, 1994:735-741.

22. Huja SS, Katona TR, Burr DB, Garetto LP, et al. Microdamage adjacent to endosseous implants subjected to bending fatigue loads. *Bone.* 25:217-222, 1999.

23. Burr DB, Martin RB, Schaffler MB, Radin EL. Bone remodeling in response to in vivo fatigue microdamage. *J Biomech.* 18:189-200, 1985.

24. Huja SS, Roberts WE. Mechanism of osseointegration: characterization of supporting bone with indentation testing and backscattered imaging. *Semin Orthod.* 10:162-173, 2004.

25. Garetto LP, Tricker ND. Remodeling of bone surrounding at the implant interface. In: Garetto LP, Turner CH, Duncan RL, Burr DB, eds. *Bridging the Gap Between Dental and Orthopaedic Implants.* Indianapolis, Ind: School of Dentistry, Indiana University, 2002:89-100.

26. Huja SS, Qian H, Roberts WE, Katona TR. Effects of callus and bonding on strains in bone surrounding an implant under bending. *Int J Oral Maxillofac Implants.* 13:630-638, 1998.

27. Huja SS, Qian H, Roberts WE, Katona TR. Stress analysis of the effects of healing and bonding of bone surrounding dental implants. Paper presented at: 98th Annual Meeting of the American Association of Orthodontists; May 1998; Dallas, Tex.

28. Hoshaw SJ, Brunski JB, Cochran GVB. Mechanical loading of Branemark implants affect interfacial bone modeling and remodeling. *Int J Oral Maxillofac Implants.* 9:345-360, 1994.

29. Herring SW, Rafferty KL. Cranial and facial sutures: functional loading in relation to growth and morphology. In: Davidovitch Z, ed. *The Biological Mechanisms of Tooth Eruption, Resorption and Replacement by Implants.* Boston, Mass: Harvard Society for the Advancement of Orthodontics, 2000:269-276.

30. Hylander WL: Stress and strain in the mandibular symphysis of primates: a test of competing hypotheses. *Am J Phys Anthropol.* 64:1-46, 1984.

31. Hylander WL, Johnson KR. In vivo bone strain patterns in the zygomatic arch of macaques and the significance of these patterns for functional interpretations of craniofacial form. *Am J Phys Anthropol.* 102:203-232, 1997.

32. Haraldson T, Carlsson GE. Bite force and oral function in patients with osseointegrated oral implants. *Scand J Dent Res.* 85:200-208, 1977.

33. Kikuchi M, Korioth TWP, Hannam AG. The association among occlusal contacts, clenching effort, and bite force distribution in man. *J Dent Res.* 76:1316-1325, 1997.

34. Huja SS. Biologic parameters that determine success of screws used in orthodontics to supplement anchorage. In: McNamara JA, ed. *Implant Anchorage in Orthodontics.* Ann Arbor, Mich: 31st Annual Moyers Symposium, 2005.

35. Kohn D, Rose C. Primary stability of interference screw fixation: influence of screw diameter and insertion torque. *Am J Sports Med.* 22:334-338, 1994.

36. Piattelli A, Trisi P, Romansco N, Emanuelli M: Histologic analysis of a screw implant retrieved from man: influence of early loading and primary stability. *J Oral Implantol.* 14:303-306, 1993.

37. Carter DR, Beaupre GS, Giori NJ, Helms JA. Mechanobiology of skeletal regeneration. *Clin Orthop Relat Res.* 355S:S41-S55, 1998.

38. Balshi TJ, Wolfinger GJ. Immediate loading of Branemark implants in edentulous mandibles: a preliminary report. *Implant Dent.* 6:83-88, 1997.

39. Brunski JB, Moccia J, Pollack SR, et al. The influence of functional use of endosseous dental implants on the tissue-implant interface, I: histological aspects. *J Dent Res.* 50:1953-1969, 1979.

40. Brunski JB. Avoid pitfalls of overloading and micromotion of intraosseous implants [interview]. *Dent Implantol Update.* 4:77-81, 1993.

41. Goodman S, Aspenberg P. Effects of mechanical stimulation on the differentiation of hard tissues. *Biomaterials.* 14:563-569, 1993.

42. Goodman S, Wang J-S, Aspenberg P. Difference in bone ingrowth after one versus two daily episodes of micromotion: experiments with titanium chambers in rabbits. *J Biomed Mater Res.* 27:1419-1424, 1993.

43. Piattelli A, Scarano A, Paolantonio M. Immediately loaded screw implant removed for fracture after a 15-year loading period: histological and histochemical analysis. *J Oral Implantol.* 23:75-79, 1997.

44. Frost HM. Wolff's law and bone's structural adapation to mechanical usage: an overview for clinicians. *Angle Orthod.* 64:175-188, 1994.

45. Huja SS, Litsky A, Beck FM, et al. Pull-out strength of monocortical screws placed in the maxillae and mandibles of dogs. *Am J Orthod Dentofacial Orthop.* 127:307-313, 2005.

46. Roberts WE, Smith RK, Zilberman Y, et al. Osseous adaptation to continous loading of rigid endosseous implants. *Am J Orthod.* 86:95-111, 1984.

47. Cook SD, Klawitter JJ, Weinstein AM. The influence of implant elastic modulus on the stress distribution around LTI carbon and aluminum oxide dental implants. *J Biomed Mater Res.* 15:879-887, 1981.

48. Wolfe LA, Hobkirk JA. Bone response to a matched modulus endosseous implant material. *Int J Oral Maxillofac Implants.* 4:311-320, 1989.

49. Hylander WL, Crompton AW. Jaw movements and patterns of mandibular bone strain during mastication in the monkey macaca fascicularis. *Arch Oral Biol.* 31:841-848, 1986.

50. Thomason JJ, Grovum LE, Deswysen AG, Bignell WW. In vivo surface strain and stereology of the frontal and maxillary bones of sheep: implications for the structural design of the mammalian skull. *Anat Rec.* 264:325-338, 2001.

51. Fontijin-Tekamp FA, Slagter AP, van't Hof MA, et al. Bite forces with mandibular implant-retained overdentures. *J Dent Res.* 77:1832-1839, 1998.

52. Schnelle M, Huja SS, Beck FM, Jaynes R. A radiographic evaluation of the availability of interradicular bone for placement of miniscrews. *Angle Orthod.* 74:832-837, 2004.

53. Albrektsson T, Lekholm U. Osseointegration: current state of the art. *Dent ClinNorth Am* 33:537-554, 1989.

54. Johansson C, Alberktsson T. Integration of screw implants in the rabbit: a 1-yr follow-up of removal torque of titanium implants. *Int J Oral Maxillofac Implants.* 2:69-75, 1987.

55. Steflik DE, Lake FT, Sisk AL, et al. A comparative Investigation in dogs: 2-year morphometric results of the dental implant-bone interface. *Int J Oral Maxillofac Implants.* 11:15-25, 1996.

56. Gotfredsen K, Berglundh T, Lindhe J. Bone reactions adjacent to titanium impants with different surface characteristics subjected to static load: a study in the dog. *Clin Oral Implants Res* 12(pt 2):196-201, 2001.

57. Prager T, Holtgrave EA. Primary stability of self-drilling and conventional screw implants for orthodontic anchorage. *J Dent Res.* 82(special issue B):B-301, 2319, 2003.

Bone Response to Loading of MiniScrew Implants

Birte Melsen, Michel Dalstra

Traditionally, dental implants used for orthodontic mechanics have been allowed to heal for a period of time in order to osseointegrate.[1-7] This was based on Brånemark's suggestion that endosseous dental implants remain unloaded for 3 months in the mandible and 6 months in the maxilla for osseointegration.[8] The rationale was based on his experience that micromotion over about 100 μm would allow fibrous tissue invasion and prevent osseointegration. It has since been demonstrated, however, that the healing period can be reduced if the loading environment is controlled. This, in combination with patient and clinician interest in completing treatment faster, has spurred much research into the immediate loading of implants. The term *immediate loading* generally refers to loads applied from minutes to several days after implant placement. In a review, Romanos[9] suggested that three factors were important for success of immediately loaded implants: (1) excellent primary stability, (2) excellent bone quality, and (3) elimination of micromotion.

Although osseointegration of endosseous dental implants largely depends on the surface roughness of the implant, miniscrew implants (MSI) used for orthodontic anchorage usually have a smooth polished surface and are therefore retained primarily via mechanical stabilization.[10-24] Most orthodontic miniscrews are loaded immediately. As is the case for dental implants, the length and diameter of the threaded body, as well the quantity and quality of bone into which the screw is inserted, determine the force level that can be applied. Both animal and human studies have been carried out. The forces applied to implants in human beings have ranged from 30 g to 250 g; however, most of these studies have applied forces after a healing period of 4 to 36 weeks. This is because the original human studies underscored the absolute necessity of longer healing times before loading in order to ensure success.[2,25,26] Subsequent animal experiments proved that shorter healing periods did not appear to compromise implant stability.[7,27] Importantly, these reports applied well-controlled forces of moderate magnitude and corroborate the successful results described in clinical case reports.[11,12,23]

LOCAL BONE STRAIN ADJACENT TO MINISCREW IMPLANTS

The mechanical stability of MSIs largely depends on the local strains generated in the bone immediately surrounding the loaded MSI. These local strains govern the processes of bony modeling and remodeling,[28,29] the outcome of which ultimately determines the mechanical competence of the bone at the bone-implant interface. This phenomenon applies to load-bearing and load-sharing implants, as well as to MSIs used for orthodontic anchorage.

The finite element (FE) method is the standard scientific model for stress/strain analysis of complex bone-implant interactions. Therefore, the authors' group developed two three-dimensional FE models to

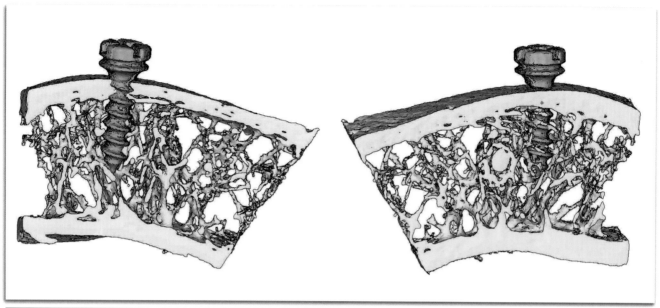

Fig. 3-1

Three-dimensional reconstruction of micro–computed tomography data with an Aarhus Anchorage screw placed in human mandible. (Reprinted from Melsen B, Verna C. Miniscrew implants: the Aarhus Anchorage System. *Semin Orthod.* 11:24-31, 2005, with permission from Elsevier.)

examine the load transfer from an MSI (Aarhus Anchorage® screw) to the surrounding bone.[30] One model was a geometrically accurate representation of the actual bone-MSI interface based on micro–computed tomography scans of an Aarhus Anchorage screw inserted in a human mandible obtained at autopsy (Fig. 3-1). In the second model, the bone from the first model was replaced by a generic rectangular block of material (Fig. 3-2). The second model was used to parametrically study the influence of cortical bone thickness and trabecular bone density on local strain distribution. The simulated cortical thickness increased from 0 to 2 mm in 0.5-mm increments, and the trabecular bone was assumed to have low, medium, or high density by assigning a Young's modulus of 50, 200, or 1000 MPa, respectively. This resulted in a total of 15 models. For both the geometrically accurate and parametric models, the same loading condition was applied (a mesially directed force of 50 g applied at the head of the screw), thereby subjecting the screw to a bending mode.

The geometrically accurate model revealed that the majority of the load transfer takes place within the cortex for a single revolution of the screw thread. This was supported upon evaluation of the micro–computed tomography scans (three-dimensional reconstruction), which revealed that the screw was fully supported in the cortex, but was only loosely supported by trabecular

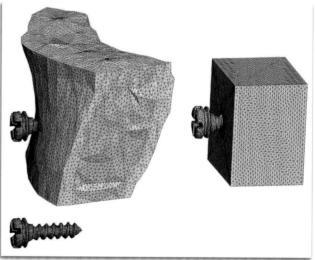

Fig. 3-2

The geometrically accurate finite element model *(left)* and the parametric model *(right)* of the Aarhus Anchorage screw and surrounding bone. The yellow elements represent the cortical bone, and the gray elements represent the trabecular bone. (Reprinted from Dalstra M, Cattaneo PM, Melsen B. Load transfer of miniscrews for orthodontic anchorage. *Orthodontics.* 1:53-62, 2004, with permission from Quintessence.)

bone (Fig. 3-1). Therefore, under the experimental loading condition, the MSI was displaced in a tipping mode with the screw apex moving in the opposite direction as the screw head, resulting in the generation of compressive stresses opposite the direction of the force. In general, the stress levels were higher in the cortical bone than in the underlying trabecular bone

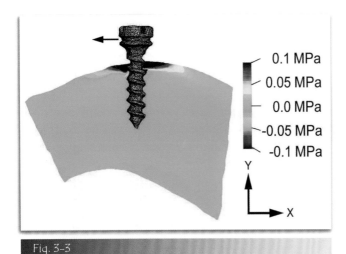

Fig. 3-3

Distribution of the mesiodistal stress (σx) in a transverse cross section of the geometrically accurate finite element model. (Reprinted from Dalstra M, Cattaneo PM, Melsen B. Load transfer of miniscrews for orthodontic anchorage. *Orthodontics.* 1:53-62, 2004, with permission from Quintessence.)

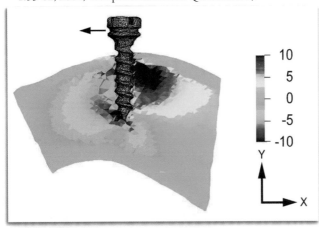

Fig. 3-4

Distribution of the mesiodistal strain (εx) in a transverse cross section of the geometrically accurate finite element model (units in microstrain). (Reprinted from Dalstra M, Cattaneo PM, Melsen B. Load transfer of miniscrews for orthodontic anchorage. *Orthodontics.* 1:53-62, 2004, with permission from Quintessence.)

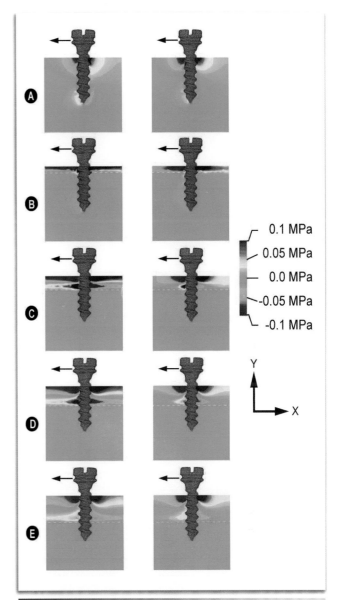

Fig. 3-5

Distribution of the transverse stress (σx) in different cortical thicknesses of the parametric model. **A,** 0.0-mm cortical thickness. **B,** 0.5-mm cortical thickness. **C,** 1.0-mm cortical thickness. **D,** 1.5-mm cortical thickness. **E,** 2.0-mm cortical thickness. Note low-density trabecular bone of 50 MPa *(left)* and high-density trabecular core of 1000 MPa *(right).* (Reprinted from Dalstra M, Cattaneo PM, Melsen B. Load transfer of miniscrews for orthodontic anchorage. *Orthodontics.* 1:53-62, 2004, with permission from Quintessence.)

(Fig. 3-3). The opposite was the case for the strain values (Fig. 3-4). Although local peak values for the strain in trabecular bone reached as high as 2465 microstrain, the general magnitude for the bone strain was 10 to 100 microstrain.

The results from the parametric model were similar to those from the geometrically accurate model. The load transfer predominantly took place in the cortex. This suggests that cortical thickness plays a significant role in the load transfer mechanism from an MSI to bone, whereas the stiffness (or density) of the trabecular bone plays a minor role (Fig. 3-5). It must be noted that similar to the geometrically accurate model, high strains in the trabecular bone occurred, particularly for low-density bone (Fig. 3-6). By plotting the peak strains that occurred in bone for all parametric models (Fig. 3-7), the strains can be compared with the bone strain window according to Frost's mechanostat theory.[28,29] Using this comparison, Frost's pathologic overload window was reached only with a thin cortex (less than 0.5 mm) overlying low-density trabecular bone. Therefore, clinicians should not insert MSIs in locations where bone quality is suspected to be poor. In these cases, initial stability would be low, probably resulting in high failure rates. For medium- or high-density trabecular bone, this danger does not exist, and the bone strain values were generally within Frost's mild overload or adapted windows.

The theoretical models described do not consider physiologic loading. The additional strains caused by physiologic loading might affect the aforementioned load transfer mechanism to some extent. In light of this, Chen and colleagues[31,32] applied FE analyses to loads transferred around dental implants used for orthodontic anchorage. They demonstrated that bone turnover surrounding osseointegrated implants could be explained by the stress/strain relationship generated during normal mandibular function and resulting from physical property differences of the bone and implant. Because of geometry differences and loading variation in distinct anatomic sites, this finding cannot be extrapolated directly to MSIs. However, the influence of physiologic loading and the difference in bone and implant stiffness is likely to play a significant role.

Another aspect of the load transfer from an MSI to the surrounding bone is the geometry of the MSI itself. The two main geometric parameters are MSI diameter and length. If the diameter is doubled, the stresses in the screw loaded under bending would decrease by a factor of 8 (Fig. 3-8). However, the strains in the surrounding bone would decrease only by a factor of 2 because the effective surface area of bone-screw contact would double. The overall deformation mode of the screw (tipping) would remain the same. Because external screw loading is of such a low magnitude, the risk of screw fracture during bending is unlikely.

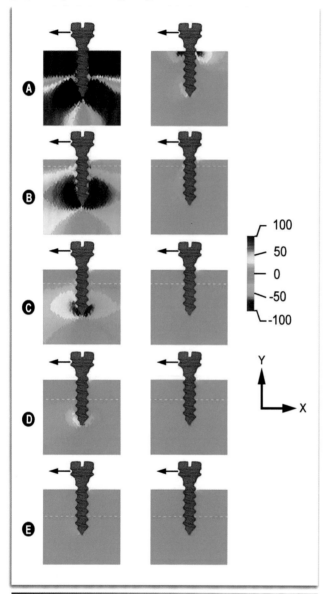

Fig. 3-6

Distributions of the transverse strain (εx) in different cortical thicknesses of the parameter model. **A,** 0.0-mm cortical thickness. **B,** 0.5-mm cortical thickness. **C,** 1.0-mm cortical thickness. **D,** 1.5-mm cortical thickness. **E,** 2.0-mm cortical thickness. Note low-density trabecular bone of 50 MPa *(left)* and high-density trabecular core of 1000 MPa *(right).* Units are in microstrain. (Reprinted from Dalstra M, Cattaneo PM, Melsen B. Load transfer of miniscrews for orthodontic anchorage. *Orthodontics.* 1:53-62, 2004, with permission from Quintessence.)

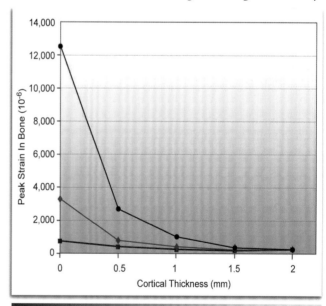

Fig. 3-7

Peak strain values occurring in the bone for the low-density *(red),* medium-density *(green),* and high-density *(blue)* trabecular bone relative to cortical thickness. The light yellow, light tan, and dark tan backgrounds represent the adapted, mild overload, and pathologic overload windows, respectively. (Reprinted from Dalstra M, Cattaneo PM, Melsen B. Load transfer of miniscrews for orthodontic anchorage. *Orthodontics.* 1:53-62, 2004, with permission from Quintessence.)

Therefore, a larger-diameter screw is not warranted. The diameter may become critical, though, during insertion and removal of the screw, when the screw is subjected to torsional loading. Upon removal, the risk of MSI fracture is higher than at insertion as a result of the increases in both bone-implant contact and local bone density. Doubling of the diameter in this case would also cause a torsional stress reduction by a factor of 8 (Fig. 3-8). For this reason, the diameters of the Aarhus Anchorage screw (1.5 and 2.0 mm) were chosen as a compromise between fracture risk and ease of insertion (see Chapter 12).

Concerning the length of the MSIs, the aforementioned FE models demonstrated that the main load transfer takes place in the cortex. The remainder of the MSI was deformed in a tipping mode. A shorter MSI would result in a lower resistance of the surrounding trabecular bone against this deformation, leading to higher bone strains. For very short MSIs, there is a potential risk that loosening could occur. With the Aarhus Anchorage screw of 7 mm in length, the bone strains are low enough to avoid this risk (Fig. 3-4).

It should also be noted that variations in mucosal thickness can theoretically give rise to similar changes in the load transfer as would changing the MSI length. For thick mucosa, the effective length of the screw in bone can be 1 to 2 mm shorter than for thin mucosa, thereby leading to increased stresses and strains in the supporting bone. The mucosa itself, whether thick or thin, offers practically no mechanical support for the miniscrew. Therefore, the tendency of the MSI to bend will be greater in thick mucosa because a larger bending moment will be present (calculated by the distance between the screw head, or point of force application, and the bony support). However, even in this case, the bending stresses should not be high enough to exceed the strength of the miniscrew.

BONE RESPONSE TO LOADED MINISCREW IMPLANTS

Although the interest in MSIs has increased recently, histologic studies evaluating bone response to implants used for orthodontic anchorage have been limited almost exclusively to dental-type implants, which are placed in the palate, the retromolar region, or the alveolar process.[4-7,31,32] Because these implants are designed for osseointegration, they are typically not loaded for the first 6 to 12 weeks or more. The bony remodeling response of immediately loaded implants or screws may be different and has been the subject of relatively few studies.[27,33-35]

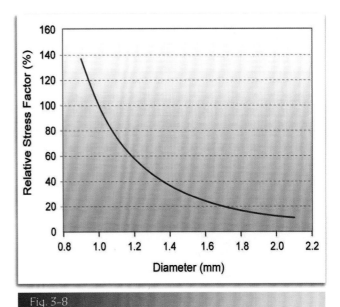

Fig. 3-8

Relative stress factor of bending/torsional stress for a miniscrew subjected to a constant bending/torsional moment relative to the diameter of the screw (set to 100% for a 1.0-mm diameter).

The initial MSI case report of Creekmore and Eklund[36] (see Chapter 1) did not discuss the biologic basis for miniscrew use. Based on experience gained from zygoma ligatures,[37] Costa and colleagues[11] began placing and immediately loading miniscrews, anticipating that screw stability was purely mechanical. To test this hypothesis, Melsen and Costa[27] studied bone-screw contact at 1, 2, 4, and 6 months following screw insertion with immediate loading.

In each of four adult male *Macaca fascicularis* monkeys, 4 titanium vanadium screws were inserted. Two were inserted into the infrazygomatic crest and 2 in the mandibular symphysis (Fig. 3-9). A total of 16 screws were placed. The screws were loaded immediately with 25- or 50-g forces to the canines. The line of action of the force was extrusive and horizontal and did not create any couples (or torsion) around the long axis of the screw. Three screws were lost during the experiment: 1 screw during insertion because of tooth contact and 2 because of infection shortly after insertion. At the end of the experiment, the screws and their surrounding bone were removed with a 5-mm trephine and were then stored in 70% alcohol. After embedding the undecalcified bone in methyl-metacrylate, 80-μm thick serial sections were cut perpendicular to the long axis of the screw according to the method of Donath and Breuner.[38] The sections were stained alternately with toluidine blue and Goldner's trichrome.

The bone response surrounding the screws was evaluated under an Olympus microscope equipped with a Zeiss® integrating reticule with equidistant lines and points. The relative extent of bone-screw contact was evaluated at a magnification of 100× by projecting a grid onto the bone section. The grid consisted of 32 radial lines extending from the center of the screw.[39] The number of intersections of the outer screw perimeter with bone contact was expressed as a percentage of the total number of intersections (Fig. 3-10).

The density of the bone adjacent to the screw was calculated by projecting a grid consisting of concentric circles onto the bone section. The inner circle coincided with the outer perimeter of the screw, and the next circle circumscribed the area within 1 mm from the outer perimeter of the screw. The grid was intersected by four equidistant lines starting from the center of the grid and dividing the bony area into four sections: one in the direction of the compressive force, one in the direction of the tensile force, and two in areas most likely subjected to shearing forces (Fig. 3-11). The relative bone volume (BV/TV %) was determined according to Parfitt and colleagues.[40] A point count method was applied, and 400 points were counted within each of the four described regions.[41]

The result of the histomorphometric analysis revealed no difference in the amount of bone-screw contact between the screws loaded with 25 or 50 g. The bone-screw contact, however, did increase over time. After 1 month of loading, 21% of the screw surface was contacted by bone, whereas the percent increased to 60% after 6 months. The variation was extreme at all time points, reflecting the original bone quantity/quality (zygoma vs. symphysis) at the insertion site.

The bone density also increased over time, initially being 8% after 1 month and increasing to 50% after 6 months. As was the case with the bone-screw contact, a variation of up to 70% was seen. Importantly, bone in each of the four quadrants around the circumference of the screw showed little variability. The bone in close contact to the mini-implant could generally be characterized as woven bone and in most cases was distinguishable from the surrounding lamellar bone. Based on this study, it appeared that the screw remained stable over time for use as an orthodontic anchorage device.

In a second similar experiment, four monkeys were included; and four mini-implants, two in the

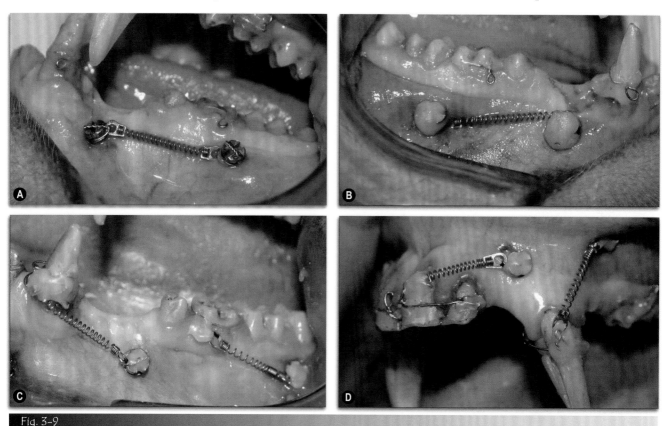

Fig. 3-9

Intraoral photographs of miniscrews placed in the maxilla and the mandible of *Macaca fascicularis* monkeys. **A,** Two mandibular miniscrews loaded against each other. **B,** Two mandibular miniscrews loaded against each other. Note composite added to prevent soft tissue irritation. **C,** Two mandibular miniscrews loaded against teeth. **D,** Two maxillary miniscrews loaded against teeth.

infrazygomatic crest and two in the mandibular symphysis, were placed in each monkey. All the mini-implants were loaded with 50 g against prosthodontic implants that had been inserted 6 months previously. The observation time was 12 weeks, after which all of the monkeys were euthanized and perfused with 70% alcohol before excising the tissue blocks containing the mini-implants and surrounding bone. Apart from the preceding, the experimental design was identical to the first study. Hygiene was controlled more carefully, and no mini-implants were lost. The result of this study confirmed the findings of the first study and added no new information.

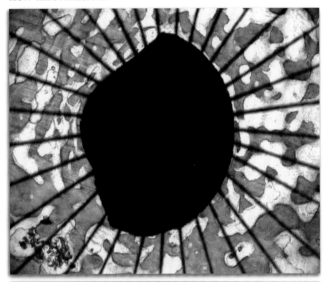

Fig. 3-10

Grid with 32 radial lines used for the determination of bone-implant contact percentage.

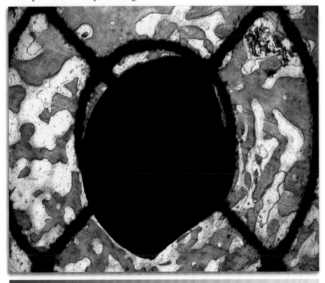

Fig. 3-11

Grid for histomorphometric evaluation of bone adjacent to the implant.

A third study was undertaken with the intention of evaluating bone turnover adjacent to the mini-implants. The study also included four monkeys (Fig. 3-12). Three months before inserting the implants, the premolars and first molars were extracted. This allowed for the insertion of four prosthodontic implants in each quadrant of each monkey. These implants were left to heal for 3 months before mini-implants were inserted in the infrazygomatic crest and mandibular symphysis. The mini-implants were loaded with 50 g immediately following placement. The study design was identical to the previous two studies, also with an observation time of 12 weeks. The purpose of the study was to evaluate the dynamic parameters of bone remodeling. The monkeys were given the fluorochrome labels calcein green and tetracycline 2 weeks and 3 days before euthanasia, respectively. The 100-µm thick sections were cut on a Leiden saw KDG 95 (MeProTech, Netherlands),

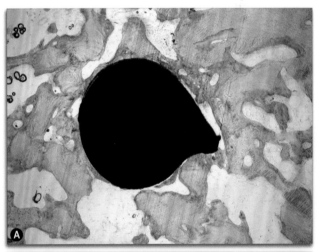

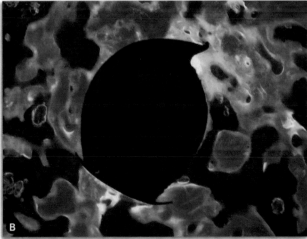

Fig. 3-12

Miniscrew placed in mandibular symphysis and loaded for 3 months. **A,** Toluidine-stained photomicrograph. Note the woven bone close to the implant surface. **B,** Photomicrograph under fluorescent light.

and the histomorphometric analysis was performed as in the first study. The dynamic variables, relative extension of erosion surface (ES/BS) and mineralizing surface/bone surface (MS/BS), were also included.

The fractional erosion surface (ES/BS) was assessed as the extent of resorption lacunae of the total surface of trabecular bone in the areas distributed. Resorption lacunae were identified as scalloped defects in the surface of the trabecular bone showing distinct erosion of the lamella system under polarized light. Fractional mineralizing surface (MS/BS) was calculated by classifying the single- and double-labeled surfaces (sLS and dLS, respectively) as a percentage of the total surface using the standard formula MS/BS = (sLS + dLS)/BS.

The results confirmed that the bone density was generally higher within 1 mm of the mini-implant surface than at a distance of more than 1 mm. The bone close to the screw was predominantly woven

bone, and the turnover was of a magnitude that made it difficult to estimate (200% to 400%). Few double labelings were found, whereas the last labeling dominated 40% to 75% of the bone surfaces within 1 mm of the screw surface (Figs. 3-13 to 3-18).

In the final study using an identical design as the previous studies, the early remodeling response from 1 to 4 weeks after loading was studied. The results are still being quantified, but preliminary findings suggest that an increased bone turnover was present after only 1 week of loading and that the initial bone density varied according to insertion site (maxilla vs. mandible). The increased bone-MSI contact and bone density appeared to be especially pronounced within the first month. The fluorochrome labeling was even more pronounced than in the previous studies. The tissue response found in these studies corroborated the findings described adjacent to both smooth and

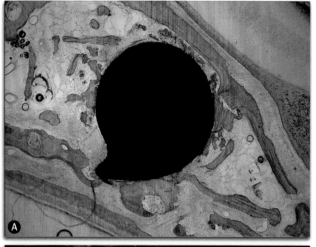

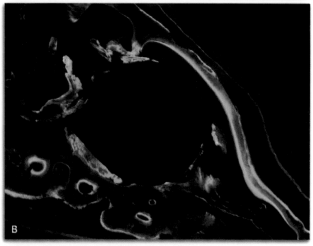

Fig. 3-13

Miniscrew placed in mandibular alveolar process between two teeth and loaded for 1 week. **A,** Toluidine-stained photomicrograph. **B,** Photomicrograph under fluorescent light.

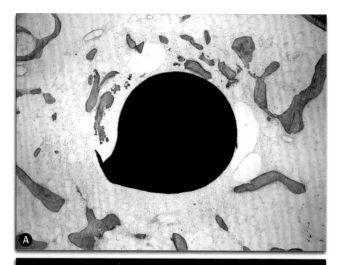

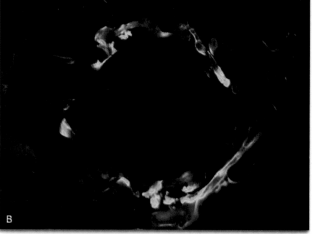

Fig. 3-14

Miniscrew placed in maxillary tuberosity area between two teeth and loaded for 1 week. **A,** Toluidine-stained photomicrograph. **B,** Photomicrograph under fluorescent light.

osseointegrated implants and seems to be independent of the loading.[32-34,37,42]

In relation to osseointegrated implants, it has been demonstrated repeatedly that the bone adjacent to the implant has been characterized as woven bone with high density. The use of fluorochrome staining has clearly demonstrated that the bone turnover adjacent to the implant is significantly increased, usually on the magnitude of 300% to 400% per year, thereby corroborating the results of Deguchi and colleagues.[7] These observations suggest that the layer of bone close to the implant never reaches a high degree of mineralization, and therefore is of a lower stiffness than the surrounding mature bone. This arrangement allows for micromovement of implants, a fact that also explains why bridges extending between tooth and an implant can be successful.

SUMMARY

The load transfer from a mini-implant to the surrounding bone depends both on the mechanical competence of the bone and the design of the mini-implant. Independent of the exact shape and size of the mini-implant, clinicians should take care not to position the implants in locations where the bone quality is poor (cortical thickness of less than 1 mm with underlying low-density trabecular bone). The loading of the screw can be initiated immediately following placement because the strain generated with the moderate forces necessary for tooth movement will be within the adaptive window and thus lead to an increase in density of the bone adjacent to the screw. However, one should remember that initial forces should be relatively low, on the magnitude of 50 g. Then, as the bone remodels around the screw over time, its stability also increases, and larger loads can be added if necessary.

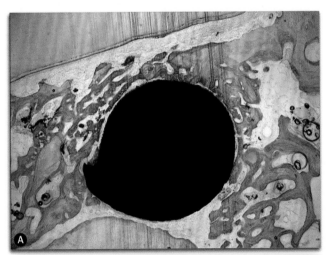

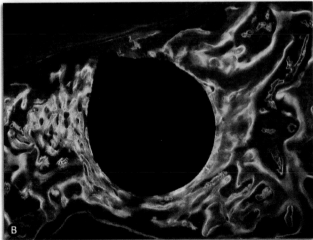

Fig. 3-15

Miniscrew placed between two teeth in mandibular alveolar process and loaded for 1 month. **A,** Toluidine-stained photomicrograph. Note the extreme remodeling activity adjacent to implant. **B,** Photomicrograph under fluorescent light.

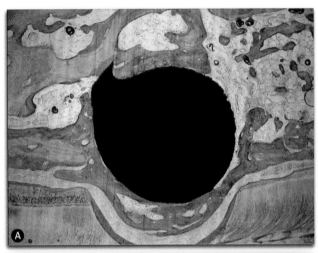

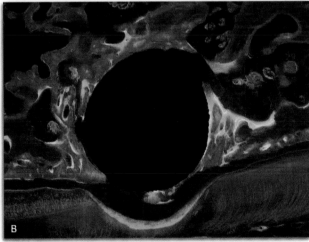

Fig. 3-16

Miniscrew placed between two teeth in mandibular alveolar process and loaded for 1 month. Note repair of root that was damaged during insertion. **A,** Toluidine-stained photomicrograph. **B,** Photomicrograph under fluorescent light.

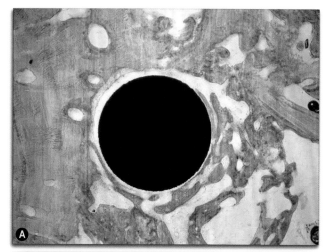

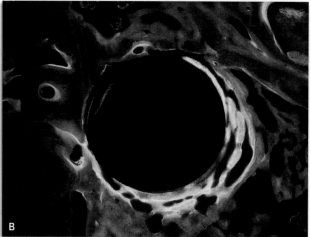

Fig. 3-17

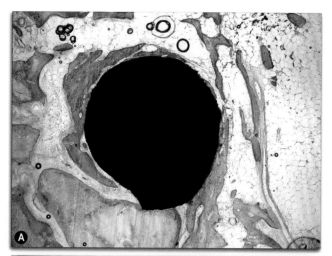

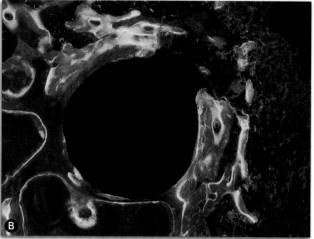

Fig. 3-18

Miniscrew placed in mandibular symphysis and loaded for 2 months. **A,** Toluidine-stained photomicrograph. Note the extreme remodeling activity adjacent to the implant. **B,** Photomicrograph under fluorescent light.

Miniscrew placed at infrazygomatic crest and loaded for 3 months. **A,** Toluidine-stained photomicrograph. Note the extreme remodeling activity adjacent to the implant. **B,** Photomicrograph under fluorescent light.

ACKNOWLEDGMENTS

This work was supported in part by Medicon Instrumente, Tuttlingen, Germany; AAO Foundation, St. Louis, Missouri; and the Aarhus University Research Foundation, Denmark.

REFERENCES

1. Roberts WE, Helm FR, Marshall KJ, Gongloff RK. Rigid endosseous implants for orthodontic and orthopedic anchorage. *Angle Orthod.* 59:247-256, 1989.
2. Roberts WE, Marshall KJ, Mozsary PG. Rigid endosseous implant utilized as anchorage to protract molars and close an atrophic extraction site. *Angle Orthod.* 60:135-152, 1990.
3. Wehrbein H, Merz BR. Aspects of the use of endosseous palatal implants in orthodontic therapy. *J Esthet Dent.* 10:315-324, 1998.
4. Wehrbein H, Merz BR, Diedrich P. Palatal bone support for orthodontic implant anchorage—a clinical and radiological study. *Eur J Orthod.* 21:65-70, 1999.
5. Wehrbein H, Yildirim M, Diedrich P. Osteodynamics around orthodontically loaded short maxillary implants: an experimental pilot study. *J Orofac Orthop.* 60:409-415, 1999.
6. Trisi P, Rebaudi A. Progressive bone adaptation of titanium implants during and after orthodontic load in humans. *Int J Periodontics Restorative Dent* 22:31-43, 2002.
7. Deguchi T, Takano-Yamamoto T, Kanomi R, et al. The use of small titanium screws for orthodontic anchorage. *J Dent Res.* 82:377-381, 2003.
8. Brånemark PI. Osseointegration and its experimental background. *J Prosthet Dent.* 50:399-410, 1983.
9. Romanos GE. Present status of immediate loading of oral implants. *J Oral Implantol.* 30:189-197, 2004.
10. Romanos GE, Toh CG, Siar CH, et al. Histologic and histomorphometric evaluation of periimplant bone subjected to immediate loading: an experimental study with *Macaca fascicularis. Int J Oral Maxillofac Implants.* 17:44-51, 2002.
11. Costa A, Raffaini M, Melsen B. Miniscrews as orthodontic anchorage: a preliminary report. *Int J Adult Orthodon Orthognath Surg.* 13:201-209, 1998.
12. Umemori M, Sugawara J, Mitani H, et al. Skeletal anchorage system for open-bite correction. *Am J Orthod Dentofacial Orthop.* 115:166-174, 1999.

13. Bernhart T, Freudenthaler J, Dortbudak O, et al. Short epithetic implants for orthodontic anchorage in the paramedian region of the palate: a clinical study. *Clin Oral Implants Res.* 12:624-631, 2001.
14. Lee JS, Park HS, Kyung HM. Micro-implant anchorage for lingual treatment of a skeletal Class II malocclusion. *J Clin Orthod.* 35:643-647, 2001.
15. Park HS, Bae SM, Kyung HM, Sung JH. Micro-implant anchorage for treatment of skeletal Class I bialveolar protrusion. *J Clin Orthod.* 35:417-422, 2001.
16. De Clerck H, Geerinckx V, Siciliano S. The Zygoma Anchorage System. *J Clin Orthod.* 36:455-459, 2002.
17. Sherwood KH, Burch J, Thompson W. Intrusion of supererupted molars with titanium miniplate anchorage. *Angle Orthod.* 73:597-601, 2003.
18. Sugawara J, Baik UB, Umemori M, et al. Treatment and posttreatment dentoalveolar changes following intrusion of mandibular molars with application of a skeletal anchorage system (SAS) for open bite correction. *Int J Adult Orthodon Orthognath Surg.* 17:243-253, 2002.
19. Bae SM, Park HS, Kyung HM, et al. Clinical application of micro-implant anchorage. *J Clin Orthod.* 36:298-302, 2002.
20. Keles A, Erverdi N, Sezen S. Bodily distalization of molars with absolute anchorage. *Angle Orthod.* 73:471-482, 2003.
21. Kyung HM, Park HS, Bae SM, et al. Development of orthodontic micro-implants for intraoral anchorage. *J Clin Orthod.* 37:321-328, 2003.
22. Maino BG, Bednar J, Pagin P, Mura P. The spider screw for skeletal anchorage. *J Clin Orthod.* 37:90-97, 2003.
23. Melsen B, Garbo D. Treating the 'impossible case' with the use of the Aarhus Anchorage System. *Orthodontics.* 1:13-20, 2004.
24. Melsen B, Verna C. Miniscrew implants: the Aarhus Anchorage System. *Semin Orthod.* 11:24-31, 2005.
25. Higuchi KW, Slack JM. The use of titanium fixtures for intraoral anchorage to facilitate orthodontic tooth movement. *Int J Oral Maxillofac Implants.* 6:338-344, 1991.
26. Garetto LP, Chen J, Parr JA, Roberts WE. Remodeling dynamics of bone supporting rigidly fixed titanium implants: a histomorphometric comparison in four species including humans. *Implant Dent.* 4:235-243, 1995.
27. Melsen B, Costa A. Immediate loading of implants used for orthodontic anchorage. *Clin Orthod Res.* 3:23-28, 2000.
28. Frost HM. Skeletal structural adaptations to mechanical usage (SATMU), I: redefining Wolff's law: the bone modeling problem. *Anat Rec.* 226:403-413, 1990.
29. Frost HM. Skeletal structural adaptations to mechanical usage (SATMU), II: redefining Wolff's law: the remodeling problem. *Anat Rec.* 226:414-422, 1990.
30. Dalstra M, Cattaneo PM, Melsen B. Load transfer of mini-screws for orthodontic anchorage. *Orthodontics.* 1:53-62, 2004.
31. Chen J, Chen K, Garetto LP, Roberts WE. Mechanical response to functional and therapeutic loading of a retromolar endosseous implant used for orthodontic anchorage to mesially translate mandibular molars. *Implant Dent.* 4:246-258, 1995.
32. Chen J, Esterle M, Roberts WE. Mechanical response to functional loading around the threads of retromolar endosseous implants utilized for orthodontic anchorage: coordinated histomorphometric and finite element analysis. *Int J Oral Maxillofac Implants.* 14:282-289, 1999.
33. Melsen B. Accroissement des possibilités therapeutiques orthodontiques a l'aide l'ancrage Aarhus: widening the orthodontics possibilities with the Aarhus Anchorage. *Journal de Parodontologie & D'Implantologie Orale.* 19:333-347, 2000.
34. Ohmae M, Saito S, Morohashi T, et al. A clinical and histological evaluation of titanium mini-implants as anchors for orthodontic intrusion in the beagle dog. *Am J Orthod Dentofacial Orthop.* 119:489-497, 2001.
35. Melsen B. Une solution alternative. *Ormco News.* 30:11-16, 2004.
36. Creekmore TD, Eklund MK. The possibility of skeletal anchorage. *J Clin Orthod.* 17:266-269, 1983.
37. Melsen B, Petersen JK, Costa A. Zygoma ligatures: an alternative form of maxillary anchorage. *J Clin Orthod.* 32:154-158, 1998.
38. Donath K, Breuner G. A method for the study of undecalcified bones and teeth with attached soft tissues: the Sage/Schliff (sawing and grinding) technique. *J Oral Pathol.* 11:318-326, 1982.
39. Melsen B, Lang NP. Biological reactions of alveolar bone to orthodontic loading of oral implants. *Clin Oral Implants Res.* 12:144-152, 2001.
40. Parfitt AM, Drezner MK, Glorieux FH, et al. Bone histomorphometry: standardization of nomenclature, symbols, and units. Report of the ASBMR Histomorphometry Nomenclature Committee. *J Bone Miner Res.* 2:595-610, 1987.
41. Gundersen HJ, Bendtsen TF, Korbo L, et al. Some new, simple and efficient stereological methods and their use in pathological research and diagnosis. *APMIS.* 96:379-394, 1988.
42. Fritz U, Diedrich P, Kinzinger G, Al-Said M. The anchorage quality of mini-implants towards translatory and extrusive forces. *J Orofac Orthop.* 64:293-304, 2003.

CHAPTER

4

Finite Element Analysis and Animal Experiments of MiniScrew Implants

Kuniaki Miyajima, Shigeru Saito, Masaru Sakai

Although dental implants have gained widespread acceptance for dental restoration and rehabilitation, their use is not widespread for orthodontic anchorage. This lack of use is primarily due to the fact that dental implants are generally 3 mm in diameter or larger and are limited to vertical placement in edentulous areas of the alveolar ridge.[1-4] More recently, other implantlike devices have been used to provide anchorage for orthodontic applications.[5-13] The most commonly used device is the miniscrew implant (MSI) because of its small size, ease of placement, inexpensive cost, variety of placement sites in the oral cavity, and ease of removal after use. Although many case reports have documented the successful implementation of these devices in providing orthodontic anchorage, few studies have provided comparative data for evaluating different MSI sizes. Therefore, our group conducted a series of mechanical and animal experiments to determine the effectiveness of different MSI sizes in providing orthodontic anchorage.

FINITE ELEMENT ANALYSIS

Finite element analysis (FEA) has been established as a valuable aid in evaluating material properties in real-world scenarios before actual use of the material.[14] The technique was first introduced in the 1950s. Since that time, FEA has been continually developed and improved. Finite element analysis is a computational method that subdivides an object into very small, finite-size elements called a finite element model

(FEM). Each element is assigned a set of characteristic equations (describing mechanical properties, boundary conditions, and imposed forces), which are then solved as a set of simultaneous equations to predict the behavior of the object. In general, the more numerous and smaller the finite elements, the more accurate the analysis. Although FEA appears complex, the fundamental principles are relatively straightforward.

The first step of any FEA is to divide the actual geometry of the experimental structure into a collection of discrete portions called finite elements. The elements are joined together by shared nodes, which connect each finite element to its surrounding finite elements. The collection of nodes and finite elements are known as the mesh. The variable to be determined in the analysis is assumed to act over each element in a predefined (e.g., quadratic) manner. The number and type of elements is chosen to ensure that the variable distribution over the whole body is adequately approximated by the combined elemental representations. After the problem has been divided into discrete units, the governing equations for each element are calculated and then assembled to give systematic equations that describe the behavior of the body as a whole.

For stress analysis, the finite element software calculates the displacements of the nodes during an applied force, and from this information the stresses and strains in the elements are determined. To prevent unlimited rigid body motion, boundary conditions are applied. To clarify the stress distribution of the applied force against the surrounding structure, FEA provides both numerical data as well as the location of applied stress as it is distributed. Therefore, both the amount and distribution of the stress applied by an MSI to its surrounding alveolar bone can be calculated using FEA. Using this information, a given MSI size can be evaluated under different loading conditions to estimate whether the implant can support a certain orthodontic force level or whether this force would cause fracture of the surrounding alveolar bone. Therefore, FEA is a valuable tool in evaluating MSI sizes prior to production and actual use.

Finite Element Model Experiment
Materials and Methods

Using COSMOS/M v1.75 software (Materialise Yokokawa Inc., Funabashi City, Japan), a virtual alveolar bone model was created. The model was 10 mm wide by 10 mm deep by 30 mm tall. For the 30 mm of height, the top 2 mm was cortical bone with the underlying 28 mm being medullary bone. A linear static module consisting of 6,293 elements and 18,879 degrees of freedom was applied. Importantly, the assumption was made that the MSI and the surrounding alveolar bone were in complete contact. Two different MSI models were tested: Model 1 was 1 mm in diameter and 5 mm in length, Model 2 was 2 mm in diameter and 15 mm in length (Fig. 4-1). For both models, a 100-g force was applied to the MSI head (4 mm above the bone surface) in three different directions: 0 (horizontal), 45 (oblique), and 90 (perpendicular) degrees relative to the bone surface. To determine the effect of point of force application in a second experiment, the force was applied to the MSI at 1, 2, and 4 mm above the alveolar surface. The mechanical properties of the FEM components are shown in Table 4-1. The MSI and alveolar bone stress distributions and deflections were calculated using the COSMOS/M linear static module.

Results

The FEM analysis revealed that the stress distributions and deflections were similar in Models 1 and 2, although the values were much larger in Model 1. In summary, the maximum stress in the alveolar bone was distributed in the cervical region, which approximates the first revolution or two of the MSI threads (Figs. 4-2 and 4-3). The maximum stress of the MSI was distributed above the alveolar bone at the top of the

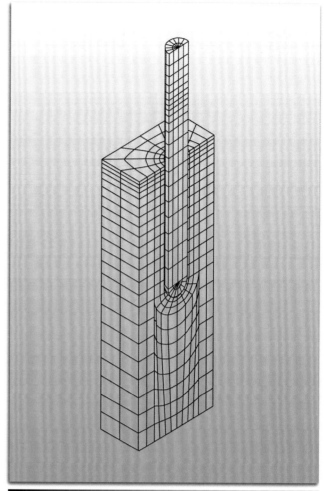

Fig. 4-1

Three-dimensional finite element model. The alveolar bone model was 10 mm wide by 10 mm deep by 30 mm tall. The Model 1 miniscrew implant (MSI) was 1.0 mm in diameter and 5 mm long. The Model 2 MSI was 2.0 mm in diameter and 15 mm long. (Reprinted with permission from Miyajima K, Saito S, Sana M, Sakai M. Three-dimensional finite element models and animal studies of the use of mini-screws for orthodontic anchorage. In: McNamara JA Jr, ed. *Implants, Microimplants, Onplants, and Transplants: New Answers to Old Questions in Orthodontics.* Ann Arbor: Center for Human Growth and Development, University of Michigan, 2005.)

MSI (Figs. 4-4 and 4-5). The deflection of the implant was seen mainly in the region lying above the surface of the alveolar bone (Figs. 4-6 and 4-7). Both the maximum stress and deflection increased in magnitude as the force level became more horizontal relative to the surface of the bone, that is, less stress at 0 degrees and more stress at 90 degrees. Stress distribution values were almost 6 times larger at 0 and 45 degrees and 3.4 times larger at 90 degrees for Model 1 (Table 4-2). When stress was evaluated relative to the point of force application above the bone surface, the higher the point of force application was above the bone, the

Table 4-1.	Mechanical Properties of Three Dimensional Finite Element Model Components	
Material	Young's Modulus	Poisson's Ratio
Cortical bone	1.4×10^4 MPa	0.30
Medullary bone	7.9×10^3 MPa	0.30
Miniscrew implant	1.1×10^4 MPa	0.30

(Reprinted with permission from Miyajima K, Saito S, Sana M, Sakai M. Three-dimensional finite element models and animal studies of the use of mini-screws for orthodontic anchorage. In: McNamara JA Jr, ed. *Implants, Microimplants, Onplants, and Transplants: New Answers to Old Questions in Orthodontics.* Ann Arbor: Center for Human Growth and Development, University of Michigan, 2005.)

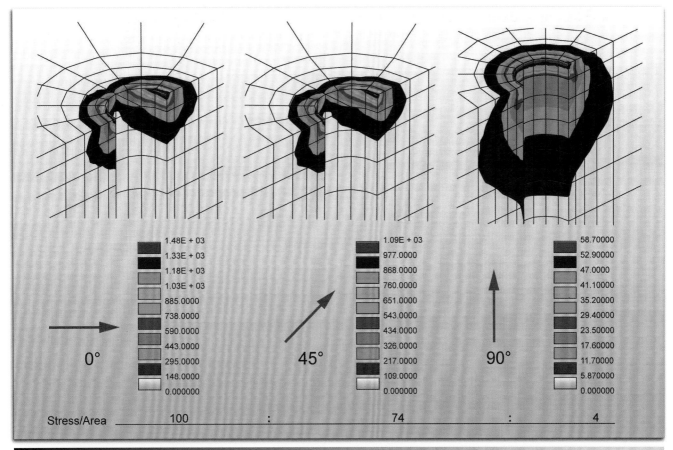

Fig. 4-2

Stress distribution in alveolar bone surrounding Model 1 MSI. Note that bone corresponding to first two threads receives the most stress when loaded horizontally and obliquely. (Reprinted with permission from Miyajima K, Saito S, Sana M, Sakai M. Three-dimensional finite element models and animal studies of the use of mini-screws for orthodontic anchorage. In: McNamara JA Jr, ed. *Implants, Microimplants, Onplants, and Transplants: New Answers to Old Questions in Orthodontics.* Ann Arbor: Center for Human Growth and Development, University of Michigan, 2005.

greater the stress. For example, when the horizontal force was applied 4 mm above the bone, the stress was 3.2 times greater than when the force was applied 1 mm above the bone (Fig. 4-8, Table 4-3).

Discussion

The results of the FEA revealed that the stress generated in the alveolar bone during force application to the MSI was about 6 times larger for Model 1 than Model 2. It should be recalled that orthodontic forces generate less than one twentieth that of masticatory forces. Therefore,

the larger stress created by the smaller MSI may not be of significant concern for bony damage. However, this stress discrepancy between different-sized MSIs should be considered. The higher stress is probably a result of decreased surface area of the smaller MSI. Smaller surface area translates to less bone-implant contact. The higher stress may also increase local microdamage around the MSI. All of this taken together may suggest using slightly larger MSIs. However, one significant benefit of small MSIs is that they are more applicable to many regions, and particularly in intraradicular and interradicular locations where larger MSIs may not be appropriate. It follows that there are risks and benefits associated with smaller and larger MSIs and that the orthodontist must weigh all factors carefully before determining the MSI of choice for any particular case.

Another important point reveled by FEA was that the more horizontal the force applied to the MSI, the larger the stress generated in both the alveolar bone and the MSI. Also apparent is that the more vertical the force applied to the MSI, the larger the area over which the stress was distributed, and consequently the stress was decreased. For example, in Model 1 (Figs. 4-2 and 4-4) when the force was oriented at 0 degrees, the stress generated was highest in both alveolar bone and the MSI but was distributed over a very small area—the first one to two threads in the bone and just above the bone in the MSI. This is in complete contrast to when the force is oriented at 90 degrees, where the stress generated was lowest in both

alveolar bone and the MSI but was distributed over a very large area—most of the length of the screw threads in the bone and along the entire length of the MSI. This may be one important reason that MSIs do not have to be osseointegrated in order to provide anchorage; that is, orthodontic force application is predominantly oriented perpendicular to the long axis of the MSI where the stress is generated primarily in the first one to two threads of the MSI in cortical bone. Importantly, this may also be why MSI length is less critical than diameter.

When considering point of force application, the further away the surface of the bone from the attachment of orthodontic force modules, the higher the stress in both the alveolar bone and the MSI. Therefore, in order to minimize these stresses, it is important to place the force module as close to the emergence from the bone surface as possible, which is not always possible because of the depth of the soft tissue through which the MSI emerges.

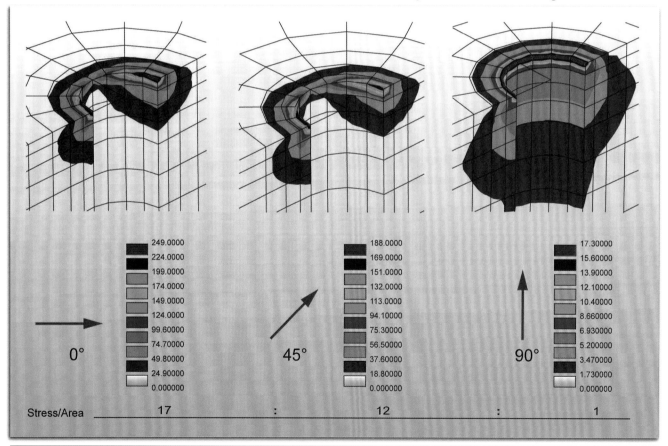

Fig. 4-3

Stress distribution in alveolar bone surrounding Model 2 MSI. Note that bone corresponding to first two threads receives the most stress when loaded horizontally and obliquely. (Reprinted with permission from Miyajima K, Saito S, Sana M, Sakai M. Three-dimensional finite element models and animal studies of the use of mini-screws for orthodontic anchorage. In: McNamara JA Jr, ed. *Implants, Microimplants, Onplants, and Transplants: New Answers to Old Questions in Orthodontics.* Ann Arbor: Center for Human Growth and Development, University of Michigan, 2005.)

ANIMAL EXPERIMENTS

Four different animal experiments were conducted; the purposes of each were as follows:

1. To evaluate stability differences between a short and a long MSI for tipping and intrusion of maxillary canines
2. To evaluate stability differences of a constant MSI size for intrusion of maxillary anterior and mandibular posterior teeth
3. To compare several different commercially available orthodontic anchorage devices
4. To evaluate age- and time-dependent differences in bone-implant contact for MSIs.

Experiment 1
Materials and Methods

Four adult beagle dogs were used for intrusion of maxillary canines. Intraoral impressions were taken to fabricate canine bands with facially soldered buttons. The bands were then cemented on both maxillary canines (Fig. 4-9). After band cementation, local infiltration was performed and a mucoperiosteal flap was raised. A 0.9-mm pilot drill was used to drill a pilot hole with saline irrigation to the depth of the corresponding MSI. The MSIs were then inserted with their accompanying screwdriver. A short MSI (3.0 mm long, 1.0 mm diameter) was placed in alveolar bone mesial to the canine on one side of the maxilla, whereas a long MSI (6.0 mm long, 1.0 mm diameter) was placed on the contralateral side (Fig. 4-10). After MSI placement, a 100-g nickel titanium closed coil spring (NiTi CCS) was immediately attached to apply a force from the MSI to the button. The animals were maintained at the Aichi-Gakuin Animal Laboratory.

Experimental records were taken at the initial surgical procedure and at the conclusion of the experiment 3 months later. The records included intraoral photographs and periapical radiographs. At the end of orthodontic intrusion, the animals were euthanized and the periimplant alveolar bone with the associated MSIs and canines was resected en bloc. The resected

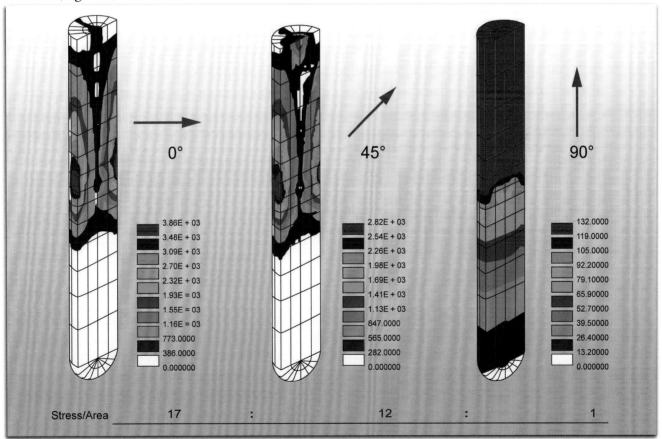

Fig. 4-4

Stress distribution in MSI Model 1. Note that the first two threads receive the most stress when loaded horizontally and obliquely and that the top of the MSI above the bone receives the most stress when loaded vertically. (Reprinted with permission from Miyajima K, Saito S, Sana M, Sakai M. Three-dimensional finite element models and animal studies of the use of mini-screws for orthodontic anchorage. In: McNamara JA Jr, ed. *Implants, Microimplants, Onplants, and Transplants: New Answers to Old Questions in Orthodontics.* Ann Arbor: Center for Human Growth and Development, University of Michigan, 2005.)

tissue blocks were prepared for standard paraffin-embedded decalcified tissue evaluation. Briefly, the blocks were fixed in 10% formalin neutral buffer solution (pH 7.4, Wako Pure Chemical, Osaka, Japan) at 4° C for 1 day and then were decalcified in a mixture of formic acid and sodium citrate at 4° C for 6 days.[15] Afterward, the specimens were embedded in paraffin, serially sectioned at a thickness of 7 to 8 μm, and stained with hematoxylin and eosin and azan.

Results

No MSI failure was seen during the 3-month experiment period for either the short or the long MSIs. Clinical measurements indicated that the canines on both sides were intruded and tipped mesially an average of 3.5 mm. The periapical radiographs revealed no significant difference in the periodontal conditions for either side (Fig. 4-11), nor was any evidence of root resorption observed.

Histologic evaluation revealed that bone-implant contact along the entire MSI surface was less than 50% for both MSI lengths. However, teeth moved without any apparent MSI mobility or failure. This suggests that complete bone-implant contact may not be required for orthodontic anchorage.

Discussion

We have previously reported using MSIs for mandibular premolar intrusion in dogs.[16,17] Although the experimental design was different from that in the present experiment, the clinical results are similar; for example, no MSI mobility, no MSI infection, minimum gingival inflammation, slight cementum resorption during intrusion, and ease of MSI removal after use. The histologic findings are also similar; for example, bone-implant contact was less than expected, but without MSI mobility or failure and with continued use through the entire experimental period.

In the present experiment the MSIs were 1.0 mm in diameter and either 3 or 6 mm in length. These data

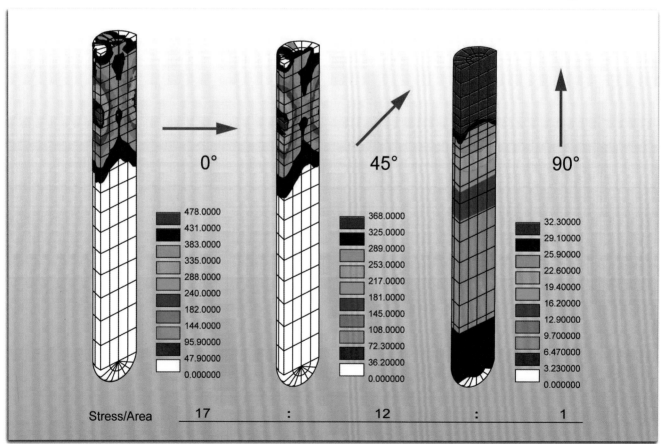

Fig. 4-5

Stress distribution in MSI Model 2. Note that the first two threads receive the most stress when loaded horizontally and obliquely and that the top of the MSI above the bone receives the most stress when loaded vertically. (Reprinted with permission from Miyajima K, Saito S, Sana M, Sakai M. Three-dimensional finite element models and animal studies of the use of mini-screws for orthodontic anchorage. In: McNamara JA Jr, ed. *Implants, Microimplants, Onplants, and Transplants: New Answers to Old Questions in Orthodontics.* Ann Arbor: Center for Human Growth and Development, University of Michigan, 2005.)

suggest that MSI length may not be a critical factor in stability or use for orthodontic force application, particularly when taken in context with the foregoing FEA data, which indicated that for loads perpendicular to the MSI long axis, that most stress is generated within the first one to two threads within cortical bone.

Experiment 2
Materials and Methods
Three adult male beagle dogs weighing 11 to 13 kg and ranging in age from 19 to 26 months were used to evaluate intrusion of maxillary anterior teeth and mandibular third premolars using MSIs. The MSIs (Sankin Industrial Company, Tokyo, Japan) were 1 mm in diameter and 4 mm in length and were made of 99.5% titanium. The animals were maintained by the Animal Laboratory at Showa University.

For maxillary intrusion, the maxillary second incisors (dogs have three incisors per side) were extracted bilaterally 8 weeks before MSI placement in all animals. Four MSIs total (two on the facial, two on the palatal) were placed in the edentulous alveolar bone of the missing second incisor site bilaterally. The two MSIs on the right side were loaded, whereas the two MSIs on the left side served as unloaded controls and as unmoving landmarks for radiographic super-imposition after intrusion.

For mandibular intrusion, no mandibular teeth were extracted. Four MSIs total (three on the facial, one on the lingual) were placed. The lingual and one facial MSI were placed in the *intraradicular* bone of the third premolar. The remaining two facial MSIs were placed in the *interradicular* bone mesial and distal to the third premolar roots. The two intraradicular MSIs were loaded to produce intrusion of the third premolar; the two interradicular MSIs served as unloaded controls and as unmoving landmarks for radiographic superimposition after intrusion.

The surgical procedure was the same for the maxillary (Fig. 4-12, *A*) and mandibular intrusion. Local infiltration was performed and a mucoperiosteal flap

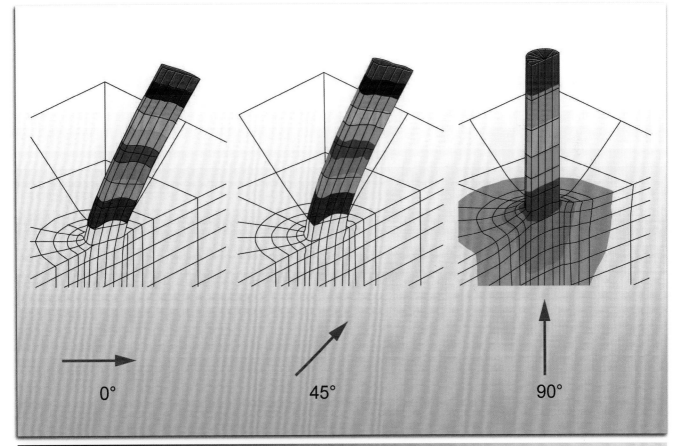

0°   45°   90°

Fig. 4-6

Deflection of MSI Model 1. Note that the largest deformation occurred at the top of the MSI for all loading directions. (Reprinted with permission from Miyajima K, Saito S, Sana M, Sakai M. Three-dimensional finite element models and animal studies of the use of mini-screws for orthodontic anchorage. In: McNamara JA Jr, ed. *Implants, Microimplants, Onplants, and Transplants: New Answers to Old Questions in Orthodontics.* Ann Arbor: Center for Human Growth and Development, University of Michigan, 2005.)

was raised. A 1.5-mm round bur was used with saline irrigation to make a pit about 1.2 mm in diameter. This was followed by a 0.9-mm pilot drill with saline irrigation to drill a pilot hole to the depth of the corresponding MSI. The MSIs were then inserted with their accompanying screwdriver, covered by the flap, and sutured closed. MSI position was documented with periapical radiographs.

For the maxilla, a pair of cast metal bridges was fabricated and cemented to the maxillary first and third incisors bilaterally. After 8 weeks of healing, the gingival tissue over all experimental MSIs was removed and an 0.011-inch ligature wire was attached to the head of the experimental MSIs to act as a hook. A NiTi CCS was then attached from the facial to the palatal MSI and looped over the top of the cast bridge on the right

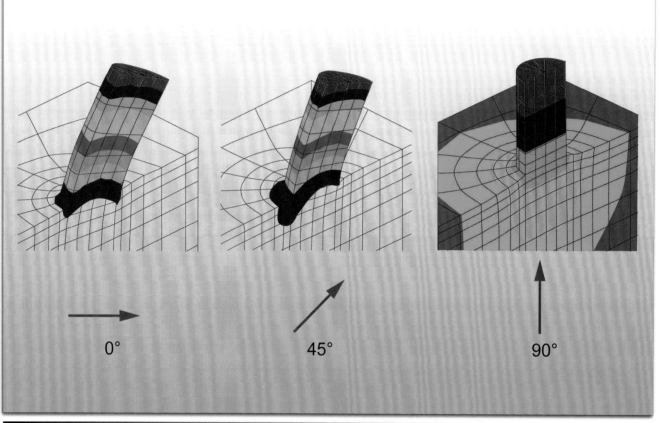

Fig. 4-7

Deflection of MSI Model 2. Note that the largest deformation occurred at the top of the MSI for all loading directions. (Reprinted with permission from Miyajima K, Saito S, Sana M, Sakai M. Three-dimensional finite element models and animal studies of the use of mini-screws for orthodontic anchorage. In: McNamara JA Jr, ed. *Implants, Microimplants, Onplants, and Transplants: New Answers to Old Questions in Orthodontics*. Ann Arbor: Center for Human Growth and Development, University of Michigan, 2005.)

Table 4-2.	Stress Distribution in Alveolar Bone and Miniscrew Implants for Different Force Orientations		
Model	Force Direction (degrees)	Stress in Alveolar Bone (g/mm)	Stress in Miniscrew Implant (g/mm)
Model 1	0	1480	3860
	45	1090	2820
	90	59	132
Model 2	0	249	478
	45	188	368
	90	17	32

Finite element analysis revealed that horizontal forces caused 25 times more stress in alveolar bone in Model 1 and 14 times more stress in Model 2 than vertical pullout forces. Horizontal forces caused 29 times more stress in MSI Model 1 and 14 times more stress in Model 2 than vertical pullout forces. (Reprinted with permission from Miyajima K, Saito S, Sana M, Sakai M. Three-dimensional finite element models and animal studies of the use of mini-screws for orthodontic anchorage. In: McNamara JA Jr, ed. *Implants, Microimplants, Onplants, and Transplants: New Answers to Old Questions in Orthodontics*. Ann Arbor: Center for Human Growth and Development, University of Michigan, 2005.)

side (Fig. 4-12, *B*). The two MSIs on the right side were loaded, whereas the two MSIs on the left side were unloaded controls. The coil spring was calibrated to produce 120 g of force, which was recalibrated biweekly.

For the mandible, the gingival tissue over all experimental MSIs was removed and an 0.011-inch ligature wire was attached to the head of the experimental MSIs to act as a hook after 8 weeks of healing. A button was bonded to the facial and lingual aspect of the third premolar cusp tip, and a NiTi CCS was attached from the facial and lingual MSIs to the facial and lingual buttons, respectively. The two MSIs in the interradicular bone were unloaded controls. The coil spring was calibrated to produce 150 g of force, which was recalibrated biweekly.

Experimental records were taken at the initial surgical procedure and biweekly thereafter until the conclusion

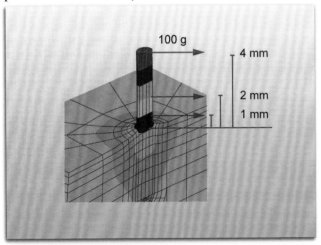

Fig. 4-8

Effect of point of force application at the MSI relative to bone surface. Note that 3.2 times more stress develops when force is applied 4 mm above bone surface for MSI Model 1. (Reprinted with permission from Miyajima K, Saito S, Sana M, Sakai M. Three-dimensional finite element models and animal studies of the use of mini-screws for orthodontic anchorage. In: McNamara JA Jr, ed. *Implants, Microimplants, Onplants, and Transplants: New Answers to Old Questions in Orthodontics.* Ann Arbor: Center for Human Growth and Development, University of Michigan, 2005.)

of the experiment. The records included dental impressions, intraoral photographs, and periapical radiographs (Figs. 4-12, *C* to *F,* and 4-13). Intramuscular injections of tetracycline (15 mg/kg) and calcein (15 mg/kg) were performed the day of MSI placement and every 4 weeks thereafter until the conclusion of the experiment.

At the end of orthodontic intrusion, the animals were euthanized and perfused with 4% para-formaldehyde and 2% glutaraldehyde in 0.05 M phosphate buffer (pH 7.4). The maxillary anterior segments with the associated MSIs and bridges and the mandibular premolar segments with the associated MSIs were resected en bloc. The bridge was removed from the maxillary teeth, and radiographs were obtained. These resected blocks were then dissected such that the MSIs and their alveolar bone were separated from the teeth and their alveolar bone. For one animal, the resected tissue containing the teeth and alveolar bone was prepared for standard paraffin-embedded decalcified tissue evaluation. Briefly, the blocks were fixed in 10% formalin neutral buffer solution (pH 7.4, Wako Pure Chemical) at 4° C for 1 day and then decalcified in a mixture of formic acid and sodium citrate at 4° C for 6 days.[15] Afterward, the specimens were embedded in paraffin, serially sectioned at a thickness of 7 to 8 μm, and stained with hematoxylin and eosin and azan.

In the maxilla, the remaining four blocks (from two animals) containing the teeth and alveolar bone (two control and two experimental) and all six blocks containing the MSIs and alveolar bone were prepared for plastic-embedded histologic analysis and backscattered electron microscopy. In the mandible, all tissue blocks were prepared for plastic-embedded histologic analysis and backscattered electron microscopy. The blocks were maintained in fixative for an additional 7 days. After washing with purified water and trimming, the specimens were dipped in Villanueva bone stain solution for 7 days under negative pressure. This solution was prepared by mixing 0.5 g Villanueva bone

Table 4-3.	Effect of Point of Force Application at Miniscrew Implant Relative to Bone Surface	
Height of Force Application	Stress in Alveolar Bone (g/mm)	Stress in Miniscrew Implant (g/mm)
1 mm	459	925
2 mm	796	1860
4 mm	1480	3860

Note that 3.2 times more stress develops when force is applied 4 mm above bone surface for MSI Model 1. (Reprinted with permission from Miyajima K, Saito S, Sana M, Sakai M. Three-dimensional finite element models and animal studies of the use of mini-screws for orthodontic anchorage. In: McNamara JA Jr, ed. *Implants, Microimplants, Onplants, and Transplants: New Answers to Old Questions in Orthodontics.* Ann Arbor: Center for Human Growth and Development, University of Michigan, 2005.)

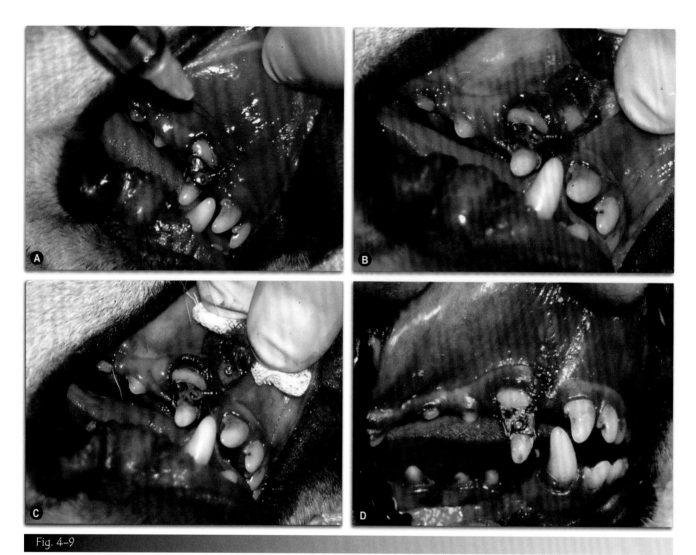

Fig. 4-9

Experimental surgical procedure. **A,** Injection of local anesthetic. **B,** Reflection of mucoperiosteal flap. **C,** Placement of MSI. **D,** Attachment of 100-g nickel titanium closed coil spring (NiTi CCS) from MSI to bracket. (Reprinted with permission from Miyajima K, Saito S, Sana M, Sakai M. Three-dimensional finite element models and animal studies of the use of mini-screws for orthodontic anchorage. In: McNamara JA Jr, ed. *Implants, Microimplants, Onplants, and Transplants: New Answers to Old Questions in Orthodontics.* Ann Arbor: Center for Human Growth and Development, University of Michigan, 2005.)

stain powder (Villanueva Bone Stain Powder, Maruto Instrument Co., Ltd., Tokyo, Japan) with 100 mL of 70% methanol. The specimens were then dehydrated and defatted with ethanol and acetone, respectively, and were embedded in polyester resin (Rigolac, Nisshin EM Co., Ltd., Tokyo, Japan). Each MSI and bone block was cross-sectioned or sagittally sectioned with a low-speed saw (Isomet, Buehler Ltd., Lake Bluff, Illinois) into 100-μm thick sections. The thickness was reduced further by polishing with waterproof abrasive paper to a thickness of less than 10 μm. These sections were then polished with 5- and 0.3-μm alumina particles on polishing cloths and were examined by fluorescence microscopy. Finally, the sections were backscattered with electrons, and scanning electron microscopic (SEM) images were

produced (Hitachi S-2500 CX; Hitachi Co. Ltd., Tokyo, Japan).

Results

For maxillary incisor intrusion, clinical measurements of study models and intraoral photographs indicated that the bridges on the right side were intruded an average of 2 mm during the 6 weeks of force application. The bridges on the control side did not show any intrusion. The periapical radiographs revealed no significant difference between the experimental and control sides for incisor periodontal conditions or periimplant bone. No root resorption was observed on periapical radiographs.

Sagittal maxillary SEM sections revealed that only a small amount of bone contacted the facial MSIs (Fig. 4-14, *A*) with more bone contacting the palatal

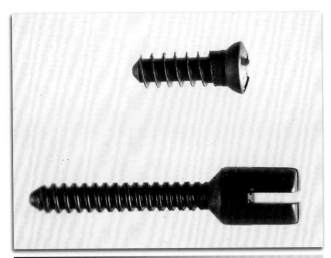

Fig. 4-10

Experimental titanium MSIs. Top MSI is 1.0 mm in diameter and 3 mm long. Bottom MSI is 1.0 mm in diameter and 6 mm long. (Reprinted with permission from Miyajima K, Saito S, Sana M, Sakai M. Three-dimensional finite element models and animal studies of the use of mini-screws for orthodontic anchorage. In: McNamara JA Jr, ed. *Implants, Microimplants, Onplants, and Transplants: New Answers to Old Questions in Orthodontics.* Ann Arbor: Center for Human Growth and Development, University of Michigan, 2005.)

MSIs. Collectively, more bone contacted the titanium surface for the loaded versus the unloaded MSIs. Fluorescence microscopy revealed active labeling of tetracycline and calcein along about 50% of the loaded MSIs (Fig. 4-14, *B*). The unloaded MSIs had little active labeling, with a slightly larger amount of labeling on the palatal compared with the facial

unloaded control MSI. Taken together, this indicates a higher bone remodeling rate around the loaded MSIs.

The maxillary SEM and fluorescence cross sections for the unloaded MSIs revealed very little bone-implant contact (Fig. 4-14, *C*). The loaded MSIs, however, had only slightly more bone-implant contact, but with a considerably higher remodeling rate as evidenced by fluorescence labeling. Interestingly, when bone-implant contact was compared by locations, the least amount of bone-implant contact was at the apex of the MSI. Also, a significant twofold increase was seen for bone-implant contact for palatal compared with facial MSIs.

For mandibular intrusion, the third premolars were intruded about 5 mm during the 16 weeks of force application (Fig 4-15, *A*). One MSI placed on the facial failed immediately after force application. It was removed and replaced 2 weeks later with a new MSI. The remaining MSIs showed no mobility.

The mandibular SEM and fluorescence cross sections for the unloaded MSIs revealed a 31% bone-implant contact (Fig. 4-15, *B* and *C*). The SEM and fluorescence sagittal sections for the loaded MSIs revealed a 34% bone-implant contact (Fig. 4-15, *D* and *E*). No significant difference was found between loaded and unloaded MSIs (Fig. 4-16). However, a significantly greater amount of bone-implant contact was found at the neck and body of the MSI compared with the apex. Also, a significant increase was seen for bone-implant contact for lingual compared with facial MSIs.

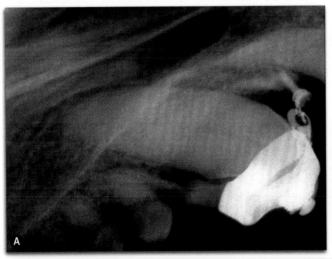
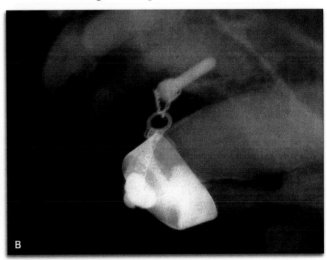

Fig. 4-11

MSI-mediated maxillary tooth movement of Experiment 1. **A,** Periapical radiograph of 3-mm long MSI after 3 months of tooth movement. **B,** Periapical radiograph of 6-mm long MSI after 3 months of tooth movement. Note that both MSI lengths were stable during 3 months of canine intrusion and tipping. (Reprinted with permission from Miyajima K, Saito S, Sana M, Sakai M. Three-dimensional finite element models and animal studies of the use of mini-screws for orthodontic anchorage. In: McNamara JA Jr, ed. *Implants, Microimplants, Onplants, and Transplants: New Answers to Old Questions in Orthodontics.* Ann Arbor: Center for Human Growth and Development, University of Michigan, 2005.)

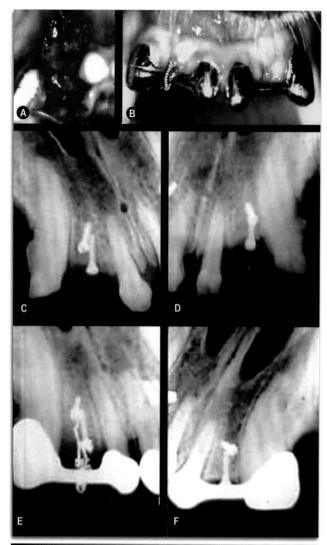

Fig. 4-12

Intrusion of maxillary incisors with MSIs. **A,** Surgical procedure with flap elevation and pilot holes between canine *(left)* and incisor *(right).* **B,** Posttreatment anterior photograph with loaded MSIs on left and unloaded MSIs on right. Note that after 6 weeks, loaded anterior bridge was intruded 2 mm. **C,** Pretreatment periapical radiograph of loaded MSIs. **D,** Pretreatment periapical radiograph of unloaded MSIs. **E,** Posttreatment periapical radiograph of loaded MSIs. **F,** Posttreatment periapical radiograph of unloaded MSIs. (Reprinted with permission from Miyajima K, Saito S, Sana M, Sakai M. Three-dimensional finite element models and animal studies of the use of mini-screws for orthodontic anchorage. In: McNamara JA Jr, ed. *Implants, Microimplants, Onplants, and Transplants: New Answers to Old Questions in Orthodontics.* Ann Arbor: Center for Human Growth and Development, University of Michigan, 2005.)

Discussion

For maxillary incisor intrusion, clinical measurements demonstrated 2 mm intrusion over 6 weeks with 120 g of force, which indicates that MSIs are capable of withstanding orthodontic forces for single-rooted teeth. Importantly, less bone-implant contact was

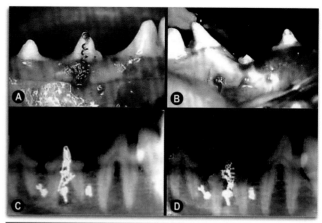

Fig. 4-13

Intrusion of mandibular third premolars by MSIs with 150-g NiTi CCS. **A,** Pretreatment left buccal photograph. **B,** Posttreatment left buccal photograph. **C,** Pretreatment periapical radiograph. **D,** Posttreatment periapical radiograph. Note 5 mm of intrusion after 16 weeks. (Reprinted with permission from Miyajima K, Saito S, Sana M, Sakai M. Three-dimensional finite element models and animal studies of the use of mini-screws for orthodontic anchorage. In: McNamara JA Jr, ed. *Implants, Microimplants, Onplants, and Transplants: New Answers to Old Questions in Orthodontics.* Ann Arbor: Center for Human Growth and Development, University of Michigan, 2005.)

seen for facial compared with palatal MSIs. There are two plausible explanations for this. First, the palatal mucosa is thicker and not mobile like the facial mucosa; therefore, healing may be better on the palatal surface. Second, more bone is present on the palatal surface than on the facial surface. Also important to note is that bone-implant contact was higher for loaded than unloaded implants, probably because MSI loading increases bone remodeling in the local bone, a point verified by the increase in tetracycline and calcein labeling of bone along the loaded MSIs compared with the unloaded MSIs.

For mandibular intrusion, clinical measurements demonstrated 5 mm of intrusion over 16 weeks with 150 g of force, which indicates that MSIs are capable of withstanding orthodontic forces for intrusion of multirooted teeth. Interestingly, bone-implant contact was similar for loaded and unloaded MSIs. This value was considerably higher at an average of 32% than that seen for maxillary MSIs (17%) and may correspond to the higher failure rate of maxillary (40%) versus mandibular (10%) MSIs. The reason may be that mandibular posterior bone is usually thicker and denser than maxillary anterior bone. As with maxillary intrusion, there was more bone-to-implant contact on the lingual compared with the facial surface.

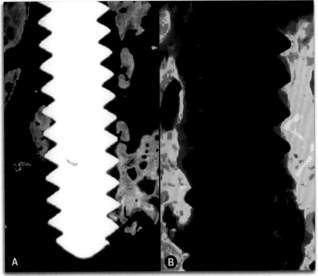

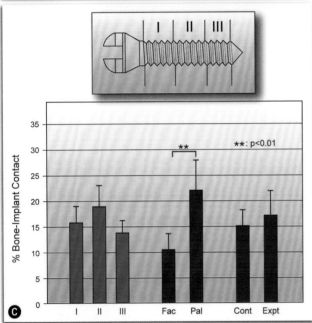

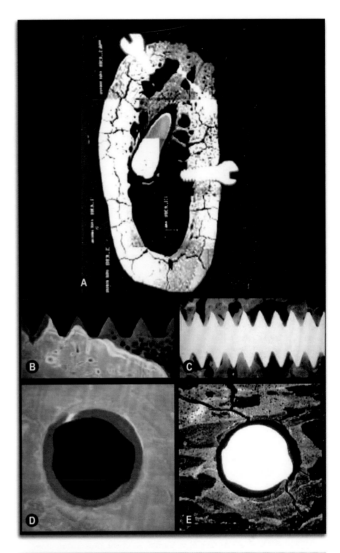

Fig. 4-14

Intrusion of maxillary incisors with MSIs. **A,** Backscattered electron photomicrograph of loaded MSI in sagittal section. **B,** Photomicrograph of loaded MSI in sagittal section (Villanueva stain). **C,** Graph demonstrating increased bone-implant contact on palatal surface relative to facial surface. *Fac* is facial, *Pal* is palatal, *Cont* is unloaded MSI, and *Expt* is loaded MSI. (Reprinted with permission from Miyajima K, Saito S, Sana M, Sakai M. Three-dimensional finite element models and animal studies of the use of mini-screws for orthodontic anchorage. In: McNamara JA Jr, ed. *Implants, Microimplants, Onplants, and Transplants: New Answers to Old Questions in Orthodontics.* Ann Arbor: Center for Human Growth and Development, University of Michigan, 2005.)

One key difference between maxillary and mandibular MSIs is that bone-implant contact was significantly higher at the top (neck and body) of the MSI compared with the apex for mandibular MSI.

Fig. 4-15

Intrusion of mandibular premolars with MSIs. **A,** Backscattered electron photomicrograph of mandible in cross section. **B,** Photomicrograph of loaded MSI in sagittal section (Villanueva stain). **C,** Backscattered electron photomicrograph of loaded MSI in sagittal section. **D,** Photomicrograph of unloaded MSI in cross section (Villanueva stain). **E,** Backscattered electron photomicrograph of unloaded MSI in cross section. (Reprinted with permission from Miyajima K, Saito S, Sana M, Sakai M. Three-dimensional finite element models and animal studies of the use of mini-screws for orthodontic anchorage. In: McNamara JA Jr, ed. *Implants, Microimplants, Onplants, and Transplants: New Answers to Old Questions in Orthodontics.* Ann Arbor: Center for Human Growth and Development, University of Michigan, 2005.)

This is likely because the top part of the MSI is in dense cortical bone, and the farther down the shaft of the MSI, the deeper into medullary bone with fewer trabeculae. The reason the same difference was not seen in the maxilla may be that maxillary cortical bone is usually thinner and less dense than mandibular bone; hence less difference exists in bone-implant between the top and bottom of the MSI.

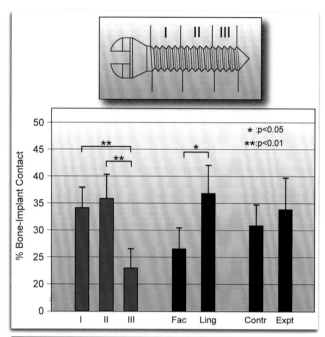

Fig. 4–16

Intrusion of mandibular premolars with MSIs. Graph demonstrates significantly more bone-implant contact in upper part of MSIs compared with tip and on lingual surface compared with facial surface. *Fac* is facial, *Ling* is lingual, *Cont* is unloaded MSI, and *Expt* is loaded MSI. (Reprinted with permission from Miyajima K, Saito S, Sana M, Sakai M. Three-dimensional finite element models and animal studies of the use of mini-screws for orthodontic anchorage. In: McNamara JA Jr, ed. *Implants, Microimplants, Onplants, and Transplants: New Answers to Old Questions in Orthodontics.* Ann Arbor: Center for Human Growth and Development, University of Michigan, 2005.)

Experiment 3
Materials and Methods

To compare commercially available temporary anchorage devices (TADs), two MSIs (Orthoanchor K-1 [Dentsply-Sankin, Japan], AbsoAnchor [Dentos, Korea], a Branemark dental implant (Nobel Biocare, Tokyo, Japan), and a custom MSI were compared. The commercial MSIs were 1.2 mm in diameter and 6 mm long. The Branemark implant was 3.75 in diameter and 7 mm long. The custom MSI was 1 mm in diameter and 4 mm long.

The mandibular third and fourth premolars were extracted, and the site allowed to heal for 8 weeks. After healing, each of the four TADs was placed into the healed extraction sites. The surgical procedure involved local infiltration and a mucoperiosteal flap. For the 1.2-mm diameter MSIs, a 0.9-mm pilot drill was used with saline irrigation to drill a pilot hole to the depth of the corresponding MSI. For the 3.75-mm diameter implant, a 3.5-mm pilot drill with saline irrigation was used to drill a pilot hole to the depth of

the implant. For the custom MSI, a 0.9-mm pilot drill with saline irrigation was used to drill a pilot hole to the depth of the implant.

After placement with their accompanying screwdrivers, each TAD was covered by the flap and sutured closed. TAD position was documented with periapical radiographs. The TADs were placed and remained unloaded for the entire experimental period. Intramuscular injections of tetracycline (15 mg/kg) were performed the day of TAD placement and every 4 weeks thereafter until the conclusion of the experiment.

After 12 weeks, the animals were euthanized and perfused with 4% paraformaldehyde and 2% glutaraldehyde in 0.05 M phosphate buffer (pH 7.4). The alveolar bone and associated MSIs were resected en bloc and were prepared for plastic-embedded histologic analysis as described in Experiment 2, except that the sagittal sections were sliced to 50-μm thicknesses. With the Villanueva bone stain, tetracycline-labeled bone stained in greenish yellow, osteoid stained red, and mineralized bone stained dark green. The calcified bone was defined as the tetracycline-stained bone combined with the mineralized bone.

Results

Although there was no significant difference in bone-implant contact between any of the four TADs evaluated, the Branemark implant demonstrated significantly more bone-implant contact than the rest of the MSIs (Fig. 4-17). When comparing the two commercially available MSIs, there was no difference in bone-implant contact (Fig. 4-18). A significant difference was found, however, between the neck and body of these MSIs and the apex, with the apex showing less bone-implant contact.

Discussion

The differences between conventional dental implants and MSIs being used for orthodontic anchorage are size, shape, and direction of force application. Dental implants range from 2.5 to 5.5 mm in diameter and 11.0 to 21.0 mm in length. MSIs, however, range from 1.0 to 2.0 mm in diameter and 3 to 15 mm in length. As suggested by the FEA data, a larger-diameter implant has a larger surface area in contact with bone, which appears to decrease the stress concentration in both the bone and the implant. The larger-diameter Branemark dental implant had significantly higher bone-implant contact than the remainder of the MSIs, which were 1.0 to 1.2 mm in diameter. These data clearly demonstrate that the amount of bone-implant

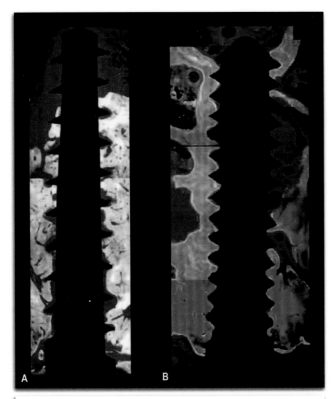

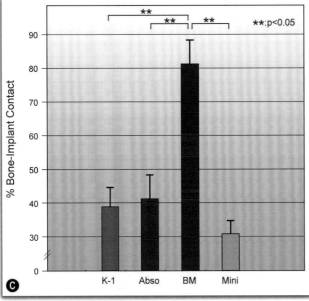

Fig. 4-17

Size-dependent differences for MSIs without force application.
A, Photomicrograph of K-1 MSI (Villanueva stain).
B, Photomicrograph of AbsoAnchor MSI (Villanueva stain).
C, Graph demonstrating that as the diameter of the MSI increased, so did bone-implant contact. (Reprinted with permission from Miyajima K, Saito S, Sana M, Sakai M. Three-dimensional finite element models and animal studies of the use of mini-screws for orthodontic anchorage. In: McNamara JA Jr, ed. *Implants, Microimplants, Onplants, and Transplants: New Answers to Old Questions in Orthodontics.* Ann Arbor: Center for Human Growth and Development, University of Michigan, 2005.)

contact depends on the size of the implant.

The two commercially available MSIs of 1.2 mm diameter were also compared. Importantly, there was no difference in bone-implant contact between the two MSIs. A significant difference was found, however, between the top (neck and body) of these MSIs and the apex, with the apex showing less bone-implant contact. Again, this is thought to be a function of the difference of the location of the top of the MSI in cortical bone and the apex in medullary bone.

Experiment 4
Materials and Methods

To evaluate age- and time-dependent differences in bone-implant contact for MSIs, three different dog ages were compared. For each age group, the MSIs were allowed to heal for 10 weeks without force application before euthanasia. The beagle dogs were divided into three groups based on age: *adolescent* was 5 to 6 months old, *adult* was 1½ years old, *aged* was 5 to 9 years old. In a second experiment, two adult dogs underwent the same protocol, but the MSIs were allowed to heal for 2, 10, or 20 weeks before euthanasia. The surgical procedure for all dogs was the same as in Experiment 3, except that in the adolescent dogs, the deciduous predecessor teeth to the third and fourth premolars were extracted at the same time as the permanent third and fourth premolars. After healing of the third and fourth premolar extraction sites, the Orthoanchor K-1 MSIs were placed and remained unloaded for the entire experimental period. Intramuscular injections of tetracycline (15 mg/kg) were performed the day of MSIs placement and every 4 weeks thereafter until the conclusion of the experiment.

After euthanasia, perfusion was performed with 4% paraformaldehyde and 2% glutaraldehyde in 0.05 M phosphate buffer (pH 7.4). The alveolar bone and associated MSIs were resected en bloc and were prepared for plastic-embedded histologic analysis as described in Experiment 3.

Results

The bone-implant contact in adult dogs was significantly greater than that in aged dogs. Bone-implant contact also was greater than that of adolescent dogs, although not to a significant degree (Fig. 4-19). For MSIs placed in adult dogs and evaluated at different healing time points following MSI placement, bone-implant contact increased from 26% after only 2 weeks of healing to about 40% for both 10 and 20 weeks of healing (Fig 4-20).

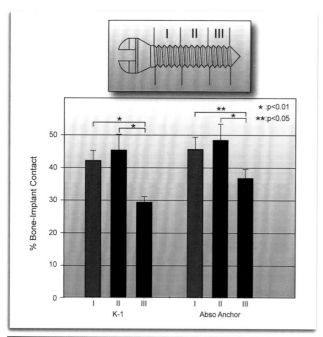

Fig. 4–18

Company-dependent difference between the K-1 and AbsoAnchor MSI implants for MSIs without force application. Although there were no differences between the MSIs, there was significantly less bone-implant contact in region III. (Reprinted with permission from Miyajima K, Saito S, Sana M, Sakai M. Three-dimensional finite element models and animal studies of the use of mini-screws for orthodontic anchorage. In: McNamara JA Jr, ed. *Implants, Microimplants, Onplants, and Transplants: New Answers to Old Questions in Orthodontics.* Ann Arbor: Center for Human Growth and Development, University of Michigan, 2005.)

Discussion

Age-dependent differences were seen in bone-implant contact for unloaded MSIs. Bone-implant contact was highest in adult dogs, followed by adolescent dogs and then aged dogs. The significant difference was observed between the adult and the aged groups. This information should be interpreted carefully, however, because the 31% bone-implant contact in the aged dogs still appears to be at a level that will allow orthodontic force application without the risk of failure.

Time-dependent differences were seen in bone-implant contact for unloaded MSIs in adult dogs. In general, bone-implant contact increased from 2 to 20 weeks, with a significant difference between the 2-week group and both the 10- and 20-week groups. Again, this information should be interpreted carefully. The 26% bone-implant contact after 2 weeks of healing still appears to be at a level that will allow orthodontic force application without the risk of failure. Moreover, immediate loading, instead of allowing MSIs to heal for any period, may increase bone remodeling and bone-implant contact much faster than delayed loading.

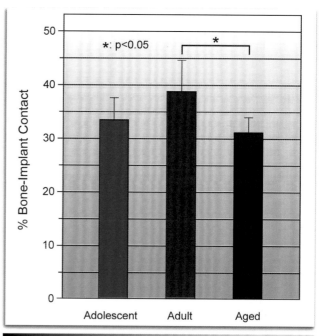

Fig. 4–19

Age-dependent differences of bone-implant contact for MSIs without force application. Note that bone-implant contact was significantly less in the aged dogs. (Reprinted with permission from Miyajima K, Saito S, Sana M, Sakai M. Three-dimensional finite element models and animal studies of the use of mini-screws for orthodontic anchorage. In: McNamara JA Jr, ed. *Implants, Microimplants, Onplants, and Transplants: New Answers to Old Questions in Orthodontics.* Ann Arbor: Center for Human Growth and Development, University of Michigan, 2005.)

SUMMARY

The purpose of this chapter was to report the findings of FEA and animal experiments conducted to evaluate MSI use. When taken together, the results suggest that the smaller the MSI diameter, the larger the stress generated in the bone and in the MSI. This may have deleterious effects on bone-implant contact and bone healing, but more detailed experiments need to be performed to understand the implications. Regardless of the diameter, the majority of the stress generated under orthodontic force applications—that is, perpendicular to the long axis of the MSI—is generated in the bone around the first one to two threads, which corresponds to cortical bone. This suggests that MSI diameter is important but that length is much less important. Point of force application is also important, because the farther the force application from the bone, the higher the stress generated. This also requires further study to understand the implications.

Although there was considerable variability, MSIs 1.0 to 1.2 mm in diameter were used for these experiments with good success. In general, bone-implant contact was higher in the mandible than the maxilla, on the

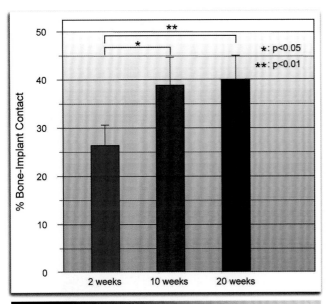

Fig. 4-20

Time-dependent differences of bone-implant contact for MSIs without force application. Note that bone-implant contact was significantly less for MSIs in place only 2 weeks compared with those placed at 10 and 20 weeks. (Reprinted with permission from Miyajima K, Saito S, Sana M, Sakai M. Three-dimensional finite element models and animal studies of the use of mini-screws for orthodontic anchorage. In: McNamara JA Jr, ed. *Implants, Microimplants, Onplants, and Transplants: New Answers to Old Questions in Orthodontics.* Ann Arbor: Center for Human Growth and Development, University of Michigan, 2005.)

palatal/lingual surface compared with the facial, and at the top compared with the apex of the MSI. This is best explained anatomically. Cortical bone in the maxilla is thinner than in the mandible, thinner on the facial than on the palatal/lingual, and thicker at the cortex than deeper in medullary bone. Loaded MSIs also had more bone-implant contact than unloaded MSIs, suggesting that static orthodontic forces stimulate bone remodeling and formation, and hence increase MSI stability, given a light force.

Finally, age appears to play a factor in that young, nongrowing adult dogs appear to have more bone-implant contact than young, growing dogs or aged, nongrowing dogs. However, the MSIs were not loaded in these dogs, making it difficult to predict success or failure rates. These age-dependent studies should be repeated using MSIs with force application to better elicit predictive age-dependent values.

REFERENCES

1. Van Roekel NB. The use of Branemark system implants for orthodontic anchorage: report of a case. *Int J Oral Maxillofac Implants.* 4:341-344, 1989.
2. Roberts WE, Helm FR, Marshall KJ, Gongloff RK. Rigid endosseous implants for orthodontic and orthopedic anchorage. *Angle Orthod.* 59:247-256, 1989.
3. Higuchi KW, Slack JM. The use of titanium fixtures for intraoral anchorage to facilitate orthodontic tooth movement. *Int J Oral Maxillofac Implants.* 6:338-344, 1991.
4. Valeron JF, Velazquez JF. Implants in the orthodontic and prosthetic rehabilitation of an adult patient: a case report. *Int J Oral Maxillofac Implants.* 11:534-538, 1996.
5. Umemori M, Sugawara J, Mitani H, et al. Skeletal anchorage system for open-bite correction. *Am J Orthod Dentofacial Orthop.* 115:166-174, 1999.
6. Kyung H, Park H, Bae S, et al. Development of orthodontic micro-implants for intraoral anchorage. *J Clin Orthod.* 37:321-328, 2003.
7. Miyawaki S, Koyama I, Inoue M, et al. Factors associated with the stability of titanium screws placed in the posterior region for orthodontic anchorage. *Am J Orthod Dentofacial Orthop.* 124:373-378, 2003.
8. Paik C, Woo Y, Boyd R. Treatment of an adult patient with vertical maxillary excess using miniscrew fixation. *J Clin Orthod.* 37:423-428, 2003.
9. Park Y, Lee S, Kim D, Lee S. Intrusion of posterior teeth using mini-screw implants. *Am J Orthod Dentofacial Orthop.* 123:690-694, 2003.
10. Park Y, Kwong O, Sung J. Uprighting second molars with micro-implant anchorage. *J Clin Orthod.* 38:100-103, 2004.
11. Saito S, Sugimoto N, Morohashi T, et al. Basic animal study of endosseous titanium implants as anchors for orthodontic tooth movement. In: Davidovitch Z, Mah J, eds. *Biological Mechanisms of Tooth Eruption, Resorption and Replacement by Implants.* Boston, Mass: Harvard Society for the Advancement of Orthodontics, 1998.
12. Saito S, Kurabayashi H, Imai S, et al. Effects of centrifugal forces on proliferation and alkaline phosphatase activity of human oral-tissue-derived cells cultured on titanium plates [in Japanese]. *Orthodontic Waves* 57:318-326, 1988.
13. Saito S, Sugimoto N, Morohashi T, et al. Endosseous titanium implants can function as anchors for mesio-distal tooth movement in the beagle dog. *Am J Orthod Dentfacial Orthop.* 118:601-607, 2000.
14. Miyajima K, Sana M. FEM analysis of mini-implants as orthodontic anchorage. In: Davidovitch Z, Mah J, eds. *Biological Mechanisms of Tooth Eruption, Resorption and Replacement by Implants.* Boston, Mass: Harvard Society for the Advancement of Orthodontics, 1998.
15. Morse A. Formic acid-sodium citrate decalcification and butyl alcohol dehydration of teeth and bone for sectioning paraffin. *J Dent Res.* 24:143-153, 1945.
16. Ohmae M, Saito S, Morohashi T, et al. A clinical and histological evaluation of titanium mini-implants as anchors for orthodontic intrusion in the beagle dog. *Am J Orthod Dentofacial Orthop.* 119:489-497, 2001.
17. Miyajima K, Saito S, Sana M, Masaru Sakai. Three-dimensional finite element models and animal studies of the use of mini-screw for orthodontic anchorage. In: McNamara JA Jr, ed. *Implants, Microimplants, Onplants and Transplants: New Answers to Old Questions in Orthodontics.* Vol 42. Ann Arbor: Center for Human Growth and Development, University of Michigan, 2005.

SECTION 3

CLINICAL BASIS

Treatment Planning for Temporary Anchorage Device Applications

Jason B. Cope, John W. Graham

As with any surgical procedure, the placement and use of orthodontic temporary anchorage devices (OrthoTADs) has the potential for the occasional complication. The best way to minimize complications is to avoid them altogether. This can be accomplished by performing a thorough clinical evaluation with diagnostic records to establish a diagnosis, which allows the subsequent formation of an ideal treatment plan. This information should be combined with an understanding of the patient's health history and disposition toward compliance before TADs are considered.

The placement of TADs for orthodontic anchorage is relatively new. Therefore, patients are generally unknowledgeable about the procedure and treatment. Considering this, patient education regarding the procedure must be clear and understandable. Visual representations, such as typodonts (Fig. 5-1) and photographs speak volumes compared with verbal explanations. Expectations of the orthodontist and patient should be addressed, and the orthodontist should obtain informed consent before the procedure (Fig. 5-2), while also maintaining constant communication throughout the treatment protocol. If, for example, a miniscrew implant (MSI) becomes mobile during treatment, the patient should have been prepared prior to placement for the protocol that will be followed to remedy the situation.

The orthodontist who chooses to place the TADs must be confident that the procedure is well within his or her skill set. If other specialists are going to be placing the

TADs, it is important that the orthodontist communicate the specific needs of the case to the specialist in order to minimize potential problems.

PATIENT EVALUATION
Health History

Because of the invasive nature of TAD placement, an evaluation above and beyond the traditional orthodontic health history review is necessary. Many complications can be avoided by attention to details in the patient's health history. The orthodontist must evaluate the patient's host defense system to determine whether special actions need to be taken to prevent complications. The orthodontist should explore immune status, history of head and neck radiation therapy, smoking history, and other factors that may compromise the patient's natural defenses.

Although placement of most TADs is a relatively bloodless procedure, the clinician must also be aware of any blood dyscrasias that may present difficulties at the time of placement and immediately postoperatively. Placement of TADs necessitates antibiotic premedication only for a patient who is at risk for bacterial endocarditis according to American Heart Association guidelines.[1]

Patient Compliance

All aspects of orthodontic treatment require some level of patient compliance; TADs are no exception. Temporary anchorage devices may be placed at virtually any age as long as adequate bone is present and the patient is compliant with instructions. Much like wearing a headgear or elastics, these devices require that the patient follow specific instructions to optimize results and minimize complications. The orthodontist should carefully evaluate the patient's ability to understand and follow instructions before making the decision to use TADs. Factors such as age, missed appointments, oral hygiene, breakages, and parental support should be a part of the screening process for determining a patient's likely success with TAD mechanics.

Indications

Some of the more common indications for TAD use are traditional malocclusions in need of additional or maximum anchorage that cannot be achieved by the teeth themselves, space closure of considerable distances—in the retraction of anterior teeth (Fig. 5-3) or protraction of posterior teeth (Fig. 5-4), preprosthetic tooth movement (Fig. 5-5), molar uprighting (Fig. 5-6), intrusion of supererupted teeth (Fig. 5-7), distalization of an end-on Class II or Class III malocclusion (Fig. 5-8), skeletal malocclusions in patients unable or unwilling to undergo surgical treatment (Fig. 5-9), occlusal cants, and maxillomandibular fixation during oral and maxillofacial surgery.

A point that deserves attention, however, is that with any new technique or device, there is always a tendency for overimplementation because of initial zeal and

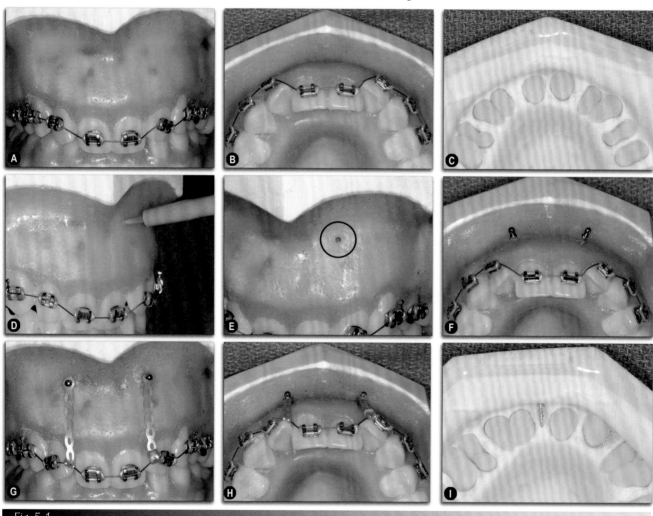

Fig. 5-1

OrthoTAD typodont model used for treatment planning, placement, and attachment of TADs, as well as patient education. The model is a clear dual-density bone with anatomic teeth and synthetic gingiva that can be incised, flapped, and sutured. **A,** Anterior photograph of prospective MSI location. **B,** Occlusal photograph of prospective MSI location. **C,** Photograph looking through the base and clear medullary bone to view tooth roots. **D,** Biopsy punch used to place punch incision in alveolar mucosa. **E,** Cleanly incised punch incision (*black circle*). **F,** Occlusal photograph of MSIs placed in sub-ANS region. **G,** Anterior photograph of MSI attachment to arch wire. **H,** Occlusal photograph of MSI attachment to arch wire. **I,** Photograph looking through the base and clear medullary bone to view MSI position relative to tooth roots. (Courtesy Dr. Jason B. Cope, Dallas, Tex. Patent pending.)

JASON B. COPE, DDS, PhD, PA
ORTHODONTICS AND DENTOFACIAL ORTHOPEDICS

OrthoTAD CONSENT AGREEMENT

Orthodontic treatment is an elective procedure. This, like any other treatment of the body, has some inherent risks and limitations. These seldom prevent treatment, but should be considered when making the decision to undergo treatment.

In orthodontic tooth movement, resistance to undesirable tooth movement is termed anchorage. Anchorage can be increased by incorporating more teeth into one segment (termed the anchorage segment), which decreases both the amount and speed with which these teeth move. Anchorage can also be increased by adding extraoral forces such as headgears, or intraoral forces such as elastics. Unfortunately, despite our efforts to build up anchorage and thereby preventing certain teeth from undesirable movement, anchorage loss is unavoidable.

An alternative solution is to utilize an orthodontic temporary anchorage device (OrthoTAD) temporarily, but rigidly placed in the upper or lower jaw bone for use as an anchor in the mouth that can be used immediately after placement. This utilizes a minimally invasive surgical approach for implant placement which diminishes the trauma and post-operative discomfort associated with traditional dental implants. These OrthoTADs allow selective tooth movement without taxing the orthodontic anchorage.

I, _____ Patient _____ / _____ Parent _____, have been informed and understand that OrthoTADs are available to certain orthodontic patients. These mini implants are small diameter (1.1 - 3.3 mm) titanium alloy screw-type dental implants or thin (0.5 - 1.0 mm) titanium plates that are placed in a patient's jaw to provide temporary anchorage of teeth. I am aware that these implants are being placed for the immediate but temporary anchorage of my teeth, and the long-term function cannot be predicted. I wish to undergo this procedure as a patient of Jason B. Cope, DDS, PhD, PA. I have requested that Jason B. Cope, DDS, PhD, PA place one or more OrthoTADs into my jaw.

I have also been fully informed by Jason B. Cope, DDS, PhD, PA that the purpose of this OrthoTAD procedure is to provide anchorage support for my upper and/or lower teeth and/or upper and/or lower jaw, and I hereby consent to the surgical insertion of OrthoTADs in my jaw by Jason B. Cope, DDS, PhD, PA. I understand that in the event the OrthoTADs implanted by Jason B. Cope, DDS, PhD, PA fail, they will be removed through a subsequent surgical procedure. I further understand that it is possible that one or more of the implants may fracture during insertion, or during the implant's life cycle, and in event a fracture were to occur, I give Jason B. Cope, DDS, PhD, PA permission and consent to leave the fractured implant in my jaw or remove it, under professional conditions and using professional judgment. It has also been explained to me that once the OrthoTADs are inserted or implanted, a recommended orthodontic treatment plan, including a program of personal oral hygiene, must be strictly followed by me and completed on schedule. I have been informed that if this schedule and plan are not carried out, the implants may fail.

I am further aware that the surgical procedure includes the insertion of the OrthoTADs in my jaw, and possibly the construction of an orthodontic appliance attached thereon. I am aware that I must return for appropriate post-operative care and evaluation on a timely basis, which will include evaluation of oral hygiene and plaque removal. I also understand that anchorage control is the primary goal of this orthodontic procedure, but that success rates vary for each patient. With that in mind, no guarantees of success have been given me by Jason B. Cope, DDS, PhD, PA or any member of his staff. He has also informed me that use of tobacco, including cigarette smoking, as well as excessive alcohol consumption, or altered sugar metabolism can affect bone/gum healing and may cause failure of the OrthoTADs.

I have further been advised that swelling, infection, bleeding, and/or pain may be associated with any surgical procedure, including the one recommended to me by Jason B. Cope, DDS, PhD, PA, and that said conditions may occur during the life of the implants. I have also been advised that temporary or permanent numbness may occur in my tongue, lips, chin, gums, or jaw as a result of this procedure, as well as the possibility of sinus involvement in the upper jaw. Jason B. Cope, DDS, PhD, PA has discussed the possibility of alternative procedures for my individual needs and has offered to answer any of my questions concerning those procedures.

I agree to follow the home care instructions of Jason B. Cope, DDS, PhD, PA, and I agree to report to Jason B. Cope, DDS, PhD, PA for regular examinations as instructed.

A

Fig. 5-2

Standard OrthoTAD consent form. **A,** Front page. **B,** Back page.

You need one or more OrthoTADs placed in your mouth. The reasons, alternatives (if any), and dangers of the planned treatment have been explained to you. We urge you to ask questions or discuss any concerns you may still have. Although problems and complications are uncommon and unpredictable, they can happen during or after surgery in any patient. Jason B. Cope, DDS, PhD, PA will do everything possible to minimize the risks, but the following are a FEW of the more common problems that can occur in any surgical case, despite the best of efforts.

INFECTION - In rare instances, an infection can put you in the hospital and even put you at risk for your life. You can become infected even when you're taking an antibiotic.

BLEEDING - Slow oozing of blood is NORMAL for 12-24 hours after surgery. Some situations, such as taking aspirin, can result in longer periods of oozing. If your bleeding is heavy or goes on for a long time, you should call us, because you may need more treatment to stop the bleeding.

NERVE DAMAGE - Some teeth are located next to nerves that give feeling to your lips, gums, and other teeth. Despite performing the most careful surgery possible, one or more nerves can get bruised or damaged during surgery, giving an area numbness that does not go away for a long time (nerves heal very slowly). In rare circumstances, it may become permanent. Jason B. Cope, DDS, PhD, PA will do everything to minimize this risk, but the risk is still there.

SINUS OPENING - Upper back teeth are next to the floor of the sinus cavities on each side, which connect with the nose. Implant placement in these locations can result in a small opening between the sinus and the mouth. If this opening doesn't heal, another operation will be needed to close the opening.

TOOTH/ROOT DAMAGE - Sometimes teeth are jammed so tightly against adjacent teeth that implant placement in these locations can cause damage to the crowns or roots of these teeth. Although this is rare, it could require the replacement of a crown, a root canal, or extraction of the tooth with replacement by a bridge or an implant/crown.

ANESTHESIA REACTIONS - You can unexpectedly react to ANY drug, ranging from getting a rash to having a life-threatening crisis. If you know of any past allergies, are taking any drugs you haven't told us about, or have any major illness you failed to write down, it's IMPORTANT you tell us now, or you may be risking your own health.

OTHER PROBLEMS - There are many other minor problems not mentioned above that can occur during or after oral surgery. No one can guarantee a perfect result, but you'll receive our best effort. We feel the expected benefits of surgery outweigh the possible risks.

To my knowledge, I have given an accurate report of my physical and mental health history. I have also reported any prior allergic or unusual reactions to drugs, food, insect bites, anesthetics, pollens, dust, blood or blood diseases, gum or skin reactions, abnormal bleeding, or any other conditions related to my health.

I have read this surgical consent form and understand the contents. I have no additional questions. Having been fully informed of the above, I hereby freely and knowingly give my informed consent to the recommended surgical procedures outlined to me by Jason B. Cope, DDS, PhD, PA and request him to place one or more OrthoTADs in my jaw for the purpose of orthodontic/orthopedic anchorage control.

_____   _____   _____
Patient's Name   Patient's Signature   Date

_____   _____   _____
Parent's Name   Parent's Signature   Date

I, Jason B. Cope, DDS, PhD, PA, certify that I have explained to the above patient the ramifications of the use of OrthoTADs to the best of my professional ability. I further certify that in my opinion, the above patient is fully informed of the risks and possible benefits of the particular surgical procedure agreed to.

_____   _____
Jason B. Cope, DDS, PhD, PA   Date

excitement. Temporary anchorage devices are not a treatment plan in and of themselves. They are simply one of many tools that orthodontists can use as a part of the final treatment plan.

Contraindications

Contraindications can be categorized as absolute and relative. Patients with absolute contraindications should not be treated with TADs at all. This includes patients with hypersensitivities, titanium allergies, localized active infection, unsuitability for surgical procedures, radiation therapy, metabolic bone disorders, bone pathologies, poor bone healing, decreased bone quality or quantity, uncontrolled periodontitis, oral mucosal pathologies, cardiovascular disease, blood dyscrasias, current/previous bisphosphonate therapy, or psychosomatic disease.

Patients with relative contraindications should be treated with TADs only if the condition can be resolved or eliminated before TAD placement and if there is a reasonable assurance that the condition will not recur during TAD treatment. Relative contraindications include poor oral hygiene, inadequate patient compliance, insufficient interradicular space, parafunctional habits, and the use of drugs, tobacco, or alcohol.

DIAGNOSTIC RECORDS

The diagnostic records required for treatment planning for OrthoTADs are identical to what an orthodontist usually acquires to make an orthodontic diagnosis. In some cases, it may be beneficial to acquire additional diagnostic aids such as a cone beam computed tomography (CT) scan. For most patients, however, the standard diagnostic materials are satisfactory. Once collected, the diagnostic materials are used to establish a definitive diagnosis so that several treatment plans, ranked from most to least ideal, can be created for presentation to and discussion with the patient before a final treatment plan is established.

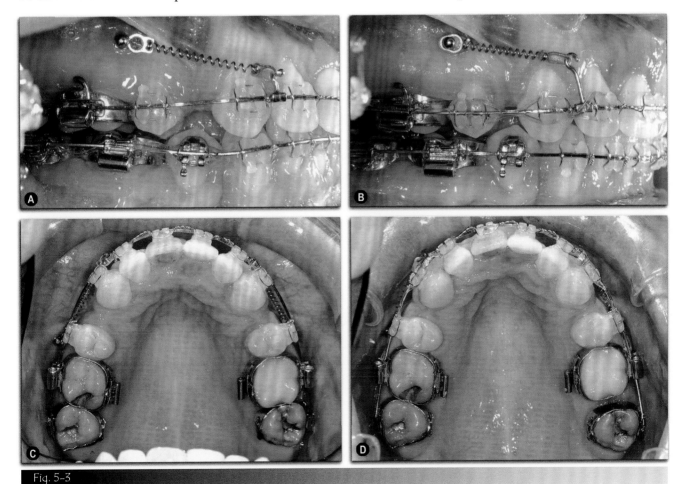

Fig. 5-3

Retraction of anterior teeth. **A,** Buccal photograph at initial TAD loading. **B,** Progress buccal photograph during retraction with new locking closed coil spring (Courtesy Dr. Jason B. Cope, Dallas, Tex. Patent pending). **C,** Occlusal photograph at initial TAD loading. **D,** Progress occlusal photograph during retraction.

After the health history, the clinical examination is usually performed. In particular, the examination should include inspection and palpation of the keratinized gingiva, alveolar mucosa, and frena attachments in the region of the planned TAD placement, as well as in the tentative line of attachment mechanics. The orthodontist should move the patient through functional movements and manually move the lips and cheeks to determine the extent of frena attachment and displacement.

Photographs should include extraoral and intraoral views. Extraoral photographs allow the orthodontist to evaluate the patients' profile and lip strain (Fig. 5-10) in combination with the lateral cephalometric radiograph to determine the need for extraction and anchorage requirements. Intraoral photographs

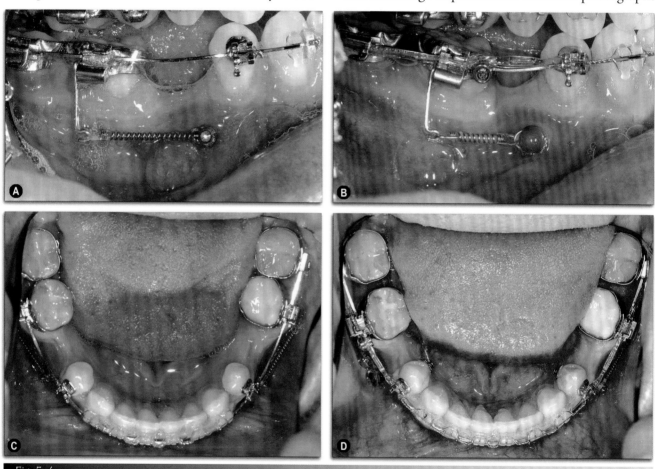

Fig. 5-4

Protraction of posterior teeth. **A,** Buccal photograph at initial TAD loading. **B,** Progress buccal photograph during protraction. **C,** Occlusal photograph at initial TAD loading. **D,** Progress occlusal photograph during protraction.

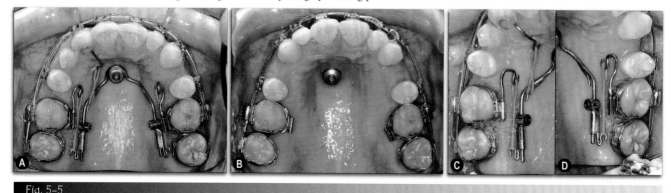

Fig. 5-5

Preprosthetic tooth movement in preparation for first premolar implants and restorations. **A,** Occlusal photograph at initial TAD loading. **B,** Occlusal photograph after dental implant site development. **C,** Right palatal mechanics. **D,** Left palatal mechanics.

provide a guide to keratinized tissue dimensions, mucogingival junction heights, and frena attachment locations (Fig. 5-11). Although photographs give a good representation of tissue dimension and location, orthodontic models are better at providing for direct measurement of soft tissues. In combination with the panoramic and periapical radiographs, the clinician can also use the models to determine the crestal bone height relative to the gingival margins or occlusal surfaces (Fig. 5-12).

The lateral cephalometric radiograph is used to establish the skeletal relationship and tooth position relative to the alveolar housing. When combined with the extraoral photographs, the lateral cephalometric radiograph can be used to evaluate the patients' profile and lip strain to determine the need for extraction and anchorage requirements (Fig. 5-13). This radiograph also allows the determination of palatal bone thickness

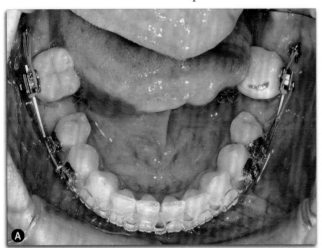

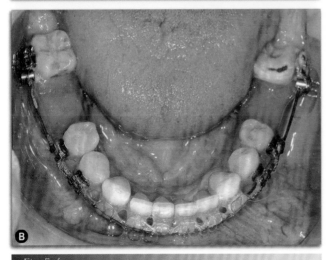

Fig. 5-6

Molar uprighting. **A,** Occlusal photograph at initial TAD loading. **B,** Occlusal photograph after molar uprighting and dental implant placement.

and root proximity relative to the symphysis. The panoramic radiograph is a good screening radiograph to determine approximate bone height, relative density, and relationships between TAD size and adjacent anatomic structures (Fig. 5-14). The panoramic radiograph can be often used without a periapical radiograph when interradicular spaces are fairly large. When root proximities appear too close on the panoramic radiograph, a periapical radiograph should be acquired because it is more specific in evaluating mesiodistal interradicular or intraradicular space and the coronoapical availability of bone stock.

In certain cases, such as for a case with an extensively pneumatized sinus, a cone beam CT may be useful. The cone beam CT is a three-dimensional radiography technique that allows the most accurate evaluation of bone morphology and density as well as the visualization of local anatomic structures (Fig. 5-15).[2,3] Moreover, cone beam CT is considerably less costly than a traditional CT scan.

TREATMENT PLANNING

Once the decision has been made that one or more TADs will be useful in accomplishing the treatment goals, several important things need to be accomplished during treatment planning to ensure that the TAD will be placed so that it can be used effectively and efficiently to accomplish the desired orthodontic or orthopedic movement without causing potential problems. First, the orthodontist must understand the anatomy of the specific TAD to be used because this will affect where and how it can be placed. Then, the orthodontist must understand what local anatomic locations can be used for TAD placement. Also of concern is the orientation of the TAD relative to the surface anatomy, as well as the emergence profile through bone and soft tissue. Considering this, the orthodontist must know what local anatomic structures must be avoided during TAD placement. Finally, the line of planned orthodontic mechanics and attachments should be considered so as to avoid soft tissue impingement.

Temporary Anchorage Device Anatomy
Miniscrew Implants
All MSIs have the same basic anatomy consisting of three parts (Fig. 5-16). Inferiorly, all MSIs have a *threaded body* to facilitate stabilization of the implant once placed. The threads themselves are oriented at an angle relative to the long axis of the implant and to the

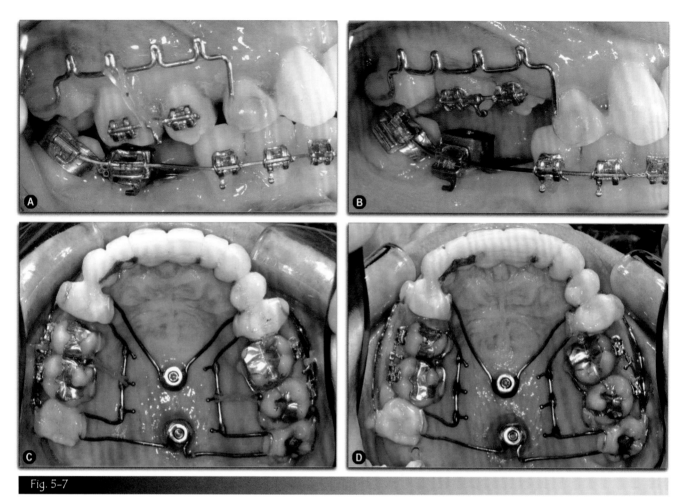

Fig. 5-7

Intrusion of supererupted teeth. **A,** Buccal photograph at initial TAD loading. **B,** Buccal photograph after overintrusion. **C,** Occlusal photograph at initial TAD loading. **D,** Occlusal photograph after overintrusion.

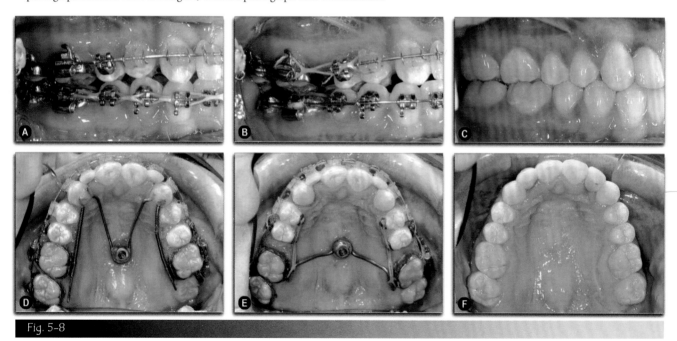

Fig. 5-8

Distalization of an end-on Class II malocclusion. **A,** Buccal photograph at initial distalization. **B,** Buccal photograph at after distalization and start of retraction. **C,** Buccal photograph after retraction. **D,** Occlusal photograph at initial distalization. **E,** Occlusal photograph after distalization and start of retraction. **F,** Occlusal photograph after retraction.

surface of the bone such that rotation against the bone surface mechanically draws the screw into the bone. The threaded body is located entirely within bone. A polished *transmucosal collar* or *neck* connects the head to the body. The collar is smooth for adaptation of soft tissue and is located transmucosally. Superiorly, all MSIs have an *abutment head* that may take on various configurations but is designed for two reasons: first, as the point of force application for screwing the implant into bone, and second, as the point of orthodontic or orthopedic force attachment. Many implant heads have holes, slots, or grooves for orthodontic force module attachment. The abutment head is located entirely within the oral cavity.

Miniplate Implants

Miniplate implants (MPIs) also consist of the three parts (Fig. 5-17). The *body* is positioned subperiosteally and

has multiple holes for bone fixation via miniscrews. The *neck* or *arm* connects the head to the body, is located transmucosally, and is usually available in several different lengths to facilitate individual anatomic variation and location of force application. The *head* is exposed within the oral cavity and is modified for attachment of orthodontic mechanics. Most plates are available in three basic shapes: T-shaped, Y-shaped, and I-shaped. A T-shaped plate can be converted to an L-shaped plate by cutting off one side of the T. It is important to understand that MPIs are nothing more than a framework that uses the holding power of one or more miniscrews in series to add more initial stability than one MSI individually, with its head serving as the bracket.

Palatal Implants

Palatal implants (PIs) are similar in design to MSIs

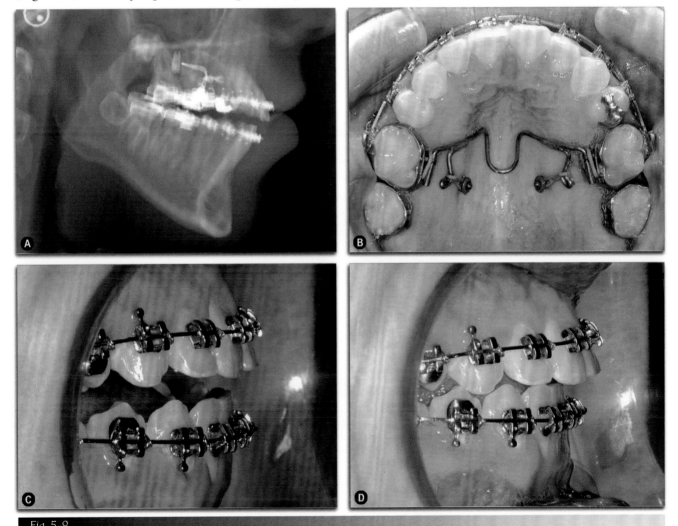

Fig. 5-9

Musculoskeletal malocclusions treated by dental intrusion. **A,** Lateral cephalometric radiograph showing high mandibular plane angle and anterior open bite. **B,** Occlusal photograph showing intrusion mechanics with new transpalatal intrusion arch (Courtesy Dr. Jason B. Cope, Dallas, Tex. Patent pending). **C,** Lateral photograph showing open bite. **D,** Lateral photograph after 4 months showing bite closing.

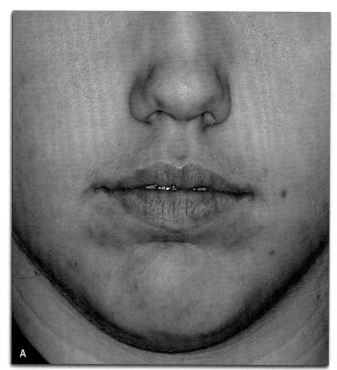
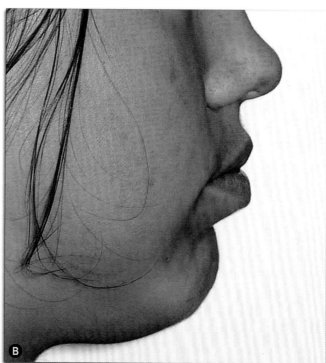

Fig. 5-10

Facial photographs to assess lip strain. **A,** Anterior. **B,** Profile. Note protrusive lips and mentalis strain.

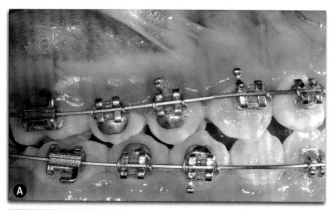
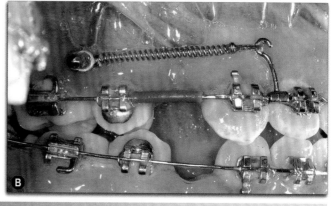

Fig. 5-11

Buccal photograph to assess soft tissue dimensions. **A,** Buccal photograph before MSI placement. **B,** Buccal photograph after MSI placement. Note MSI placed so that attachments pass below frenum.

(Fig. 5-18). Inferiorly, all PIs have a *threaded body* to facilitate stabilization of the implant once placed. The threaded body is located entirely within bone and has a self-tapping or cutting flute cut in its apex, which is usually flat and not tapered, thereby necessitating a pilot hole with a complete osteotomy preparation as with a traditional dental implant. Like the MSIs, a polished *transmucosal collar* or *neck* connects the head to the body. Superiorly, all PIs have an *abutment head* that may take on various configurations. The primary difference is that PIs, like dental and retromolar implants, have some type of cap that is screwed onto the abutment head for attachment of orthodontic mechanics, usually by soldering, after an initial period of healing for osseointegration.

Placement Locations

Although it may not be readily apparent, TADs (particularly MSIs) can be placed just about anywhere in the oral cavity where there is adequate bone for fixation. Temporary anchorage devices can be placed in the maxilla or mandible. However, several factors must be considered: (1) the orientation of the TAD relative to the bony surface, (2) the emergence of the TAD through the soft tissues, (3) the appropriate TAD length, and (4) how the TAD will be attached to the orthodontic appliances. In addition, it is important to place TADs where they will not impinge on the underlying soft tissues.

Angulation

Miniscrew implants can be placed in one of two orientations relative to the bone surface: perpendicular or oblique (Fig. 5-19). For perpendicular placement, the MSI is oriented at a 90-degree angle relative to the bone surface. For oblique placement, the MSI is oriented at an angle of greater or lesser than 90 degrees relative to the bone surface.

The perpendicular orientation is the preferred method when possible. This angle gives the operator the most control when placing a drill-free MSI because there is less opportunity for the screw apex to slide on the bone surface during initial perforation of the outer bone layer. The main reasons not to place the MSI at a perpendicular angle to the bone surface include proximity to adjacent structures such as roots, soft tissue emergence, or surgical access. In cases for which an inadequate amount of interradicular bone is present, the orthodontist can create more bone by moving the teeth or place the MSI at an oblique angle relative to the long axis of the teeth. Oblique placement in this situation places the apex of the MSI in a more apical location, which is where more interradicular space is available. Further, if the desired placement location would cause the MSI to emerge through mobile mucosa, then the MSI can be placed obliquely so that the abutment head emerges closer to the mucogingival junction. Finally, if surgical access will not allow ideal perpendicular placement, then the orthodontist can accept an oblique orientation, if the mechanics will not be negatively affected, or find another location.

It should be recalled that the dental literature has shown that placement of dental implants in nonkeratinized tissue does not necessarily predispose an implant to failure.[4,5] The absence of keratinized tissue around dental implants may increase the susceptibility of the periimplant region to plaque-induced tissue destruction,[6] but this does not mean that MSI placement in alveolar mucosa is an absolute contraindication. It simply means that closer attention must be paid to hygiene procedures. Further, the mucosa apical to the mucogingival junction is not as mobile as the mucosa in the depth of the vestibule. Placement of an MSI 2 to 3 mm apical to the mucogingival junction is not nearly as problematic as

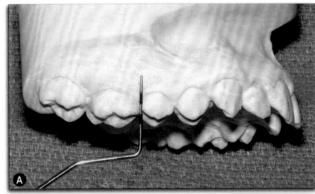

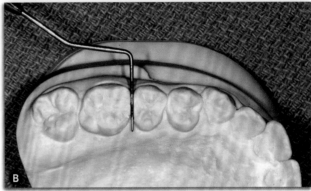

Fig. 5-12

Models to determine bone height and width. **A,** Measure crestal bone height relative to gingival margins or occlusal surfaces. **B,** Measure alveolar bone width at approximate level of MSI placement.

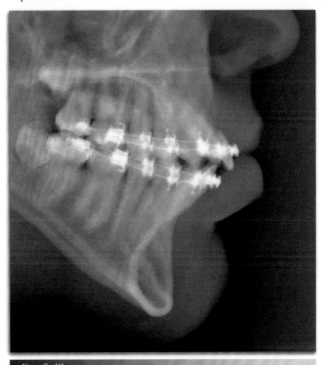

Fig. 5-13

Lateral cephalometric radiograph to assess lip strain, incisor angulation, and alveolar base relationships. Note protrusive incisors, lips, and mentalis strain.

placing an MSI 10 to 12 mm apical to the mucogingival junction.

Another important point should be clarified. Some clinicians have suggested that Tweed's anchorage preparation philosophy could be applied to MSI placement orientation. Basically, Tweed's philosophy[7] suggested that distally tipping the crown of the lower molars before Class II elastic wear enhanced anchorage by creating a *tent peg effect*. This seems logical; however, the same is not the case for MSIs. A tent peg is effective at holding down a tent because it is oriented at a 45-degree angle relative to the tent; a traditional tent peg is a smooth tapered peg. An MSI, however, is screw shaped. For example, the Ortho Implant (see Chapter 9) has a modified buttress thread form (Fig. 5-20). The lead in angle is at 45 degrees to the shaft, and the trailing angle is 90 degrees to the shaft. The trailing angle creates a butt-joint interface with the bone to prevent screw backout. The trailing angle actually acts as a tent peg, *without* having to angle the screw relative to the bone surface. Moreover, recent evidence[8] suggests that if a screw is to be oriented at all, it should actually be oriented toward the direction of the force rather than away from it, which is exactly opposite of what logic suggests. Angling the MSI in this way places the 90-degree trailing angle in a position to resist screw pullout (Fig. 5-21).

Soft Tissue Emergence

Two different methods have been advocated concerning MSI emergence through the soft tissues: *open* and *closed*. The *open method*

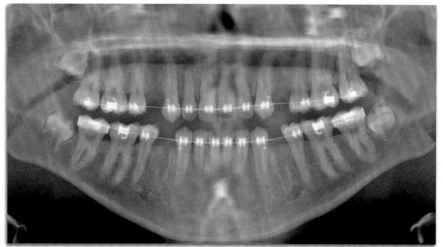

Fig. 5-14

Panoramic radiograph to assess approximate bone height, relative density, and relationships of local adjacent anatomic structures.

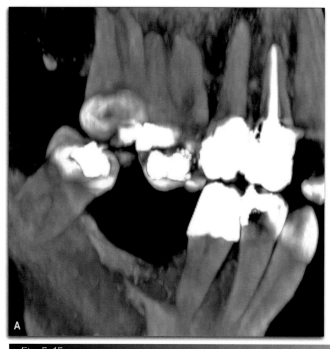

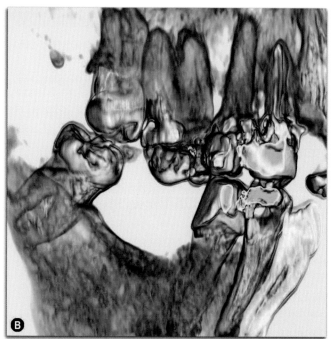

Fig. 5-15

Cone beam CT is a three-dimensional radiograph technique that allows the most accurate evaluation of bone morphology and density and the visualization of local anatomic structures. **A,** Radiograph view. **B,** Three-dimensional view. (Images taken with ILUMA Ultra Cone Beam CT, courtesy Dr. Ron Bulard, IMTEC Imaging, LLC, Ardmore, Okla.)

involves placing the TAD and allowing the abutment head to pass through the soft tissue and reside within the oral cavity (Fig. 5-22). Kyung and colleagues[9] suggest that the open method is best for MSIs in keratinized gingiva but that the closed method should be used with alveolar mucosa. To date, however, we have not found the closed method to be necessary. The *closed method* has been advocated in cases in which anatomic constraints necessitate TAD placement in

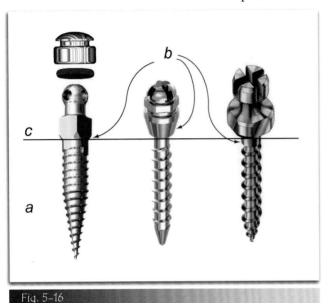

Fig. 5-16

MSI anatomy. *(a)* Threaded body, *(b)* transmucosal collar or neck, and *(c)* abutment head.

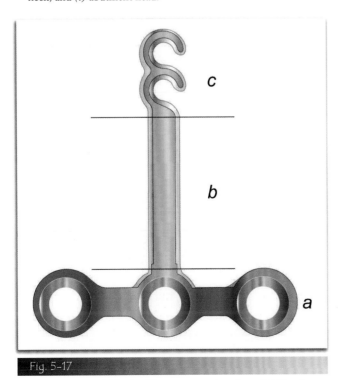

Fig. 5-17

MPI anatomy. *(a)* Body, *(b)* transmucosal neck, and *(c)* head.

alveolar mucosa or in thick soft tissue. For more on the closed method, the reader is referred to Chapter 13. In these cases, there is more risk of soft tissue overgrowth and potential infection, so a true incision is made and a flap is reflected to expose the surgical site. The TAD is placed, followed by ligature attachment to the abutment head and twisting enough ligature length to leave several millimeters exposed out of the mucosa after soft tissue closure. The soft tissue is sutured closed, leaving the twisted ligature wire sufficiently exposed for orthodontic attachment.

Temporary Anchorage Device Length

Determining MSI length is another critical factor that should be based on soft tissue thickness and bone thickness (cortical bone plus medullary bone up to but not including the contralateral cortex). Recall that most MSIs have a tapered, threaded apex leading up to the full-diameter thickness. The most critical aspect is that the full-diameter threaded body completely traverse the outer cortex, not the tapered apex of the threaded body. Recent evidence suggests that the majority of MSI primary stability comes from the cortical bone, with little stability coming from the medullary bone.[10] Theoretically, medullary bone serves more as a stabilizer in cases in which primary stability

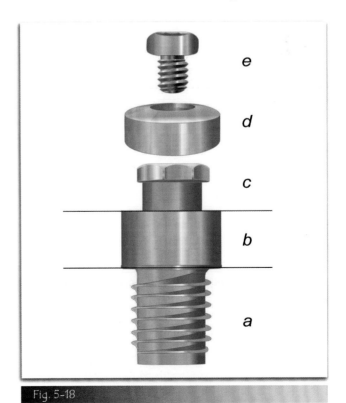

Fig. 5-18

PI anatomy. *(a)* Threaded body, *(b)* transmucosal collar or neck, *(c)* abutment head, *(d)* bonding cap, and *(e)* retention screw.

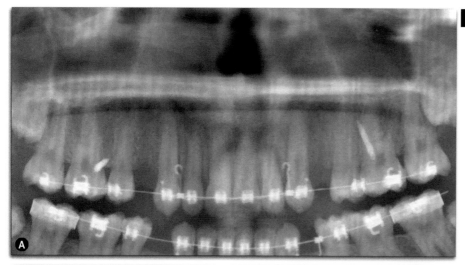

Fig. 5-19

MSI placement orientations. **A,** Panoramic radiograph. Note that inadequate interradicular bone stock was available between the maxillary left second premolar and first molar for perpendicular placement, so the MSI was placed at an oblique angle relative to the long axes of the teeth. **B,** MSI oriented perpendicular to bone surface. **C,** Anterior photograph showing perpendicular orientation *(left)* and oblique orientation *(right)*. **D,** MSI oriented oblique to bone surface.

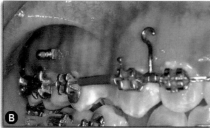
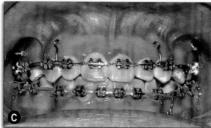
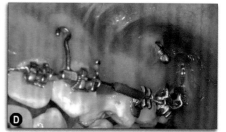

is not gained in the cortex, which would allow the implant to shift or tip in the direction of the force. In this scenario, presumably the apex of the screw would tip away from the force and engage medullary bone, thereby stabilizing the implant. Considering this, use of the longest MSI possible is not necessary.

Direct measurements taken from the diagnostic models can be combined with direct clinical measurements and approximate values from the radiographs to aid in determining the appropriate MSI length and placement location relative to the interproximal contact. If the soft tissue is greater than about 1.5 mm thick, then a longer MSI may be required because the abutment head may be too close to the soft tissue or possibly even submerged (Fig. 5-23, *A*). To have part of the threaded body traverse the soft tissue is not a problem as long as the part of the MSI that resides in the outer cortex is not tapered and adequate hygiene protocols are followed (Fig. 5-23, *B*).

Attachment Mechanics

The first step in evaluating a case for TAD use is a careful vector analysis to identify ideal device placement. It is important to recognize that although some cases will rely on TADs alone, many cases will use traditional orthodontic anchorage in combination with TADs. In general, the orthodontist should consider three main factors simultaneously: TAD

location, specific biomechanics involved, and local anatomic structures around which the attachments will pass. After determining one or more possible TAD locations, the orthodontist should evaluate the biomechanics. For example, consider a case with a Class II molar relationship and anterior maxillary crowding.

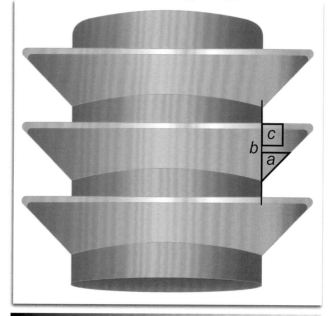

Fig. 5-20

Modified buttress thread form. Note the lead in angle *(a)* is 45 degrees to the long axis of the screw shaft *(b)*. The trailing angle *(c)* is 90 degrees to the shaft.

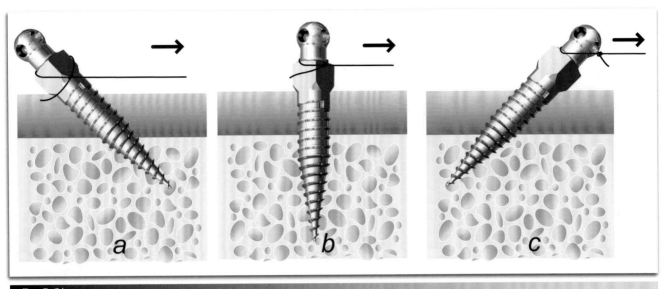

Fig. 5-21

MSI placement orientations. *(a)* Forty-five degrees opposite force application is worst orientation. *(b)* Ninety degrees from force application is better orientation. *(c)* Forty-five degrees toward force application is best orientation.

After bilateral maxillary first premolar extractions, the anterior segment will be retracted maximally with a hook attached between the canines and lateral incisors (Fig. 5-24, *A*). First, the anteroposterior position of the MSI should be selected. The MSI will be placed between the second premolar and first molar, if there is enough room. If not, then space will be made, the insertion angle changed, or another location selected. Second, the vertical position should be selected. In order to determine this, however, it should be known whether pure translation or facial or lingual root torque is desired during retraction. For pure translation, the MSI and the retraction hook should be placed at the level of the center of resistance of the anterior six-tooth segment, which will be about 7 mm apical to the arch wire level (Fig. 5-24, *B*). For lingual root torque, the MSI should be placed as coronally as possible and the retraction hook should be long enough so that the force passes apical to the center of resistance (Fig. 5-24, *C*). For lingual crown torque, the MSI should be placed at or slightly apical to the center of resistance of the anterior segment and the retraction hook should be short so that the force passes coronal to the center of resistance (Fig. 5-24, *D*). After considering the foregoing, the last factor to address is local anatomy. The two most common problems in this situation are frena attachments and the natural curvature of the bone and soft tissue when traveling from the posterior to the anterior aspect of the arch. If the closed coil retraction spring from the MSI to the retraction hook will impinge on either, the mechanics should be altered

to avoid these structures or another plan designed. Based on the foregoing example, it should become readily apparent that attachment mechanics should be determined on a case by case basis.

Maxilla

In the maxilla, several intraalveolar and extraalveolar locations are available for TAD placement (Fig. 5-25). Intraalveolar sites include the alveolar bone itself. Specifically, the TAD can pass from the facial or palatal cortices into the medullary bone intraradicularly or interradicularly. Extraalveolar sites include the zygomatic buttress region located superior to the mesiobuccal cusp of the first molar, the sub–anterior

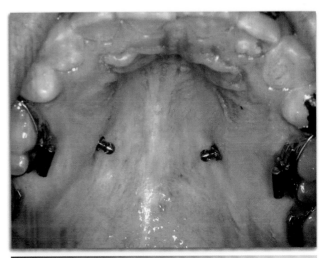

Fig. 5-22

Open method of MSI placement. Note that entire abutment head lies outside the gingiva.

nasal spine (sub-ANS) region above the incisors, or in the palatal bone. In the palate, TADs can be placed anterolaterally, parasagittally to the midpalatal suture, in the midpalatal suture for nongrowing individuals, or in the maxillary tuberosity.

When evaluating locations for TAD placement, the overriding qualification must always be cortical bone thickness. Recent evidence suggests that the majority of primary stability comes from the cortex,[10] specifically where the threads engage the cortical bone. Although cortical bone thickness varies from patient to patient, certain sites provide rather consistent cortical bone thicknesses.[9]

One of the most reliable maxillary buccal cortical sites is found mesial to the first molar. Bone stock in this location is consistently found to average 3 to 4 mm of mesiodistal interradicular cortical width at a level 5 to 8 mm apical to the cementoenamel junction (CEJ).[11] This is followed by the interradicular space between the canine and the lateral incisor. Recent

evidence demonstrates that the thickest bone in these areas is located more than halfway down the root length.[11] This is important, because many clinicians may feel that the best location for TAD placement is through attached gingiva so as to avoid potential soft tissue inflammation. However, the data suggest that it may not be possible to place an MSI through attached gingiva and still have enough bone stock for primary stability.

The sub-ANS area provides the dense cortical bone of the inferior piriform rim. However, this site is also subject to irritation from TADs because of the labial frenum and mobility of the upper lip. It may therefore be more appropriate to move laterally to the interradicular space between the lateral incisor and canine. Bone stock there is generally sufficient, and two well-placed MSIs may provide better biomechanics for intruding the maxillary incisors. The maxillary tuberosity has also been cited as a possible location for the distalization of molars.[9] However, the combination

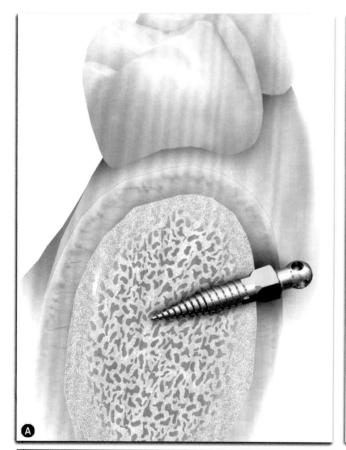 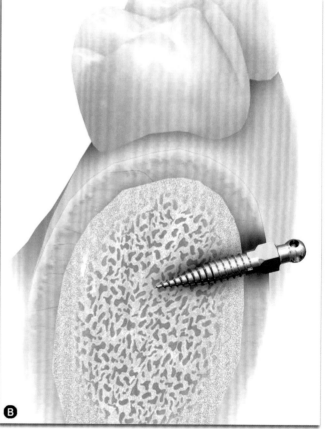

Fig. 5-23

Schematic cross section showing final MSI position. **A,** Full 1.8-mm diameter in cortex but too much of head is embedded in soft tissue, which will lead to soft tissue irritation when the orthodontic attachments are connected. **B,** Full 1.8-mm diameter in cortex and part of threads in gingiva because of gingival thickness but with at least half of the square head outside the gingiva, which minimizes soft tissue irritation.

of difficult access and high ratio of cancellous bone to cortical bone in this area limits its usefulness.

The palatal aspect of the maxilla provides multiple sites for TAD placement. The alveolar interradicular sites mirror their corresponding buccal counterparts yet have slightly more available bone because of single palatal roots compared with the same teeth having two facial roots. The midpalatal area provides considerably more cortical bone than the alveolus. In the midpalate, midsagittal placement is suitable in nongrowing adults; however, nongrowing children should have MSIs placed parasagittally instead.

Another maxillary extraalveolar location for MSI or MPI placement is the zygomatic buttress, which is the sweeping arc of bone palpable high in the maxillary vestibule adjacent to the first and second molars. More than 80% of the zygomatic bone is cortical bone, with an average thickness of 4.5 mm.[12,13] Implants placed in this area are surprisingly unobtrusive and cause little if any discomfort or irritation. When placing a zygomatic implant, the clinician must be mindful of the maxillary sinus. A slight medial MSI trajectory is usually acceptable. However, in the case of an overly pneumatized sinus, a more vertical MSI trajectory may be necessary yet still provide excellent anchorage. Particularly in the zygomatic region, MSI length determination should take into consideration the

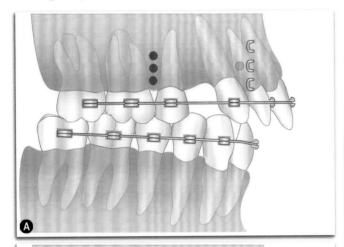

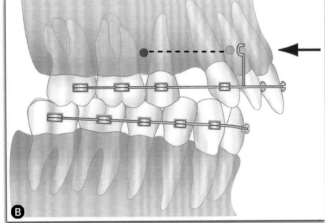

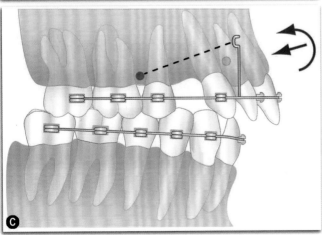

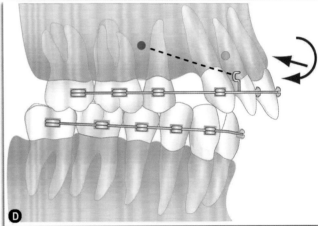

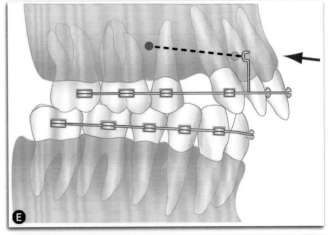

Fig. 5-24

Typical Class II maximum retraction case. **A,** Scenario after extraction with different implant levels *(green)*, hook attachment levels *(gray)*, and an assumed center of resistance *(tan)*. **B,** Mechanics for pure translation. **C,** Mechanics for increasing lingual root torque. **D,** Mechanics for increasing lingual crown torque. **E,** Mechanics for simultaneous intrusion with retraction.

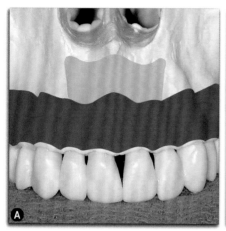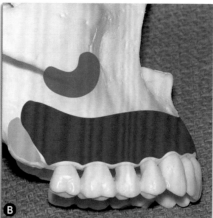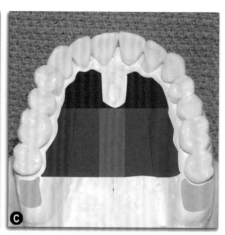

Fig. 5-25

Maxillary placement locations. **A,** Anterior facial alveolar ridge *(purple)* and sub-ANS region *(tan).* **B,** Posterior facial alveolar ridge *(purple),* zygomatic ridge *(blue),* and maxillary tuberosity *(tan).* **C,** Anterolateral palate *(maroon),* midpalate *(green),* parasagittal midpalate *(blue),* posterior palatal alveolar ridge *(purple),* and maxillary tuberosity *(tan).*

amount of soft tissue that will be traversed by the MSI so that the abutment head resides in the oral cavity without soft tissue irritation.

Mandible

In the mandible, several intraalveolar and extraalveolar locations are available (Fig. 5-26). Although the facial and lingual surfaces of the alveolar bone are candidates, the lingual aspect is difficult to access and is in a location that predisposes it to premature failure because of the activity of the tongue musculature. Good cortical bone is available in several extraalveolar locations. Anteriorly, the symphysis can be readily accessed; however, soft tissue irritation may occur after TAD placement. The ascending ramus, retromolar area, and the external oblique ridge offer excellent sites as well.

One of the most reliable mandibular buccal cortical sites is found mesial to the first molar. Bone stock in this location is consistently found to average 3 to 4 mm of mesiodistal interradicular cortical width at a level 4 to 5 mm apical to the CEJ.[11] However, because the cortex is dense and thick, a pilot hole is often required for MSI insertion. This site is followed by the interradicular space between the canine and the lateral incisor. Although the symphysis region provides dense cortical bone, this region is also subject to irritation from TADs due to the labial frenum and lower lip movement. It may therefore be more appropriate to move laterally to the interradicular space between the lateral incisor and canine.

Another extraalveolar location for MSI placement is the posterior mandible. In this region are three distinct sites. Miniscrew implants or MPIs can be placed obliquely in the external oblique ridge lateral to the first and second molars for intrusion or retraction

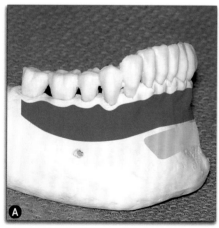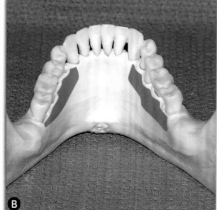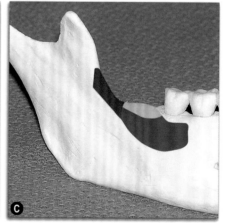

Fig. 5-26

Mandibular placement locations. **A,** Anterior and posterior facial alveolar ridge *(blue)* and symphysis region *(tan).* **B,** Posterior lingual alveolar ridge *(green).* **C,** External oblique ridge *(purple),* ascending ramus *(maroon),* and retromolar region *(tan).*

mechanics. Similarly, the ascending ramus or the retromolar region can be used for retraction or molar uprighting. Because all of these sites have dense, thick cortical bone, a pilot hole is often required.

Local Anatomic Structures

Several anatomic structures within the oral cavity should be avoided during TAD placement. These structures include major nerves and vessels, the maxillary sinus, and tooth roots. Although most TAD placement avoids these structures, a thorough knowledge of the local anatomy is required prior to surgically placing any object in the oral cavity.

Neurovascular Structures

Nasopalatine nerves and vessels. The nasopalatine nerves and vessels are terminal branches of the pterygopalatine vessels and nerves.[14,15] These nerves and vessels course along the roof of the nasal cavity and track down along the anterior extent of the nasal septum. As they arrive at the floor of the nasal cavity, they dive down into the incisive canal, which gives passage to the roof of the mouth via the incisive foramen. The incisive foramen is located in the midline of the palate, approximately 10 mm posterior to the maxillary central incisors (Fig. 5-27). These nerves and vessels provide sensory innervation and blood to the palatal mucosa of the premaxillary segment. Avoidance of these structures requires that any TAD placement in the anterior palate be lateral to the midline.

Greater palatine nerves and vessels. The greater palatine nerves and vessels descend through the

pterygopalatine canal and exit onto the posterior palate via the greater palatine foramen, usually located 10 mm toward the palatal midline, just distal to the second molar (Fig. 5-27).[14,15] These nerves and vessels supply sensory innervation and blood to the posterior hard palate and a portion of the soft palate. Temporary anchorage device placement on the posterior palate should not be placed in the region of the greater palatine foramen. The midline of the posterior palate is generally free of major neurovascular anatomy.

Apical nerves and vessels. The maxillary dentition receives its innervation from nerve rootlets that originate from the maxillary nerve.[14,15] The anterior, middle, and posterior superior alveolar nerves enter individual tooth roots at the apices, with the anterior superior alveolar nerve branching from the infraorbital nerve and the middle and posterior superior nerves originating directly from the maxillary nerve. The blood supply of the maxilla comes from apical branches of the maxillary artery, with the posterior superior alveolar artery supplying molars and premolars and the remaining dentition receiving arterial branches from the infraorbital artery. All mandibular teeth are innervated by the inferior alveolar branch of the mandibular nerve after it enters the mandibular foramen (Fig. 5-28). The blood supply of the mandible comes from apical branches of the inferior alveolar artery, also a branch of the maxillary artery.

Mental nerve. Anteriorly, the inferior alveolar nerve exits the mandibular canal via the mental foramen as the mental nerve, usually between the mandibular

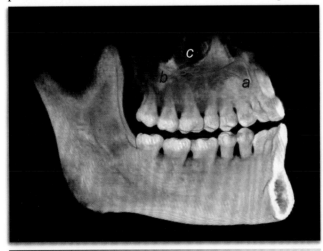

Fig. 5-27

Maxillary nerves and vessels. *(a)* Nasopalatine nerves and vessels emerge through the incisive foramen. *(b)* Greater palatine nerves and vessels emerge through the greater palatine foramen. *(c)* Maxillary sinuses are air-filled spaces within the maxillary bones. (Courtesy Drs. James Mah and Craig Cheung.)

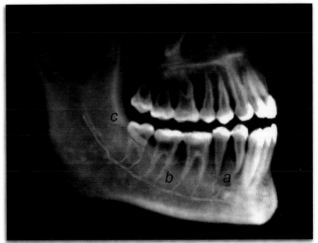

Fig. 5-28

Mandibular nerves and vessels. *(a)* The mental nerve emerges through the mental foramen. *(b)* Apical nerves and vessels enter the tooth roots at the apices. *(c)* The lingual nerve can pass through the retromolar triangle. (Courtesy Drs. James Mah and Craig Cheung.)

premolar roots at the level of the apices (Fig. 5-28).[14,15] Placement of a TAD in this region should be coronal to the mental foramen.

Lingual nerve. The lingual nerve passes between the ramus and the medial pterygoid muscle. The nerve parallels the inferior alveolar nerve, deviating at the level of the mandibular canal and running deep to the pterygomandibular raphae. At a point near the root apices of the mandibular third molar, the lingual nerve courses medially toward the base of the tongue (Fig. 5-28). The primary location of possible lingual nerve impingement for TAD placement is the lingual aspect of the retromolar region.[14,15]

Maxillary Sinuses

The maxillary sinuses are air-containing spaces that occupy the maxillary bone bilaterally (Fig. 5-27).[16] The maxillary sinus is the largest of the paranasal sinuses and is described as a four-sided pyramid with the base lying vertically on the medial surface and forming the lateral nasal wall. The apex extends laterally into the zygomatic process of the maxilla. The roof of the sinus is also the floor of the orbit. The posterior wall extends to the maxillary tuberosity. Anterolaterally, the sinus extends to the first premolars or canines. The floor of the sinus forms the base of the alveolar process.

The maxillary sinus is a stratified squamous epithelium-lined cavity that receives its innervation from branches of the maxillary division of the trigeminal nerve; specifically, the greater palatine nerve and branches of the infraorbital nerve.[14,15] The blood supply of the maxillary sinus is provided by the branches of the internal maxillary artery, including the infraorbital artery, lateral branches of the sphenopalatine artery, the greater palatine, and alveolar arteries. When placing TADs in the maxilla, there is always a chance that the MSI might perforate the maxillary sinus. This chance is increased if pneumatization of the sinuses is noted in the preoperative radiographic evaluation. The most concerning sequelae following a sinus perforation are postoperative maxillary sinusitis and formation of a chronic oroantral fistula.[16] The diagnosis and treatment of this problem is described in detail in Chapter 8.

Maxillary sinus evaluation is important when TADs are to be placed in the maxilla. Young patients tend to have robust amounts of bone around their maxillary sinuses with several exceptions. Mouth breathers and Class III skeletal patterns tend to have maxillary hypoplasia that may be demonstrated on cephalometric evaluation.[17-19] This includes hypoplasia of maxillary

bone itself, a consideration which must be kept in mind when placing MPIs and mini fixation screws between and above maxillary roots. Edentulous areas in the posterior maxilla, regardless of age, may increase the likelihood of sinus pneumatization. In these instances, alternative screw placement positions should be considered to avoid sinus perforation.

Tooth Roots

As described earlier, maxillary and mandibular teeth receive their sensory innervation and their blood supply through small, terminal neurovascular bundles that enter each canal at or near the apex of the roots. Of all the potential complications that are possible with TAD placement, possibly the most feared is placement of an MSI into a tooth root. Amazingly, there is a paucity of literature regarding this subject.[20-25]

If during the operative procedure, the clinician does not feel a "drop" into the medullary space as the MSI advances, or the MSI simply stops advancing altogether, the clinician can assume that the MSI may be contacting the root. Sudden onset of dental pain during the advancement of the MSI also indicates that the screw has probably contacted the root structure of an adjacent tooth. This mandates MSI removal followed by redirection away from the root. This is usually the only step that is necessary in this instance; however, the tooth should be evaluated during routine follow-up appointments.

A particular concern is root location, not only to avoid primary root damage during placement but also to avoid secondary root damage by placing the MSI in the path of active root movement. In an effort to avoid direct root impingement, the clinician may inadvertently place MSIs directly in the path of a tooth root that is to be moved. This could arrest tooth movement or cause pressure necrosis or root resorption.

Soft Tissue and Hard Tissue Variation

Another important factor in determining where to place TADs in the oral cavity is the depth of soft tissue and bone in various regions. The soft tissues can be categorized as masticatory mucosa or alveolar mucosa.[26] Masticatory mucosa is a keratinized mucosa designed to handle the mechanical forces and surface abrasion that occur during mastication. Masticatory mucosa is found in two main locations: the hard palate and gingiva surrounding the teeth. Keratinized gingiva starts at the crest of the alveolar bone and continues apically to the mucogingival junction. The reason keratinized gingiva is bound tightly to the alveolar bone is that the mucosa is attached directly to the periosteum of the underlying bone with no intervening submucosa. This attachment is often referred to as mucoperiosteum. The alveolar mucosa is a nonkeratinized lining mucosa that starts at the mucogingival junction and continues apically to the depth of the vestibule. This mucosa is mobile because of its intervening submucosal layer between the mucosa and periosteum. An important note is that alveolar mucosa is less mobile closer to the mucogingival junction than in the depth of the vestibule.

Similarly, bone within the oral cavity can be categorized based on location: alveolar bone or basal bone. Alveolar bone is that bone of the jaws containing the sockets (alveoli) for the teeth.[27] Alveolar bone is composed of an outer cortical plate of bone, an inner medullary bone, and a specialized bundle bone lining the alveolus. Basal bone is the bone that lies apical to the teeth; it also has an outer cortical plate of bone and an inner medullary bone. As would be expected, OrthoTADs can be placed in alveolar and basal bone. And because alveolar bone is covered with masticatory and alveolar mucosa, it follows that TADs may be located in masticatory or alveolar mucosa. It is, therefore, important for the clinician to have a good understanding of the average depths of all types of soft tissue and bone within the oral cavity.[28] For a detailed description on intraoral bony and soft tissue depths, the reader is referred to Chapter 7.

Timing of Temporary Anchorage Device Placement

Several authors have advocated allowing the soft tissue to heal for 1 to 2 weeks before loading a TAD.[29-31] This, however, is unnecessary unless an extensive flap is laid or a TAD designed to be osseointegrated is placed. For example, most PI manufacturers advocate a 6- to 12-week healing period for osseointegration prior to loading. In addition, many MPIs are placed with a more extensive flap, which may cause more extensive swelling. Surgical placement of most MSIs does not involve more than a biopsy punch, which results in little to no postoperative swelling.

Perhaps a more critical factor is local bone healing, not so much for trauma caused by MSI placement but for other procedures performed in a similar time frame. For example, extraction of a tooth leaves a bony void. The body immediately mounts a response to fill the void and reestablish the bony contour. This detailed biologic response has frequently been referred to as fracture healing; however, this is not accurate. Fracture healing is a specific cascade of events that occurs under *mechanically unstable* conditions, as when a bone is fractured into two or more discontinuous segments. What actually occurs following extraction is more analogous to large cortical bone defect repair, in which cortical bone defects are filled in initially by a blood clot that is subsequently reorganized into callus tissue in which an initial scaffold of woven bone is formed. This is followed by reinforcement by parallel-fibered and/or lamellar bone. After a lag of several weeks, Haversian remodeling begins on the avascular areas of the socket wall and the newly formed tissue in the extraction site.[32] Osseous regeneration starts approximately 3 weeks after extraction and is completed after 4 to 6 months.[33-36] By the end of the first week, osteoclasts appear at the alveolar ridge and start to smooth the alveolar margin via resorption.[37] This regressive restructuring is most pronounced in the first 4 weeks after extraction and then gradually declines until the fifth month.[38]

Considering the foregoing, as well as the regional acceleratory phenomenon associated with bony trauma,[39-41] it is likely that a regional osteopenia occurs at sites adjacent to recent extraction sites. This can be explained as follows: As the body begins to infuse the extraction site with nutrients and cells to remove necrotic tissue and begin to build osteoid that is subsequently mineralized, it borrows minerals from adjacent bone, leading to a regional osteopenia. This may weaken adjacent bone and predispose MSIs placed simultaneously with dental extractions to inadequate primary stability and premature failure. In this scenario, it may be advisable to place the MSI several weeks before tooth extraction or to wait 6 to 10 weeks after extraction for MSI placement.

SUMMARY

Like all successful adjunct modalities in orthodontics, TADs will only be as good as the presurgical evaluation, diagnosis, treatment planning, patient cooperation, biomechanics analysis, and clinical techniques. As the orthodontist becomes more comfortable in the evaluation and placement of TADs, more clinical applications will become readily apparent. The addition of skeletal anchorage to the orthodontist's armamentarium provides the beginning of a new and exciting age in a profession that has heretofore been subjugated to Newton's third law.

REFERENCES

1. Dajani AS, Taubert KA, Wilson W, et al. Prevention of bacterial endocarditis: recommendations by the American Heart Association. *Circulation.* 96:1274-1275, 1997.

2. Danforth R, Dus I, Mah J. 3-D volume imaging for dentistry: a new dimension. *CDA J.* 31:817-823, 2003.

3. Nakajima A, Sameshima G, Arai Y, et al. Two- and three-dimensional orthodontic imaging using limited cone beam-computed tomography. *Angle Orthod.* 75:895-903, 2005.

4. Adell R, Lekholm U, Rockler B, Branemark PI. A 15-year study of osseointegrated implants in the treatment of the edentulous jaw. *Int J Oral Surg.* 10:387-416, 1981.

5. Albreksson T, Zarb GA, Worthington D, Eriksson R. The long-term efficacy of currently used dental implants: a review and proposed criteria of success. *Int J Oral Maxillofac Implants.* 1:11-25, 1986.

6. Warrer K, Buser D, Lang NP, Karring T. Plaque-induced peri-implantitis in the presence or absence of keratinized mucosa. *Clin Oral Implants Res.* 6:131-138, 1995.

7. Tweed C. *Clinical Orthodontics.* St Louis, Mo: CV Mosby, 1966.

8. Pickard M. *Effect of Mini-Screw Orthodontic Implant Orientation on Implant Stability and Resistance to Failure at the Bone-Implant Interface* [dissertation]. Dallas, Tex: Department of Orthodontics, TAMUSHSC—Baylor College of Dentistry; 2004.

9. Kyung HM, Bae SM, Park HS, et al. Microimplant anchorage (MIA) in orthodontics: various application sites and their considerations. In: McNamara JA Jr, ed. *Implants, Microimplants, Onplants, and Transplants: New Answers to Old Questions in Orthodontics.* Ann Arbor: Center for Human Growth and Development, University of Michigan, 2005:69-88.

10. Dalstra M, Cattaneo PM, Melsen B. Load transfer of miniscrews for orthodontic anchorage. *Orthodontics.* 1:53-62, 2004.

11. Schnelle MA, Beck FM, Jaynes RM, Huja S. A radiographic evaluation of the availability of bone for placement of miniscrews. *Angle Orthod.* 74:830-835, 2004.

12. Francischone CE, Padovani CR, Branemark PI. Zygomatic bone: anatomic bases for osseointegrated implant anchorage. *Int J Oral Maxillofac Implants.* 20:441-447, 2005.

13. Cheung LK, Zhang Q, Wong MCM, Wong LLS. Stability consideration for internal maxillary distractors. *J Craniomaxillofac Surg.* 31:142-148, 2003.

14. Clemente CD. The neck and head. In: Clemente CD, ed. *Anatomy: A Regional Atlas of the Human Body.* Philadelphia, Pa: Lea & Febiger, 1987:574-624.

15. Kendell BD. Applied surgical anatomy of the head and neck. In: Fonseca RJ, Walker RV, Betts N, Barber H, eds. *Oral and Maxillofacial Trauma.* Philadelphia, Pa: WB Saunders, 1997: 247-307.

16. Schow S. Odontogenic diseases of the maxillary sinus. In: Peterson L, Ellis E III, Hupp J, Tucker MR, eds. *Contemporary Oral and Maxillofacial Surgery.* St Louis, Mo: Mosby-Year Book, 1993:465-482.

17. Epker BN, Stella JP, Fish LC. Class III dentofacial deformities secondary to maxillary deficiency. In: Epker BN, Stella JP, Fish LC, eds. *Dentofacial Deformities, Integrated Orthodontic and Surgical Correction.* St Louis, Mo: Mosby, 1996:734-748.

18. Arat ZM, Iseri H, Arman A. Differential diagnosis of skeletal open bite based on sagittal components of the face. *World J Orthod.* 6:41-50, 2005.

19. Bresolin D, Shapiro PA, Shapiro GG, et al. Mouth breathing in allergic children: its relationship to dentofacial development. *Am J Orthod Dentofacial Orthop.* 83:334-240, 1983.

20. Fabbronni G, Aabed S, Mizen K, Starr DG. Transalveolar screws and the incidence of dental damage: a prospective study. *Int J Oral Maxillofac Surg.* 33:442-446, 2004.

21. Farr DR, Whear NM. Intermaxillary fixation screws and tooth damage. *Br J Oral Maxillofac Surg.* 40:84-85, 2002.

22. Coburn DG, Kennedy DWG, Hodder SC. Complications with intermaxillary fixation screws in the management of fractured mandibles. *Br J Oral Maxillofac Surg.* 40:241-243, 2002.

23. Borah GL, Ashmead D. The fate of teeth transfixed by osteosynthesis screws. *Plast Reconstr Surg.* 97:726-729, 1996.

24. Jones DC. The intermaxillary screw: a dedicated bicortical bone screw for temporary intermaxillary fixation. *Br J Oral Maxillofac Surg.* 37:115-116, 1999.

25. Majumdar A, Brook IM. Iatrogenic injury caused by intermaxillary fixation screws. *Br J Oral Maxillofac Surg.* 40:84, 2002.

26. Squier C, Finkelstein M. Oral mucosa. In: Ten Cate A, ed. *Oral Histology: Development, Structure, and Function.* St Louis, Mo: Mosby-Year Book, 1998:345-385.

27. Ten Cate A. Periodontium. In: Ten Cate A, ed. *Oral Histology: Development, Structure, and Function.* St Louis, Mo: Mosby-Year Book, 1998:253-288.

28. Costa A, Pasta G, Bergamaschi G. Intraoral hard and soft tissue depths for temporary anchorage devices. *Semin Orthod.* 11:10-15, 2005.

29. Liou EJ, Pai BCJ, Lin JC. Do miniscrews remain stationary under orthodontic forces? *Am J Orthod Dentofacial Orthop.* 126:42-47, 2004.

30. Cheng SJ, Tseng IY, Lee JJ, Kok S-H. A prospective study of the risk factors associated with failure of mini-implants used for orthodontic anchrorage. *Int J Oral Maxillofac Implant.* 19:100-106, 2004.

31. Park HS, Kwon OW, Sung JH. Uprighting second molars with micro-implant anchorage. *J Clin Orthod.* 38:100-103, 2004.

32. Schenk RK, Hunkizer EB. Histologic and ultrastructural features of fracture healing. In: Brighton CT, Friedlaender G, Lane JM, eds. *Bone Formation and Repair.* Rosemont, Ill: American Academy of Orthopedic Surgeons, 1994:117-146.

33. Amler M. The time sequence of tissue regeneration in human extraction wounds. *J Oral Surg.* 27:309-318, 1969.

34. Amler M. The age factor in human extraction wound healing. *J Oral Surg.* 35:193-197, 1977.

35. Amler M, Johnson P, Salman I. Histological and histochemical investigation of human alveolar socket healing in undisturbed extraction wounds. *J Am Dent Assoc.* 61:32-44, 1960.

36. Simpson H. The healing of extraction wounds. *Br Dent J.* 126:550-557, 1969.

37. Schröder HE. *Pathobiologie Oraler Srukturen.* Basel, Switzerland: Karger, 1983.

38. Lam R. Contour changes of the alveolar processes following extractions. *J Prosthet Dent.* 10:25-32, 1960.

39. Frost HM. The biology of fracture healing: an overview for clinicians, II. *Clin Orthop.* 294-309, 1989.

40. Frost HM. The biology of fracture healing: an overview for clinicians, I. Clin Orthop. 283-293, 1989.

41. Frost HM. The regional acceleratory phenomenon: a review. Henry Ford Hosp Med J. 31:3-9, 1983.

Biomechanics of Temporary Anchorage Devices

Joong-Ki Lim, Cheol-Ho Paik

Biomechanics is one of the most critical components of orthodontic mechanotherapy. However, with the advent of the straight wire system, it has become far too easy to forget about centers of resistance, centers of rotation, lines of force, and the like. In lieu of critically analyzing the biomechanical systems with which we work, most orthodontists think at the level of the occlusal plane because that is where the arch wires lay. In light of the recent introduction of temporary anchorage device (TAD) technology, with its inherent ability to alter and more predictably control lines of force relative to the center of resistance of teeth, this line of thinking will have to change. It is important then to reconsider biomechanics as it relates to orthodontic tooth movement in general, and the application of biomechanics to orthodontics in combination with TADs in particular.

SINGLE FORCE ORTHODONTICS

A static equilibrium is formed when an orthodontic force is applied to a tooth. This means that the tooth does not move immediately at the time the orthodontic force is applied. Therefore, an equal and opposite reactive force works against the applied force. Furthermore, the sum of the moments developed from all directions equals zero ($\Sigma F = 0$, $\Sigma M = 0$).

Two types of orthodontic force systems are a statically determinate system and a statically indeterminate system. In a statically determinate system, the forces and moments applied to the active and reactive components

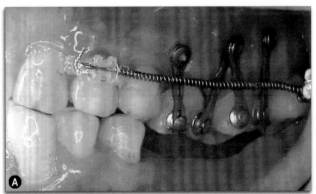

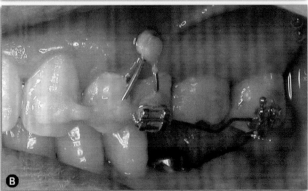

Fig. 6-1

Intrusion of supererupted molars. **A,** Statically determinate system. Intrusive forces applied from miniscrews to molars via a single point contact. **B,** Statically indeterminate system. Intrusive force applied from second premolar bracket via a step bend to the second molar. The second premolar was stabilized indirectly by the miniscrew. Note that because no single point contact is applied to the second molar for intrusion, the system became a two-couple system (couple at the second premolar and molar brackets), making it difficult to determine the force magnitude and net moment direction.

can be easily quantified because they are easily recognizable (Fig. 6-1, *A*). In a statically indeterminate system (Fig. 6-1, *B*), the forces and moments are too complex to analyze. Therefore, only the direction of net moments and approximate net force levels can be determined in an indeterminate system.[1]

Because the orthodontic force applied using TADs is a single force, a statically determinate system can be built to accurately measure the forces and moments of the moving teeth. Even when a single force is applied by the TADs in continuous arch mechanics (where all the forces and moments cannot be analyzed), the tooth movement can be predicted more easily because there is no reactive force.

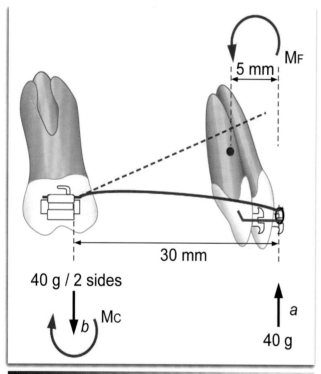

Fig. 6-2

Intrusion arch for deepbite correction: one-couple system. An intrusion arch made from rectangular wire fits into a rectangular tube on the molars and is tied to a single point contact at the incisor segment. If the arch wire is activated by pulling it down and tying it to the incisor segment so that it delivers a 40-g intrusion force *(a;* 10 g per tooth, 20 g per side), and if the distance from the molar tube to the point of attachment is 30 mm, each molar will feel a 20-g extrusive force *(b)* in reaction and a 600 g-mm moment (M_C = 20 g × 30 mm) to tip the crown distally. At the incisor segment the force will create a 200 g-mm moment (M_F = 40 g × 5 mm) to rotate the incisor crowns facially. M_C is couple moment; M_F is third-order moment. (Redrawn from Proffit WR: Mechanical principles in orthodontic force control. In: Proffit WR, Fields HW Jr, eds. *Contemporary Orthodontics,* 3rd ed. St Louis, MO: Mosby, 2000:349-352; with permission from Elsevier.)

Statically Determinate System: One-Couple System

A typical one-couple system used in orthodontics is a cantilever spring where one side is inserted into a bracket or tube and the other side makes a single point contact (Fig. 6-2).[1,2] A force and a moment (M_C = couple moment created by activating the arch wire) develop at the site where the arch wire is inserted; whereas only a force develops at the site of single point of force application. The magnitude and direction of the force and moment created can be analyzed, comprising the statically determinate system. This means that tooth movement can be accurately predicted.

For orthodontic treatment using miniscrews, a determinate force system is possible because a force is applied with a single point contact. For example, when comparing intrusion of upright maxillary anterior teeth using a palatal compared with a facial appliance, it is difficult to develop a facial crown flaring moment with a palatal appliance because the forces pass closer to the center of resistance (Fig. 6-3).[3]

When a single intrusive force is applied from a miniscrew in the facial alveolar ridge, a third-order moment is created to move the crown facially. Therefore, a statically determinate system is formed when the anterior segment is isolated and the center of resistance is accurately identified, then the direction and size of the third-order moment (M_F) can be accurately measured (Fig. 6-4). Unlike a conventional intrusion spring, side effects caused by a reactive force do not appear with miniscrews because they are immovable absolute anchorage.

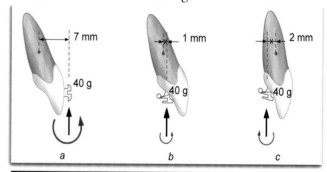

Fig. 6-3

Comparison of palatal and facial appliance. *(a)* Intrusive force of 40 g is applied at a facial bracket 7 mm anterior to the center of resistance, causing a counterclockwise moment of 280 g-mm (40 g × 7 mm) moving the crown facially. *(b)* Intrusive force of 40 g is applied at a lingual bracket 1 mm anterior to the center of resistance, causing a counterclockwise moment of 40 g-mm (40 g × 1 mm) moving the crown facially only slightly. *(c)* For an upright incisor, an intrusive force of 40 g is applied at a lingual bracket 2 mm posterior to the center of resistance, causing a clockwise moment of 80 g-mm (40 g × 2 mm) moving the crown lingually.

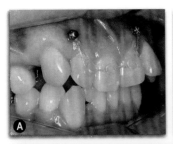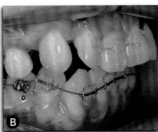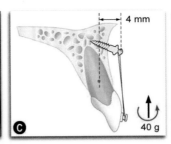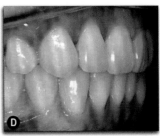

Fig. 6-4

Intrusion of upright incisors using miniscrews. **A,** Initial lateral overjet photograph of intrusive force (40 g per side) applied from the miniscrews to the incisor brackets. **B,** Progress lateral overjet photograph after 2 months of intrusion. **C,** Diagram illustrating counterclockwise crown flaring moment of 160 g-mm because the force is applied 4 mm anterior to center of resistance. Note that the teeth moved further forward, the moment becomes larger because the teeth are further forward of the center of resistance. **D,** Posttreatment lateral overjet photograph showing proper inclination of maxillary incisors.

Statically Indeterminate System: Two-Couple System

In contrast to the one-couple system, a two-couple system is formed when a rectangular arch wire is actually inserted into the bracket slot instead of it being tied above or below the brackets at the anterior component of the intrusion arch. In so doing, a couple moment develops within the bracket in the incisor segment.[4,5] This creates a statically indeterminate system where the magnitude and direction of the net force and net moment can only be approximated. A typical example of this system is the Rickett's utility arch for intrusion of the incisors (Fig. 6-5). The magnitude of the vertical force changes according to the amount of torque bent into the arch wire at the incisor segment. This, however, is difficult to measure.

Continuous arch mechanics is another typical example of a statically indeterminate system. A continuous arch forms complex multiple couples and forces because all of the teeth are tied into the bracket slots. Moreover, a new force system is created with even minuscule tooth movements. Therefore, it is impossible to accurately measure the force and moment applied to each tooth. When a single force is applied from a TAD, the exact force and moment cannot be measured because the force module is tied to a continuous arch wire. The outcome of the specific orthodontic tooth movement can be predicted, however, because the reactive force does not have to be considered (Fig. 6-6).

Action vs. Reaction

One of the factors that makes orthodontic treatment difficult is Newton's third law of motion, which states, "for every action, there is an equal and opposite reaction." For example, when the mandibular left second molar is in crossbite and is to be uprighted with a lingual arch, a reactive force and moment are created at the right second molar (Fig. 6-7, *A*). If crossbite elastics are added between the upper and lower second molars, the molars become extruded as a result of an undesirable vertical component from the elastic force (Fig. 6-7, *B*).

When a TAD is used instead, there is no reactive force to consider, and Newton's third law of motion can be disregarded. This means that the only consideration is how to apply the orthodontic force from the TAD to the tooth via the force module. For example, a crossbite can be corrected using a miniscrew without using the conventional methods (Fig. 6-8). In this way, the molar is moved horizontally without any unwanted side effects to the adjacent teeth. The lower molar undergoes simultaneous buccal movement and intrusion, thereby avoiding relative extrusion and bite opening of the anterior teeth during crossbite correction.

ANTERIOR RETRACTION USING TEMPORARY ANCHORAGE DEVICES

In extraction treatment, TADs act as absolute anchorage that do not move, and the types of tooth movement possible are determined based primarily on the location of the implant. In the following section, anterior retraction is explained using TADs with sliding mechanics on a continuous arch wire.

Temporary Anchorage Device Force Systems

Accurate calculation of the force and moment applied to a tooth using continuous arch mechanics is impossible. However, a free-body diagram is possible for analytical purposes if the anterior segment is isolated (Fig. 6-9). Using a miniscrew, the orthodontic force is a single force where the line connecting the miniscrew to the arch wire hook becomes the line of action, which shows both magnitude and direction. The type of tooth movement is determined by where the line of

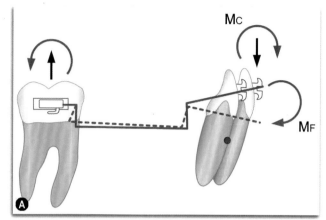

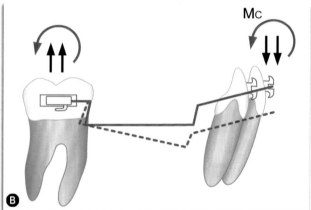

Fig. 6-5

Intrusion arch for deep bite correction: two-couple system. An intrusion arch made from rectangular wire fits into a rectangular tube on the molars and is tied into the brackets on the incisors. When this is done, the precise magnitude of forces and couples cannot be known. **A,** Activating the utility arch by placing it in the brackets creates the intrusion force, with a reactive force of the same magnitude on the anchor molar and a couple to tip its crown distally. At the incisors a moment to tip the crowns facial (M_F) is created by the distance of the brackets anterior to the center of resistance, and an additional moment in the same direction is created by the couple within the bracket (M_C) as the inclination of the wire is changed when it is brought to the brackets. The moment of this couple cannot be known, but it is clinically important because it affects the magnitude of the intrusive force. **B,** Placing a torque bend in the utility arch creates a moment to bring the crown lingually, controlling the tendency for the teeth to tip facially as they intrude, but it also increase the magnitude of the intrusive force on the incisor segment and the extrusive force and couple on the molar. (Redrawn from Proffit WR: Mechanical principles in orthodontic force control. In: Proffit WR, Fields HW Jr, eds. *Contemporary Orthodontics.* 3rd ed. St Louis, MO: Mosby, 2000:349-352; with permission from Elsevier.)

action passes relative to the center of resistance of the segment that is being moved.

Controlled Tipping

Controlled tipping is possible when the line of action between the miniscrew and arch wire hook is located incisal to the center of resistance of the anterior teeth

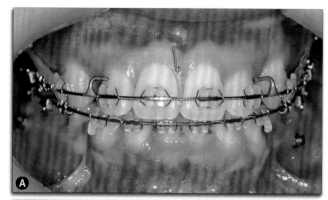

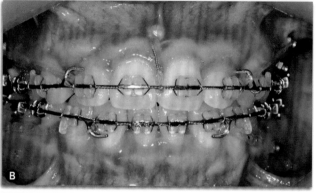

Fig. 6-6

Anterior intrusion using a miniscrew and a continuous arch wire. **A,** A miniscrew was placed in the sub–anterior nasal spine region, and a single intrusion force was applied to the arch wire. **B,** An intrusive force was created by the miniscrew placed facial to the center of resistance, thereby causing intrusion and flaring of the incisors.

(Fig. 6-10, *A*). In this case, the appropriate location of the miniscrew is just above the cementoenamel junction in the buccal alveolar bone between the maxillary second premolar and first molar. The arch wire hook is short, so the force has a predominantly horizontal component (retraction force) and only a slight vertical component (intrusion force).

Torque control can be incorporated to the anterior teeth through additional arch wire bending. An accentuated curve of Spee can be added when incisor intrusion is needed to reduce maxillary incisor display. When incisor display is to be maintained or increased, a lingual root torque bend is placed in the anterior portion of the arch wire. When significant incisor intrusion is desired because of a significant gummy smile, the miniscrew would be placed high in the buccal alveolar bone (Fig. 6-10, *B*). The vertical component (intrusion force) is increased by placing the miniscrew in the buccal alveolar bone mesial to the maxillary second premolar. In addition, the arch wire hook is directed incisally for the desired line of action.

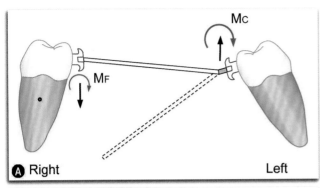

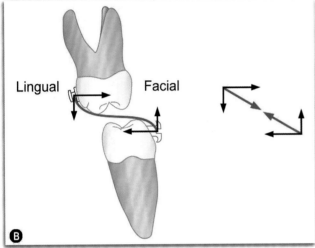

Fig. 6-7

Crossbite correction using conventional methods. **A,** A lingual arch is used to upright a lingually tipped mandibular left second molar. A one-couple system would form when buccal crown torque is applied to the left second molar, and the arch wire in the right second molar is rounded to prevent torque application and apply only a single force to the right molar. When the lingual arch is activated by placing it into the bracket, a moment (M_C) is created, displacing the crown buccally, and an extrusive force develops to satisfy the static equilibrium. An intrusive force is created lingual to the center of resistance of the right molar, resulting in a third-order moment (M_F) torquing the molar crown lingually. This causes undesirable intrusion and lingual tipping of the right second molar. **B,** Crossbite elastics worn to correct the left crossbite cause an undesirable extrusive force at the molars, possibly causing anterior bite opening.

Bodily Movement

Direct translation is possible when both the miniscrew and the arch wire hook are level with the center of resistance of the anterior teeth (Fig. 6-11). If the arch wire hook cannot be extended to the level of the center of resistance, then an accentuated curve of Spee and/or a lingual root torque bend can be placed in the arch wire in order to increase the counterclockwise moment in the anterior teeth and attempt to maintain bodily movement.

Root Movement

To achieve root movement, the line of action must pass apical to the center of resistance (Fig. 6-12). The arch wire hook should be extended maximally into the vestibule but without causing soft tissue irritation, and the miniscrew should be placed as low in the buccal alveolar bone as possible. Accentuated curve of Spee and/or a lingual root torque bend can also be added into the arch wire to increase root movement. One limitation with labial appliances is the potential for soft tissue trauma with the long arch wire hook (lever arm). The lever arm, however, can usually be extended sufficiently from lingual appliances. Therefore, root movement may be more easily obtained when a miniscrew is inserted in the lingual alveolar bone and is used in combination with lingual appliances (Fig. 6-13).

Systematic Approach for Proper Temporary Anchorage Device Placement

An orthodontic force using a miniscrew is a single force without a reactive force; thus tooth movement is easily predicted and monitored even when applied to a statically indeterminate system, that is, a continuous arch wire. True "single force orthodontics" becomes possible by knowing the center of resistance of the segment to be moved and deriving an equation between the type of tooth movement (center of rotation) and the single force created from the miniscrew. Therefore, it is theoretically possible to achieve tooth movement (i.e., controlled tipping and translation) by placing the miniscrew at a site determined using a specific equation and applying a single force to the segment to be moved.

Center of Resistance of Maxillary Anterior Teeth

Vanden Bulcke and colleagues[6,7] examined the center of resistance of the maxillary anterior teeth using a dry human skull. They reported that the anteroposterior position of the center of resistance is distal to the first premolar and the vertical position is 7 mm apical to the interproximal bone level.

Pedersen and colleagues[8] used a human cadaver and reported that the anteroposterior position of the center of resistance is 3 mm posterior to the distal surface of the canine and the vertical position is 6.5 mm apical to the bracket position. Fig. 6-14 shows a comparison of the two results.[9]

Center of Rotation (Types of Tooth Movement)

Bodily movement (translation) occurs when a single force is applied to the center of resistance of a tooth. For translation, the center of rotation of tooth movement is at infinity. When a single force is applied apical to the center of resistance, root movement occurs, whereas

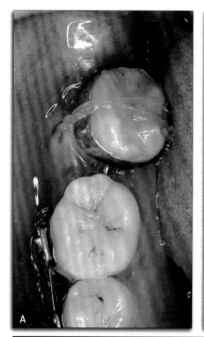
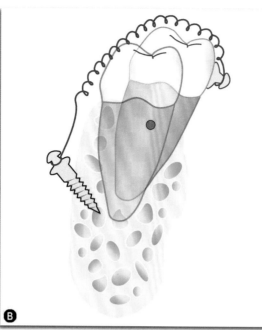
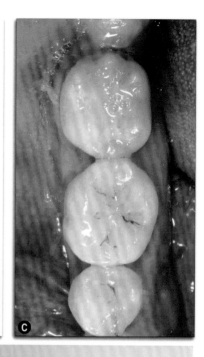

Fig. 6-8

Crossbite correction using a miniscrew. **A,** Pretreatment occlusal photograph of lower right second molar in complete crossbite with the upper molar. An elastic chain was extended from a miniscrew in the facial cortical bone to the lingual surface of the band. **B,** Diagram of mechanics simultaneously to intrude and move the molar bucally. **C,** Posttreatment occlusal photograph of uprighted molar. Note that traumatic occlusion caused by premature contact is avoided because of intrusive force.

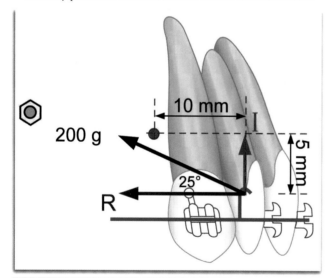

Fig. 6-9

Free-body diagram of anterior retraction using a miniscrew. Miniscrew is placed between maxillary first molar and second premolar. A 200-g force is applied to the arch wire hook. This force can be divided into an intrusive component *(I)* and a retraction component *(R)*. From the arch wire hook to the center of resistance, the vertical distance is 5 mm and the anteroposterior distance is 10 mm. Each component and its moment is calculated as follows: component forces: I = 200 g × sin 25 degrees = 84.6 g; R = 200 g × cos 25 degrees = 181.2 g; moment (M$_F$): clockwise moment = R × 5 mm = 906 g-mm; counterclockwise moment = I × 10 mm = 846 g-mm; net moment = clockwise moment 60 g-mm (906 g-mm – 846 g-mm). This means that when a 200-g force is applied to the miniscrew through an arch wire hook, a 181.2-g retraction force and an 84.6-g intrusive force, as well as a 60 g-mm lingual crown tipping moment, are created.

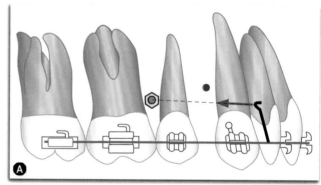

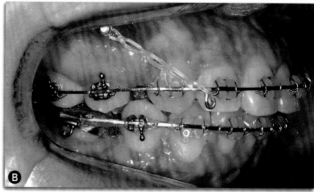

Fig. 6-10

Controlled tipping of anterior teeth using a miniscrew. **A,** Diagram showing line of action from miniscrew to hook passing incisal to center of resistance of anterior teeth. **B,** Buccal photograph of miniscrew inserted into buccal alveolar bone between maxillary first and second premolar to increase intrusive force.

tipping occurs when a single force is applied occlusally. Fig. 6-15 shows the center of rotation relative to different types of tooth movement. Fig. 6-16 shows the center of rotation of a tooth before and after movement.[10]

Interrelationship between the C_{RES}, C_{ROT}, and Force (a × b = σ²)

Nagerl and colleagues[11] derived the following equation for the relationship between center of resistance (C_{RES}), center of rotation (C_{ROT}), and applied force (F) using the upper canine with a simulated periodontal ligament: $a\ (F \sim C_{RES}) \times b\ (C_{RES} \sim C_{ROT}) = \text{Constant}\ (\sigma^2)$.

They reported on the "general theory of tooth movement" in which the product of two distances (*a*, the distance from the center of resistance to the point of force application, and *b*, the distance from the center of resistance to the center of rotation) is constant (Fig. 6-17). The values of the constant (σ^2) can be obtained experimentally (Table 6-1). This value is affected by the force direction, root morphology, and alveolar bone level.[12]

One variable can be calculated when the values of the constant (σ^2) and two variables are known. This means that the position of the force can be determined when the center of resistance of the tooth or tooth segment is known and the types of tooth movement (center of rotation) can be defined. The desired tooth movement can be obtained when the miniscrew is placed at the desired location at one end of the line of action with a force applied to the tooth at the other end.

For example, Fig. 6-18 shows the point of force application in a patient where the desired treatment result was to retract the maxillary anterior teeth 7 mm, and change the upper incisor relationship from 120 to 100 degrees relative to sella-nasion.

Obviously, it is difficult to accurately predict tooth movement when using a continuous archwire. Moreover, applying σ^2 is limited clinically because it is determined experimentally from the maxillary canine rather than being the value obtained from all six maxillary anterior teeth. It can, however, at least provide guidelines for the proper positioning of miniscrews.

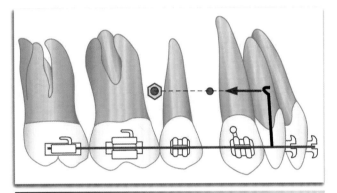

Fig. 6-11

Translation of anterior teeth using a miniscrew. The miniscrew and the arch wire hook should be placed at the level of the center of resistance and parallel to the occlusal plane.

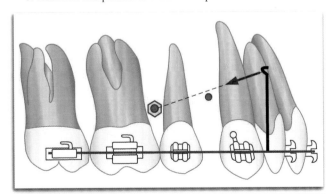

Fig. 6-12

Root movement of anterior teeth using a miniscrew. Relative to the anterior center of resistance, the arch wire hook should extend maximally above and the miniscrew placed below, respectively. When it is impossible to extend the hook above the center of resistance, increased curve of Spee may be bent into the arch wire to increase root movement.

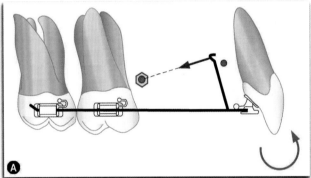

A

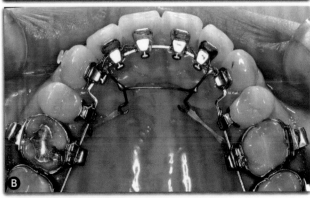

B

Fig. 6-13

Root movement of anterior teeth using a lingual miniscrew and lingual lever arm. **A,** Diagram of miniscrew in lingual alveolar bone with lingual appliance and lever arm placed as apical as possible in order to locate the line of action apical to the center of resistance, thereby making root movement possible. **B,** Occlusal photograph of lingual miniscrew and lever arm.

The following are some characteristics of orthodontic treatment using TADs:

1. Single force: The orthodontic force using a TAD is a single force that can be predicted. Tooth movement can be understood and easily controlled without complex biomechanics. However, all tooth movement cannot be achieved using a single force. Therefore, an additional force system might be required.

2. No reactive force: TADs provide absolute anchorage without being affected by an orthodontic force so that a reactive force and moment relative to the applied force do not occur. Therefore, it is possible to apply an orthodontic force without serious complications.

3. Statically determinate: When a single force from a TAD is applied to a single tooth or an isolated segment, a statically determinate force system becomes possible where the applied force and consequent moment can be accurately calculated. Tooth movement can be predicted more easily, even with continuous arch mechanics, because the orthodontic force from a TAD is a single force without a corresponding reaction force.

4. Systematic mechanical application: In contrast to traditional orthodontic treatment mechanics, the line of action can be controlled using TADs. Hence, a systematic approach is needed to apply TADs at the appropriate sites in order to achieve the desired tooth movement (Fig. 6-19).

CLINICAL APPLICATION

Multiple applications of TADs are possible, depending on the direction of desired tooth movement and the location of the TAD. Applications can be grouped into four main categories. To facilitate the selection of appropriate appliance design, each category is subdivided further based on the three planes of space (Fig. 6-20).

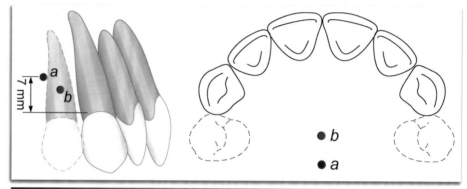

Fig. 6-14

Comparison of the position of the centers of resistance with fixation of the anterior teeth. (a) From study by Vanden Bulcke and colleagues[6,7]; (b) from study by Pedersen and colleagues.[8] (Redrawn from Matsui S, Caputo AA, Chaconas SJ, Kiyomura H. Center of resistance of anterior arch segment. *Am J Orthod Dentofacial Orthop.* 118:171-178, 2000; with permission from Elsevier.)

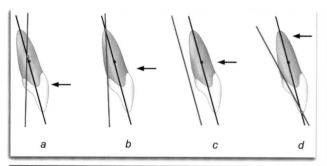

Fig. 6-15

Single force application and the changes in center of rotation. Note that center of rotation is red and the center of resistance is black. (a) Uncontrolled tipping (M:F = 0:1) occurs when a single force (arrow) is applied well below the center of resistance. (b) Controlled tipping (M:F = 5:1) occurs when a single force is applied slightly below the center of resistance. Note that the center of rotation is at the root apex. (c) Translation (M:F = 10:1) occurs when a single force is applied through the center of resistance. (d) Controlled root movement (M:F = 12:1) occurs when a single force is applied well above the center of resistance. Note that the center of rotation is at the incisal edge. M:F is Moment to Force ratio.

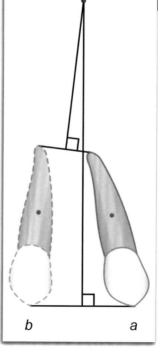

Fig. 6-16

Center of rotation of a tooth. Points *a* and *b* represent the cusp tip before and after movement, respectively. A line has been drawn connecting these points. At the midpoint of this line a perpendicular has been constructed. The point at which this perpendicular line intersects any other perpendicular line constructed in a similar manner (the apex is selected as the other point) is the center of rotation. (Redrawn from Smith RJ, Burstone CJ. Mechanics of tooth movement. *Am J Orthod.* 85:294-307, 1984; with permission from Elsevier.)

Type I is for anteroposterior tooth movement, type II is for vertical tooth movement, type III is for transverse tooth movement, and type IV is for applications that do not involve tooth movement. The Venn diagram of the malocclusion proposed by Proffit[13] has been modified to illustrate the classification of miniscrew applications.

Type I: Anteroposterior Tooth Movement

Type I TAD applications are designed for anteroposterior tooth movement and are divided further into four categories: (1) absolute anchorage, (2) distalization of the entire dentition, (3) molar distalization, and (4) mesial tooth movement.

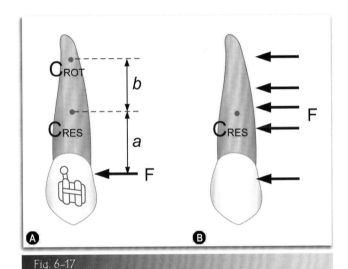

Fig. 6-17

General theory of tooth movement. **A,** The general theory of tooth movement states that the product of the distances *a* and *b* equals a constant (σ^2), $a \times b = \sigma^2$. **B,** σ^2 is a constant, provided that the single forces are parallel and act in the same plane. Any of the individual forces shown in **B** produces the same σ^2. C_{RES}, Center of resistance; C_{ROT}, center of rotation. (Redrawn from Nagerl H, Burstone CJ, Becker B, et al. Centers of rotation with transverse forces: an experimental study. *Am J Orthod Dentofacial Orthop.* 99:337-345, 1991; with permission from Elsevier.)

I-A: Absolute Anchorage

The term *anchorage,* in its orthodontic application, is defined as "resistance to unwanted tooth movement." When maximum retraction is needed, reinforcement of anchorage can be obtained by adding teeth within the same arch to the anchor unit, or by using elastics

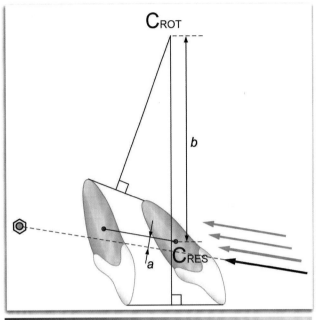

Fig. 6-18

Interrelationship between the C_{RES}, C_{ROT}, and force ($a \times b = \sigma^2$). Two points (root apex and incisal edge) are selected before *(right tooth)* and after *(left tooth)* tooth movement. The two points are then connected from one time period to the other. The point of intersection is the center of rotation *(red dot)* when a perpendicular line is drawn from the center of this line. When the distance *b* is measured from the center of resistance to the center of rotation (C_{RES} to C_{ROT} = 45 mm), the distance *a* from the center of resistance to the force (F to C_{RES} = 2.7 mm) can be calculated using the formula $a \times b = \sigma^2$, or $2.7 \times 45 = 123.7$ mm, which corresponds to palatal movement of the canine (Table 6-1). Based on this diagram, the miniscrew was placed on an extension of the calculated line of action and a single force was applied.

Table 6-1.	Position of Center of Resistance (C_R), σ^2 Values, and Force Direction			
Force Direction	C_R	C_R/L	σ^2 (cm^2)	σ^2/L^2
Labial	6.9	0.35	1.029	0.257
Distolabial	5.4	0.27	1.009	0.252
Distal	6.4	0.32	0.869	0.217
Distopalatal	6.6	0.33	1.028	0.257
Palatal	6.1	0.31	1.237	0.309
Mesiopalatal	6.9	0.35	0.885	0.221
Mesial	7.0	0.35	0.909	0.227
Mesiolabial	8.3	0.42	0.985	0.246

Modified from Nagerl H, Burstone CJ, Becker B, et al. Centers of rotation with transverse forces: an experimental study. *Am J Orthod Dentofacial Orthop.* 99:337-345, 1991; with permission from Elsevier. Center of resistance is measured from a uniform alveolar crest. Average standard deviation for C_R was 0.25 mm. Average standard deviation for σ^2 was 0.033 cm^2.

from the opposite arch. Additional resistance can be obtained with an extraoral device such as a headgear. With miniscrews, sufficient anchorage is provided to

withstand the reciprocal force produced by the retraction forces of the anterior teeth (Fig. 6-21). In this context, absolute anchorage refers to the need for complete retraction of anterior teeth into an extraction space without the posterior teeth moving forward at all.

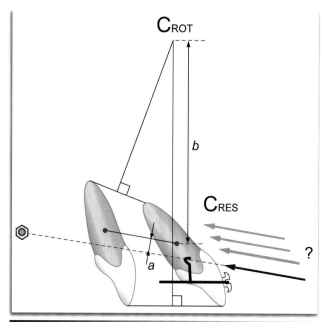

Fig. 6-19

Systemic mechanical application of miniscrew implants. First, determine C_{ROT}. Second, determine C_{RES}. Third, draw line of action. Fourth, determine miniscrew implant position and hook height. Fifth, verify tooth movement clinically.

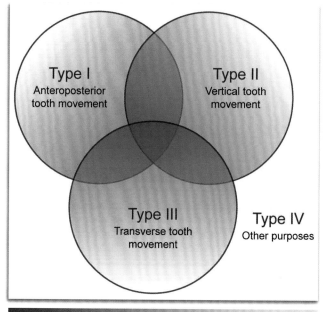

Fig. 6-20

Classification system for orthodontic miniscrew applications.

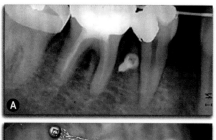
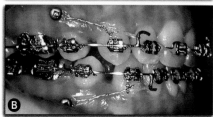
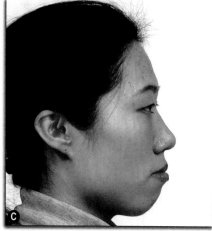
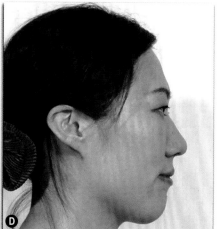

Fig. 6-21

A 22-year-old Korean woman had bidentoalveolar protrusion, severe lip protrusion, and mentalis strain on lip closure. Four first premolars were extracted. **A,** Periapical radiograph of miniscrew placed in interdental alveolar bone between second premolars and first molar. **B,** Right buccal photograph of active tiebacks[14] placed between soldered arch wire hooks and miniscrews for extraction space closure. **C,** Pretreatment facial profile photograph. **D,** Posttreatment facial profile photograph. Note that lip protrusion is greatly reduced. **E,** Cephalometric superimposition shows minimal change in molar position with maximal retraction of anterior teeth.

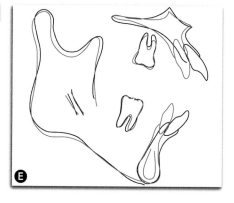

I–B: Distalization of the Entire Dentition

The entire dentition can be distalized using a TAD without the adjunctive use of an extraoral appliance. Miniscrews can be placed in the midpalatal area or in the buccal alveolar bone area to distalize the entire maxillary dentition (Fig. 6-22). For distalization of the mandibular dentition, miniscrews can be placed in the buccal alveolar bone or in the retromolar area. A greater amount of distal movement of the mandibular teeth is possible by placing miniscrews in the retromolar area where there is no concern for root interference (Fig. 6-23). For miniscrews placed in interdental bone, the total amount of distal movement is limited by root proximity. A miniscrew placed in the retromolar area should be located slightly buccal to the center of retromolar triangle. Depending primarily on the thickness of soft tissue, the miniscrew can be placed directly through the mucosa with its head exposed (open method) or placed beneath the mucosa with an emerging steel ligature hook (closed method) for force application (See Chapters 5 and 13). The term *retromolar knob* has been used to refer to a miniscrew placed in the retromolar area for distalization of the entire mandibular dentition (Fig. 6-24).

I–C: Molar Distalization

Molar distalization is used commonly in maxillary crowding cases with end-on Class II malocclusions. Traditional methods of molar distalization tend to cause unwanted movement of anterior teeth, however. Even with successful distalization, the initial arch length gained is frequently lost in the course of retracting the anterior teeth. With miniscrews, these shortcomings are overcome because the posterior teeth cannot slip forward (Fig. 6-25).

I–D: Mesial Tooth Movement

Mesial movement of posterior teeth is difficult to attain without any concomitant distal movement of anterior teeth because of inadequate anchorage. Miniscrews can be used to overcome this limitation and provide absolute anchorage for mesial movement of posterior teeth (Fig. 6-26).

Type II: Vertical Tooth Movement

Type II TAD applications are designed for vertical tooth movement and are divided further into three categories: (1) intrusion of the entire dentition, (2) various types of molar intrusion, and (3) various types of anterior intrusion. Because the need for tooth extrusion is much less common, the foregoing classification is related only to intrusion.

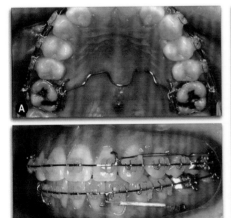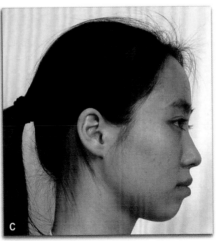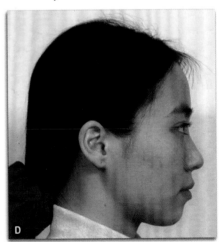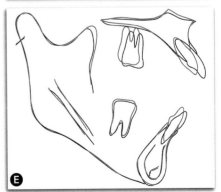

Fig. 6-22

An 18-year-old Korean woman had upper protrusion with mild mentalis strain on lip closure. Three miniscrews were placed: one in the midpalate and one between the right and left mandibular second premolars and first molars. **A,** Maxillary occlusal photograph showing traction force applied between midpalatal miniscrew and transpalatal bar to distalize maxillary dentition. **B,** Left buccal photograph showing traction force applied from miniscrews to soldered arch wire hooks in mandibular arch. **C,** Pretreatment facial profile photograph. **D,** Posttreatment facial profile photograph. Note improvement of lip protrusion with distal movement of upper and lower dentitions. **E,** Cephalometric superimposition shows distal movement of entire dentition.

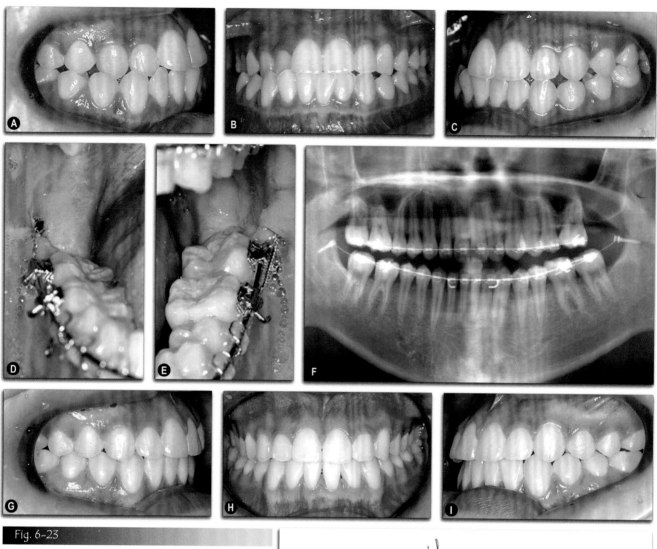

Fig. 6-23

A 16-year-old Korean girl had a skeletal Class III malocclusion and a large mandibular asymmetry. **A,** Pretreatment right buccal photograph. Note buccal crossbite. **B,** Pretreatment anterior photograph. Note midline deviation. **C,** Pretreatment left buccal photograph. **D,** Right occlusal photograph at initial miniscrew loading. Note steel ligature wire tied to retromolar knob (miniscrew head) to facilitate distal movement of mandibular dentition. **E,** Left occlusal photograph at initial miniscrew loading. **F,** Panoramic radiograph showing position of miniscrews. **G,** Posttreatment right buccal photograph. **H,** Posttreatment anterior photograph. Note alignment of dental midlines. **I,** Posttreatment left buccal photograph. **J,** Cephalometric superimposition shows distal movement of entire mandibular dentition and normal overjet.

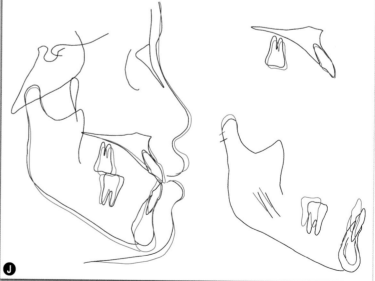

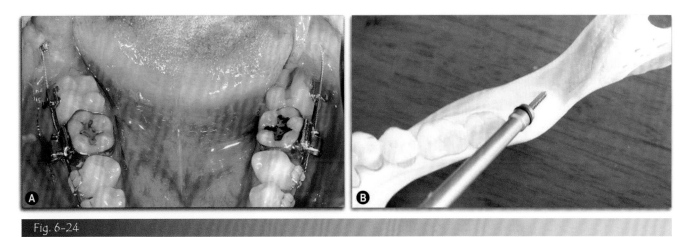

Fig. 6-24

Retromolar miniscrew implant position. **A,** The miniscrew head can be exposed *(left)* or submerged under mucosa *(right)* when placed in the retromolar area. **B,** Intraorally, palpation of the outer aspect of the oblique ridge helps to locate the optimal area for miniscrew placement. The most favorable placement site is slightly buccal to the center of the retromolar triangle.

II-A: Intrusion of the Entire Dentition

Control of the vertical dimension is probably the single most important factor in the correction of the hyperdivergent case. With effective intrusion of the entire maxillary arch, the mandible is allowed to rotate in an upward and forward direction, resulting in reduction of the anterior facial height (Fig. 6-27).[15]

II-B: Intrusion of Posterior Teeth

Although intrusion of anterior teeth is possible by using posterior teeth as anchorage, intrusion of posterior teeth is difficult because of inadequate dental anchorage. By using miniscrews as anchorage, intrusion of posterior teeth in both the maxilla and the mandible is possible (Fig. 6-28).

II-C: Intrusion of Anterior Teeth

In high-angle cases with a deep overbite and/or gummy smile, overbite reduction can occur only by the intrusion of the anterior teeth, without extruding the posterior teeth unless surgical intervention is planned. A miniscrew placed in the sub–anterior nasal spine region can be used for absolute intrusion of the upper anterior teeth. The miniscrew can be placed in one of two ways: either into the oral cavity or submerged under the soft tissue. This is often determined by the height of the labial frenum (Fig. 6-29). Miniscrew placement in the mandibular midline requires more care, however, because there is minimal interdental bone between the incisor roots.

Type III: Transverse Tooth Movement

Type III TAD applications are designed for transverse tooth movement and are divided further into two categories: (1) unilateral arch width correction and (2) dental midline correction.

III-A: Unilateral Transverse Tooth Movement

A miniscrew can be used for unilateral transverse tooth movement. This is accomplished by incorporating the TAD into traditional mechanics. For example, a transpalatal arch may be used to expand the upper arch with a unilateral crossbite. In this case, a miniscrew would be placed on the side opposite the crossbite to minimize expansion of that side (Figs. 6-30 and 6-31).

III-B: Correction of Dental Midline

Intermaxillary elastics are commonly used to align upper and lower dental midlines by applying an elastic force from one direction in one arch and in the opposite direction in the other arch. With this approach, however, both the upper and lower arches move. If the problem exists in only one arch, then a miniscrew can be used to slide the entire arch and midline in that direction (Fig. 6-32).

Type IV: Other Tooth Movement

Type IV TAD applications are designed for uses that do not involve tooth movement. Several applications are possible. In patients without orthodontic appliances, miniscrews can be used as replacements for surgical hooks with intermaxillary splint wiring during orthognathic surgery. In this case, the miniscrews are placed into the buccal cortical bone in interradicular locations (Fig. 6-33).[16] These same miniscrews can be used for intermaxillary fixation after jaw surgery using either steel ligatures or rubber elastics (Fig. 6-34).

REFERENCES

1. Proffit WR. Mechanical principles in orthodontic force control. In: Proffit WR, Fields HW Jr, eds. *Contemporary Orthodontics.* 3rd ed. St Louis, MO: Mosby, 2000:349-361.
2. Lindauer SJ, Isaacson RJ. One-couple orthodontic appliance systems. *Semin Orthod.* 1:12-24, 1995.
3. Scuzzo G, Takemoto K. Biomechanics and comparative biomechanics. In: Scuzzo G, Takemoto K, eds. *Invisible Orthodontics.* Carol Stream, IL: Quintessence, 2003:55-59.
4. Davidovitch M, Rebellato J. Two-couple orthodontic appliance systems utility arches: a two-couple intrusion arch. *Semin Orthod.* 1:25-30, 1995.
5. Isaacson RJ, Rebellato J. Two-couple orthodontic appliance systems: torquing arches. *Semin Orthod.* 1:31-36, 1995.
6. Vanden Bulcke MM, Dermaut LR, Burstone CJ, et al. The center of resistance of anterior teeth during intrusion using the laser reflection technique and holographic interferometry. *Am J Orthod Dentofacial Orthop.* 90:211-220, 1986.
7. Vanden Bulcke MM, Burstone CJ, Sachdeva RCL, et al. Location of the center of resistance for anterior teeth during retraction using the laser reflection technique. *Am J Orthod Dentofacial Orthop.* 91:375-384, 1987.
8. Pedersen E, Isidor F, Gjessing P, et al. Location of centers of resistance for maxillary anterior teeth measured on human autopsy material. *Eur J Orthod.* 13:452-458, 1991.

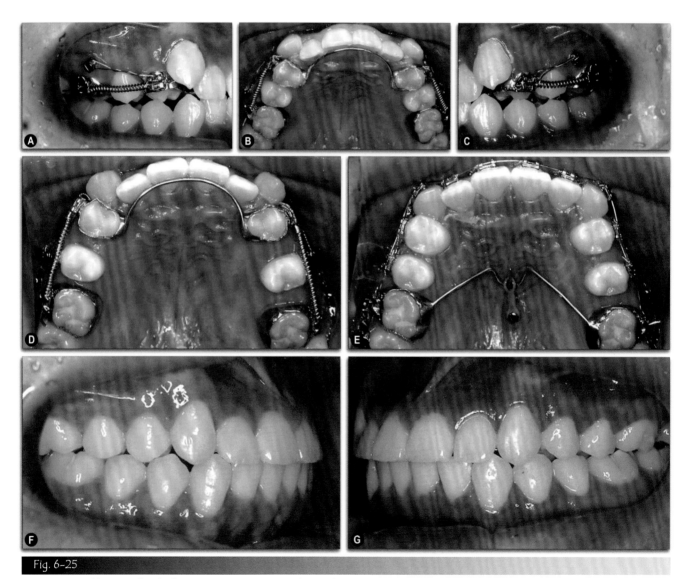

Fig. 6-25

An 11-year-old Korean boy had severe upper anterior crowding and a full Class II molar relationship. His parents insisted on nonextraction treatment; therefore, molar distalization was planned to resolve anterior crowding. **A,** Right buccal photograph at initial miniscrew loading. Note miniscrews placed between second premolar and first molar and used indirectly to stabilize the palatal arch. **B,** Maxillary occlusal photograph at initial miniscrew loading. Note that palatal wire was banded to first premolars. **C,** Left buccal photograph at initial miniscrew loading. **D,** Maxillary occlusal photograph after 12 months of miniscrew loading. **E,** Maxillary occlusal photograph showing palatal arch replaced by transpalatal arch. Note new miniscrew placed in midpalate with distal force applied to stabilize molars as anterior teeth were retracted. **F,** Posttreatment right buccal photograph. **G,** Posttreatment left buccal photograph. Note overcorrected Class I molar relationship.

9. Matsui S, Caputo AA, Chaconas SJ, Kiyomura H. Center of resistance of anterior arch segment. *Am J Orthod Dentofacial Orthop.* 118:171-178, 2000.
10. Smith RJ, Burstone CJ. Mechanics of tooth movement. *Am J Orthod* 85:294-307, 1984.
11. Nagerl H, Burstone CJ, Becker B, et al. Centers of rotation with transverse forces: an experimental study. *Am J Orthod Dentofacial Orthop.* 99:337-345, 1991.
12. Choy KC, Pae EK, Park YC, et al. Effect of root and bone morphology on the stress distribution in the periodontal ligament. *Am J Orthod Dentofacial Orthop.* 117:98-105, 2000.
13. Proffit WR. The development of a problem list. In: Proffit WR, Fields HW Jr, eds. *Contemporary Orthodontics.* 2nd ed. St Louis, MO: Mosby-Year Book, 1993:177.
14. McLaughlin RP, Bennett JC, Trevisi HJ. Space closure and sliding mechanics. In: *Systemized Orthodontic Treatment Mechanics.* Edinburgh, Scotland: Mosby, 2001:254-258.
15. Paik CH, Woo YJ, Boyd RL. Treatment of an adult patient with vertical maxillary excess using miniscrew fixation. *J Clin Orthod.* 37:423-428, 2003.
16. Paik CH, Woo YJ, Kim J, et al. Use of miniscrews for intermaxillary fixation of lingual-orthodontic surgical patients. *J Clin Orthod.* 36:132-136, 2002.

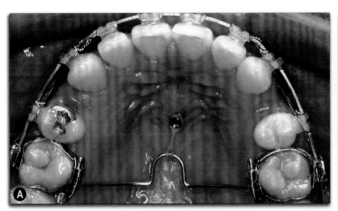 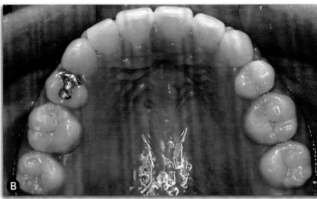

Fig. 6-26

Maxillary protraction mechanics. **A,** Maxillary occlusal photograph showing miniscrew placed in anterior midpalate to serve as stationary anchorage to translate two premolars and four molars mesially into extraction sites. **B,** Maxillary occlusal photograph showing mesial movement of posterior teeth without moving the anterior teeth posteriorly after 10 months of treatment.

(Figs. 6-27 to 6-34 continued on next page)

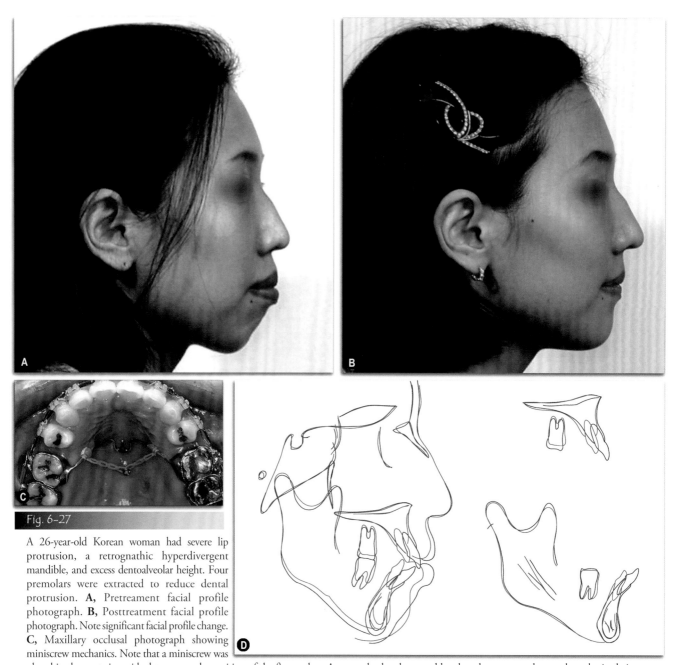

Fig. 6-27

A 26-year-old Korean woman had severe lip protrusion, a retrognathic hyperdivergent mandible, and excess dentoalveolar height. Four premolars were extracted to reduce dental protrusion. **A,** Pretreament facial profile photograph. **B,** Posttreatment facial profile photograph. Note significant facial profile change. **C,** Maxillary occlusal photograph showing miniscrew mechanics. Note that a miniscrew was placed in the posterior midpalate area at the position of the first molars. A transpalatal arch was soldered to the upper molars, and an elastic chain was stretched between the palatal arch and the midpalatal miniscrew. The transpalatal arch was offset from the palate to prevent impingement of the palatal soft tissue as the molars intruded. **D,** Cephalometric superimposition showing autorotation of mandible resulting from upper molar intrusion.

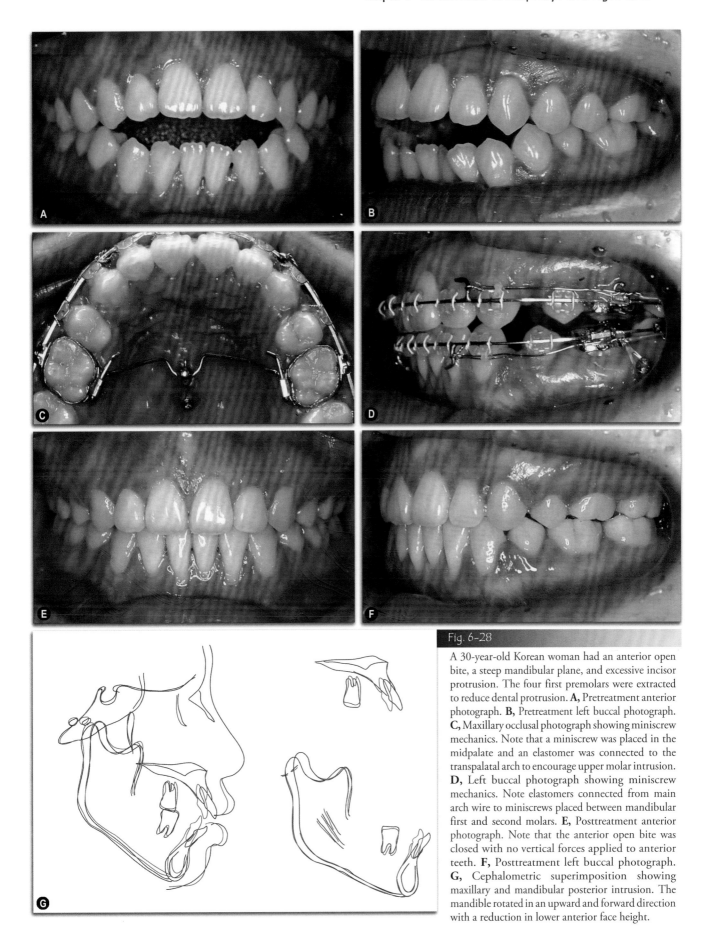

Fig. 6-28

A 30-year-old Korean woman had an anterior open bite, a steep mandibular plane, and excessive incisor protrusion. The four first premolars were extracted to reduce dental protrusion. **A,** Pretreatment anterior photograph. **B,** Pretreatment left buccal photograph. **C,** Maxillary occlusal photograph showing miniscrew mechanics. Note that a miniscrew was placed in the midpalate and an elastomer was connected to the transpalatal arch to encourage upper molar intrusion. **D,** Left buccal photograph showing miniscrew mechanics. Note elastomers connected from main arch wire to miniscrews placed between mandibular first and second molars. **E,** Posttreatment anterior photograph. Note that the anterior open bite was closed with no vertical forces applied to anterior teeth. **F,** Posttreatment left buccal photograph. **G,** Cephalometric superimposition showing maxillary and mandibular posterior intrusion. The mandible rotated in an upward and forward direction with a reduction in lower anterior face height.

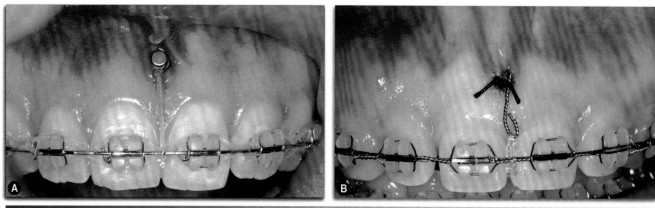

Fig. 6-29

Miniscrew emergence into oral cavity. **A,** Open technique. Miniscrew head is exposed when labial frenum is located so that its movement will not interfere with the miniscrew. **B,** Closed technique. Miniscrew is placed under mucosa, and only steel ligature (tied to miniscrew) is exposed intraorally. This is often necessary adjacent to a heavy frenum attachment.

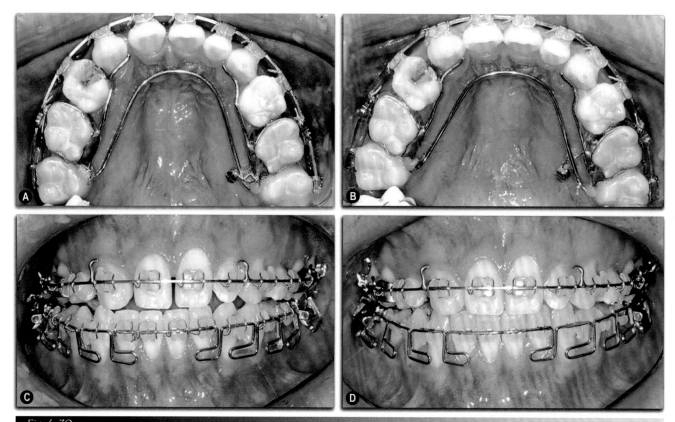

Fig. 6-30

Unilateral maxillary expansion. **A,** Maxillary occlusal photograph at initial miniscrew loading. Note W-arch cemented for upper arch expansion (on patient's right side). The left arm of the W-arch side of the arm was ligated to the miniscrew to prevent left side expansion and achieve unilateral expansion on the right. **B,** Maxillary occlusal photograph at completion of miniscrew loading. Note asymmetry of W-arch after correction. **C,** Anterior photograph at initial miniscrew loading. Note crossbite on patient's right side. **D,** Anterior photograph at completion of miniscrew loading. Note normal buccal overjet.

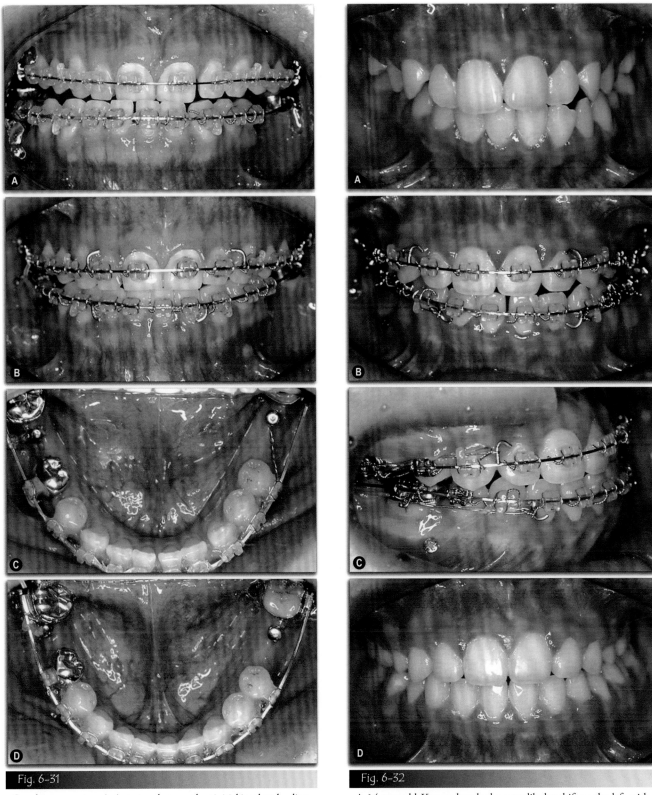

Fig. 6-31

Fig. 6-32

Crossbite correction. **A,** Anterior photograph at initial implant loading. Note anterior and right posterior crossbite. **B,** Anterior photograph after crossbite correction. Note optimal buccal overjet by constriction of right mandibular posterior teeth. **C,** Mandibular occlusal photograph at initial implant loading. Note initial position of miniscrews in edentulous area for unilateral arch constriction and distal movement of mandibular teeth. **D,** Mandibular occlusal photograph after crossbite correction. Note final miniscrew positions.

A 14-year-old Korean boy had a mandibular shift to the left with dental midline deviation. **A,** Pretreatment anterior photograph. Note left midline shift. **B,** Anterior photograph at initial miniscrew loading. **C,** Right buccal photograph at initial miniscrew loading. Note miniscrew placed between mandibular right first and second premolars to shift the lower dental midline to right. **D,** Posttreatment anterior photograph. Note midline and mandibular asymmetry correction.

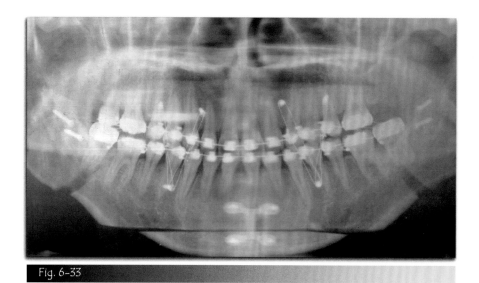

Fig. 6-33

Miniscrews placed in facial alveolar bone used for intermaxillary wire fixation after orthognathic surgery.

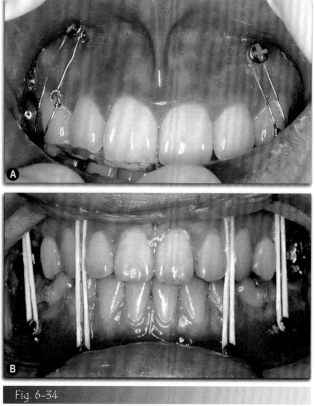

Fig. 6-34

Intermaxillary fixation. **A,** Steel ligature fixation, **B,** Elastic fixation.

Intraoral Hard and Soft Tissue Dimensions for Temporary Anchorage Device Placement

Antonio Costa

Temporary anchorage devices[1] (TADs) are useful in orthodontic cases in which patients do not have a sufficient number of teeth to provide traditional dental anchorage[2,3] or for esthetic reasons.[4] One limitation to these devices, however, is the anatomy underlying the superficial soft tissues, as well as individual anatomic variation. This makes it difficult to consistently place devices without the risk of damaging adjacent interalveolar vital structures. The interalveolar spaces increase in buccolingual width[5] from the cementoenamel junction to the apical region. Some authors[6-8] have suggested only placing TADs in the apical regions because there is a decreased risk of touching tooth roots. This, however, usually means that the TADs will be located in mobile mucosa, which may predispose the TADs to inflammation and subsequent failure. To clarify what sites might be candidates for TAD placement, this project was designed to identify both intraalveolar and extraalveolar sites for TAD placement and to establish some hard and soft tissue thickness guidelines within the oral cavity.

STUDY DESIGN

Intraalveolar Bone Dimension

In a study of human skulls, a group of 20 white male skulls of European descent were acquired from the Human Anatomy Institute at the University of Siena in Italy. The age range was 20 to 40 years old. Seven interradicular regions of interest (ROI) in both the maxillary and mandibular arches were chosen to study the intraalveolar hard tissue dimensions. Mesiodistal bone interradicular widths were measured mesial to each tooth with an Absolute Digimatic Caliper (Mitutoyo, West Point Business Park, Andover, Hampshire, United Kingdom; resolution 0.01 mm). The measurements for all 14 ROIs were taken perpendicular to the occlusal plane. At each horizontal ROI (between each extracted tooth socket), a measurement was taken at the alveolar crestal, midroot, and apical bone levels (Fig. 7-1). All measurements were taken twice and were averaged (Table 7-1).

Extraalveolar Bone Dimension and Mucosal Depth

In a separate study of clinical patients, a group of 20 white males with normal maxillomandibular relationships (ANB = 2 degrees ± 2 degrees) were chosen. This was a subgroup of patients who had been selected for TAD placement based on anchorage requirements and who consented to be participants in the study. The age range was 20 to 40 years old. Ten extraalveolar ROIs in the oral cavity were chosen to study the hard and soft tissue dimensions. The terminology for the anatomic ROI was based on standard definitions[9] but was modified slightly to narrow the ROI for clarity.

Bone depths were quantified using volumetric CT scans (NewTom, QR Srl, Verona, Italy). The settings were as follows: scan time of 75 seconds; time of distribution ray, 36 seconds; 110 kV; 15 mA. The measurements for all 10 ROI, except the retromolar area and the midpalatal region, were taken in transaxial sections at 45 degrees (maxilla) or 30 degrees (mandible) relative to the long axis of the adjacent teeth.[12] In the retromolar area and in the midpalatal region, the measurement was taken parallel to the long axis of the

adjacent molar. In the upper and lower canine fossae and in the submaxillary fossa an addition measurement perpendicular to the occlusal section was recorded (Table 7-2).

For each bone depth data set at all of the ROIs evaluated, a chart was constructed to determine whether TADs of lengths ranging from 4 mm to 12 mm, in 2-mm increments (4, 6, 8, 10, and 12 mm), would have rested completely within the available bone of the patient population studied or would have perforated the contralateral bony cortex. The data were pooled according to ROI and were expressed as the number of perforations out of a total of 20 patients, as well as the percentage of perforations (Table 7-3).

Soft tissue depth[10,11] was recorded by piercing the mucosa with a 32-gauge mesotherapy needle (Biotekne; Gallini Mirandola, Modena, Italy) until the attached rubber stop rested on the mucosa. The distance between the stop and the end of the needle was measured by an Absolute Digimatic Caliper. In regions of mobile alveolar mucosa, the depth was measured by stretching the soft tissues taught. All measurements were taken 3 times and were averaged (Table 7-2).

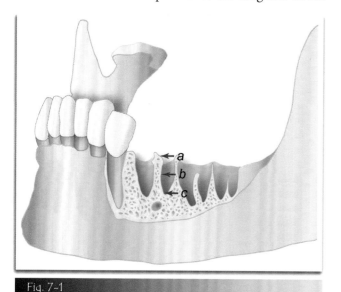

Fig. 7-1

Intraalveolar bone measurements. Mesiodistal interradicular bone widths were measured at the alveolar crest level *(a)*, the midroot level *(b)*, and the apical level *(c)*.

Table 7-1.			Mesiodistal Interradicular Bone Width									
						Bone Width (mm)						
		Coronal Third				Middle Third				Apical Third		
	Min	Max	Mean	SD	Min	Max	Mean	SD	Min	Max	Mean	SD
MAXILLA												
Central incisor	0.27	2.32	1.12	0.87	1.30	5.99	3.76	1.48	3.07	8.59	6.12	1.53
Lateral incisor	0.23	3.51	1.08	1.37	0.6	4.2	1.92	0.76	1.30	4.64	2.94	0.94
Canine	0.53	2.13	1.63	2.03	0.68	4.36	2.52	1.02	0.51	9.60	3.0	1.38
First premolar	0.28	5.00	1.07	1.05	0.86	3.91	2.36	0.48	1.09	5.21	3.45	1.05
Second premolar	0.32	3.19	1.14	0.83	0.71	4.20	2.16	1.14	0.99	6.63	3.45	1.54
First molar	0.33	4.57	1.17	0.96	0.82	4.46	2.24	0.85	1.05	7.08	4.6	1.86
Second molar	0.28	2.37	1.22	0.87	1.21	5.83	2.74	1.32	0.79	5.28	3.38	1.19
MANDIBLE												
Central incisor	0.17	3.0	1.0	0.76	0.81	5.87	2.22	1.14	0.62	3.47	1.63	0.69
Lateral incisor	0.24	1.53	0.72	0.32	1.24	7.28	3.41	1.45	1.13	4.17	2.65	0.80
Canine	0.25	1.68	0.79	0.35	0.58	2.89	1.78	0.64	0.97	5.80	3.76	1.24
First premolar	0.01	1.81	0.81	0.50	0.64	3.31	2.17	0.67	1.20	5.55	3.98	0.83
Second premolar	0.23	2.73	1.12	0.72	0.86	4.64	2.55	1.08	1.94	6.08	4.13	1.16
First molar	0.24	6.83	1.56	1.7	1.01	6.50	2.6	1.28	1.67	7.61	4.38	1.61
Second molar	0.33	2.37	1.38	1.17	0.53	4.91	2.85	1.35	1.13	7.28	4.6	1.86

Anatomic Regions of Interest
Maxillary Facial

Incisive fossa: limited distally by the canine eminence, inferiorly by the apices of the incisors, and superiorly by the nasal cavity (Fig. 7-2)

Canine fossa: limited mesially by the canine eminence, inferiorly by the apex of the first premolar and superiorly by the medial portion of the maxillary sinus and the projecting zygomatic process (Fig. 7-3)

Infrazygomatic ridge: limited distally by the zygomatic ridge, inferiorly by the apex of the mesial root of the first molar, and superiorly by the medial portion of the maxillary sinus and the projecting zygomatic process (Fig. 7-4)

Maxillary Palatal

Premaxillary region: paramedial area of the premaxillary region of the palate limited laterally by the incisors and canine roots and medially by the incisive foramen (Fig. 7-5)

Midpalatal region: limited anteroposteriorly between the first and second premolars and medially by the midpalatal suture (Fig. 7-6)

Mandibular Facial

Symphysis: limited bilaterally by the canine eminences, inferiorly by the mental tubercles, and superiorly by the incisor apices (Fig. 7-7)

Canine fossa: limited mesially by the canine eminence, distally by the mental foramen, superiorly by the first premolar apex, and inferiorly by the mandibular inferior border (Fig. 7-8)

Anterior external oblique ridge: limited laterally by the external oblique ridge and medially by the facial bone of the second molar (Fig. 7-9)

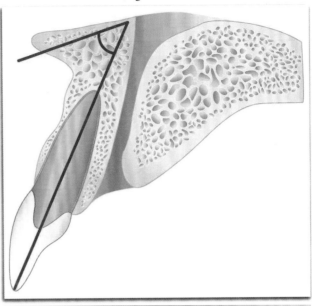

Fig. 7-2

Transaxial diagram of incisive fossa. Note insertion angle was at 45 degrees relative to tooth long axis.

Table 7-2.	Bone and Soft Tissue Depths							
	Bone Depth (mm)				Mucosal Depth (mm)			
	Min	Max	Mean	SD	Min	Max	Mean	SD
MAXILLA								
Incisive fossa	4.3	9.6	7.22	1.40	2.0	3.8	2.83	0.46
Canine fossa	5.9	11.0	8.57	1.26	1.4	2.7	2.15	0.30
Canine fossa*	5.9	8.2	6.95	0.72				
Infrazygomatic ridge	2.7	4.4	3.64	0.54	2.1	2.9	2.57	0.18
Premaxillary region	7.1	13.1	10.57	1.57	2.8	4.2	3.38	0.45
Midpalatal region	4.2	7.3	5.81	0.85	2.3	3.8	3.06	0.45
MANDIBLE								
Symphysis	12.0	16.0	13.5	1.40	1.9	3.4	2.65	0.35
Canine fossa	5.9	13.0	9.97	2.40	1.8	3.0	2.56	0.36
Canine fossa*	6.6	8.8	7.66	0.60				
Anterior external oblique ridge	9.4	15.5	11.65	1.53	1.5	3.2	2.43	0.47
Retromolar area	11.0	16.0	13.55	1.23	2.3	4.0	3.02	0.44
Submaxillary fossa	9.4	14.0	11.28	1.15	1.5	2.8	2.10	0.35
Submaxillary fossa†	3.5	4.9	4.02	0.41				

*Measurement taken distal to canine eminence and perpendicular to occlusal plane.
†Measurement taken distal to first premolar root and perpendicular to occlusal plane.

Table 7-3.					Risk of Contralateral Cortex Perforation for Incremental Increases in TAD Length					
	Temporary Anchorage Device Length (mm)									
	4 mm		6 mm		8 mm		10 mm		12 mm	
	No. Perf.	%	No. Perf.	%	No. Perf.	%	No. Perf.	%	No. Perf.	%
MAXILLA										
Incisive fossa	0/20	0	4/20	20	13/20	65	20/20	100	20/20	100
Canine fossa	0/20	0	1/20	5	6/20	30	17/20	85	20/20	100
Canine fossa*	0/20	0	1/20	5	17/20	85	20/20	100	20/20	100
Infrazygomatic ridge	14/20	70	20/20	100	20/20	100	20/20	100	20/20	100
Premaxillary region	0/20	0	0/20	0	1/20	5	6/20	40	15/20	75
Midpalatal region	0/20	0	12/20	60	20/20	100	20/20	100	20/20	100
MANDIBLE										
Symphysis	0/20	0	0/20	0	0/20	0	0/20	0	0/20	0
Canine fossa	0/20	0	0/20	0	6/20	30	8/20	40	15/20	75
Canine fossa*	0/20	0	0/20	0	13/20	65	20/20	100	20/20	100
Anterior external oblique ridge	0/20	0	0/20	0	0/20	0	3/20	15	14/20	70
Retromolar area	0/20	0	0/20	0	0/20	0	0/20	0	1/20	5
Submaxillary fossa	0/20	0	0/20	0	0/20	0	3/20	15	12/20	60
Submaxillary fossa†	10/20	50	20/20	100	20/20	100	20/20	100	20/20	100

*Measurement taken distal to canine eminence and perpendicular to occlusal plane.
†Measurement taken distal to first premolar root and perpendicular to occlusal plane.

Retromolar area: limited mesially by the distal surface of the second molar, laterally by the external oblique ridge, and superiorly by the ascending ramus (Fig. 7-10)

Mandibular Lingual

Submaxillary fossa: limited anteroposteriorly between the roots of the first and second premolars (parallel to the tooth long axis), superiorly by the apices of the premolars, and inferiorly by the mandibular inferior border (Fig. 7-11)

RESULTS
Intraalveolar Bone Dimension

In the maxilla, the mean value of the crestal bone width ranged from 1.07 to 1.63 mm. The greatest width was located between the lateral incisor and canine. The remainder of the measurements were less than 1.22 mm. For the midroot bone, the mean value of the bone width ranged from 3.76 to 1.92 mm. The greatest width was located between the central incisors, whereas the narrowest width was located between the central and lateral incisors. For the apical bone, the mean value of the bone width ranged from 2.94 to 6.12 mm. The greatest width was located between the central incisors. The second greatest width was located between the second premolar and first molar.

In the mandible, the mean value of the crestal bone width ranged from 0.72 to 1.56 mm. The greatest widths were located mesial to the first and second molars. The remainder of the measurements were less than 1.12 mm. For the midroot bone, the mean value of the bone width ranged from 1.78 to 3.41 mm. Other than mesial to the lateral incisors, the greatest widths were located posteriorly—mesial to the molars and second premolar. For the apical bone, the mean value of the bone width ranged from 1.63 to 4.38 mm. The greatest widths were located posteriorly—mesial to the molars and second premolar.

Extraalveolar Bone Dimension and Mucosal Depth
Maxillary Facial

Incisive fossa: The mean value of the mucosal depth was 2.83 mm. The mean value of the bone depth was 7.22 mm. If TADs had been placed, all of the 4-mm TADs would have resided completely within bone. For the 6-mm and 8-mm TADs, 20% and 65% would have perforated the contralateral cortex, respectively. All of the 10-mm and 12-mm TADs would have perforated the contralateral cortex.

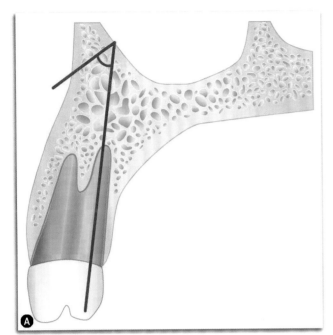

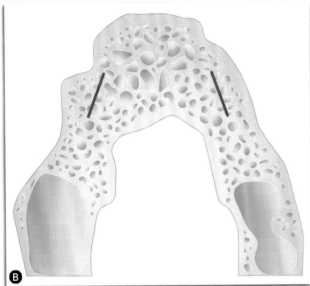

Fig. 7-3

Transaxial diagram of maxillary canine fossa. **A,** Note insertion angle was at 45 degrees relative to tooth long axis. **B,** Occlusal view showing location of slice *(red line)*.

Canine fossa: The mean value of the mucosal depth was 2.15 mm. The mean value of the bone depth was 11.0 mm. If TADs had been placed, all of the 4-mm TADs would have resided completely within bone. For the 6-mm and 8-mm TADs, only a small number would have perforated the contralateral cortex: 5% and 30%, respectively. The majority of the 10-mm and 12-mm TADs would have perforated the contralateral cortex.

The mean value of the bone depth perpendicular to the occlusal plane was 6.95 mm. If TADs had

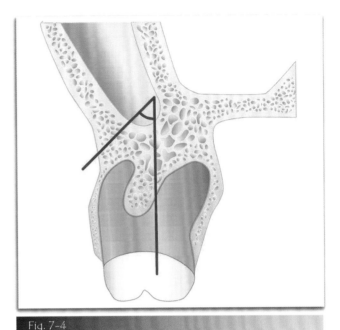

Fig. 7-4

Transaxial diagram of infrazygomatic ridge. Note insertion angle was at 45 degrees relative to tooth long axis.

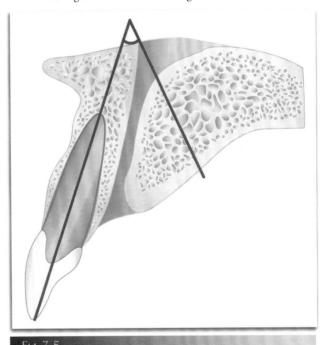

Fig. 7-5

Transaxial diagram of premaxillary region. Note insertion angle was at 45 degrees relative to tooth long axis.

been placed, all of the 4-mm TADs would have resided completely within bone, and only 5% of the 6-mm TADs would have perforated the contralateral cortex. The 8-mm TADs, however, would have perforated the contralateral cortex 85% of the time. All of the 10-mm and 12-mm TADs would have perforated the contralateral cortex.

Infrazygomatic ridge: The mean value of the

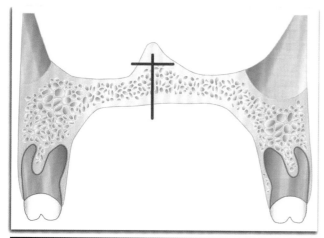

Fig. 7-6

Transaxial diagram of midpalatal region. Note insertion angle was parallel to tooth long axis.

mucosal depth was 2.57 mm. The mean value of the bone depth was 3.64 mm. Because the bone depth was much smaller, almost all of the TADs placed in this region would have perforated the contralateral cortex.

Maxillary Palatal

Premaxillary region: The mean value of the mucosal depth was 3.38 mm. The mean value of the bone depth was 10.57 mm. If TADs had been placed, only a small minority of the 4-, 6-, or 8-mm TADs would have perforated the contralateral cortex. A larger number of the 10-mm (40%) and 12-mm (75%) TADs would have perforated the contralateral cortex.

Midpalatal region: The mean value of the mucosal depth was 3.06 mm. The mean value of the bone depth was 5.81 mm. If TADs had been placed, all of the 4-mm TADs would have resided completely within bone. The remainder of the TADs would have perforated the contralateral cortex.

Mandibular Facial

Symphysis: The mean value of the mucosal depth was 2.65 mm. The mean value of the bone depth was 13.5 mm. If TADs had been placed, all of the TADS, regardless of length, would have resided completely within bone.

Canine fossa: The mean value of the mucosal depth was 2.56 mm. The mean value of the bone depth was 9.97 mm. If TADs had been placed, all of the 4-mm and 6-mm TADs would have resided completely within bone. For the 8-mm and 10-mm TADs, only 30% and 40% would have perforated the contralateral cortex, respectively. For the

Fig. 7-7

Transaxial diagram of symphysis. Note insertion angle was at 30 degrees relative to tooth long axis.

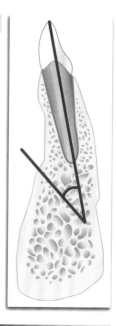

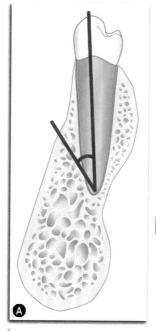

A

Fig. 7-8

Transaxial diagram of mandibular canine fossa. **A,** Note insertion angle was at 30 degrees relative to tooth long axis. **B,** Occlusal view showing location of slice *(red line)*.

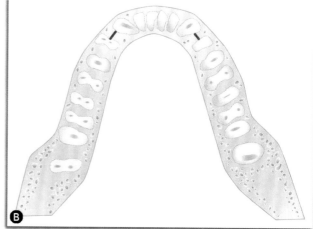

B

12-mm TADs, 75% would have perforated the contralateral cortex.

The mean value of the bone depth perpendicular to the occlusal plane was 7.66 mm. If TADs had been placed, all of the 4-mm and 6-mm TADs would have resided completely within bone. For the rest of the TADs, the majority would have perforated the contralateral cortex.

Anterior external oblique ridge: The mean value of the mucosal depth was 2.43 mm. The mean value of the bone depth was 11.65 mm. If TADs had been placed, all of the 4-mm, 6-mm,

8-mm, and 85% of the 10-mm TADs would have resided completely within bone. For the 12-mm TADs, 70% would have perforated the contralateral cortex.

Retromolar area: The mean value of the mucosal depth was 3.02 mm. The mean value of the bone depth was 13.55 mm. If TADs had been

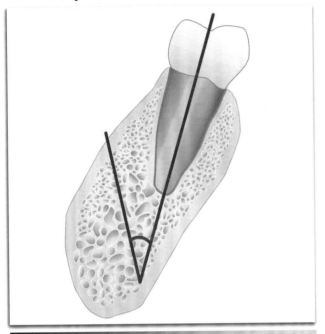

Fig. 7-9

Transaxial diagram of anterior external oblique line. Note insertion angle was at 30 degrees relative to tooth long axis.

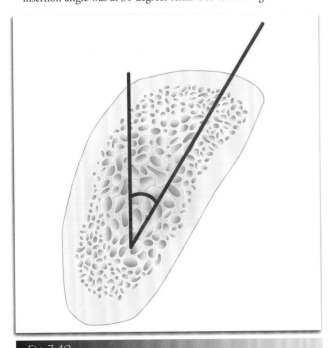

Fig. 7-10

Transaxial diagram of retromolar area. Note insertion angle parallel to tooth long axis.

placed, only one of the 12-mm TADs would have perforated the contralateral cortex.

Mandibular Lingual

Submaxillary fossa: The mean value of the mucosal depth was 2.1 mm. The mean value of the bone depth was 11.28 mm. The mean value of the bone depth perpendicular to the occlusal plane was 4.02 mm. If TADs had been placed, all of the 4-, 6-, and 8-mm TADs would have resided completely within bone. Only 15% of the 10-mm and 60% of the 12-mm TADs would have perforated the contralateral cortex.

The mean value of the bone depth perpendicular to the occlusal plane was 4.02 mm. If TADs had

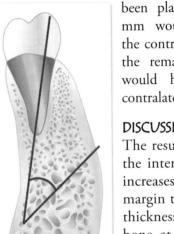

been placed, half of the 4-mm would have perforated the contralateral cortex. All of the remaining TAD lengths would have perforated the contralateral cortex.

DISCUSSION

The results demonstrate that the interalveolar bone width increases from the alveolar margin to the apical tip. The thickness of the interalveolar bone at the crestal and the midroot levels suggest that these locations are generally insufficient for the placement of TADs because the mean

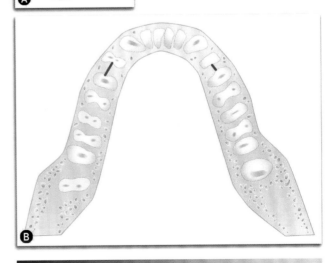

Fig. 7-11

Transaxial diagram of submaxillary fossa. **A,** Note insertion angle was at 30 degrees relative to tooth long axis. **B,** Occlusal view showing location of slice *(red line).*

values are usually less than 4 mm,[12] whereas the bone width at the apical level is more sufficient to host TADs. Using panoramic radiographs, however, Schnelle and colleagues[13] suggested that several specific midroot sites often have sufficient bone for miniscrew implant (MSI) placement. The most common site was between the second premolar and first molar, which is an ideal location for en masse retraction of anterior teeth in extraction cases.

In the anterior maxilla the interradicular bone dimensions suggest that two specific sites may be applicable to TAD placement: between the roots of the central incisors and between the lateral incisor and canine. This can be explained by the common distal tip of the central incisors and mesial tip of the lateral incisors, which provide more interradicular bone mesial to the central incisors and distal to the lateral incisors. These two sites would be applicable for MSI placement for delivery of an intrusive force in correcting and deep bite. One concern, however, that may prevent the placement of an MSI between the central incisor roots is the maxillary frenum, because it might cause soft tissue problems around the MSI. The posterior maxillary data suggest that TADs can generally be placed consistently in the apical region mesial to the second molar and premolars because of the average mesiodistal bone width of approximately 3.5 mm.

The anterior mandibular measurements generally preclude placement of MSIs because the measurement from the crest of the alveolar ridge to the apical region is generally less than 2.5 mm. One alternative, if an MSI is needed in this area, might be to angle the MSI apically upon placement in order to minimize potential contact with the tooth roots. The posterior mandibular data indicate that an MSI can be placed in the apical region between all posterior teeth because the measurements are all 4 mm or greater.

It is important to interpret this data with caution. It should be recalled that the data are pooled and averaged. The information is valuable in that it provides general guidelines of bone widths. However, just as it is common for maxillary lateral incisors to be tipped mesially toward the central incisors, thereby providing ample bone for MSI placement distal to the lateral incisors, it is possible that the lateral incisors present with a distal tip and hence provide more bone stock mesial to the lateral incisors for MSI placement. If sufficient bone is not available for MSI placement without the risk of MSI-root contact, it is always possible to move the roots apart before MSI placement.

The use of volumetric computed tomography[14] provides a method to presurgically analyze the inclination and depth of planned TAD insertion. Additionally, the amount of radiation exposed to the patient is less than with other types of tomography.[15,16] The data herein suggest that ample amounts of bone are available in extraalveolar bone for placing TADs, which would minimize the risk of hitting tooth roots.[17,18] In some instances, placing TADs in these areas may allow force placement closer to the center of resistance of the tooth.[19] However, one potential problem of placing TADs in extraalveolar bony sites is the lack of keratinized mucosa available; that is, that if placed extraalveolarly, the TAD will lay in mobile alveolar mucosa, possibly causing problems.[20,21]

The results indicate that TADs of specific lengths should be considered for each ROI available. For example, any length TAD up to 12 mm can be safely placed in the bone of the symphysis, whereas TADs up to 10 mm can be placed safely in the retromolar area. However, the data from the 20 patients herein suggest that the incisive fossa, the maxillary canine fossa, and the midpalatal region should have TADs of 4 mm placed. Although these data are important in providing guidelines, it must be stressed that the data are derived from only 20 patients and that considerable individual variation exists within and between patients. Therefore, each patient should be evaluated for different TAD lengths in all ROIs.

When considering the soft tissues associated with TAD placement, it is important to determine the type of soft tissue, whether keratinized masticatory mucosa or mobile alveolar mucosa, in which the TAD will reside. Although it is possible for TADs to be placed in mobile mucosa, the mucosa often covers the abutment component of the TAD, making it difficult to alter orthodontic mechanics during treatment without a minor surgical uncovering procedure.

SUMMARY

The results demonstrate that for intraalveolar MSI placement, the more apical the MSI is placed, the better. In addition, several extraalveolar regions available for the placement of TADs in length ranging from 4 mm to 12 mm. For extraalveolar sites in general, TADs 4 mm to 6 mm in length are safe in most regions. However, individual patient variation dictates that individual evaluation of bone depth occur in all patients. Because many of these extraalveolar regions are covered by mobile masticatory mucosa, soft tissue inflammation and coverage may occur over the TADs.

REFERENCES

1. Kanomi R. Mini-implant for orthodontic anchorage. *J Clin Orthod.* 1:763-767, 1997.
2. Melsen B, Petersen J K, Costa A. Zygoma ligatures: an alternative form of maxillary anchorage. *J Clin Orthod.* 32:154-158, 1998.
3. Daimaruya T, Nagasaka H, Unemori M, et al. The influences of molar intrusion on the inferior alveolar neurovascular bundle and root using the skeletal anchorage system in dogs. *Angle Orthod.* 71:60-70, 2001.
4. Costa A, Dalstra M, Melsen B. L'Aarhus Anchorage System. *Ortognatodonzia Italiana.* 9:480-489, 2000.
5. Costa A, Levrini L, Tagliabue A. Osteointegrazione negli impianti come ancoraggio ortodontico. *Ital J Oral Implantol.* 2:133-139, 2000.
6. Costa A, Gnech G, Doldo T, Giorgetti R. Value of the intralveolar bone thickness for the insertion of orthodontic anchorages. Paper presented at: XVII Annual Meeting SIDO; October 1-4, 2003; Florence, Italy.
7. Borah GL, Ashmead D. The fate of teeth transfixed by osteosynthesis screw. *Plast Reconstr Surg.* 97:726-729, 1996.
8. Kyung HM, Park HS, Bae SM, et al. Development of orthodontic micro-implants of intraoral anchorage. *J Clin Orthod.* 37:321-328, 2003.
9. Moore KL. The head. In: Moore KL, ed. *Clinically Oriented Anatomy.* 2nd ed. Baltimore: Williams & Wilkins, 1985:794-982.
10. Wara-aswapati N, Pitiphat W, Chandrapho N, et al. Thickness of palatal masticatory mucosa associated with age. *J Periodontol.* 72:10, 2001.
11. Costa A, Doldo T, Giorgetti R. Evaluation of oral tissue thickness for the insertion of orthodontic implants (abstract). *Eur J Orthod.* 25:429, 2003.
12. Park HS, Bae SM, Kyung HM, et al. Micro-implant anchorage for treatment of skeletal Class I bialveolar protrusion. *J Clin Orthod.* 35:417-422, 2001.
13. Schelle M, Beck FM, Jaynes R, Huja SS. A radiograph evaluation of the availability of bone for placement of miniscrews. *Angle Orthod.* 74:832-837, 2004.
14. Siewerdscn JH, Jaffray DA. Cone-beam computed tomography with a flat-panel imagery. *Med Phys.* 26:2635-2647, 1999.
15. Mozzo P, Procacci C, Tacconi A, et al. A new volumetric CT machine for dental imaging based on the cone beam technique: preliminary results. *Eur Radiol.* 8:1558-1564, 1998.
16. Hassfeld S, Streib S, Stahl H, et al. Low-dose-computertomographie des kiefernochens in der praimplantologischen. *Diagnostik Mund Kiefer Gesichts Chir.* 2:188-193, 1998.
17. Ohmae M, Saito S, Morohashi T, et al. A clinical and histological evaluation of titanium mini-implants as anchors for orthodontic intrusion in the beagle dog. *Am J Orthod Dentofacial Orthop.* 119:489-497, 2001.
18. Unemori M, Sugawara J, Mitani H, et al. Skeletal anchorage system for open-bite correction. *Am J Orthod.* 115:166-174, 1999.
19. Costa A, Raffaini M, Melsen B. Miniscrew as orthodontic anchorage: a preliminary report. *Int J Adult Orthodon Orthognath Surg.* 3:201-209, 1998.
20. Melsen B, Costa A. Immediate loading of implants used for orthodontic anchorage. *Clin Orthod Res.* 3:23-28, 2000.
21. Costa A. Impianti a vite come ancoraggio ortodontico. *Mondo Ortod* 6:481-886, 2001.

CHAPTER 8

Potential Complications with OrthoTADs: Classification, Prevention, and Treatment

John W. Graham, Jason B. Cope

The current enthusiasm for orthodontic temporary anchorage devices (OrthoTADs) has encouraged a great number of orthodontists to get involved in this fast-growing and challenging field. Most, however, are not formally trained in the placement and use of TADs and have treated few cases. This situation may initially result in a high number of complications, which may inaccurately lead to the presumption that the procedure is ineffective. This false assumption, fortunately, may be disproved by understanding proper placement techniques. As has been demonstrated in numerous case reports, OrthoTAD placement is predictable and stable.[1-5] However, implementation of the procedure by clinicians without adequate training in the basic biologic and biomechanical fundamentals germane to OrthoTADs may lead to less-than-ideal treatment results or even complications.

Often when a new technique, procedure, or appliance is developed, the developers, being involved from the beginning, understand all too well the possible pitfalls encountered during implementation. This may create the illusion for others that the procedure is technically simple. The difference is experience. To quote James Boswell, "Men are wise in proportion, not to their experience, but to their capacity for experience."

Experience can be gained three ways. First, it can be ascertained indirectly by obtaining fundamental knowledge before the fact. Second, it can be *borrowed* by learning from the success and failures of other experiencing complications firsthand. This chapter was written to cover the first two by presenting basic facts about anatomy, TADs, and biomechanics and by reporting the complications of others as reported in the literature. In so doing, the hope is that the complications experienced firsthand will be significantly minimized. In addition, a classification system of TAD-related complications is outlined.

TERMS AND DEFINITIONS

A review of the TAD-related literature reveals several types of definitions of complications ranging from any unwanted event during treatment such as minor pain,[6] cheek irritation,[7] swelling/pain after flap closure,[8] soft tissue inflammation,[6-8] and screw tipping or migration[4] to problems that change the outcome of treatment such as soft tissue overgrowth,[10] periimplant infection,[11] screw failure caused by rotational forces,[12] screw loosening,[6,8,11] screw failure,[10] plate loosening,[13] root shortening,[14] and intrusion-associated root resorption.[14-17] The former suggests that even expected (but unwanted) sequelae such as temporary postoperative edema or discomfort should be considered complications. The latter may actually narrow the group of complications to only those that produce unexpected problems. In clinical practice, however, identical complications (i.e., inadequate cortical purchase) may seriously affect the treatment outcome in one patient and minimally affect the treatment outcome in another patient. Alternatively, some minor short-term problems such as soft tissue impingement may produce

In order to more clearly define the scope of complications pertaining to OrthoTADs, we have defined the terms *problem* and *complications* for use herein. A problem is a state of difficulty that needs to be resolved.[18] Put another way, a problem is an occurrence during treatment that was not expected or predicted based on the treatment plan. If the problem is not identified or solved, then it will most likely progress into a complication. A complication is a pathologic process or event occurring during a disease that is not an essential part of the disease; it may result from the disease or from independent causes.[19] In this instance, the "disease" is malocclusion. Fortunately, with OrthoTADs, complications are infrequent, and when they do occur, they are rarely significant.

Interestingly, there is often no direct relationship between problems and complications; similar problems can create different complications. Moreover, a single problem may possibly result in several complications. For example, an inaccurately used drill bit may leave an over enlarged pilot hole, with clinically imperceptible miniscrew implant (MSI) mobility, which when immediately loaded with too high a force level may cause MSI tipping or migration that may allow soft tissue impingement by the attachment mechanics.

It is important to pay attention to any problem that occurs during the course of treatment, even when this problem might initially seem insignificant. For example, slight soft tissue erythema and irritation around an MSI may not seem cause for concern, particularly because most orthodontists are all too familiar with appliance-associated gingivitis. This localized inflammation adjacent to an MSI, however, has worse potential because the MSI perforates the soft tissue and cortical bone and resides within the medullary bone. The orthodontist should address this problem immediately by vigorous oral hygiene protocols, chlorhexidine rinses, and more frequent follow-up appointments. If left unchecked, this problem could progress into a soft tissue infection that could progress to osteomyelitis.

POTENTIAL PROBLEMS
Problems that occur during TAD procedures can be divided into two major groups: (1) clinician- or auxiliary-related problems and (2) patient-related problems. The first group can be further subdivided into three categories: (1) primary or strategic problems, (2) secondary or tactical problems, and (3) technical problems.

Primary, or strategic, problems occur during treatment planning and may include incorrect indications for TADs, unrealistic treatment objectives, or inappropriate patient selection. This includes patients who are psychologically unprepared for TADs or who cannot implement the normal hygiene procedures required during TAD treatment. Other strategic problems include the selection of inappropriate biomechanics or inadequate force level calculation for tooth movement.

Secondary, or tactical, problems usually result from an inadequate attempt to correct a developing complication. This type of problem often results in a new pathologic condition (secondary complication) that sometimes is more difficult to correct than the initial complication. An example would be inadequate adjustment of the moment arm length (tactical problem) to correct upper incisor torque problems during retraction (initial complication), which in turn had developed because of an inadequately calculated anterior segment center of resistance (strategic problem) during treatment planning. This may lead to premature anterior contact upon jaw closure, fremitus, incisor wear, and dental pain.

Technical problems are those that are made during a surgical procedure, application of attachment mechanics, or execution of tooth movement procedures. Technical problems are usually a direct result of insufficient training and/or lack of experience. An example of a technical problem would be inaccurate placement of the TAD, leading to inadequate biomechanics of orthodontic force attachments, inaccurate tooth movement, possible soft tissue impingement, or even damage to an adjacent tooth root. In addition, this group includes technical problems associated with TAD defects or fracture.

Patient-related problems are those that may be attributed to poor compliance or failure to follow instructions (inadequate oral hygiene [Fig. 8-1], playing with the TADs or attachment mechanics with the tongue or fingers [Fig. 8-2], or engaging in activities that may damage the TAD or mechanics). Patient-related problems are often directly related to insufficient patient/parent education and may occur because of strategic problems during treatment planning.

POTENTIAL COMPLICATIONS
The complications that may occur during OrthoTAD use may be grouped into four categories: (1) bone, (2) tooth, (3) soft tissue, and (4) biomechanics.

Bone

Inadequate Primary Stability

Research has clearly demonstrated that primary stability is critical for temporary anchorage devices. Primary stability refers to the movement, or the lack thereof, of a TAD upon initial placement. A lack of primary stability almost routinely leads to overt TAD mobility, with subsequent failure. Recent evidence suggests that the majority of primary TAD stability comes from cortical bone, with lesser

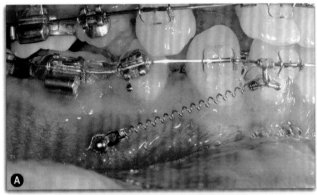

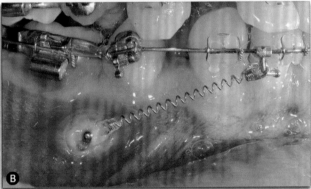

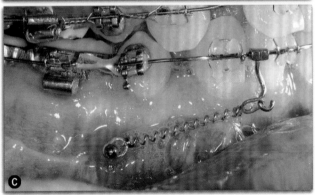

Fig. 8-1

Patient with poor oral hygiene/inflammation. **A,** MSI upon initial placement and activation. **B,** MSI after 8 weeks of activation. Note poor oral hygiene and inflammation around MSI head. **C,** MSI after 10 weeks of activation. Note that ideal oral hygiene and chlorhexidine rinse completely resolved

stability coming from medullary bone.[20] This group of complications basically results from inadequate cortical bone around the TAD. Causes of inadequate primary stability can be divided into three major categories: (1) inadequate bone stock, (2) pilot hole overenlargement, and (3) pilot drill overheating.

Upon placement an MSI should have at least 0.5 to 0.75 mm of available bone stock around its circumference. If not, the MSI has an increased risk of failure. Recently, several authors have provided data outlining predictable intraalveolar and extraalveolar sites that provide adequate bone stock for TAD placement (see Chapter 7).[21-23] If an MSI is placed in a region of questionable cortical bone thickness or density, such as adjacent to a pneumatized sinus or a recent extraction site, and the screw feels even subtly mobile, then the orthodontist should consider a new location. Miniscrew implant mobility is a certain predictor of soft tissue irritation, which may increase the chance of infection. Because most TADs are intended to be placed and loaded at the same visit, the clinician should be confident that the miniscrew has adequate cortical bone purchase and exhibits no mobility. If mobility is present at the time of placement, it will never get better but will most certainly get worse. The TAD should be relocated immediately.

Another reason for inadequate primary stability is an overdrilled pilot hole.[24,25] This problem is more probable in thin cortical and soft cancellous bone.[26,27] The main reason for hole overenlargement is inability to hold the handpiece stable and perpendicular to the bone surface during drilling. Any angular movement other than straight up-and-down during drilling will enlarge the pilot hole and minimize the tight fit of the MSI in the pilot hole.

Excessive trauma during implant surgery is considered an important cause of implant failure.[28,29] During a pilot hole osteotomy, most of the energy not used in the cutting process is transformed into heat. The amount of heat depends on the drill flute geometry,[30,31] the sharpness of the cutting tool,[32] the pressure applied,[32] the duration of the cutting action,[29,33] the cooling technique,[34,35] the speed of the drill,[36,37] and bone density.[38] These factors are important because heat production leading to a temperature rise above 47° C for more than 1 minute negatively affects living bone[39] and compromises its regeneration.[40] It follows that placing a pilot hole for TADs can generate enough

the pilot hole undergo necrosis, followed by remodeling. This results in the hole getting larger, which may lead to decreased stability of the TAD. Importantly, this is a delayed complication that occurs 1 to 3 weeks after placement. The probability increases in the posterior mandible where cortical bone is thicker and denser than most locations in the oral cavity. Complications in this area are best avoided by using drill-free screws or by using copious irrigation with brief, intermittent pressure during pilot hole placement.

Insufficient Bone Plate Adaptation

For miniplate implants (MPIs), a well-formed plate is essential to avoiding complications. Intimate plate-to-bone contact is critical for two major reasons: first, complete miniscrew engagement is only possible if the plate is flush with the bone it contacts; and second, any "dead space" created by an ill-adapted bone plate will provide space for hematoma formation and a possible environment for infection. The clinician must take the time to adapt the bone plate completely to fit the individual osseous anatomy while ensuring that the holes for screw placement are away from tooth roots and sinuses.

Implant Mobility

Implant mobility can be divided into two periods: immediate and delayed. Immediate mobility upon placement also is referred to as inadequate primary stability as covered before. Delayed mobility, which occurs days to months after placement, is a separate entity. This type of mobility is usually caused by implant overloading or by epithelial ingrowth.

Implant overloading is caused by force levels applied to the implant that exceed the functional loading capacity of the bone-to-implant interface. Although it might be assumed that orthodontic force levels are the only cause of this type of mobility, other factors should be considered. Patient manipulation with the fingers or tongue can also overload the bone-to-MSI interface (Fig. 8-2). A traumatic accident, such as getting hit in the face with a ball can also dislodge an MSI. Not all mobile MSIs must be removed. Miniscrew implants with subtle, not frank, mobility of −1 (using the periodontal mobility score)[41] need not be removed. If the MSI is stable enough to be loaded by orthodontic forces without frank mobility, it can most often be left in place. If the MSI is considerably mobile, it should be removed and replaced because mobility can lead to other problems such as patient discomfort. Soon after an MSI becomes mobile, the surrounding periimplant tissues may become irritated and inflamed. This inflammation is not only painful to the patient but also sets the stage for infection.

Epithelial ingrowth is also possible, which would undermine any remaining mechanical purchase. This is different from the placement of a traditional dental implant, for which the gingiva and periosteum is reflected prior to placement. When a drill-free MSI is placed, it is pushed through gingiva and periosteum, possibly introducing epithelial cells into the bone-to-screw interface. A key to the success in using MSIs may be immediate loading. Immediate loading creates pressure at the bone-to-implant interface, thus preventing epithelial ingrowth. If a TAD is not loaded immediately, epithelial ingrowth may occur between the bone and the implant, thereby leading to mobility that may worsen with time. One must keep this concept in mind when applying an elastic material to the TAD for activation. If the orthodontist allows the patient to go too long between visits with elastic thread or chain,

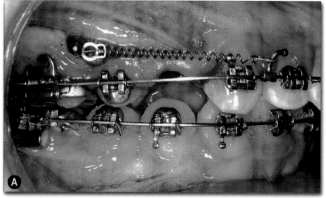
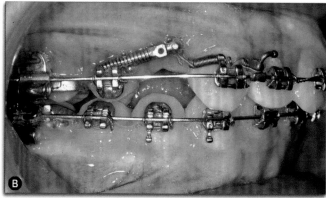

Fig. 8-2

Patient-induced MSI failure. **A,** Buccal photograph of initial MSI placement during first premolar extraction. **B,** Buccal photograph of MSI 6 weeks after placement. Patient "did not realize" there was a problem.

the potential exists for loss of implant tension, followed by epithelialization of the bone-to-implant interface. Patients must be educated before leaving the office with a TAD that they must be aware of MSI mobility and must contact the orthodontist at once if recognized.

Once the clinician confirms frank implant mobility, the loose MSI should be removed immediately. The orthodontist should choose an alternate site located away from any inflammation and place a new MSI. If no alternate location is readily available, the patient should be sent home with a chlorhexidine rinse protocol, and the clinician should attempt reimplantation after tissue irritation has subsided and the hole is filled by new bone.

Oroantral Communication

During placement of TADs in the maxilla, there is always a chance that the miniscrew might perforate the maxillary sinus. This chance is increased if pneumatization of the sinuses is noted in the preoperative radiographic evaluation. The most concerning sequelae following a sinus perforation are postoperative maxillary sinusitis and formation of a chronic oroantral fistula. The probability that either of these two sequelae will occur is related to the size of the communication. The diagnosis of a perforation is best performed by having the patient blow through the nose gently with the nostrils pinched together. If bubbling of air is visualized at the site of the suspected perforation, then a diagnosis of sinus perforation is established. An alternative test is to hold a mouth mirror over the suspected communication and have the patient gently breathe through the nose. If the mirror fogs, then a diagnosis of sinus perforation is established. If the communication is 2 mm or less, then no further management is required other than routine postoperative observation and sinus precautions.[42] This is usually the case because most current MSIs available are less than 2 mm in diameter.

Sinus precautions help ensure that an adequate blood clot is formed and its integrity is maintained. Precautions include avoidance of nose blowing, sucking on straws, drinking of carbonated beverages, and smoking. Although not routinely necessary, the clinician may prescribe an antibiotic, a nasal decongestant, and an oral decongestant. The primary reason for these medications is to prevent maxillary sinusitis by antibiotic prophylaxis and maintenance of ostium patency.

Should the communication be between 2 and 6 mm, then a figure-eight suture over the site is recommended should be followed. Any oroantral communication greater that 6 mm should be considered for flap coverage by an oral and maxillofacial surgeon.

Temporary Anchorage Periimplantitis (TAP)

Periimplantitis has been studied extensively since the advent of osseointegrated implants. It is appropriate to include a discussion of periimplantitis at this juncture because of the nature of the MSI location in bone. However, to label infections involving the bone surrounding miniscrews as periimplantitis is a misnomer. *Periimplantitis* is defined as the pathologic changes confined to the surrounding hard and soft tissues adjacent to an osseointegrated implant.[43] The diagnosis of periimplantitis is confirmed by a gradual loss of bone around an osseointegrated implant documented via probing depths and serial radiographs. Because no such osseointegration takes place with most TADs and their removal is usually less than 12 months after initial placement, a term that is more applicable to TADs in orthodontics is needed. For the purposes of this discussion the term *temporary anchorage periimplantitis,* or TAP, will be used to properly differentiate this phenomena from true periimplantitis.

Much like periimplantitis, TAP may result from anaerobic bacterial infection between the bone-to-miniscrew interface. Although periimplantitis results in progressive attachment loss (not an issue with TADs), localized bone loss may occur with TAP, resulting in progressive miniscrew mobility and pain. Radiographic evidence may not be helpful in these situations, given the brief nature of the TAD role in an orthodontic treatment plan. As such, the clinician must identify the potential existence of TAP by clinical evaluation and move forward with appropriate TAP treatment.

In the instance of periimplantitis, great efforts are made to salvage an osseointegrated implant with a questionable future. Fortunately, TADs do not require such heroic efforts. Once identified, the miniscrew that has TAP should be removed. Antibiotic therapy generally is not indicated; however, several days of chlorhexidine rinses should be instituted to aid in resolving any associated inflammation. Whether to place a new miniscrew immediately following the removal of the affected miniscrew is left to the judgment of the clinician. Certainly, allowing the periodontal tissues time to heal before placing another miniscrew

Tooth

Root Impingement

Of all the potential complications that are possible with TAD placement, the most feared seems to be placement of a miniscrew into a tooth root. There is a paucity of literature regarding this subject, however, and only a few studies may shed light on the topic. In a study by Borah and Ashmead,[44] 387 consecutive facial fractures were examined for teeth transfixed by osteosynthesis screws. The incidence of root impingement per screw was 0.47% (13 transfixed teeth per 2,340 screws). The results suggested that mandibular teeth were more at risk for screw impingement than maxillary teeth by a ratio of 10:3. Posterior teeth were more at risk than anterior teeth. Interestingly, none of the impinged teeth developed any documented periapical abscess during follow-up. None of the patients in the study were required to undergo endodontic treatment or surgical apicoectomy to any of the impinged teeth. The conclusion was that impingement of tooth roots by osteosynthesis screws during fracture fixation does not appear to adversely affect the survival of affected teeth. In fact, the authors suggest that if the periodontal ligament (PDL) or cementum was contacted, but without disruption of the apical neurovascular bundle or frank invasion of the pulp canal, the chance of devitalization was minimal. Further, the authors noted that teeth that were transfixed generally did not become infected and did not appear to require extraction more often than similar adjacent teeth. A comparable study by Fabbroni and colleagues[45] found similar results.

Careful planning and determination of the precise implant location, radiographic survey evaluation, and clinical examination can minimize the risk of root impingement. If during the operative procedure, the clinician does not feel a "drop" into the medullary space as the drill bit or miniscrew continues to advance, the clinician should assume the root is being encountered. Another sign that a root is being contacted is failure of the screw to advance despite adequate operator pressure. Indication that a root has been contacted mandates miniscrew removal followed by redirection away from the root (Fig. 8-3). This is the only step that is necessary in this instance, and the involved tooth should be observed during routine follow-up. To place an Ortho Implant (IMTEC Corp., Ardmore, Oklahoma) directly into a tooth root, even with the drill-free property of the screw, is nearly impossible (Fig. 8-4). Furthermore, the placement protocols call for a mere perforation of the cortical plate

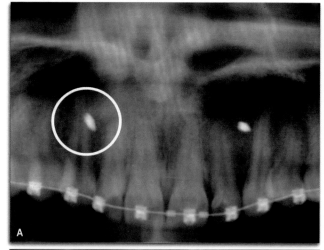

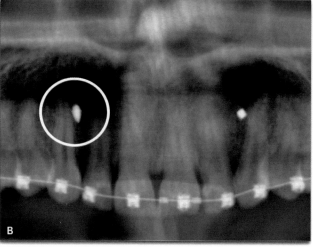

Fig. 8-3

MSI placement positions adjacent to tooth roots. **A,** Panoramic radiograph taken after patient complained of diffuse pain on the right side of her face. Note MSI position relative to the canine root (*white circle*). **B,** Panoramic radiograph taken immediately after removal and redirection of right miniscrew (*white circle*), which left the patient pain free.

when the pilot hole is drilled. Care not to extend the pilot hole further into the bone should minimize the chance to contact an adjacent tooth with the drill.

In case the PDL or cementum is contacted, the most frequent concern is that the tooth may undergo ankylosis. Evidence by Tsukiboshi and colleagues[46] and others[47] suggests that this is not likely. Tsukiboshi and colleagues[46] suggest that deficits of PDL on the root surface are repaired by new attachment, which is defined as regeneration and attachment of PDL tissue to a root surface that lost PDL pathologically or mechanically. The mechanism of new attachment is by formation of connective tissue between exposed root surface and surrounding tissue (bone and gingival connective tissue) by proliferation of cells derived from the PDL around the exposed root surface with addition

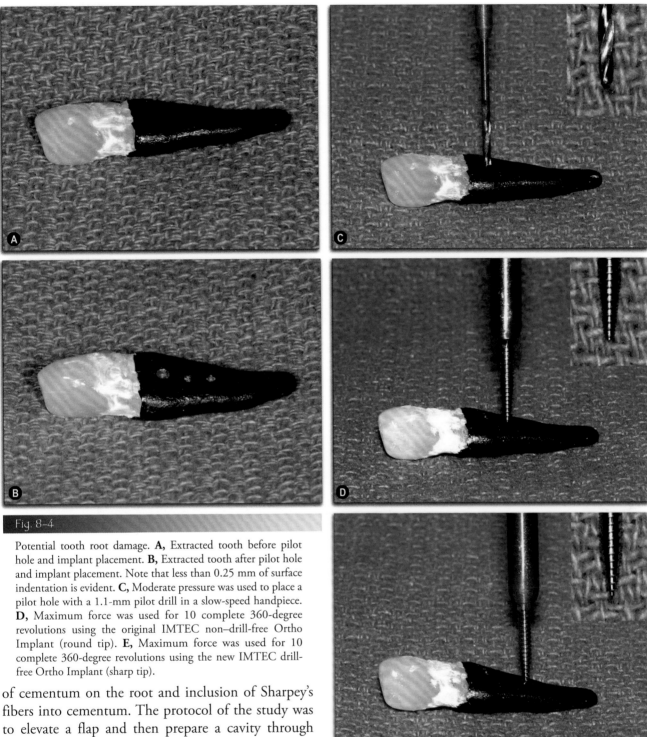

Fig. 8-4

Potential tooth root damage. **A,** Extracted tooth before pilot hole and implant placement. **B,** Extracted tooth after pilot hole and implant placement. Note that less than 0.25 mm of surface indentation is evident. **C,** Moderate pressure was used to place a pilot hole with a 1.1-mm pilot drill in a slow-speed handpiece. **D,** Maximum force was used for 10 complete 360-degree revolutions using the original IMTEC non–drill-free Ortho Implant (round tip). **E,** Maximum force was used for 10 complete 360-degree revolutions using the new IMTEC drill-free Ortho Implant (sharp tip).

of cementum on the root and inclusion of Sharpey's fibers into cementum. The protocol of the study was to elevate a flap and then prepare a cavity through bone, PDL, cementum, and into dentin. Over the first 3 to 9 days, the PDL proliferated from the ruptured PDL tissue. From 14 to 21 days, new PDL tissue filled the cavity; new cementum was deposited on dentin, and bone was deposited on the socket wall. From 21 to 28 days, bony healing progressed. Then over 60 to 470 days, the cavity was repaired by new cementum and PDL with the PDL space eventually being reestablished.

Most important was vitality of the PDL. The other factors were the deficit size on the root and the distance of the cavity from the socket wall. Andreasen and Kristerson[47] found that up to 2 mm width of PDL loss on the root surface can be repaired by new attachment without ankylosis. An increase

Soft Tissue

Soft Tissue Tearing

Careful attention is sufficient to avoid most soft tissue injuries. With the vast majority of TAD placements, little or no soft tissue manipulation is required. If a miniscrew is to be placed in an area that is covered by attached gingiva, an indirect approach may be used to avoid the likelihood of soft tissue trauma. After anesthetizing the area, the clinician uses a slow-speed drill to puncture the attached gingiva and cortical bone. Upon completion of this procedure, the clinician places the miniscrew without any further tissue manipulation. Some have suggested using a sterile tissue punch to remove attached gingiva and periosteum, followed by a slow-speed drill to perforate the cortical plate.

If a drill-free miniscrew is used, then the clinician inserts the screw through the attached gingiva and manually screws it into the cortical bone without the aid of a drill (Fig. 8-5). This is the simplest method of miniscrew placement but requires bone thin enough to facilitate penetration by the miniscrew alone. Mandibular cortical bone, 3 mm or more thick, may prove in some instances to be too dense to allow drill-free insertion of a miniscrew.

There may be cases in which a miniscrew needs to be placed in a location that is covered by unattached gingiva. In this instance, it is necessary to utilize a sterile tissue punch to remove mucosa and periosteum. If a tissue punch is not used, the mucosa has a tendency to wrap around the drill or MSI during insertion, causing needless soft tissue trauma.

Miniplate implant use requires a mucoperiosteal flap to provide adequate adaptation of the miniplate. The most common injury in flap procedures is tearing of the flap itself. Tearing is usually a by-product of inadequate flap size, requiring retraction for visualization that is beyond the ability of the tissue to withstand. To prevent tearing of a mucoperiosteal flap, the operator must visualize how much access will be necessary to place the MPI and then make the flap large enough to accommodate such access. Retraction forces should always be minimal, and the clinician should inspect the edges of the incision frequently for tears. If a flap tear should occur, the flap should be carefully repositioned, such that adequate suturing may be performed without placing the flap under tension.

Improper Temporary Anchorage Device Emergence

Evaluation of the location of the terminal attachment of a TAD and its relationship to the desired force vector is critical. If, for instance, one is using an MPI and it is properly adapted to the bone, but the plate fails to emerge from the flap as desired or is in the incorrect location for the required biomechanics, then the clinician should remove the plate and reposition it. It is important to ensure that after an MPI is placed in an ideal location and position, the flap is sutured such that the terminal attachment hole is completely visible to allow proper engagement after surgery. The same is true for miniscrew placement. One must be sure that if the miniscrew is traversing soft tissue, such as in the area of the zygomatic buttress, it is long enough to have strong cortical engagement and adequate emergence into the oral cavity.

Another aspect of emergence that must be addressed is the local tissue irritation that a high-profile TAD may cause. If the TAD emergence profile is too prominent, then significant irritation to adjacent soft tissue structures may occur. For example, MSIs placed between the maxillary lateral incisors and canines for anterior segment intrusion may inadvertently embed themselves in the soft tissue of the upper lip (Fig. 8-6). This situation may be initially treated conservatively with chlorhexidine rinses and liberal application of orthodontic wax, but removal of the miniscrews may be required if the irritation and swelling persist.

Soft Tissue Impingement

Once biomechanical activation is initiated following the placement of a TAD, evaluation of the local soft tissues and their relationships to elastics, open coil springs, and the like is critical. Soft tissues that are adjacent not only to the TAD itself but also to auxiliary mechanical devices are subject to trauma and irritation (Fig. 8-7). Careful visualization of all soft tissues after active mechanics have been initiated is important to the ultimate success of TADs. Patients should be aware of what has been attached to the TAD and how to evaluate any discomfort they might have subsequent to placement and activation. For instances in which soft tissue impingement occurs, auxiliaries such as hooks, arms (Fig. 8-8), or ligatures may be used to redirect or relieve gingival pressure created during TAD use.

Temporary Anchorage Periimplant Mucositis (TAM)

As the name suggests, periimplant mucositis is a localized infection of the marginal tissues surrounding TADs. This is a reversible inflammatory change that is analogous to gingivitis and is primarily an inflammatory disorder caused by plaque accumulation.[48] Once proper hygiene is established, the inflammation

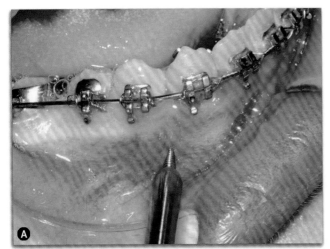

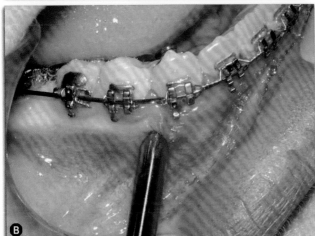

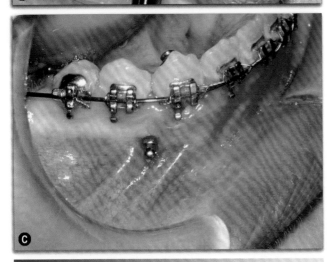

Fig. 8-5

Standard placement of a drill-free screw through attached gingiva. **A,** Buccal photograph of initial MSI placement after topical anesthetic application. **B,** Buccal photograph upon completion of MSI placement. **C,** Buccal photograph of final MSI position.

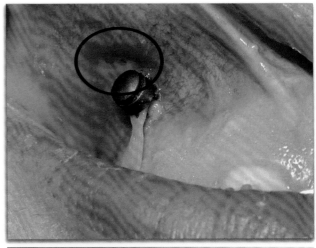

Fig. 8-6

MSI-induced soft tissue trauma. Two days after MSI placement, the patient returned with soft tissue ulceration (*black circle*) from MSI placement high in the vestibule.

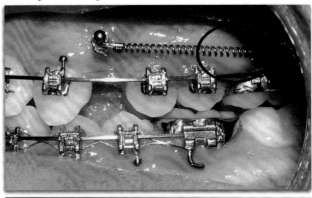

Fig. 8-7

MSI attachment–induced soft tissue trauma. The NiTi spring placed from the MSI to protract the maxillary molar caused gingival blanching (*black circle*), indicating undue pressure on the soft tissues.

the inflammation does not subside within several days. The inflammation should be addressed immediately, however, because Cheng and colleagues[11] suggest a bacterial role in the failure of orthodontic MSIs.

Soft Tissue Infection

Although relatively uncommon, localized infections caused by TAD placement and activation can and do occur. The placement of TADs to facilitate orthodontic mechanics requires increased clinical examination for the presence of mobility and infection. Fortunately, infections related to TADs are easy to recognize and treat. Locally, the signs and symptoms of pain, swelling, surface erythema, pus formation, and TAD mobility are possible. Recall that not all of the clinical signs of infection need to be

resolves without any permanent bone or tissue damage. Implant removal in these cases is not necessary unless

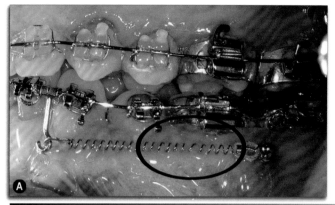 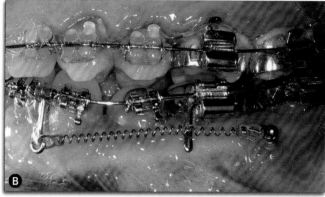

Fig. 8-8

Correction of MSI attachment–induced soft tissue trauma. **A,** The NiTi spring placed from the MSI to retract the mandibular anterior teeth had embedded into the gingival tissue. Note the overgrowth of tissue around the closed coil spring (*black circle*). **B,** The simple addition of an auxiliary wire lifts the coil spring away from the gingiva and corrects the problem.

this instance, the orthodontist's clinical judgment must guide the course of therapy.

Slight erythema and discomfort immediately adjacent to a TAD indicates the early signs of localized infection. If caught early enough, placing a patient on a regimen of chlorhexidine gluconate rinses for 5 to 7 days, along with proper hygiene instruction, is sufficient to ameliorate the infection (Fig. 8-9). If the infection persists for more than 10 days or even worsens, it becomes imperative to remove the TAD to allow for infection resolution and complete tissue healing. The orthodontist must determine whether to prescribe oral antibiotics in the face of a TAD-related infection. Frank pus, increasing pain, fever, malaise, and other signs of a progressive infection indicate the need for antibiotics. Upon resolution of the active infection, the clinician may choose a suitable alternative location for TAD placement and place a new implant. Added diligence on the part of the orthodontist is necessary for a patient who has experienced a TAD-related infection; frequent visits and examinations are prudent in order to avoid further infections.

Neurovascular Impingement

As discussed in Chapter 5, a solid understanding of the neurovascular anatomy within the oral cavity should prevent any neurovascular impingement. Fortunately, miniscrews are small, and if vascular damage does occur, treatment is straightforward. If excessive, continuous bleeding is noted immediately upon insertion of the miniscrew or drill bit, the clinician should remove the screw and apply direct pressure until hemostasis is achieved. Once the bleeding has stopped, another location may be chosen and the procedure continued.

The patient will note nerve impingement as continued discomfort after the effects of the local anesthetic have ended. In this situation the clinician should anesthetize the area once again and remove and redirect the miniscrew. This is the same protocol as for tooth root impingement. Nerve impingement is rarely an issue when using topical anesthetic alone or with local infiltration. With these techniques, the PDL and tooth roots are not anesthetized, allowing the patient to sense the discomfort before PDL contact or root impingement. Often the patient will describe a diffuse pain involving the ipsilateral side of MSI placement (Fig. 8-3).

Biomechanics
Undesirable Tooth Movement

A well-thought-out vector analysis is critical to TAD success. Unwanted intrusive or extrusive movements are common with TADs unless careful attention is paid to the vectors and forces involved. Molar intrusion may introduce unwanted tipping or crown torque unless proper counterforces are used to prevent such problems. If, for example, a TAD is used in the buccal cortex to intrude a maxillary molar, a force must be placed on the lingual via another TAD, or the molars must be stabilized by a transpalatal arch to prevent unwanted buccal crown torque. Retraction of anterior tooth segments may be subject to intrusive forces or to excessive palatal crown torque. If intrusion is not part of the treatment plan, auxiliaries must be used to place the TAD force vector closer to the center of rotation, thus inducing a translational movement of the segment.

Temporary Anchorage Device Interference

When TADs are used to assist in dental intrusion, it is important to evaluate the anticipated path of the

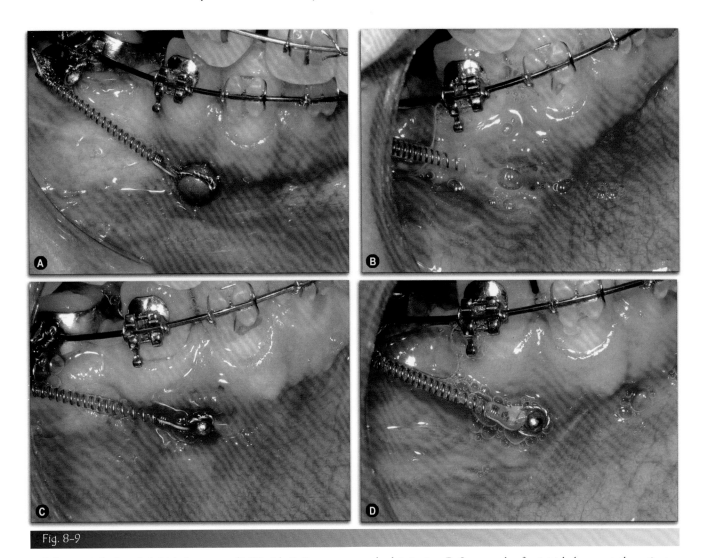

Fig. 8-9

Soft tissue infection. **A,** Initial placement of MSI with O-Cap to prevent cheek irritation. **B,** Seven weeks after initial placement, the patient returned with a soft tissue infection caused by embedding of the closed coil spring into the gingiva and excessive pressure caused by sleeping habits. **C,** The O-Cap was removed, the site was well-irrigated, oral hygiene procedures were reviewed, and chlorhexidine and antibiotics were prescribed for 10 days. **D,** Seven days later the infection was resolved without the need for MSI removal.

tooth in question. Often, in an attempt to optimally locate a TAD for intrusion, the body of the implant is placed directly in the path of the tooth. Progression of the intrusive movement will obviously be arrested, and continued forces on the tooth may contribute to iatrogenic root resorption.

Critical evaluation before TAD placement is also necessary to avoid the need for moving the anchor during therapy because of loss of mechanical advantage; for example, not placing an MSI far enough away from a tooth to provide ample distance for continuous activation. If a miniscrew is placed too close to a tooth that must be intruded, there may be a point in treatment that the miniscrew can no longer provide anchorage. In fact, the MSI itself may interfere with the mechanics of the movement (Fig. 8-10).

Temporary Anchorage Device Fracture

Although infrequent, the chance for miniscrew fracture always exists during the placement procedure. When the miniscrew fractures at the level of the bone, making removal difficult, it may be appropriate to leave the miniscrew in place. The clinician should choose another site adjacent to the fractured screw and place a new miniscrew. In this instance, a postoperative radiograph will rule out root impingement as the cause for the miniscrew fracture. If the root has been contacted or penetrated by the fractured miniscrew, removal of the remnant is necessary to avoid any possible sequelae. If the miniscrew is difficult to remove, a small, round bur can be used to create a trough around the exposed miniscrew remnant, allowing adequate access for

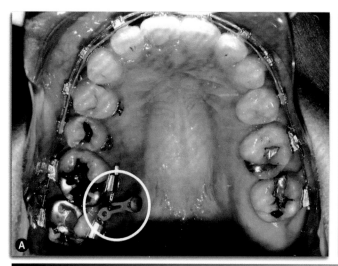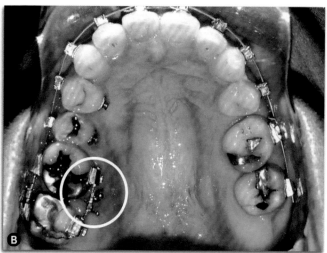

Fig. 8-10

MSI interference with tooth movement. **A,** Initial palatal photograph of MSI used for maxillary molar intrusion (*white circle*). **B,** Progress palatal photograph of MSI used for maxillary molar intrusion. Note the relationship of the palatal MSI relative to the arch wire (*white circle*). The MSI impeded further intrusion and so had to be removed and replaced more apically to allow continued intrusion.

On occasion, implant fracture may occur postoperatively during the course of TAD activation. The protocol for this situation is the same as if the fracture occurred during placement. If the miniscrew remnant is accessible, the clinician can remove it and place a new miniscrew in a different location. If the miniscrew remnant is difficult to remove, it may be left in place.

It is important to attempt to identify any possible causes of miniscrew fracture such as occlusal forces, eating of inappropriate foods, and parafunctional habits so that a repeat fracture does not occur. The clinician must educate the patient as to the potential for screw fracture and what protocol will be followed should it occur.

TIME-RELATED CLASSIFICATION OF COMPLICATIONS

It is also useful to organize a discussion of complications by the time of their recognition. The classic division of surgical complications into intraoperative (early) and postoperative (late) distinctions might not be as applicable to the placement of OrthoTADs. Temporary anchorage device placement and subsequent activation extends the umbrella of time under which definitions and divisions of complications apply. This temporal distinction requires the expansion of the clinician's awareness, such that the TAD is placed with the end in mind. Therefore we prefer to group TAD complications into six temporal categories: (1) intraoperative (TAD placement), (2) postoperative (immediately after placement and during initial mechanical activation),

(3) orthodontic mechanics activation, (4) TAD removal, (5) posttreatment healing, and (6) late complications. This classification will assist the clinician in choosing the most appropriate course of correction to avoid further deviation from the original treatment plan.

Anesthesia Complications

Before discussing complications that happen during the TAD placement procedure, it is important to discuss potential complications with the administration of local anesthesia. Although anesthetic requirements are minimal for the routine placement of most TADs, anesthetic complications are still a potential cause for concern. Examination of every possible anesthetic complication that may occur is beyond the scope of this text, yet a brief overview is included for completeness.

Although difficulty in obtaining enough anesthesia for a given procedure in dentistry is always a potential problem, the opposite is true for most TAD placements. The goal of anesthesia for the placement of TADs is to obtain anesthesia of the periosteum and supraperiosteal soft tissues immediately adjacent to the location where the miniscrew will be placed. A supraperiosteal injection at or near the tooth roots of maxillary teeth may often result in pulpal anesthesia. Pulpal anesthesia may prevent the patient from sensing discomfort when a miniscrew is inadvertently directed into the vicinity of the PDL or tooth root. Similarly, avoiding anesthesia of the lingual alveolar surface when introducing a miniscrew on the buccal alveolar surface will allow the patient to sense when a miniscrew or drill has been placed too deep and contacts the contralateral cortex. Care should also be taken when placing miniplates in the maxilla, because the increased anesthetic requirement when placing multiple screws makes pulpal anesthesia more likely.

Aspiration is appropriate with the administration of any injection. Positive aspiration with this type of local administration is negligible, but possible (less than 1%).[50] The requirement for much smaller amounts of anesthetic significantly reduces the risk for overdose, yet practitioners must always be mindful of the amount of local anesthetic delivered. This is especially true for small children. The advent of powerful, topical local anesthetics may further reduce the amount of anesthetic introduced into the vasculature, adding to the safety of the procedure.[51-53]

Anesthetics with vasoconstrictors introduce another aspect of potential complications when being given in larger doses, or when introduced into the vasculature. Fortunately, most TAD procedures require such small amounts of anesthetic that adverse reactions are unlikely. Clearly, patients with cardiovascular compromise must be carefully evaluated and observed when using any vasoactive compounds with local anesthesia. Aspiration upon injection and a thorough understanding of anatomy should help to prevent any untoward events.

Intraoperative Complications

Intraoperative complications usually develop as a result of poor treatment planning, inattention to miniscrew angulation during placement, failure to appreciate and execute proper emergence of the abutment head, and failure to evaluate and confirm primary stability. These complications are generally preventable but upon recognition are easily correctable. The patient should be made aware that the placement of TADs is a dynamic process, much like placing an orthodontic bracket, which is subject to constant and ongoing evaluation and adjustment.

Postoperative Complications

During the postoperative period, the clinician should pay special attention to two critical factors: primary stability and local tissue response. After several days, the clinician should evaluate the patient and examine the TAD carefully. Several questions should be answered: Is the TAD stable in cortical bone? Is the emergence of the terminal end of the TAD compatible with the surrounding tissues? Are there any areas of ulcerations that might need addressing? Is the auxiliary appliance attached in such a manner that it is stable and free of

that the capability of maintaining excellent hygiene in the area of the TAD? Are the surrounding teeth and tissues pain free? These are a few of the questions that a thoughtful clinician must note in the postoperative follow-up examination.

Orthodontic Mechanics Activation Complications

Complications during activation are intuitive and include three main concerns. First is whether the TAD is stable or demonstrates subtle mobility such that it is to the point at which the TAD is no longer beneficial? Second is whether any soft tissue ulceration or damage is present from improper emergence and impingement by auxiliaries? Finally is whether the biomechanical demands of the case are being met by the addition of the TAD? The clinician should address all of these concerns and answer them in an honest and straightforward manner to allow remedy if necessary.

Temporary Anchorage Device Removal Complications

By definition, TADs must be removed at some point during a patient's orthodontic therapy. For this reason the clinician must address complications during TAD removal. After the TAD has fulfilled its role in the orthodontic treatment plan it should be expeditiously removed. Although the vast majority of patients tolerate miniscrew removal without anesthesia of any kind, some patients may require administration of local anesthetic before the removal procedure. Certainly, the removal of miniplates requires anesthesia because a flap elevation over the plate is required.

Should miniscrew fracture occur at the time of removal, the orthodontist should remove the remnant if it is readily accessible. Leaving the remnant in place is acceptable if it proves too difficult to remove or extensive bone damage would occur during removal. At times, soft tissue will migrate over the head of a miniscrew, requiring administration of local anesthesia and limited gingival curettage to expose the hardware.

As with miniplate placement, removal demands an adequate mucoperiosteal flap to provide visualization and access. Upon removal of a miniplate, the clinician should irrigate the site copiously and reapproximate the flap and secure it via several resorbable sutures. Antibiotic therapy need not be initiated, but a course of chlorhexidine rinses immediately following hardware removal is beneficial.

Posttreatment Complications

Posttreatment healing complications likely relate to

then the site of removal is small and rarely develops complications. If persistent pain, swelling, or drainage occurs after MSI removal, chlorhexidine rinses for 5 days will normally resolve any localized infection.

If, however, MPIs were used, posttreatment healing occasionally may occur with minor complications. Gravity provides welcome drainage to most maxillary incisions; hence MPIs placed and removed in the mandible necessitate greater scrutiny. Should pain, fluctuance, purulent drainage, swelling, or other signs of infection arise in the posttreatment healing period, careful evaluation and possible referral to an oral and maxillofacial surgeon may be necessary.

Sinus perforation is a finding that may not present itself until TAD removal. If sinus perforation is suspected, the clinician needs to evaluate the possible fistula and treat it as described previously. However, if the TAD originally perforated the sinus and remained in place for several months before removal, it is likely that no sequelae will ensue. Most probably, if a perforation existed initially, the TAD plugged the perforation, and over time the sinus membrane healed over the apex of the TAD. Recently, Diamaruya and colleagues[16] experimentally intruded molars and premolars into the maxillary sinuses of dogs. In samples in which the premolars had intruded, the root apex of the second premolars penetrated the bony floor of the nasal cavity. As the premolars intruded, the nasal mucosa was lifted and a thin epithelial layer covered the root apex. In the 7-month groups, the bone formation occurred abundantly around the premolar root in the direction of the root apices. A thin bony layer covered the root apex of intruding molars.

In other studies, investigators attempted to insert implants into the maxillary alveolar bone in dogs until the nasal floor was penetrated. The results of the study demonstrated that the hard and soft tissues around the penetrating implants were covered with connective tissue and coated with respiratory mucosa[54] and did not show any signs of adverse tissue reaction at the resolution level of the radiograph.[55] After surgical removal of the sinus mucosa, the denuded sinus lining was reepithelialized by a flattened ciliated epithelium on lamina propria displaying fibrosis and lacking serous glands.[56] The number of vessels in the regenerated mucosa significantly increased, and there was no difference in blood flow between the operated cavities and their control sides.[57] These results suggest that even after perforation of a sinus, if the perforation is plugged

with a TAD for a period of time, tissue regeneration, including alveolar bone, could occur to reestablish normal periodontal conditions.

Late Complications

Late complications almost exclusively belong to the teeth themselves. Progressive pain and sensitivity to pressure may indicate that a tooth root was penetrated by the TAD and that pulpal damage has ensued. If proper procedures are followed during the planning and placement of TADs, this unfortunate circumstance is not likely to go unnoticed until after removal of the TAD, but all significant tooth pain in the area of a recent TAD removal should be thoroughly investigated.

Ankylosis is rare with TAD use because of the small size of the TADs. As mentioned before in this chapter, PDL breeches less than 2 mm usually do not progress to ankylosis. If ankylosis is suspected, the clinician should take periapical radiographs to examine the PDL and should perform and document a thorough examination. The clinical relevance of single tooth ankylosis in an adult is likely minimal but should be monitored for internal or external resorption.

THE LEARNING CURVE

As with any new procedure, a learning curve accompanies the placement and use of TADs. Fortunately, the placement procedure is straightforward. The greatest leap of faith that a practitioner must make is in the placement of the first 5 to 10 TADs. Any misplacements or complications that may be encountered along the way will only prove to increase the clinician's confidence and understanding.

Complications associated with proper TAD use are infrequent and usually minor. Proper treatment planning, tempered with appropriate clinical judgment, will avoid almost all potentially serious complications. As mentioned previously, most problems encountered with TADs prove to be more of a nuisance than anything else.

SUMMARY

The relatively new introduction of temporary skeletal anchorage to the orthodontic world opens up an entirely new era of biomechanics. Naturally, because of the invasive nature of this treatment modality, clinicians may hesitate to introduce TADs into their routine practice. Fortunately, there is a paucity of case reports on complications caused by the placement and use of these devices. In the coming years, more case reports and randomized studies will likely demonstrate that the benefits of TADs far outweigh the potential risks, thus allowing the orthodontist to expand the scope of treatment options for all patients.

REFERENCES

1. Bae SM, Park HS, Kyung HM, et al. Clinical application of micro-implant anchorage. *J Clin Orthod.* 36:298-302, 2002.
2. Bantleon HP, Bernhart T, Crismani AG, Zachrisson BU. Stable orthodontic anchorage with palatal osseointegrated implants. *World J Orthod.* 3:109-116, 2002.
3. Chung K, Kim S-H, Kook Y. C-Orthodontic microimplant for distalization of mandibular dentition in Class III correction. *Angle Orthod.* 75:119-128, 2004.
4. Erverdi N, Tosun T, Keles A. A new anchorage site for the treatment of anterior open bite: zygomatic anchorage—case report. *World J Orthod.* 3:147-153, 2002.
5. Hong R-K, Heo J-M, Ha Y-K. Lever-arm and mini-implant system for anterior torque control during retraction in lingual orthodontic treatment. *Angle Orthod.* 75:129-141, 2004.
6. Branemark PI, Breine U, Adell R, et al. Intra-osseous anchorage of dental prostheses, I: experimental studies. *Scand J Plast Renconstr Surg.* 3:81-100, 1969.
7. Erverdi N, Keles A, Nanda R. The use of skeletal anchorage in openbite treatment: a cephalometric evaluation. *Angle Orthod.* 74:381-390, 2004.
8. Miyakawa S, Koyama I, Inoue M, et al. Factors associated with the stability of titanium screws placed in the posterior region for orthodontic anchorage. *Am J Orthod Dentofacial Orthop.* 124:373-378, 2003.
9. Liou EJ, Pai BCJ, Lin JC. Do miniscrews remain stationary under orthodontic forces? *Am J Orthod Dentofacial Orthop.* 126:42-47, 2004.
10. Park HS, Lee SK, Kwon OW. Group distal movement of teeth using microscrew implant anchorage. *Angle Orthod.* 75:510-517, 2005.
11. Cheng SJ, Tseng IY, Lee JJ, Kok S-H. A prospective study of the risk factors associated with failure of mini-implants used for orthodontic anchorage. *Int J Oral Maxillofac Implants.* 19:100-106, 2004.
12. Costa A, Raffaini M, Melsen B. Miniscrews as orthodontic anchorage: a preliminary report. *Int J Adult Orthodon Orthognath Surg.* 13:201-209, 1998.
13. Sugawara J, Nishimura M. Mini bone plates: the skeletal anchorage system. *Semin Orthod.* 11:47-56, 2005.
14. Sugawara J, Baik U, Umemori M, et al. Treatment and posttreatment dentoalveolar changes following intrusion of mandibular molars with application of a skeletal anchorage system (SAS) for open bite correction. *Int J Adult Orthodon Orthognath Surg.* 17:243-253, 2002.
15. Ari-Demirkaya A, Masry MA, Erverdi N. Apical root resorption of maxillary first molars after intrusion with zygomatic skeletal anchorage. *Angle Orthod.* 75:633-639, 2005.
16. Daimaruya T, Takahashi I, Nagasaka H, et al. Effects of maxillary molar intrusion on the nasal floor and tooth root using the skeletal anchorage system in dogs. *Angle Orthod.* 73:158-166, 2003.
17. Daimaruya T, Nagasaka H, Umemori M, et al. The influence of first molar intrusion on the inferior alveolar neurovascular bundle and root using the skeletal anchorage system in dogs. *Angle Orthod.* 71:60-70, 2001.

19. Kleinedler S. *The American Heritage® Stedman's Medical Dictionary.* Boston, Mass: Houghton Mifflin Co, 2002.
20. Dalstra M, Cattaneo PM, Melsen B. Load transfer of miniscrews for orthodontic anchorage. *Orthodontics.* 1:53-62, 2004.
21. Schnelle MA, Beck FM, Jaynes RM, Huja S. A radiographic evaluation of the availability of bone for placement of miniscrews. *Angle Orthod.* 74:830-835, 2004.
22. Costa A, Pasta G, Bergamaschi G. Intraoral hard and soft tissue depths for temporary anchorage devices. *Semin Orthod.* 11:10-15, 2005.
23. Poggio PM, Incorvati C, Velo S, Carano A. Safe zones: a guide for miniscrew positioning in the maxillary and mandibular arch. *Angle Orthod.* 76:191-197, 2006.
24. Heidemann W, Gerlach KL, Grobel KH, Kollner HG. Drill free screws: a new form of osteosythesis. *J Craniomaxillofac Surg.* 26:163-168, 1998.
25. Heidemann W, Terheyden H, Gerlach KL. Analysis of the osseous/metal interface of drill free screws and self-tapping screws. *J Craniomaxillofac Surg.* 29:69-74, 2001.
26. Nunamaker DM, Perren SM. Force measurements in screw fixation. *J Biomech.* 9:669-675, 1976.
27. Phillips JH, Rahn BA. Comparison of compression and torque measurements of self-tapping and pre-tapped screws. *Plast Reconstr Surg.* 83:447-456, 1989.
28. Lundskog J. Heat and bone tissue: an experimental investigation of the thermal properties of bone tissue and threshold level for thermal injury. *Scand J Plast Renconstr Surg.* 6:5-75, 1972.
29. Albrektsson T, Eriksson R. Thermally induced bone necrosis in rabbits: relation to implant failure in humans. *Clin Orthop.* 195:311-312, 1985.
30. Jacobs C, Pope M, Berry J, Hoagland F. A study of the bone machining process: orthogonal cutting. *J Biomech.* 7:131-136, 1974.
31. Wiggins K, Malkin S. Drilling of bone. *J Biomech.* 9:553-559, 1976.
32. Adell R, Lekholm U, Branémark PI. Surgical procedures. In: Branémark PI, Zarb GA, Albreksson T, eds. *Tissue Integrated Prostheses: Osseointegration in Clinical Dentistry.* Chicago, Ill: Quintessence, 1985:211-232.
33. Ågren E, Arwill T. High speed or conventional dental equipment for the removal of bone in oral surgery, III: a histologic and microradiographic study on bone repair in the rabbit. *Acta Odontol Scand.* 26:223-246, 1968.
34. Eriksson R, Albreksson T. Heat caused by drilling cortical bone: temperature measured in vivo in patients and animals. *Acta Odontol Scand.* 55:629-631, 1984.
35. Lavelle C, Wedgewood D. Effect of internal irrigation on frictional heat generated from bone drilling. *J Oral Surg.* 38:499-503, 1980.
36. Bolla E, Muratore F, Carano A, Bowman S. Evaluation of maxillary molar distalization with the distal jet: a comparison with other contemporary methods. *Angle Orthod.* 72:481-494, 2002.
37. Costich E, Youngblood P, Walden J. A study of the effect of high speed rotary instruments on bone repair in dogs. *Oral Surg Oral Med Oral Pathol.* 17:563-571, 1964.
38. Yacker M, Klein M. The effect of irrigation on osteotomy depth and bur diameter. *Int J Oral Maxillofac Implants.* 11:634-638, 1996.
39. Eriksson R, Albreksson T. Temperature threshold level for

40. Thompson H. Effect of drilling into bone. *J Oral Surg.* 16:22-30, 1958.

41. Fleszar T, Knowles J, Morrison E, et al. Tooth mobility and periodontal therapy. *J Clin Periodontol.* 6:495-505, 1980.

42. Schow S. Odontogenic diseases of the maxillary sinus. In: Peterson L, Ellis E III, Hupp J, Tucker MR, eds. *Contemporary Oral and Maxillofacial Surgery.* St Louis, Mo: Mosby-Year Book, 1993:465-482.

43. Goldberg M. Control and prevention of infection in the surgical patient. In: Topazian RG, Goldberg MH, Hupp JR, eds. *Oral and Maxillofacial Infections.* Philadelphia, Pa: WB Saunders, 2002:468-483.

44. Borah GL, Ashmead D. The fate of teeth transfixed by osteosynthesis screws. *Plast Reconstr Surg.* 97:726-729, 1996.

45. Fabbronni G, Aabed S, Mizen K, Starr DG. Transalveolar screws and the incidence of dental damage: a prospective study. *Int J Oral Maxillofac Surg.* 33:442-446, 2004.

46. Tsukiboshi M, Asai Y, Nakagawa K, et al. Wound healing in transplantation and replantation. In: Tsukiboshi M, ed. *Autotransplantation of Teeth.* Tokyo, Japan: Quintessence, 2001:21-56.

47. Andreasen JO, Kristerson L. The effect of limited drying or removal of the periodontal ligament: Periodontal healing after replantation of mature permanent incisors in monkeys. *Acta Odontol Scand.* 29:1-13, 1981.

48. Pontoriero R, Tonelli M, Carnevale G, et al. Experimentally induced peri-mucositis: a clinical study in humans. *Clin Oral Implants Res.* 5:254-259, 1994.

49. Peterson L. Principals of surgical and antimicrobial infection management. In: Topazian RG, Goldberg MH, Hupp JR, eds. *Oral and Maxillofacial Infections.* Philadelphia, Pa: WB Saunders, 2002:99.

50. Malamed S. Anatomical considerations. In: Malamed SF, ed. *Handbook of Local Anesthesia.* St Louis, Mo: Mosby, 1990:142-159.

51. Keim R. Managing orthodontic pain. *J Clin Orthod.* 38:641-642, 2004.

52. Donaldson D, Gelesky S, Landry R, et al. A placebo-controlled multi-centred evaluation of an anaesthetic gel (Oraqix) for periodontal therapy. *J Clin Periodontol.* 30:171-175, 2003.

53. Samaras CD. Noninjectable anesthetics: haven't got time for the pain. *Contemp Esthet Restor Pract.* 8:44-46, 2004.

54. Geiger S, Pesch H. Animal experimental studies on the healing around ceramic implantation in bone lesions in the maxillary sinus region. *Dtsch Zahnarztl Z.* 32:396-399, 1977.

55. Branemark P, Adell R, Albrektsson T, et al. An experimental and clinical study of osseointegrated implants penetrating the nasal cavity and maxillary sinus. *J Oral Maxillofac Surg.* 42:497-505, 1984.

56. Norlander T, Forsgren K, Kumlien J, et al. Cellular regeneration and recovery of the maxillary sinus mucosa: an experimental study in rabbits. *Acta Otolaryngol Suppl.* 492:33-37, 1992.

57. Forsgren K, Otori N, Stierna P, Kumlien J. Microvasculature, blood flow, and vasoreactivity in rabbit sinus mucosa after surgery. *Laryngoscope.* 109:562-568, 1999.

SECTION 4

MiniScrew Implant Systems

CHAPTER 9

The Ortho Implant System

Jason B. Cope, Robert J. Herman

IMTEC ORTHO IMPLANT

The Ortho Implant® (IMTEC Corp., Ardmore, Oklahoma) is a recently developed miniscrew implant (MSI) designed for enhancing orthodontic anchorage. The Ortho Implant is 1.8 mm in diameter and is available in 6-, 8-, or 10-mm lengths. The dimensions allow placement in a wide variety of intraoral locations, which permits the addition of stable anchorage in the treatment of many different malocclusions. Placement and removal of the Ortho Implant is technically simple and can be accomplished by the orthodontist.

The size of traditional dental implants restricts the locations in which they can be placed for orthodontic anchorage. To overcome this limitation, many different orthodontic temporary anchorage devices (OrthoTADs) have been developed specifically for use in orthodontics. One variety of TAD, the MSI, has substantially smaller dimensions than dental implants. The IMTEC Ortho Implant was developed by modifying the established IMTEC Sendax Mini Dental Implant (MDI) system specifically for use as an adjunctive orthodontic anchorage device. The Sendax MDI is a titanium alloy (Ti6Al4V) 1.8-mm diameter screw-shaped implant with a square head for insertion and an O-Ball retentive mechanism for attachment of implant-retained overdentures (Fig. 9-1).[1,2] The Sendax MDI system has been in use since 1998 and is accepted by the Food and Drug Administration for long-term use in denture

Simplicity of use and integration into the daily orthodontic practice were the primary goals when designing the Ortho Implant. With those goals in mind, only one head design and one diameter with three different lengths were chosen. Three different lengths are available to facilitate placement in different locations within the oral cavity based on gingival thickness and bony depth.

Threaded Body Design

The threaded body is self-drilling and self-tapping (thread-forming), thereby eliminating the necessity of placing a pilot hole. It is not, however, thread-cutting because it does not have a cutting flute at the apex that cuts or taps the bone during placement. In lieu of a thread-cutting flute, the apical 4 mm is tapered from 0.1 mm to the full 1.8 mm (Fig. 9-2) so that bone is compressed in and around the screw threads during advancement instead of the cutting and removing of bone common with other self-tapping screws.[3] In addition, the Ortho Implant is one of the few MSIs available with a modified buttress thread form, which minimizes screw backout or pullout (see Chapter 5). The outer diameter is 1.8 mm with a core diameter of 1.6 mm. Three threaded lengths are available: 6, 8, and 10 mm (Fig. 9-3). The surface is machine-polished to minimize osseointegration but allow bone apposition.

Transmucosal Collar Design

The transmucosal collar is 1.0 mm tall. The surface is

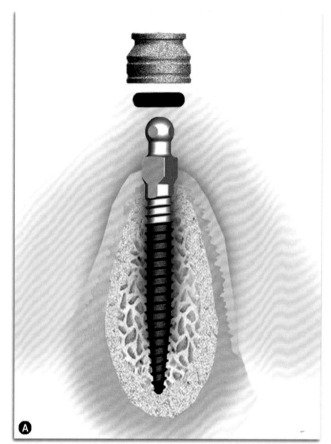

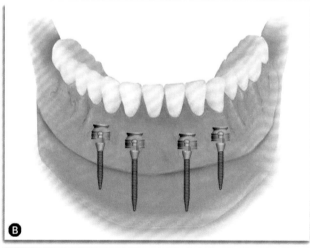

Fig. 9-1

IMTEC Sendax Mini Dental Implant system. **A,** Mini dental implant. **B,** MDI-retained overdenture.

thereby creating a seal between the oral cavity and the underlying bone. This also minimizes the risk of temporary anchorage device periimplantitis, or TAP (see Chapter 8).

Abutment Head Design

The abutment head of most MSIs is round, hexagonal, or octagonal with a Phillips (+) head. The slotted head is used for MSI placement and/or for rectangular wire

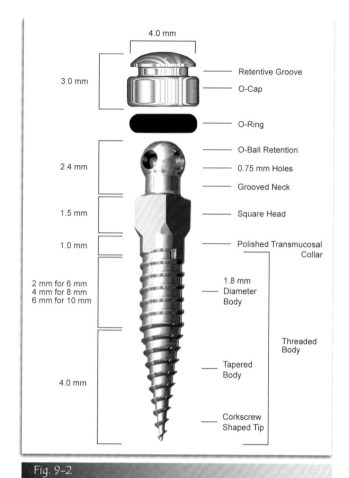

Fig. 9-2

IMTEC Ortho Implant.

attachment, whereas the hexagonal- or octagonal head can also be used for MSI placement. For these MSIs, the force for screwing the MSI into bone is applied at the most coronal aspect of the MSI (Fig. 9-4).

The weakest part of an MSI is the grooved neck that lies between the transmucosal collar and the abutment head.[4] The neck is where ligatures, power chains, or other force modules are often attached. Many MSIs also have one or two holes in the neck for passing ligatures or power thread. This construction often compromises the strength of the neck, which for most MSIs, lies below the level where the force is applied to screw the MSI into the bone. When considering the foregoing, it becomes apparent that excessive forces applied to the head of an MSI during placement may damage or fracture the head from the body of the implant at the neck. This is of particular concern in thick cortical bone.[5]

To avoid this, the head of the Ortho Implant is designed more like a dental implant than a miniscrew and is placed by applying force to the square head. Because the square head is apical to the grooved neck and the O-Ball where orthodontic forces are applied,

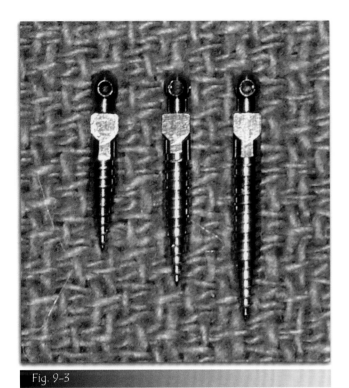

Fig. 9-3

Available Ortho Implant lengths are *(left to right)* 6, 8, and 10 mm.

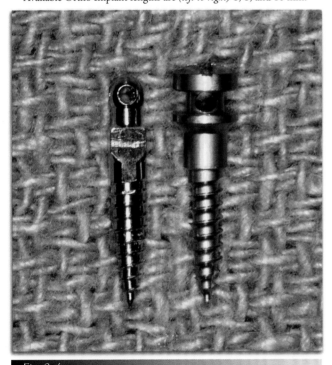

Fig. 9-4

Miniscrew implant abutment head designs. Insertion force is delivered to square head *(left)* and round head *(right)*. Note the weakest aspect of each screw is the small neck between head and body.

there is little risk of fracturing the Ortho Implant upon insertion. The square head is 1.5 mm tall. The grooved

at 90 degrees to each other and perpendicular to the long axis of the screw. The Ortho Implant can be attached to through the holes in the O-Ball or around the grooved neck. The O-Ball makes the system universally adaptable; it serves as one component in a ball and socket joint, the other being the Ortho Cap.

Ortho Cap Design

The Ortho Cap (O-Cap) is a stainless steel abutment component with an internal O-ring or gasket that locks in place around the O-Ball (Fig. 9-5). The O-Cap can be placed and removed with little effort but is stable enough that a patient cannot inadvertently dislodge it. The beauty of the O-Cap is that if the clinical situation warrants, it can be placed to suppress the soft tissues and prevent mucosal overgrowth, a situation not uncommon with other MSI systems. A groove is located around the circumference of the O-Cap so that ligatures, elastics, or power chain can be attached directly to the O-Cap. And because the O-Cap is made of stainless steel, it can be soldered to, thereby allowing different attachments to be fabricated.

TREATMENT PLANNING

Once the decision has been made that one or more TADs will be useful in accomplishing the treatment goals, several important things need to be accomplished during treatment planning to ensure that the TAD will be placed so that it can be used effectively and efficiently to accomplish the desired orthodontic or orthopedic movement without causing potential problems. First, the orthodontist must understand the anatomy of the specific TAD to be used because this will affect where and how it can be placed. Then, the orthodontist must understand what local anatomic locations can be used for TAD placement. Also of concern is the orientation of the TAD relative to the surface anatomy and the emergence profile through bone and soft tissue. Considering this, knowing what local anatomic structures must be avoided during TAD placement is also critical. Finally, the line of planned orthodontic mechanics and attachments must be considered so as to avoid soft tissue impingement. The reader is referred to Chapter 5 for review.

Of particular concern with the Ortho Implant is how the MSI is placed and removed. It should be recalled that the force for placing the Ortho Implant is applied to the square head. In doing so, the screw driver tip must be placed over and around the entire between the square head and any adjacent structures so that the tip of the screw driver can be placed over the head for engagement and removal (Fig. 9-6).

PRESURGICAL ORTHODONTICS

Completion of an initial phase of treatment prior to the placement of the Ortho Implant is frequently necessary. Because MSIs can be loaded with orthodontic forces immediately after placement, there is no advantage to placing the MSIs until they are needed. The objective of presurgical orthodontics depends largely on the general objectives of the treatment plan. Complete leveling and aligning of the arches before implant placement is usually necessary. This would be the case for premolar extraction followed by maximum anterior dental retraction via sliding mechanics on a continuous arch wire. However, in a skeletal anterior open bite with different anterior and posterior maxillary occlusal plane levels, leveling and aligning the maxillary arch before MSI-based posterior intrusion may actually exacerbate the malocclusion and make the open bite worse. Another reason for presurgical orthodontics is correction of root angulations in cases where teeth lie in the desired location of MSI placement such that placement would increase the risk of root impingement.

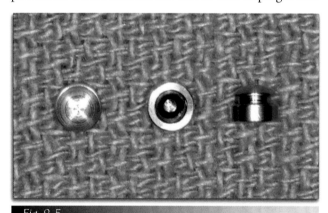

Fig. 9-5
Ortho Cap for placement around the O-Ball of the Ortho Implant.

It therefore becomes apparent that the need for presurgical orthodontics should be determined on a case by case basis.

SURGICAL PROCEDURE

The surgical armamentarium (Fig. 9-7, A) for Ortho Implant placement includes cotton pliers, a violet-colored mucosal marking pen, a periodontal probe with a rubber endodontic stopper, a curved explorer, a mouth mirror, Oraqix® topical anesthetic (Dentsply Pharmaceutical, York, Pennsylvania), the stainless steel O-Caps, the appropriate length Ortho Implants, a 1.5-mm soft-tissue biopsy punch, 2 × 2-inch cotton gauze, cotton rolls, the LT-Driver with adapter tips (Under Dog Media, Dallas, Texas), and the Ortho Driver. Items that may be necessary in certain cases include a syringe, needle, and anesthetic; a 1.1-mm pilot drill; a No. 2 round bur latch-grip; and a slow-speed latch-grip contra-angle handpiece (Fig. 9-7, B).

The surgical procedure is as follows (Cope Placement Protocol™):

1. Patient brushes teeth to remove plaque and debris. Chlorhexidine has been shown to interact with detergents and fluoride in toothpaste.[6] Therefore, the patient should rinse vigorously with water after brushing and before rinsing with chlorhexidine or should use no toothpaste at all.
2. Patient rinses with 15 mL of 0.12% chlorhexidine gluconate for 30 seconds. Chlorhexidine has been shown to provide antimicrobial activity during rinsing.[7]
3. Apply Oraqix® anesthetic topically (Fig. 9-8). Oraqix is a 2.5% lidocaine and 2.5% prilocaine topical periodontal anesthetic that provides profound soft tissue and periosteal anesthesia.[8,9] Oraqix has limited anesthetic effect on bone and tooth roots via absorption. So similar to extraction of teeth, the patient will feel pressure, but not pain, unless the periodontal ligament (PDL) or tooth root is contacted, in which case the orthodontist needs to know so that the orientation angle of the Ortho Implant can be altered prior to root damage.

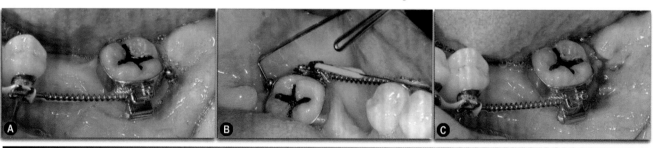

Fig. 9-6
Ortho Implant without enough space for removal. **A,** Distalized second molar is contacting O-Ball with no space for screwdriver engagement of the square head. **B,** A separator is ligated anteriorly to compress the periodontal ligament so that an 0.028-inch stainless steel wire can be used to unscrew the Ortho Implant. **C,** Photograph after Ortho Implant removal.

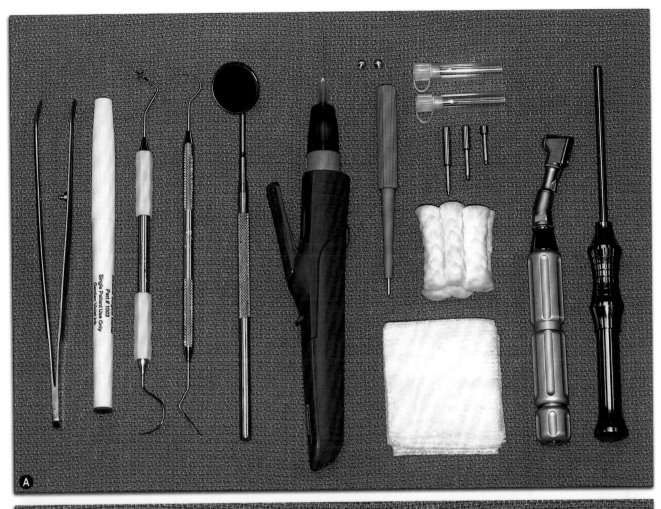

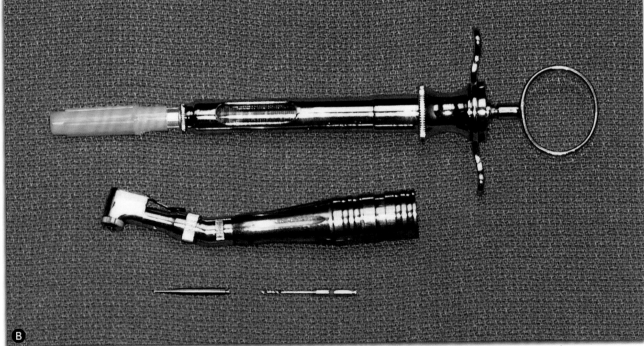

4. Apply local anesthetic (optional). In certain locations such as the retromolar region or palate, the soft tissue is so thick that topical anesthetic simply cannot be

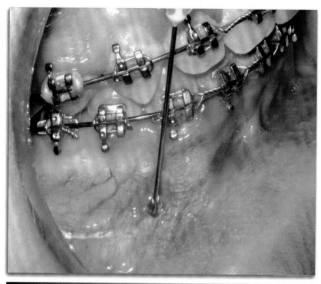

Fig. 9-8

Topical anesthesia using Oraqix. Note that the flat syringe tip is not for injection but rather is the manufacturer's system of choice for anesthetic delivery into a periodontal defect.

absorbed through the entire thickness of the gingiva to reach the periosteum. These same locations often have thicker or denser cortical bone, whereby the patient may feel more pressure upon MSI placement. In these situations and in overly apprehensive patients, localized injection of local anesthetic may be beneficial.

5. Determine the Ortho Implant insertion site. Several methods are available to mark the insertion site. It is important to place the Ortho Implant in locations with a minimum of 0.5 mm of bone around the circumference of the Ortho Implant.

a. The simplest method is to use a panoramic or periapical radiograph with direct clinical visualization to identify the site (Fig. 9-9).

b. A modification of this approach is to use the lateral end of an explorer firmly to indent the outline of the roots into the soft tissues before using direct clinical visualization to identify the site (Fig. 9-10). The violet mucosal marker can also be used to mark the site.

c. A clear vacuum-formed stent can be fabricated on the patient's cast. Identify the site on the plastic stent with a permanent marker, and then drill a hole into the stent. Insert a 0.044-inch tube into the hole at the proper orientation, and then use cold-cured acrylic to attach the tube (Fig. 9-11).

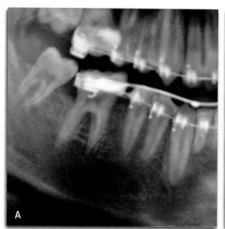
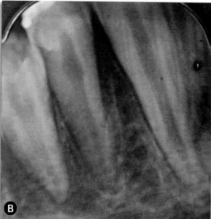
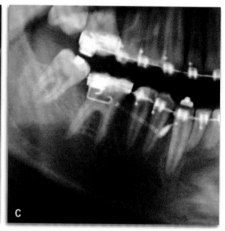

Fig. 9-9

Radiographic evaluation. **A,** Preoperative panoramic radiograph to determine placement location in adequate bone stock. **B,** Preoperative periapical radiograph to confirm placement location in adequate bone stock. **C,** Postoperative panoramic radiograph showing good placement.

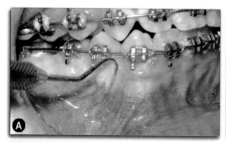
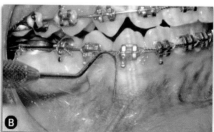
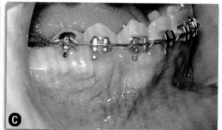

Fig. 9-10

Curved end of explorer used to indent outline of root surface in gingiva. **A,** Explorer outlining mesial edge of first premolar root. **B,** Explorer outlining distal edge of canine root. **C,** Resulting indentation possible because of tissue turgor pressure.

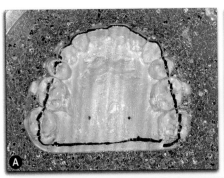 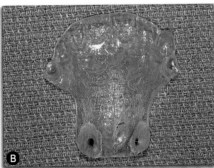 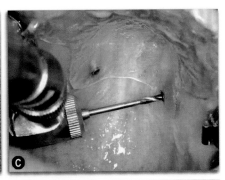

Fig. 9–11

Vacuum-formed stent used to locate desired MSI placement location. **A,** A 0.5-mm plastic vacuum-formed stent on working model with Ortho Implant sites marked. **B,** Stent trimmed to cover lingual surfaces of teeth and 0.044-inch tubes inserted at proper orientation. **C,** Sterile stent used to place pilot holes.

    d. Take panoramic or periapical x-rays with a polyvinyl siloxane partial occlusal stent and a loop-ended metal wire extending to the planned site. The wire can be bent and adjusted until the appropriate site is identified.

6. Perform bone sounding with periodontal probe to measure soft tissue thickness. Probe a marked periodontal probe with an endodontic stopper through the soft tissue in the planned Ortho Implant location until bone is contacted. At this point, the stopper rests on the soft tissue. Then remove the probe and record the soft tissue thickness from the periodontal probe (Fig. 9-12).

7. Determine Ortho Implant length based on both soft tissue thickness and bone thickness. The Ortho Implant length is determined more by the soft tissue thickness than by the bony thickness (cortical bone plus medullary bone up to but not including contralateral cortex). The most critical aspect is that the full 1.8-mm diameter threaded body should reside within the outer cortex, with the tapered part of the threaded body in the medullary bone. Usually, direct measurements taken from the diagnostic models (Fig. 9-13) can be combined with direct clinical measurements and approximate values from the radiographs to aid in determining the appropriate Ortho Implant length and placement location relative to the interproximal contact.

    If the soft tissue is greater than 1.5 mm thick, a longer Ortho Implant is required. For example, the 6-mm

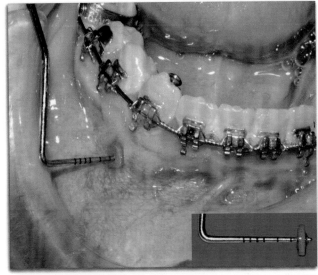

Fig. 9–12

Bone sounding with periodontal probe to determine gingival thickness.

Ortho Implant has 4-mm of taper and 2 mm of the full 1.8-mm diameter threaded body (Fig. 9-14; Table 9-1). The 2 mm of the full 1.8-mm diameter should reside in the cortex. So if the soft tissue is more than 1.5 mm, then the neck of the Ortho Implant will be too close to the soft tissue or possibly even submerged. Therefore, a

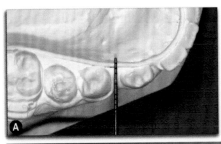 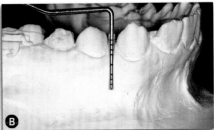 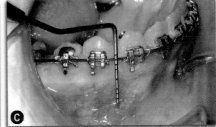

Fig. 9–13

Determine Ortho Implant length and location. **A,** Alveolar width is estimated directly from model and subtracting gingival thickness from bone sounding. **B,** Vertical height is estimated directly from model and compared with the radiographs. **C,** Intraoral location is determined from radiograph and model measurements.

longer Ortho Implant should be used. For part of the threaded body to traverse the soft tissue is not a problem as long as the part of the Ortho Implant that resides in the outer cortex is not tapered. Table 9-2 lists the most common locations for each Ortho Implant length.

8. Place punch incision with 1.5-mm soft tissue biopsy punch (optional). The soft tissue punch is necessary

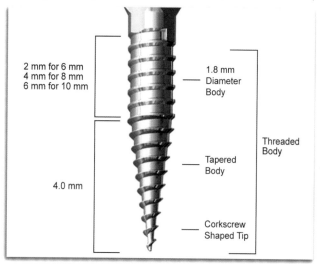

2 mm for 6 mm
4 mm for 8 mm
6 mm for 10 mm

4.0 mm

1.8 mm Diameter Body

Tapered Body

Threaded Body

Corkscrew Shaped Tip

Fig. 9-14

Ortho Implant threaded body dimensions.

Table 9-1.	Threaded Body Dimensions	
Threaded Implant Length (mm)	Tapered Length (mm)	1.8-mm Diameter Length (mm)
6	4	2
8	4	4
10	4	6

Table 9-2.	Common Ortho Implant Locations*
Length (mm)	Implant Location
6	Facial surface maxillary/mandibular alveolar ridge mesial to second premolar, maxillary sub–anterior nasal spine region, mandibular symphysis
8	Facial surface maxillary/mandibular alveolar ridge distal to second premolar, parasagittal midpalate
10	Maxillary tuberosity or zygomatic buttress, posterior or lateral palate, ascending ramus, retromolar region, external oblique ridge

* Use this only as a guide because soft tissue and bone thicknesses vary from patient to patient.

only in cases where the Ortho Implant will penetrate through alveolar (mobile) mucosa. This should be done whether a pilot hole is used or not. A punch incision is not necessary through keratinized gingiva. Place the punch directly over the implant site and perpendicular to the bone surface, and then push it through the soft tissue until the bone is contacted (Fig. 9-15). Once the bone is contacted, rotate the punch against the bone surface three complete 360-degree revolutions to cleanly incise the tissue. If the tissue is cleanly incised, it usually remains in the head of the punch. If not, it can be removed with a curette, hemostats, or small cotton forceps. In some cases, if the patient experiences sensitivity with the punch, additional topical anesthetic can be applied to the exposed surface of the mucosa and periosteum.

9. Place pilot notch with No. 2 round bur or pilot hole with 1.1-mm pilot drill bit (optional). Drilling a pilot hole is not necessary in most cases. The drill-free Ortho Implant will perforate the cortex as it is screwed into the bone with the O-Driver. However, in certain locations where cortical bone is thicker or denser, such as the posterior mandible or palate, simply drilling a pilot notch or pilot hole may be helpful and quicker. Two different methods for doing this use a slow-speed contra-angle handpiece.

a. Pilot notch: Use the No. 2 round bur to create a notch about 1.0 mm in depth, which is just deep enough to allow the Ortho Implant apex to "bite" into the bone upon insertion.

b. Pilot hole: Use the 1.1-mm drill bit to perforate the cortex only (Fig. 9-16). As the pilot hole is being drilled, the clinician will feel the drill bit "drop" into the medullary bone from the cortex. As soon as this "drop" is felt, drilling should stop. Unlike with traditional dental implants, a complete osteotomy to the full threaded length is not only unnecessary but also contraindicated. Only the cortex should be perforated.

For either method the bur should be used at 500 to 800 rpm with physiologic saline irrigation (5° C) to prevent overheating of the bone. Drilling should take place intermittently and without undue pressure so that the tip of the bur or drill bit can cool down. It is critical to drill the bur or drill bit into the bone consistently at the exact same axis in order to prevent hole overenlargement because this would prevent primary stability of the Ortho Implant.

10. Insert Ortho Implant with O-Driver or contra-angle LT-Driver. Remove the white cap from the sterile vial. While holding the white cap in one hand, place the O-Driver or LT-Driver over the O-Ball and around the square head so that the O-ring tightly holds the Ortho Implant in the O-Driver (Fig. 9-17) or LT-Driver (Fig. 9-18). The O-Driver is applicable to most locations. The LT-Driver is usually more applicable

in the retromolar regions for implants placed vertically, in the anterior palate for implants placed vertically, and in the posterior palate for implants placed laterally.

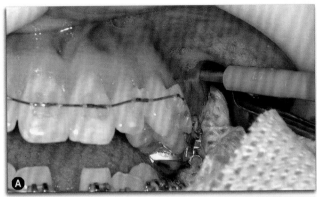

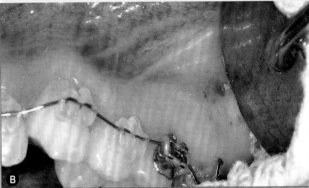

Fig. 9-15

Soft tissue punch incision procedure. **A,** Biopsy punch is placed over alveolar mucosa and then is rotated as it is pushed against the bone. **B,** This results in a 1.5-mm window in the tissue with cleanly incised margins and minimal bleeding.

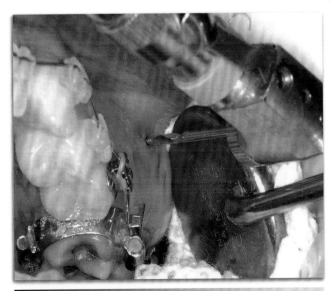

Fig. 9-16

Pilot hole procedure for perforating the cortex only. Note that the alveolar mucosa is maintained under tension by the mouth mirror to prevent its being wrapped around the pilot drill bit.

Place the tip of the Ortho Implant against the bone or in the pilot notch or pilot hole at the proper orientation and screw it clockwise into the bone with firm seating pressure at the base of the handle as the O-Driver is rotated with the fingers (Fig. 9-19). If the LT-Driver is used, twist the base of the handle clockwise into the bone with firm seating pressure applied with the thumb or palm of the contralateral hand (Fig. 9-20).

As the Ortho Implant is screwed into the bone, the resistance of the bone will most likely begin to increase. This occurs more often in the mandible than in the maxilla. It is important to recall that bone is viscoelastic and will expand in response to internal pressure.[5] Therefore, when placing an Ortho Implant in dense bone (usually posterior mandible), it may be appropriate to screw the Ortho Implant until pressure increases considerably and then stop, allowing the bone to expand around the Ortho Implant for 10 to 20 seconds before continuing. This respite should be repeated as often as necessary and is usually required only for the range from 2 to 4.0 mm of the tapered body (Table 9-3). After the tapered body is through the cortex and the full 1.8-mm diameter body begins to enter the bone, the bone is no longer required to expand to accommodate the increasing diameter; therefore, the pressure remains relatively constant and respites are usually no longer required. Insert the Ortho Implant until the polished collar engages the outer cortex or the square head penetrates the soft tissue by no more than 0.5 mm (Fig. 9-21).

At the end of Ortho Implant placement, the inferior aspect of the square head (polished transmucosal collar) should contact the bone surface with the entire O-Ball, neck, and part of the square head located supramucosally (Box 9-1). Because the primary stability of the Ortho

Table 9-3.	Respites for Ortho Implant Placement*	
	Section of Implant Body	Respite
	0-2 mm	Usually no respites required
	2-4 mm	Respites usually required in dense bone
	4+ mm	Usually no respites required

* Measurements start at apex.

Box 9-1.	Ortho Implant Placement Checklist

The 1.8-mm diameter body should be in the cortex.
The tapered apex should be in medullary bone.
The apex should not touch the contralateral cortex.
The variable is primarily in the soft tissue depth.

Implant comes from the cortex, it is also important to have the entire cortex traversed by the 1.8-mm diameter body with the tapered end in medullary bone. The Ortho Implant must be stable upon initial placement or should be placed in an alternate location.

11. Place O-Cap to suppress alveolar (mobile) mucosa (optional). With some MSI systems the alveolar mucosa will grow over the head of the implant. This, however, is rarely a problem with the Ortho Implant. There are 4 reasons for placing the O-Cap:

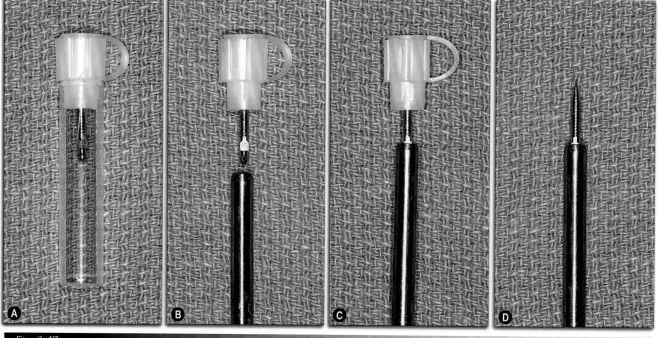

Fig. 9-17

Ortho Implant pickup procedure with O-Driver. **A,** The sterile vial is removed from the blister pack. **B,** The cap is removed from the vial, and the O-Driver tip is aligned over the square head. **C,** The O-Driver tip engages the square head and unscrews the Ortho Implant. **D,** Ortho Implant is ready for placement.

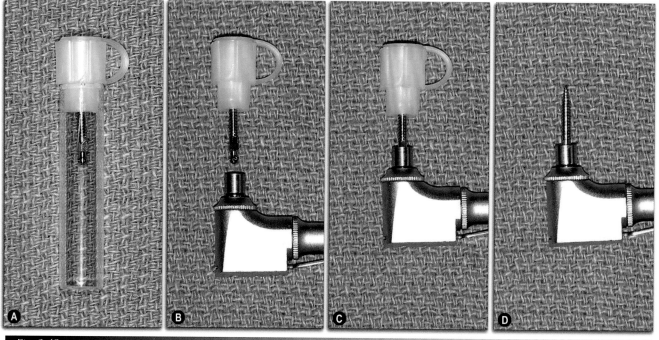

Fig. 9-18

Ortho Implant pickup procedure with LT-Driver. **A,** The sterile vial is removed from the blister pack. **B,** The cap is removed from the vial, and the LT-Driver tip is aligned over the square head. **C,** The LT-Driver tip engages the square head and unscrews the Ortho Implant. **D,** Ortho Implant is ready for placement.

a. The O-Cap suppresses alveolar mucosa and prevents soft tissue overgrowth of the O-Ball (Fig. 9-22, *A* and *B*).

b. When in place, the groove on the O-Cap is 1.0 mm higher and 1.5 mm lateral to the Ortho Implant neck, which in certain cases is beneficial to prevent the orthodontic attachment mechanics from impinging the soft tissue (Fig. 9-22, *C* and *D*).

c. Because the O-Ball is so small, it may actually feel sharp to some patients in certain circumstances (i.e., when placed laterally in the alveolar bone anteriorly). In these cases, because the O-Cap is larger, it makes the emergence profile feel smoother to the patient (Fig. 9-22, *E* and *F*).

d. Because the O-Cap is made of stainless steel, various attachments can be soldered to it, thereby making the Ortho Implant even more versatile (Fig. 9-22, *G* and *H*). It is important to note that the force must pass through the long axis of the Ortho Implant for single Ortho Implants. If two O-Caps are soldered together in series, this is not as critical because the rotational tendency is no longer present.

Also, because the Ortho Implant is a modification of the Sendax MDI system, the components of that system can also be used for orthodontic anchorage (Fig. 9-23). For example, in the case of an Ortho Implant placed in the palate, the impression cap is placed on the implant clinically for impression acquisition. The laboratory analog is then placed in the impression cap and the impression poured in stone to create a working model. Next, the O-Cap is placed on the analog to fabricate an implant-supported appliance by soldering attachments or by incorporating acrylic around the O-Cap. The appliance is then seated clinically and activated.

It is important to understand the dimensions of the Ortho Implant and the O-Cap in cases where two implants may be placed side by side. In this case, if the O-Caps will be used, the implants must be a minimum of 5.0 mm apart (center to center) or the O-Caps will be too close together to fit on the abutment heads (Fig. 9-24).

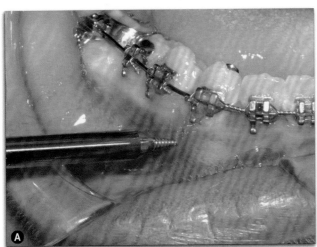

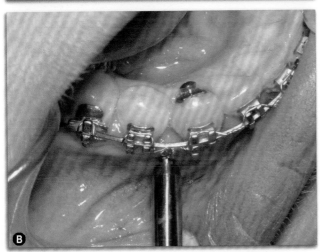

Fig. 9-19

Ortho Implant placement procedure with O-Driver. **A,** Ortho Implant tip is aligned vertically and horizontally according to gingival indentations. **B,** Horizontal angulation is verified from the occlusal aspect.

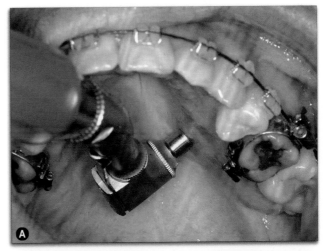

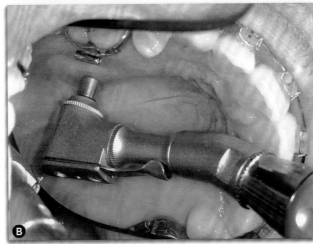

Fig. 9-20

Ortho Implant placement procedure with LT-Driver. **A,** Ortho Implant tip is aligned vertically and horizontally in pilot hole at proper angulation. **B,** Horizontal angulation is verified from the occlusal aspect.

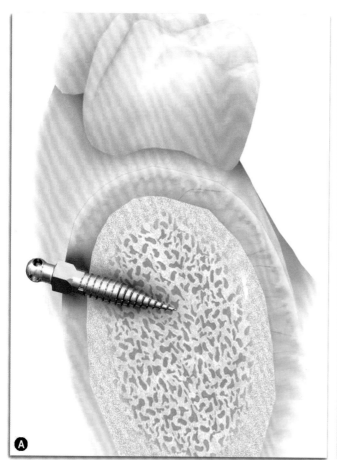

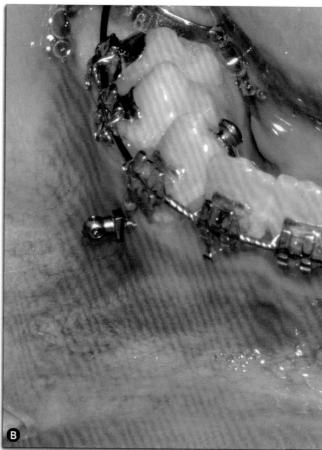

Fig. 9–21

Final position of Ortho Implant. **A,** Schematic cross section showing full 1.8-mm diameter in cortex and part of threads in gingiva because of gingival thickness but with at least half of the square head outside the gingiva. **B,** Final position of Ortho Implant clinically.

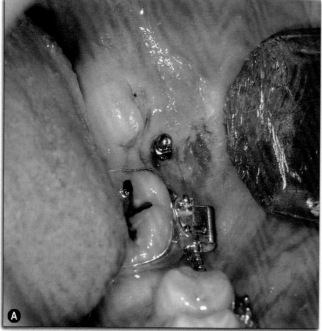

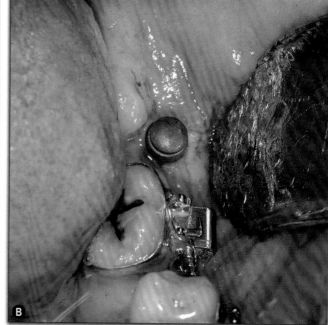

Fig. 9–22

Ortho Cap uses. **A,** Ortho Implant surrounded by mobile retromolar soft tissue. **B,** O-Cap placed to prevent mucosal overgrowth. *(continued)*

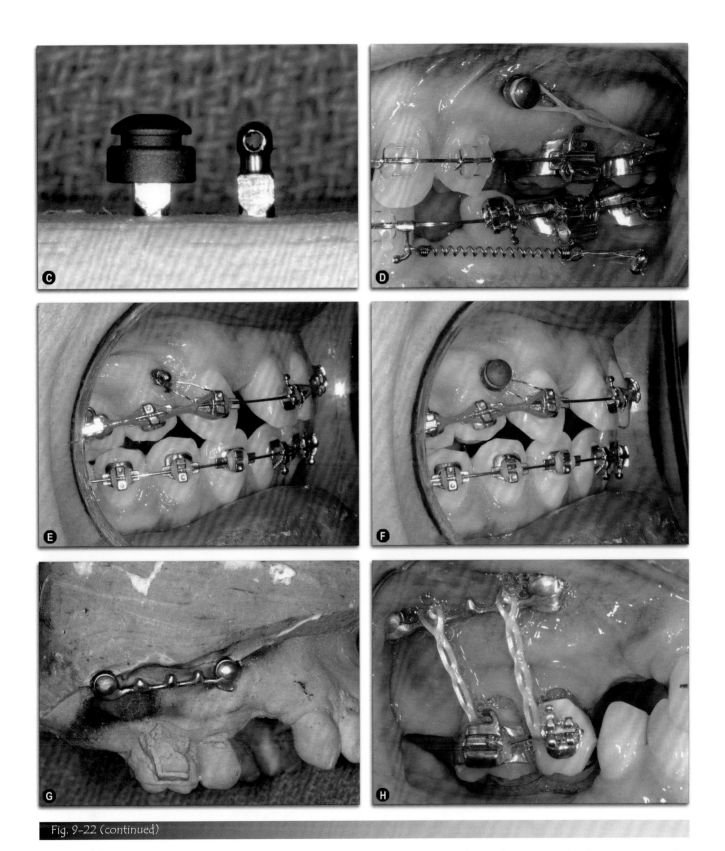

Fig. 9-22 (continued)

C, O-Cap groove is located 1.0 mm higher and 1.5 mm lateral compared with Ortho Implant neck. **D,** O-Cap placed to prevent gingival impingement by powerchain. **E,** O-Ball head may feel sharp in the arc of the canine region. **F,** O-Cap placed to make emergence profile feel smooth. **G,** Two O-Caps soldered together with an 0.032-inch stainless steel wire. **H,** Right buccal photograph with soldered O-Caps in place.

ORTHODONTIC MECHANICS

After placement, the Ortho Implant can be loaded immediately. There is no need to wait days or weeks to load for soft tissue or bony healing. Attachment mechanics can be placed directly through the 0.030-inch holes (Fig. 9-25, *A*), around the implant neck

> ### Box 9-2. Ortho Implant Postoperative Instructions
>
> - Take 800 mg ibuprofen immediately, and then 400 mg as needed for dental discomfort.
> - Rinse with 15 mL of 0.12% chlorhexidine gluconate for 30 seconds twice a day for 10 days.
> - Rinse with 15 mL of 0.12% chlorhexidine gluconate for 30 seconds as needed for periimplant erythema thereafter.
> - Do not play with the Ortho Implant with fingers or tongue.
> - Do not eat anything hard, chewy, or sticky in the vicinity of the Ortho Implant.
> - Call if Ortho Implant or orthodontic attachments become loose or for any other concerns.

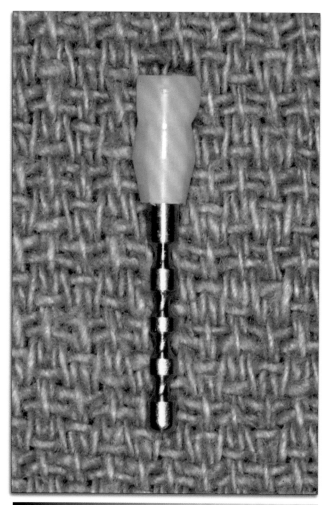

Fig. 9-23

Mini dental implant laboratory analog *(bottom)* and impression cap *(top)*.

(Fig. 9-25, *B*), around a cotter pin placed through the 0.030-inch holes (Fig. 9-25, *C*), around the groove in O-Cap if placed (Fig. 9-25, *D*), or to attachments soldered to the O-Cap itself. Postoperative pain is negligible, and at most 800 mg of ibuprofen is administered. Postoperative antibiotics for prophylactic reasons are not necessary unless the patient otherwise would be covered under the American Heart Association guidelines. Box 9-2 lists the Ortho Implant postoperative instructions.

Anterior Retraction

When implants are planned as anchorage for retraction, a variety of mechanisms exist to apply the desired force directly to the anterior segment. Depending on the vertical placement of the implants, retraction can be combined with intrusion of the anterior segment. Maximum anchorage is a primary indication of MSIs in premolar extraction cases. When it is desired to maximize the retraction of maxillary anterior teeth into space gained by extraction, the Ortho Implant can be placed laterally in the alveolar ridge mesial to the first molar. The vertical height of placement depends on the desired movement of the anterior segment. A more apical placement would cause intrusion during retraction, whereas a more coronal placement would be used for more pure translation without a vertical component. Nickel titanium springs can be ligated to the head of the implant and attached to the arch wire by a crimpable hook (Fig. 9-26). However, the eyelet of most manufacturers is too small to fit over the O-Ball.

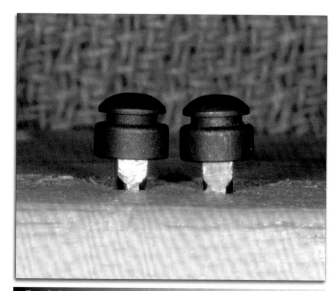

Fig. 9-24

Inter–O-Cap distance. Note that two Ortho Implants with O-Caps in place must be at least 5.0 mm apart.

To overcome this, the first author has developed a special closed coil spring that locks onto the head of the O-Ball so that it does not have to be ligated and the patient cannot inadvertently dislodge it.

Arch Distalization

Mechanics for entire arch distalization can be designed to pull or push the arch distally. In pulling mechanics the implants must be placed posteriorly so that ample

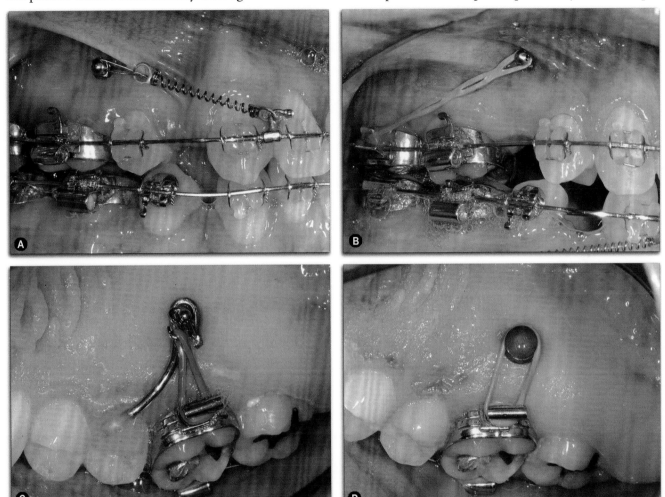

Fig. 9-25

Methods of attachment. **A,** Directly through the 0.030-inch holes. **B,** Around the implant neck. **C,** Around a cotter pin placed through the 0.030-inch holes. **D,** Around the groove in O-Cap.

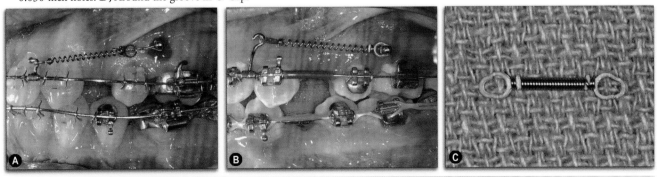

Fig. 9-26

Anterior retraction. **A,** A short crimpable hook lies below the center of resistance, which will result in decreasing crown torque during retraction. **B,** A longer crimpable hook will be closer to the center of resistance, which will result in translation without decreasing crown torque during retraction. **C,** New closed coil spring design that fits over the Ortho Implant and then locks in place so that it cannot be dislodged by the patient. (Courtesy Dr. Jason B. Cope, Dallas, Tex. Patent pending.)

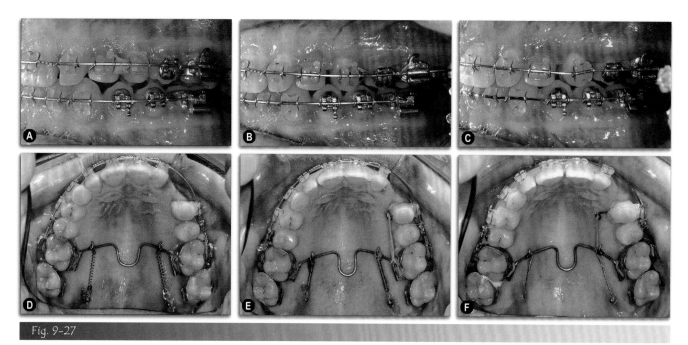

Fig. 9-27

Arch distalization with pulling mechanics. **A,** Buccal photograph at initial Ortho Implant placement. **B,** Buccal photograph after molar distalization. **C,** Buccal photograph at Ortho Implant removal after premolar retraction. Total Ortho Implant duration was 7 months. **D,** Occlusal photograph at initial Ortho Implant placement. **E,** Occlusal photograph after molar distalization. **F,** Occlusal photograph at Ortho Implant removal after premolar retraction. Note that after molar retraction was complete, the closed coil springs were replaced with ligatures for premolar retraction.

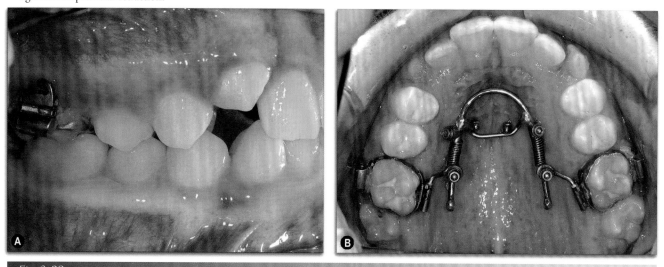

Fig. 9-28

Arch distalization with pushing mechanics. **A,** Buccal photograph at initial Ortho Implant placement and loading with Distal Jet. **B,** Occlusal photograph at initial Ortho Implant placement and loading with Distal Jet. Note photographs were taken in maximum intercuspation.

distance exists for active mechanics (Fig. 9-27). The active mechanics can be power chain, power thread, or closed coil springs. In pushing mechanics the implants must be placed more anteriorly. Several different distalizing appliances can be incorporated. The implant-supported Distal Jet (American Orthodontics, Sheboygan, Wisconsin) is a relatively hygienic appliance that locates the force through the approximate center of resistance of the molars and is simple to activate (Fig. 9-28).

Posterior Protraction

Ortho Implants used for protraction require additional consideration. This is particularly of concern when protracting molars. Recall that when retracting the six anterior teeth en masse from a facially placed MSI, there is no rotational tendency around the center of resistance because the anterior teeth lie in an arc and are constrained by the arch wire. When protracting molars from a facially placed MSI along a straight arch wire, the force passes facial and superior to the center

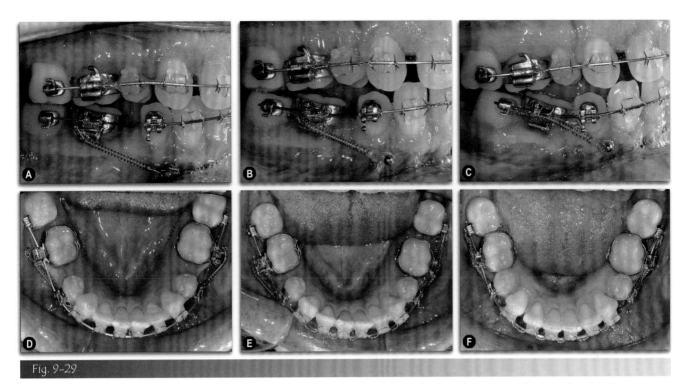

Fig. 9-29

Posterior protraction with facial mechanics only. **A,** Buccal photograph at initial Ortho Implant placement and loading. Note that force passes above the molar center of resistance. **B,** Buccal photograph after 3 months of loading. **C,** Buccal photograph after 7 months of loading. Note tipped molars and exacerbation of curve of Spee. **D,** Occlusal photograph at initial Ortho Implant placement and loading. **E,** Occlusal photograph after 3 months of loading. **F,** Occlusal photograph after 7 months of loading. Note distal out rotation of second (terminal) molars.

of resistance. This can result in the crown tipping anteriorly (Fig. 9-29, *A* to *C*) and a distal out rotational tendency, particularly if the force is attached to a terminal molar (Fig. 9-29, *D* to *F*). Even if the tooth is constrained by the arch wire, the rotational tendency presumably increases friction and slows protraction. In these situations, use a full-sized rectangular stainless steel arch wire (rounded posteriorly to ease sliding mechanics). In addition, the force should pass through the center of rotation on the facial, and a light force should also be applied on the lingual (Fig. 9-30). The lingual force is not necessarily for protraction but simply to minimize any rotational tendency and decrease friction.

Molar Uprighting

Traditional mechanics use posteriorly directed forces or uprighting springs to distalize and upright mesially tipped molars. Unfortunately, this usually causes relative extrusion of molars, placing them in traumatic occlusion with the opposing molars, potentially leading to periodontal problems. Ortho Implants make molar uprighting relatively simple, especially if they are placed below the bracket position of the tipped molar. Although it may seem logical to line up the implant along the lateral occlusal plane in line with the arch wire,

this is usually in a location that causes trauma to the soft tissues during mastication and so should be avoided (Fig. 9-31). Ideally, the implant should be placed distal to the tipped molar and in line with the central fossa. The molar is pulled distally and intruded simultaneously, thereby preventing extrusion. It is important to incorporate extra arch wire with a hook bent to prevent the molar from sliding off of the arch wire.

Molar Intrusion

For single supererupted teeth, molar intrusion is relatively simple. An implant can be placed on both the facial and palatal surfaces (Fig. 9-32) or just on the facial surface. The reason it is possible to place an implant on the facial surface only is due to root surface area. Recall that maxillary molars have two facial roots and only one palatal root. This means that if the anatomy warrants only one implant, it is better to err on the facial because the root surface area is larger. If the implant were placed on the palatal only where root surface is less, then less resistance would be offered and the tooth would tend to tip palatally as it is intruded.

Posterior Intrusion

When an Ortho Implant is used to address vertical problems in the maxilla, the implant can be placed in the facial alveolar bone or in the palatal alveolar bone. The problem with placing an MSI in facial alveolar bone is that usually it cannot be placed high enough to avoid soft tissue problems associated with the height of the vestibule and still have enough attachment length for intrusion mechanics. In addition, the teeth tend to tip facially, causing the palatal cusps to drop and exacerbate

the open bite (Fig. 9-33). An alternative would be to place the MSI in the zygomatic ridge; however, the soft tissues are still difficult to manage in this region. Perhaps the best location for MSI placement in hyperdivergent skeletal open bite case being treated by dental intrusion is in the palatal bone, but only if the patient does not have a

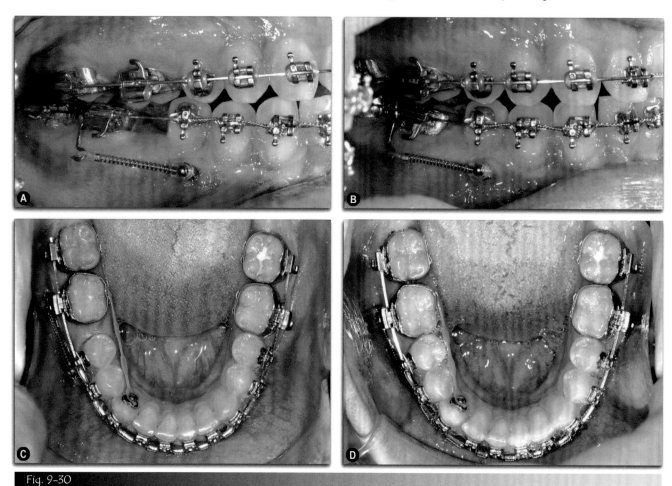

Fig. 9-30

Posterior protraction with facial and lingual mechanics. **A,** Buccal photograph at initial Ortho Implant placement and loading. Note that force passes close to molar center of resistance. **B,** Buccal photograph after 8 weeks of loading. **C,** Occlusal photograph at initial Ortho Implant placement and loading. Note light lingual powerchain placed for antirotation. **D,** Occlusal photograph after 8 weeks of loading.

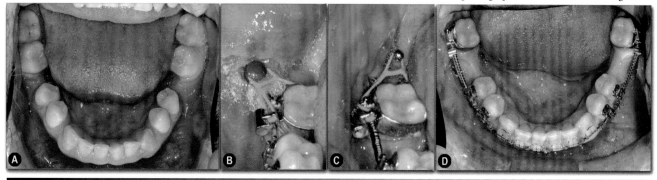

Fig. 9-31

Molar uprighting. **A,** Pretreatment occlusal photograph. Note tipped molars. **B,** Improper Ortho Implant location in line with appliances. **C,** Proper Ortho Implant location in line with central fossa. **D,** Progress occlusal photograph after 5 months of molar uprighting with Ortho Implants.

narrow intermolar width. These patients characteristically have a high palatal vault such that placement of an MSI at the junction of the palatal bone and palatal alveolar ridge is high enough for intrusion mechanics (Fig. 9-34). Moreover, these patients usually have hanging lingual cusps that need more intrusion than the facial cusps.

REMOVAL PROCEDURE

Ortho Implant removal is indicated after its use for anchorage and tooth movement is complete. In certain cases of molar intrusion for open bite correction, it may be beneficial to leave the unloaded Ortho Implant in place for several months after active

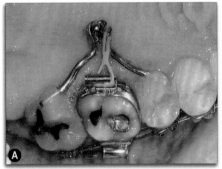
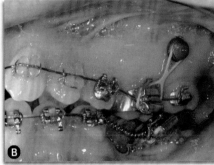
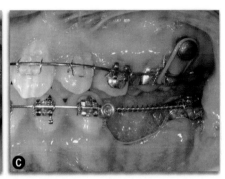

Fig. 9-32

Molar intrusion. **A,** Occlusal photograph of palatal Ortho Implant at initial loading. **B,** Buccal photograph of Ortho Implant at initial loading. **C,** Buccal photograph of Ortho Implant after 7 months of loading. Note overintrusion of first and second molars. Photographs taken in maximum intercuspation.

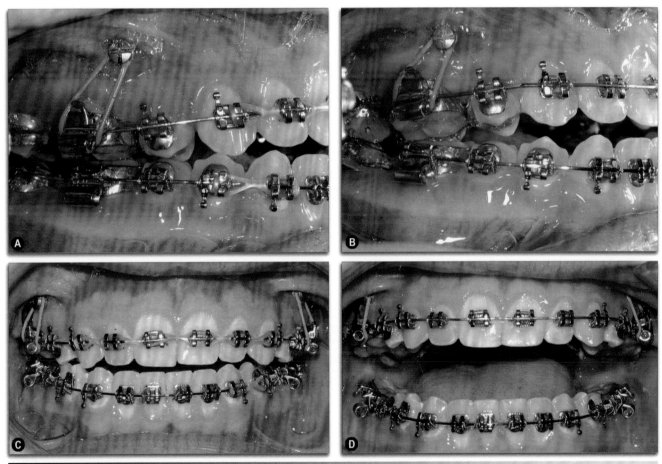

Fig. 9-33

Posterior intrusion using facial mechanics. **A,** Buccal photograph at initial Ortho Implant placement and loading. **B,** Buccal photograph after 3 months of loading. Note that the palatal cusps are hanging down. **C,** Anterior photograph at initial Ortho Implant placement and loading. **D,** Anterior photograph after 3 months of loading. Note that the palatal cusps are hanging down.

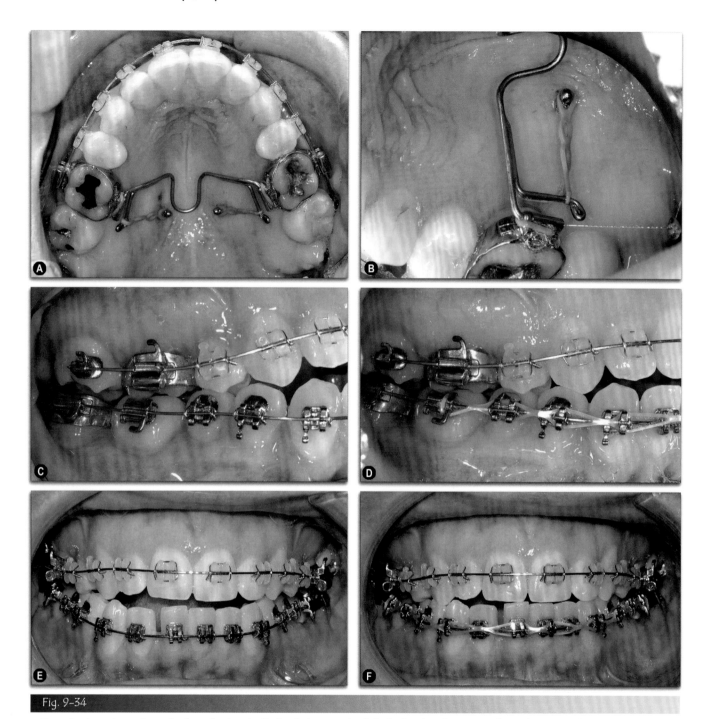

Fig. 9-34

Posterior intrusion using palatal mechanics. **A,** Occlusal photograph of Ortho Implant location and attachment mechanics. **B,** Close-up photograph of Ortho Implant location and attachment mechanics (Courtesy Dr. Jason B. Cope, Dallas, Tex. Patent pending). **C,** Buccal photograph at initial Ortho Implant placement and loading. **D,** Buccal photograph after 8 weeks of loading. Note that the palatal cusps are more seated. **E,** Anterior photograph at initial Ortho Implant placement and loading. **F,** Anterior photograph after 8 weeks of loading. Note that the overbite has closed somewhat.

use in the event that dental relapse occurs. Ortho Implant removal occurs without topical or local anesthetic by simply unscrewing the Ortho Implant. Topical anesthetic may be indicated in cases where the soft tissue has slightly overgrown the square head in order to anesthetize the superficial soft tissues as they are compressed during square head engagement for

Ortho Implant removal. No pain is associated with the Ortho Implant removal; therefore, analgesics are not indicated. Upon Ortho Implant removal, no treatment is indicated and no sutures are warranted. The soft tissue and bone heal uneventfully within 3 to 7 days (Fig. 9-35).

An important note is that removal of an Ortho

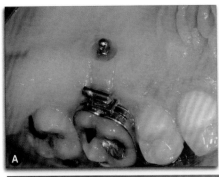
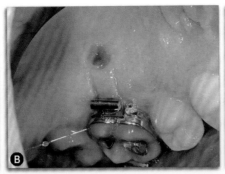
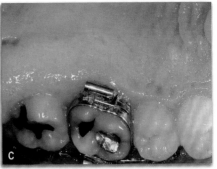

Fig. 9-35

Ortho Implant removal. **A,** The O-Cap is removed. Note the slight depression and erythema where the O-Cap suppressed the soft tissue. **B,** The Ortho Implant is unscrewed without any anesthesia. **C,** After 8 weeks, it is difficult to determine where the Ortho Implant was located.

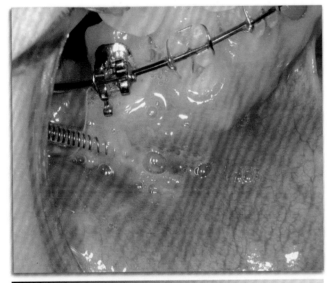

Fig. 9-36

A rare complication seen with the Ortho Implant is soft tissue overgrowth. In this case the Ortho Implant was not removed but the site was irrigated and cleaned, and the patient was prescribed clindamycin for 8 days and chlorhexidine twice daily for 14 days. (See CR-MSI 16 for details.)

Implant is not necessary during loading (if in place more than a month) with subtle mobility (periodontal mobility score of –1). As long as the Ortho Implant is clinically stable and usable with no frank mobility, there is no indication for removal. Removal of a stable Ortho Implant with localized soft tissue infection also is not necessary. Ortho Implant removal is indicated only in cases with frank mobility, infection that does not respond to antibiotic therapy within 2 to 3 weeks, or of infection with suppuration.

POTENTIAL COMPLICATIONS

The complications associated with the Ortho Implant, or any TAD system, predominately lie in the potential for iatrogenic placement, inadequate bone support, poor patient compliance, and poor soft tissue response. The stability of an MSI has been shown to be related to the health of the soft tissues surrounding it.[10] Infection or inflammation is associated with greater potential for implant loss. After placement, the soft tissue is tender and may present erythematously, but infection is rarely seen. In those cases in which inflammation occurs, proper oral hygiene and chlorhexidine rinses twice daily are usually sufficient to prevent any more serious problems. Infection or purulence requires definitive management with an appropriate antibiotic, such as amoxicillin or clindamycin. In addition to infection, the soft tissue has the potential to grow over the abutment head (Fig. 9-36). The O-Cap can be used to suppress the soft tissues and prevent overgrowth. This is usually only the case in alveolar mucosa as opposed to keratinized gingiva. If the soft tissue does cover the abutment head, the head is easily exposed with topical anesthesia and a scalpel.

SUMMARY

The Ortho Implant system is an excellent adjunct to provide stable, bone-based anchorage for the application of orthodontic mechanical force systems. The Ortho Implant is applicable for enhancing anchorage in a wide variety of malocclusions because of its small dimensions and ease of placement and use. The placement procedure has been simplified so that in most instances, no injections, flaps, or pilot holes are required. Placing the Ortho Implant is a simple procedure that can be performed by the orthodontist or can be referred to an oral surgeon, periodontist, or general dentist. After use, the Ortho Implant is also easily removed without anesthesia or complications.

REFERENCES

1. Minsk L. Interim implants for immediate loading of temporary restorations. *Compend Contin Educ Dent.* 22:186-196, 2001.

2. Balkin B, Steflik DE, Naval F. Mini-dental implant insertion with the auto-advance technique for ongoing applications. *J Oral Implantol.* 27:32-37, 2001.

3. Ernberg J, Asnis S. Materials and manufacturing of orthopedic bone screws. In: Asnis S, Kyle R, eds. *Cannulated Screw Fixation: Principles and Operative Techniques.* New York, NY: Springer, 1996:1-14.

4. Heidemann W, Gerlach KL, Grobel KH, Kollner HG. Drill free screws: a new form of osteosynthesis. *J Craniomaxillofac Surg.* 26:163-168, 1998.

5. Sowden D, Schmitz JP. AO self-drilling and self-tapping screws in rat calvarial bone: an ultrastructural study of the implant interface. *J Oral Maxillofac Surg.* 60:294-299, 2002.

6. Barkvoll P, Rolla G, Svendsen A. Interaction between chlorhexidine digluconate and sodium lauryl sulfate in vivo. *J Clin Periodontol.* 16:592-595, 1989.

7. Turkum M, Ozata F, Uzer E, Ates M. Antimicrobial substantivity of cavity disinfectants. *Gen Dent.* 53:182-186, 2005.

8. Donaldson D, Gelesky S, Landry R, et al. A placebo-controlled multi-centred evaluation of an anaesthetic gel (Oraqix) for periodontal therapy. *J Clin Periodontol.* 30:171-175, 2003.

9. Friskopp J, Nilsson M, Isaacson G. The anesthetic onset and duration of a new lidocaine/prilocaine gel intra-pocket anesthetic (Oraqix) for periodontal scaling/root planing. *J Clin Periodontol.* 28:453-458, 2001.

10. Miyakawa S, Koyama I, Inoue M, et al. Factors associated with the stability of titanium screws placed in the posterior region for orthodontic anchorage. *Am J Orthod Dentofacial Orthop.* 124:373-378, 2003.

10

The Ortho Anchor MiniScrew

Paul M. Thomas

Proper diagnosis and treatment planning are understood to be paramount to providing an optimal orthodontic treatment result. An integral component of this process is anchorage management. Anchorage, or resistance to unwanted tooth movement, provides a means of quantitatively evaluating the amount of desired tooth movement relative to the desired outcome. Traditionally, if maximum tooth movement were required, multiple teeth may have been grouped together and pitted against a few teeth undergoing tooth movement. Alternatively, intraoral or extraoral auxiliaries may have been incorporated to prevent anchorage loss. The latter of these strategies largely depended on patient compliance, which if inadequate, led to less than ideal results.

Because of lack of complete success with traditional mechanics, there has been increasing interest in establishing absolute anchorage with implantable devices over the last 25 years. Although clinician interest in this approach has grown exponentially in the last decade, the idea is not new. In their 1945 paper, Gainsforth and Higley[1] reported the concept of basal bone anchorage via orthopedic bone screws placed in the mandibular ramus. Today, although a multitude of companies have introduced a variety of implantable devices, there are four basic approaches to implantable anchorage (see Chapter 1). These are osseointegrated dental implants, modified bone screws, modified bone plates, and anatomically specific miniaturized dental implants (i.e., palatal and retromolar implants). In the mutilated dentition, osseointegrated implants provide excellent anchorage and, with the appropriate planning and placement, can subsequently be incorporated into the final prosthetic treatment. The remaining three categories are intended to be temporary and are removed upon completion of orthodontic mechanics.

THE ORTHO ANCHOR MINISCREW

The evolution of the Ortho Anchor™ miniscrew implant (MSI) began in 1998 with the development of a prototype for use in a dog study. Because of the limited utility, the expense, and protocol/armamentarium complexity of the palatal implants, our goal was to develop an approach that was simple, flexible, minimally invasive, and cost-effective and that would allow immediate loading. The first prototype was based on a specialized bone screw intended for maxillomandibular fixation without the use of arch bars or interdental wiring (Fig. 10-1). The double-flanged head was kept to prevent soft tissue overgrowth and allow easy attachment of elastic chain. The threaded body was changed to 1.5 mm in diameter by 10 mm in length with an 0.028-inch hole machined through the abutment head for attachment of springs or orthodontic wires.

With awareness that skeptics might doubt the absolute stability of an anchorage miniscrew, the initial pilot study evaluated the failure rate as well as any positional changes relative to tantalum bone markers (Fig. 10-2). One of the six miniscrews failed. Of those remaining, none exhibited movement or mobility during the 7 months of tooth movement. Furthermore, histologic sections of the bone-screw interface (Fig. 10-3) demonstrated an appearance similar to that seen with osseointegrated titanium implants.[2]

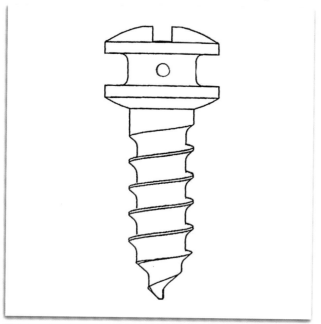

Fig. 10-1

The original engineer's sketch of the Ortho Anchor miniscrew from 1998.

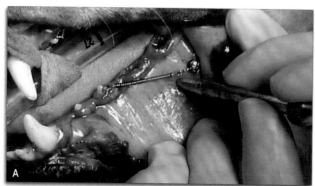

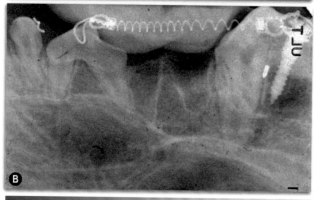

Fig. 10-2

Initial Ortho Anchor pilot study. **A,** Placement of a tantalum bone marker at the onset of tooth movement with the Ortho Anchor prototype. **B,** Standardized periapical radiographs and the tantalum markers used to document lack of Ortho Anchor movement.

The initial MSI design was modified based on observations during the pilot study. The final MSI is manufactured in several configurations as part of the Ortho Anchor kit (Fig. 10-4, *A*). The overall MSI lengths are 10 and 12 mm with the threaded body being 6 or 8 mm in length and 1.5 or 2.0 mm in diameter (Fig. 10-4, *B* and *C*). The Ortho Anchor miniscrews are self-tapping and are placed with a self-retaining cross-drive screwdriver (Fig. 10-5). The MSI can be loaded immediately with 150 to 175 g of force

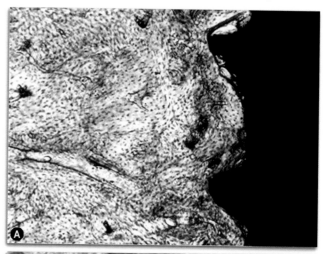

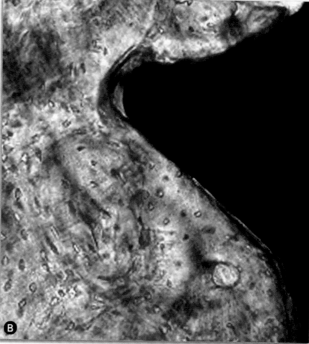

Fig. 10-3

Histologic examination of pilot study Ortho Anchors. **A,** Photomicrograph revealed no osteoclastic activity at the miniscrew surface. **B,** Higher-power photomicrograph demonstrates bone adaptation to the titanium miniscrew similar to that seen with osseointegrated implants. Note that mature bone with secondary osteons is evident.

applied at a right angle to the path of MSI placement. The load limit is 600 g, which is more than 3 times the recommended therapeutic force level.

TREATMENT PLANNING

The Ortho Anchor is intended for direct and indirect anchorage applications. The miniscrew was designed for interradicular placement from the facial surface of the maxillary or mandibular alveolus with bicortical engagement being desirable. Although mandibular lingual placement is technically feasible, the supramucosal projection may cause tongue irritation. A general goal is to place the miniscrew in a location where it will provide the optimum vector of force application yet not contact adjacent teeth or interfere with the planned tooth movement. For example, if used to assist with space closure in retraction or protraction applications, placement in the extraction space may compromise the force vector and the total amount of tooth movement possible. A more desirable placement site may be an interproximal location one or two teeth away from the space to be closed (Fig. 10-6).

If the Ortho Anchor is used as an alternative to a palatal implant, two screws placed lateral to the suture are recommended. These can then be used to stabilize a transpalatal bar for indirect anchorage. For example, the transpalatal bar and screw heads can be interconnected with quick-cure methyl methacrylate for maximum stability.

Using MSIs, possible tooth movement includes protraction, retraction, intrusion, or extrusion of single or multiple-tooth units (Fig. 10-7). Forces should be applied through the center of the screw head. Activation vectors that might result in reciprocal tortional forces may result in further screw tightening or loosening depending on the vector. To resist the reciprocal response, two screws can be used together with the arch wire or a separate wire passing through the machined hole in both screwheads.

Panoramic, bite-wing, or periapical radiographs are needed before placement to establish the interradicular bone stock (Fig. 10-8). Following administration of local anesthesia, calipers can be used to determine the ridge width and appropriate screw length with either measurements from the study model or direct measurements of bicortical dimension. Measurements also can be taken using the patient's study models. Care should be taken to note the position of the maxillary antrum and the course of the inferior alveolar canal on the panoramic radiograph. Use of transalveolar screws,

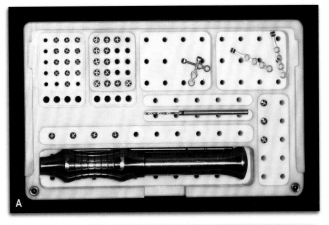

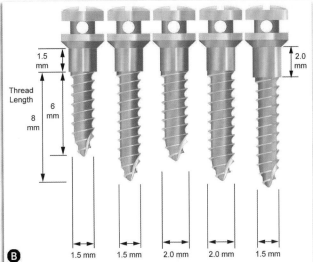

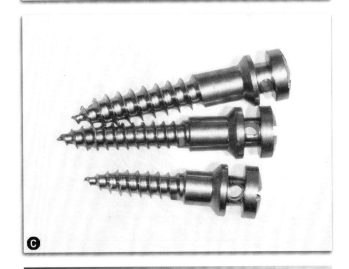

Fig. 10-4

Ortho Anchor kit. **A,** The kit is autoclavable and has compartments for the miniscrews, the screw driver, pilot drills, C-tubes (see Chapter 20), and C-plates (see Chapter 19). **B,** The Ortho Anchor miniscrew is available in several different threaded body lengths, transmucosal collar lengths, and diameters. **C,** A sample of the Ortho Anchor in 2.0-mm *(top)* and 1.5-mm *(bottom)* diameters. Note gold color is due to titanium anodizing process.

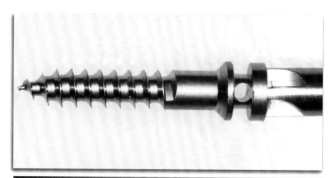

Fig. 10-5

The Ortho Anchor miniscrews are cross-drive and self-retaining.

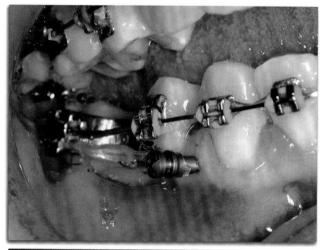

Fig. 10-6

Placement of Ortho Anchor for molar protraction. The location of the Ortho Anchor miniscrew introduces an intrusive component with protraction. Although intrusion is often a desired component of protraction, if it is to be avoided, the MSI should be located several teeth distant to the teeth undergoing movement in order to minimize the intrusive vector.

such as the Ortho Anchor, is restricted in patients having a large sinus that extends around the roots of maxillary posterior teeth. In these cases, a modified bone plate with monocortical screws or a palatal implant is indicated. Likewise, placement in the maxillary tuberosity may be less successful because the bone quality is often inadequate for use in miniscrew anchorage.

PRESURGICAL ORTHODONTICS

The need for presurgical orthodontics depends on the anticipated application and the nature of the malocclusion. If there is appreciable crowding and minimal interproximal space, some initial alignment and root paralleling may be necessary prior to placement of the MSI. Likewise, preliminary alignment may better position groups of teeth for consolidation in an indirect application (Fig. 10-9). The optimum site for placement may be more obvious after the preliminary orthodontics.

SURGICAL PROCEDURE

Placement of the Ortho Anchor can be easily accomplished in 5 to 10 minutes using local anesthetic infiltration. Articaine may be the local anesthetic of choice because of its decreased half-life and increased potential for bone penetration compared with other local anesthetics. Because no specialized surgical skills are required, the miniscrews can be placed either by the orthodontist, a surgeon, or the patient's general dental practitioner. If a clinician other than the orthodontist places the MSI, the desired location needs to be clearly communicated. Undesirable soft tissue inflammation can be minimized or avoided by placing the MSI at the

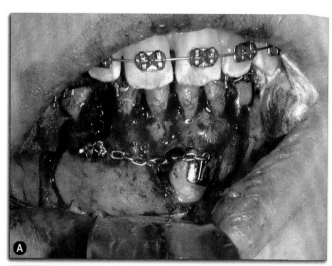

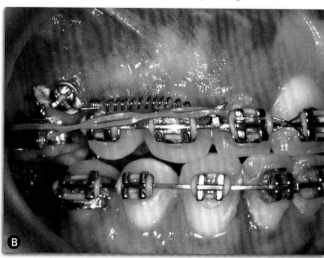

Fig. 10-7

Ortho Anchor applications for single or multiple tooth units. **A,** Ortho Anchor used to retrieve impacted mandibular canine that would otherwise be unsalvageable. **B,** Ortho Anchor used for en masse retraction of premolar-to-premolar segment with no concern for anchorage loss.

mucogingival junction. Tissue thickness is the primary consideration when selecting the appropriate height of transmucosal collar. Although no incision is necessary, the transmucosal portion of the screw may seat more easily if the overlying soft tissue is removed with a No. 8 round bur.

The Ortho Anchor is self-tapping and therefore requires no pilot hole (Fig. 10-10). If the cortical bone is dense and/or thick, perforation of the cortex with a 1.0-mm twist drill may aid in starting screw insertion. Placement should be perpendicular to the cortical plate unless angulation vertically would allow engagement of a greater amount of bone. Although chlorhexidine mouth rinse can be used to decrease the intraoral microbial content and assist with local hygiene for several days after MSI placement, antibiotics are not routinely prescribed postoperatively. Once any soft tissue sensitivity has diminished, gentle brushing with

a soft nylon brush is recommended to prevent the accumulation of debris and/or calculus (Fig. 10-11).

The Ortho Anchor is intended for immediate loading. Although differing protocols are advocated by various authors, there are few well-controlled published studies evaluating the optimum force level or timing of force application, either delayed or immediate. Some reports suggest immediate loading,[3-5] whereas others suggest a delay of several weeks before force application.[6,7] Miyawaki and colleagues[8] found no relationship between failure rate and immediate loading. Considering the above, there is no apparent benefit to delayed loading of MSIs until it is demonstrated that immediate loading leads to increased failure.

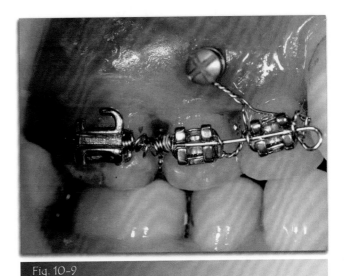

Fig. 10-9

Ortho Anchor used for indirect anchorage by stabilizing first premolar to indirectly distalize the second premolar and first molar.

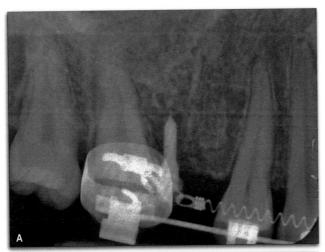

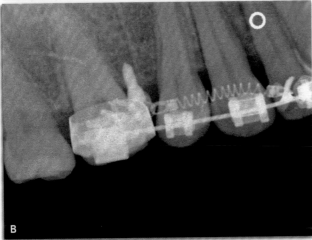

Fig. 10-8

Radiographs used to estimate interradicular bone stock. **A,** Pretreatment periapical radiograph. **B,** Posttreatment periapical radiograph.

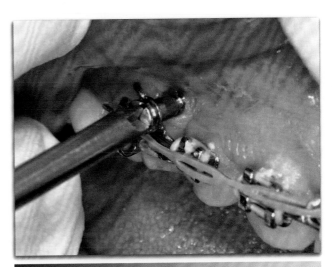

Fig. 10-10

Ortho Anchor placement requires no incision and typically no pilot hole.

ORTHODONTIC MECHANICS

The Ortho Anchor can be used for either direct or indirect anchorage (see Chapter 1). Elastic chain and superelastic nickel titanium coil springs are easily attached for use in direct anchorage applications with sliding mechanics (Fig. 10-12). The 0.028-inch hole in the screw head allows placement of an arch wire for frictionless closing loop mechanics (Fig. 10-13). The intended load is 150 to 175 g of force, which is well below the materials capability of the titanium miniscrew. The active force level needed for tooth movement and, accordingly, the reactive force against the MSI can be reduced by variations in bracket design and the approach to mechanotherapy. For example, the use of tip-edge brackets[9] or self-ligating brackets would reduce frictional forces[10] and decrease the load on the MSI. Placing the Ortho Anchor above the base arch for protraction or retraction also applies an intrusive component. As the point of force application is moved away from the MSI, the amount of intrusion decreases due to the geometry of the force vectors.

REMOVAL PROCEDURE

Removal of the Ortho Anchor is simply the reverse of the placement procedure. Removal is actually easier since topical anesthesia only is often adequate to perform the procedure. This should not be surprising because our orthopedic colleagues routinely remove larger skeletal devices such as fixator screws, Kirchner wires, and Steinmann pins without the use of anesthesia. To allay patient apprehension, however, some form of anesthesia

should be offered. The defect left by miniscrew removal needs no further management and heals quickly much like an extraction site (Fig. 10-14).

POTENTIAL COMPLICATIONS

Screw loosening with subsequent failure is the most likely complication. A false sense of security can result from reading the reports of animal research. The

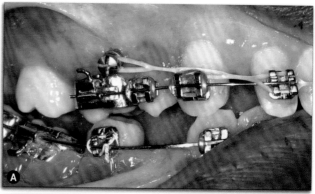
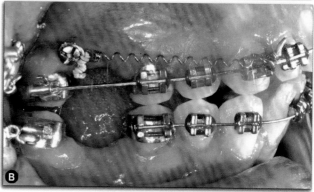

Fig. 10-12

Ortho Anchor attachments for sliding mechanics. **A,** The double-headed design allows easy application of elastic chain for retraction. **B,** Superelastic nickel titanium coil springs can be attached with wire ligatures to the 0.028-inch hole in the head for retraction.

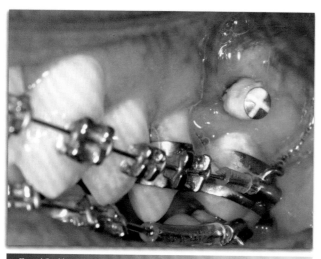

Fig. 10-11

Hygiene for the Ortho Anchor should be the same as for the remaining teeth. Inadequate hygiene can lead to debris accumulation, which can affect the stability of the device.

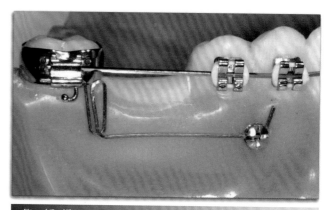

Fig. 10-13

Ortho Anchor attachment for frictionless mechanics. An arch wire is passed through the 0.028-inch hole and cinched to activate protraction loops.

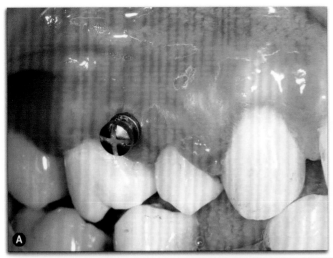
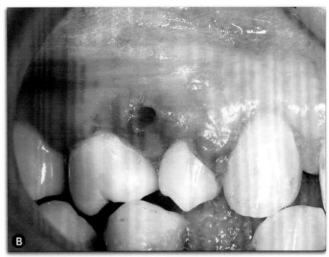

Fig. 10-14

Ortho Anchor removal procedure. **A,** Very little soft tissue inflammation is associated with Ortho Anchor use if placed at mucogingival junctions and maintained with good hygiene. **B,** Ortho Anchor removal leaves a small defect that heals quickly without further treatment.

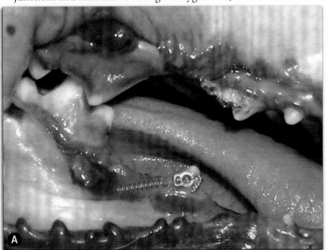
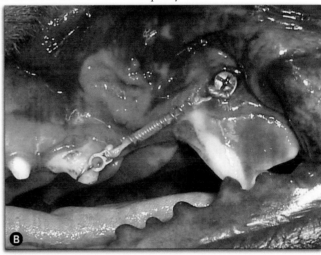

Fig. 10-15

Potential complications. **A,** The pilot study forecast the problems when placing MSIs in unattached mucosa. Although the soft tissue inflammation/hypertrophy was accentuated by lack of regular hygiene in the dog model, similar problems occur in human patients. **B,** Placement of the Ortho Anchor in attached gingiva minimizes the soft tissue inflammation, even in this dog model with no regular oral hygiene.

literature describing clinical application lists failure rates between 10% and 30%.[11,12] Failure appears highest with the smaller-diameter miniscrews (1.0 to 1.5 mm).[8] Accordingly, it would seem prudent to use MSIs with a diameter of 1.5 mm to 2.0 mm and length sufficient to allow bicortical engagement. Other potential complications include infection, root damage at placement, or screw fracture during the course of treatment. Although there was no report of infection, Miyawaki and colleagues[8] found that inflammation of the periimplant soft tissue was associated with an increased risk of failure. This problem is exacerbated when the device is placed in mobile mucosa (Fig. 10-15). No mention of root damage or screw fracture was found in the literature reviewed.

SUMMARY

There has been a significant increase in the available implantable anchorage devices and the level of interest over the last decade. These devices reduce or eliminate the need for patient compliance during orthodontic mechanotherapy. Instead, the patient's efforts can be concentrated on hygiene and care of the orthodontic appliance system. Ideally, an implantable anchorage device should be economical, minimally invasive, tissue compatible, easily placed and removed, immediately loadable, and easily applied in a variety of biomechanical schemes. In the event of failure, there should be minimal downside for either the patient or clinician. The Ortho Anchor miniscrew meets these criteria and allows tooth movement that would be difficult if not impossible with traditional anchorage strategies.

ACKNOWLEDGMENTS

This research was supported in part by KLS Martin Surgical, LLP, Jacksonville, Florida.

REFERENCES

1. Gainsforth BL, Higley LB. A study of orthodontic anchorage possibilities in basal bone. *Am J Orthod Oral Surg.* 31:406-417, 1945.

2. Forrister MR. *Implantable Devices as Orthodontic Anchorage: A Pilot Study* [master's thesis]. Department of Orthodontics, University of North Carolina at Chapel Hill; 2000.

3. Gelgor IE, Buyukyilmaz T, Karaman AI, et al. Intraosseous screw-supported upper molar distalization. *Angle Orthod.* 74(6):838-850, 2004.

4. Freudenthaler JW, Haas R, Bantleon HP. Bicortical titanium screws for critical orthodontic anchorage in the mandible: a preliminary report on clinical applications. *Clin Oral Implants Res.* 12(4):358-363, 2001.

5. Costa A, Raffainl M, Melsen B. Miniscrews as orthodontic anchorage: a preliminary report. *Int J Adult Orthodon Orthognath Surg.* 13(3):201-209, 1998.

6. Deguchi T, Takano-Yamamoto T, Kanomi R, et al. The use of small titanium screws for orthodontic anchorage. *J Dent Res.* 82(5):377-381, 2003.

7. Liou EJ, Pai BC, Lin JC. Do miniscrews remain stationary under orthodontic forces? *Am J Orthod Dentofacial Orthop.* 126(1):42-47, 2004.

8. Miyawaki S, Koyama I, Inoue M, et al. Factors associated with the stability of titanium screws placed in the posterior region for orthodontic anchorage. *Am J Orthod Dentofacial Orthop.* 124(4):373-378, 2003.

9. Rocke RT. Employing Tip-Edge brackets on canines to simplify straight-wire mechanics. *Am J Orthod Dentofacial Orthop.* 106(4):341-350, 1994.

10. Redlich M, Mayer Y, Harari D, Lewinstein I. In vitro study of frictional forces during sliding mechanics of "reduced-friction" brackets. *Am J Orthod Dentofacial Orthop.* 124(1):69-73, 2003.

11. Cheng SJ, Tseng IY, Lee JJ, et al. A prospective study of the risk factors associated with failure of mini-implants used for orthodontic anchorage. *Int J Oral Maxillofac Implants.* 19(1):100-106, 2004.

12. Fritz U, Ehmer A, Diedrich P. Clinical suitability of titanium microscrews for orthodontic anchorage-preliminary experiences. *J Orofac Orthop.* 65(5):410-418, 2004.

The Temporary Orthodontic Mini Anchorage System

Axel Bumann, James Mah

Reliable anchorage is crucial in clinical orthodontics. Conventionally, anchorage has been controlled by teeth, bone, dental implants, and extraoral appliances.[1] A loss of anchorage during treatment can have deleterious effects on the ultimate orthodontic treatment outcome.[2] Recent clinical studies have demonstrated molar distalization with noncompliance distalization appliances ranging from 1.4 to 5.7 mm. These same appliances, however, allowed anterior anchorage loss from 24% to 68%.[3]

Another study by Kinzinger and colleagues[4] showed anterior anchorage loss of 30% with a modified pendulum appliance. In an attempt to overcome these limitations, several authors have used miniscrews and mini-implants to avoid these problems.[5-20] Although miniscrews are economic and simple to insert and remove, little scientific data other than clinical case reports are available concerning success rates and predictability.[20-21] Therefore, the aim of this chapter is to introduce the Temporary Orthodontic Mini Anchorage System (*tomas*™ pin; Dentaurum Inc., Newtown, Pennsylvania) as an absolute anchorage tool in orthodontic anchorage.

THE *tomas* PIN

The *tomas* pin is a specific system for compliance-independent absolute anchorage in orthodontics that comes packaged as a complete kit (Fig. 11-1). The kit contains all the necessary instrumentation to place and use the pin (Fig. 11-2). The *tomas* pin belongs to the group of miniscrew implants (MSIs) with a cross slot head. The pin is made of grade 5 titanium alloy (TiAl6V4)—the standard material for titanium dental implants and fixation screws—and comes packaged in a sterile blister pack (Fig. 11-3). Both Food and Drug Administration approval in the United States and

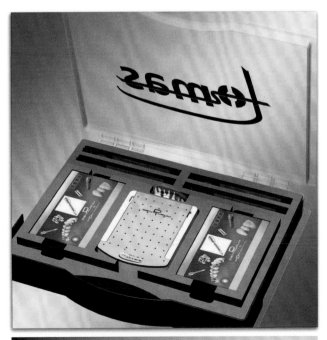

Fig. 11-1

The temporary orthodontic mini anchorage system. The case contains the *tomas* tray (*gold lid*), four biopsy punches (*in upper slots*), four *tomas* pins (*blue boxes*), and a demo model.

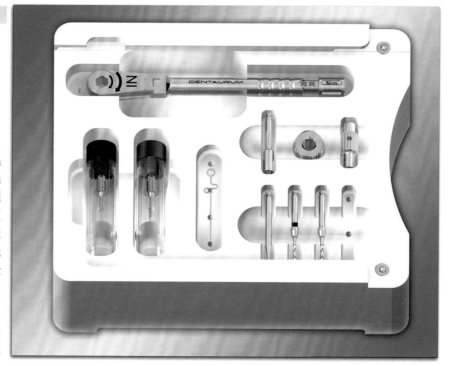

The *tomas* tray with an 8-mm tomas pin *(blue lid)*, a 10-mm *tomas* pin *(green lid)*, a locator, a 1.0-mm round bur, a 1.1-mm drill *(red collar)*, a 1.2-mm drill, a driver, a wheel, an applicator, and a torque ratchet. The entire tray is autoclavable.

the CE mark in Europe have been attained. The pins are available in two lengths: 8 (Fig. 11-4, *A*) and 10 mm (Fig. 11-4, *B*). Any MSI can be divided into three functional parts (Fig. 11-5): a threaded body, a transmucosal collar, and an abutment head.

Threaded Body Design

Two threaded lengths are available: 8 and 10 mm. Origianlly, 6- and 12-mm lengths were also available. However, 5 years of clinical experience revealed that the 8- and 10-mm lengths are sufficient to cover the daily demands in orthodontics. The core diameter (not including the threads) is 1.2 mm, and the external diameter (including the threads) is 1.6 mm. The pitch, or distance between two threads, is 0.9 mm, which allows for optimum bone apposition. The nontreated surface is machine-polished to prevent osseointegration but allow bone apposition.

The threads of the screw are similar to most of the currently available orthodontic MSIs. Typically there are only minor differences in length, diameter, and geometry of the thread design between various manufacturers. The threaded body is self-tapping but not drill-free. One important feature is that the thread stops 1 mm short of the collar. The smooth surface of the transmucosal collar helps to reduce the probability of bacterial invasion into the underlying bone.

Transmucosal Collar Design

The transmucosal collar of the tomas pin has a height of 2.0 mm. The shape is slightly conical with a diameter of 2.0 mm at the bottom and 2.75 mm at the top. The surface is polished to a high gloss and allows for intimate adaptation of the gingiva, thereby reducing the risk of temporary anchorage device periimplantitis (TAP). The shape of the collar also helps to minimize any postoperative bleeding, which is caused by incising the gingiva with the enclosed biopsy punch.

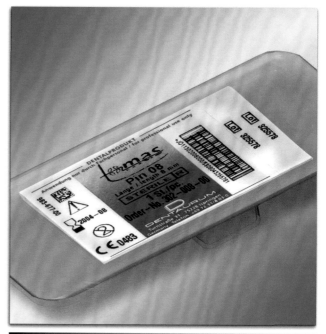

Sterile blister pack for *tomas* pin delivery. The back has two stickers with lot numbers for documentation in the patient's file.

Abutment Head Design

Both the height and the diameter of the abutment head are 2.3 mm, which is the smallest head of the currently available MSIs with a cross slot. Two cross slots are incorporated into the head. The cross slots are oriented at 90 degrees to each other and perpendicular to the long axis of the screw. They have a dimension of

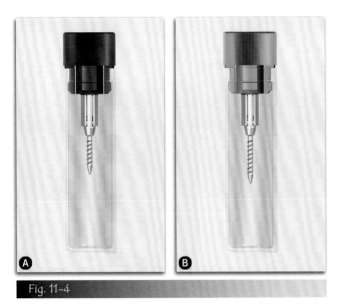

Fig. 11-4

Sterile glass vials containing the *tomas* pin. **A,** Blue lid with 8-mm pin. **B,** Green lid with 10-mm pin.

0.022 inch, which enables the orthodontist to work with 0.018- and 0.022-inch prescriptions. Because orthodontists are used to working with slots, the *tomas* pin is easy to handle and allows for a wide variety of mechanical attachment schemes.

An undercut area is located just below the cross slots and has a height of 0.4 mm and a depth of 0.2 mm. The undercut allows for fixation of a rectangular wire into the slots with light-cured acrylic resin, thereby avoiding ligatures. This saves chair time and hygiene and minimizes soft tissue inflammation.

Advantages of the *tomas* pin include a small diameter, 8- and 10-mm lengths, a head designed like a bracket, intimate gingival adaptation, versatility of use, and three-dimensional control of tooth movement with rectangular wires.

TREATMENT PLANNING

The standard orthodontic diagnostic records are used for treatment planning with the *tomas* pin. In cases of buccal placement, clinical findings, models, and radiographs (panoramic and periapical) are usually sufficient to plan treatment. The specific position of the pin depends mainly on three parameters: keratinized gingival height, crestal alveolar bone height, and interradicular space.

Our preferred location for the *tomas* pin is between the roots of the premolars, but other positions are also possible (Fig. 11-6). The entry point should be at the mucogingival junction. The width of bone between the roots of the premolars should be a minimum of 2.6 mm (1.6 mm for the pin diameter plus 0.5 mm on

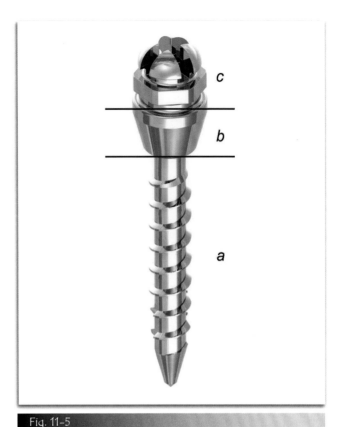

Fig. 11-5

The *tomas* pin has three functional parts: *(a)* threaded body; *(b)* transmucosal collar; and *(c)* abutment head.

each side). The alveolar bone height combined with the keratinized gingival height determines the threaded length and the angulation of the *tomas* pin. The position of the *tomas* pin is determined by the specific mechanics planned.

In lieu of using direct visualization for placement, it is also possible to use the locator instrument. The locator is a stainless steel wire with a loop at one end. First, adapt the locator to the model in the planned location (Fig. 11-7). Next, transfer the locator to the mouth and take a periapical radiograph using the parallel technique.

PRESURGICAL ORTHODONTICS

The amount of presurgical orthodontics depends primarily on the treatment plan. In most patients, presurgical orthodontic treatment is not needed. However, when excess space exists in the premolar region, it may be beneficial to close the space first to prevent movement of a tooth root into a placed pin. Likewise, if inadequate interradicular space exists, it is necessary to either open space or change root angulations to prevent potential root damage during placement.

SURGICAL PROCEDURE

The surgical procedure can be divided in three phases: presurgical preparation, surgical placement, postsurgical loading.

Presurgical Preparation

All necessary instruments should be in position in the *tomas* tray in their proper locations, and the planned number of *tomas* pins should be placed in an upright position in the prefabricated holes (Fig. 11-8). The orthodontic assistant sterilizes the *tomas* tray as well as an instrument tray with two mouth mirrors, an explorer, cotton pliers, a small excavator, a low-volume evacuator, a 20-mL irrigation syringe, and endodontic pin-removing pliers used only in the event of a broken pin (No. DA297R; Aesculap, Tuttlingen, Germany). In addition to the foregoing, the assistant dispenses chlorhexidine mouth rinse, prepares a syringe with 1.8 mL of lidocaine with 1:100,000 epinephrine, gathers a surgical drape (100 × 120 cm), and lays out sterile gloves. Before surgery, the patient rinses for 1 minute with the chlorhexidine solution. Subsequently, the orthodontist administers local anesthetic by infiltration at the proposed location of the pin. Usually, 0.2 to 0.3 mL of lidocaine is sufficient to anesthetize the mucosa for the surgical procedure. If the *tomas* pin is placed on the buccal, no anesthesia is desired on the palatal or lingual side. Local infiltration anesthesia is used almost exclusively. This has the advantage of avoiding profound block anesthesia, which may increase patient acceptance. Another advantage of this procedure is that the periodontal ligament (PDL) and palatal/lingual periosteum and mucosa are not anesthetized, which allows the patient to give feedback in the event the pin is in close proximity to the PDL, root, or opposite cortex. After these preparatory steps are performed, cover the patient's head with a surgical drape and initiate the surgical procedure.

Surgical Placement

The chairside procedure starts by marking the exact anatomic position of the *tomas* pin intraorally. The panoramic radiograph is usually sufficient to determine the final position (Fig. 11-9). For more specific determination, use the locator adapted to the model during treatment planning. The locator is adapted to the teeth with the wire circle over the planned pin location. Take a periapical radiograph until the locator hole is in the correct position between the roots. The circle of the locator marks the precise spot where the

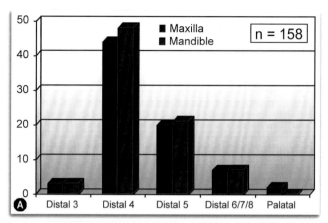

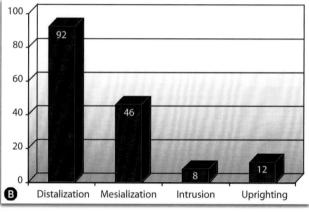

Fig. 11-6

Placement location and uses of 158 *tomas* pins. **A,** The preferred location was between the first and second premolars. **B,** Most common clinical indications for *tomas* pins.

gingiva is to be punched. Ideally, the path of the x-ray beam should be perpendicular to the proposed implant site; however, unpublished experimental studies have shown that angulation errors are in the range of ±10 degrees, which may be inadequate for accurate placement of MSIs. The most common placement method, however, is direct visualization without the use of a periapical radiograph or the locator.

After determining the ideal pin position, lightly press the soft tissue biopsy punch against the gingiva to slightly indent the epithelium. This results in a circular impression, which can then be evaluated from different angles. If the circle is in the correct position, replace the punch over the circle and press it firmly against the cortical bone while turning 360 degrees 3 times to incise the underlying gingiva and periosteum completely (Fig. 11-10, *A*). Subsequently, remove the gingival cutout with a small excavator. Cleanly incised gingival margins are important and allow for smooth gingival adaptation to the collar of the *tomas* pin. Next, center mark the cortical bone with a 1.0-mm

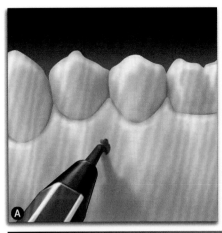 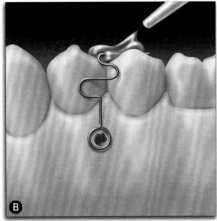 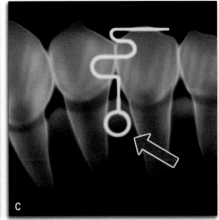

Fig. 11-7

Locator use to determine the optimal location of the *tomas* pin. **A,** Mark the desired position on the model. **B,** Adapt the prefabricated locator to the model. **C,** Expose periapical radiograph with the locator placed intraorally.

Fig. 11-8

tomas tray prepared for the surgical procedure. All tools and pins are placed upright for easy access.

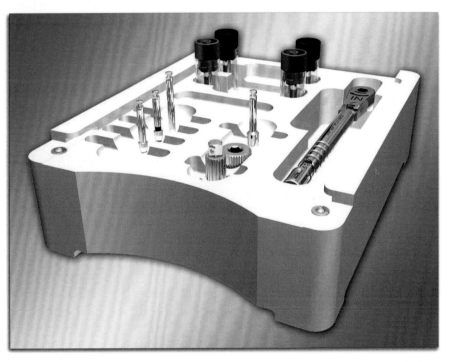

round bur followed by the pilot drill (Fig. 11-10, *B* to *D*). Two pilot drills are available. The 1.1-mm drill (red collar) is intended for the less dense bone in the upper jaw, and the 1.2-mm drill usually is used for the more dense bone in the lower jaw. In most cases, however, the 1.1-mm drill is used for both jaws. The drilling orientation is almost always perpendicular to the cortical bone surface. If the alveolar bone is less than 8 mm wide, angulate the pilot drill slightly to allow for a more diagonal implant position. This prevents contact with the contralateral cortex.

Use the pilot drill at a speed of 800 to 1000 rpm under constant sterile saline irrigation. Higher speeds, especially in the absence of irrigation, will lead to bone damage, usually overheating the bone surface. The most favorable handpieces are speed- and moment-controlled motors. Our preference is the INTRAsurg 300 plus (KaVo Dental Corp., Lake Zurich, Illinois).

After finishing the pilot hole, select the glass vial with the correct pin length (blue, 8 mm; green, 10 mm) and remove the lid (Fig. 11-10, *E*). The lid of the vial also functions as the initial placement device, enabling the orthodontist to avoid any contact with

the threads of the sterile *tomas* pin. Use the lid to rotate the pin 2 to 3 revolutions into the pilot hole until initial bony engagement is accomplished (Fig. 11-10, *F*). Placement can be completed with any one of four methods: manually with the applicator (Fig. 11-11, *A*), manually with the applicator and wheel (Fig. 11-11, *B*), manually with the applicator and torque ratchet (Fig. 11-11, *C*), or machine driven with a moment-controlled motor (Fig. 11-11, *D*).

Initially, the orthodontist should use only the applicator or the applicator combined with the torque ratchet, which gives better tactile sense of bone quality. The torque ratchet is limited to 20 N-cm, thereby avoiding the potential of breaking the tomas pin during placement (Fig. 11-12).

Unpublished experimental studies show that the pin can withstand approximately 30 N-cm of shear force before breakage. Therefore, the recommended limitation of 20 N-cm provides a safety margin of 30%. Once the torque level reaches 20 N-cm, the handle of the torque ratchet "breaks" to indicate a torque level of 20 N-cm. If the *tomas* pin is not seated completely at this point, the orthodontist can remove it and replace it with a shorter pin. Alternatively, the orthodontist can unscrew the pin two to three revolutions before advancing the pin back into the bone to complete placement. If the pin is placed with the driver, a moment-controlled motor is necessary. The settings for the motor unit should be 20 N-cm with a speed setting of 11 to 25 rpm. In the final position, the soft tissue collar should be surrounded by gingiva with the abutment head lying outside the gingiva (Fig. 11-13).

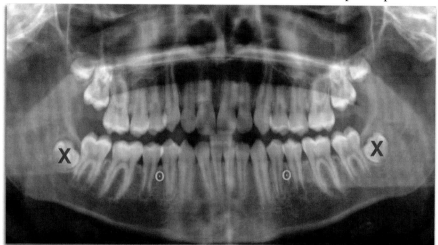

Fig. 11-9

Panoramic radiograph after planning the appropriate pin position *(circles)* for distalization of the posterior teeth. The wisdom teeth will be removed before treatment *(Xs)*.

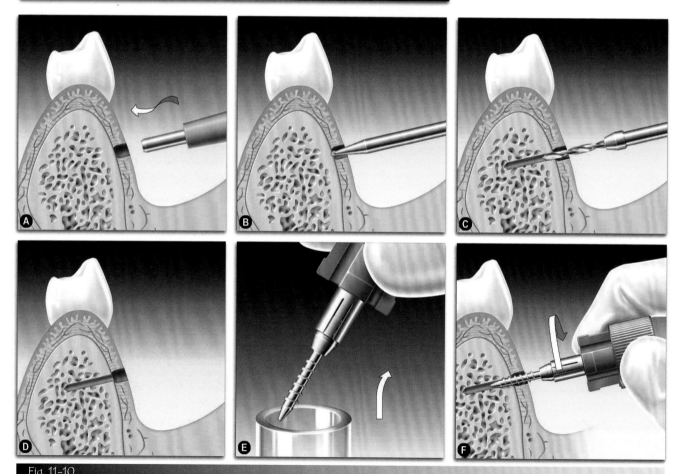

Fig. 11-10

Placement of the *tomas* pin. **A,** Punch incision in gingiva. **B,** Center drilling the cortical bone with the round bur. **C,** Drilling the pilot hole. **D,** Pilot hole complete. **E,** Pin removal from vial. **F,** Initial pin placement with lid.

Based on experience with more than 200 *tomas* pins, no antibiotics, antiinflammatory drugs, or analgesics are necessary. After the surgical procedure, connect the *tomas* pin to the orthodontic appliance (Fig. 11-14). The pin can be loaded immediately with forces up to 250 g. Stabilization of the wire in the head, for direct or indirect anchorage, is achieved by applying composite resin (Heliosit Orthodontic; Ivoclar Vivadent, Ellwangen, Germany) around the wire and the undercut. The composite holds the wire in the slot and, because of its smooth cured surface, minimizes gingival irritation (Fig. 11-15).

Postsurgical Loading

In the event that a patient experiences pressure or hypersensitivity while clenching, observe the patient in

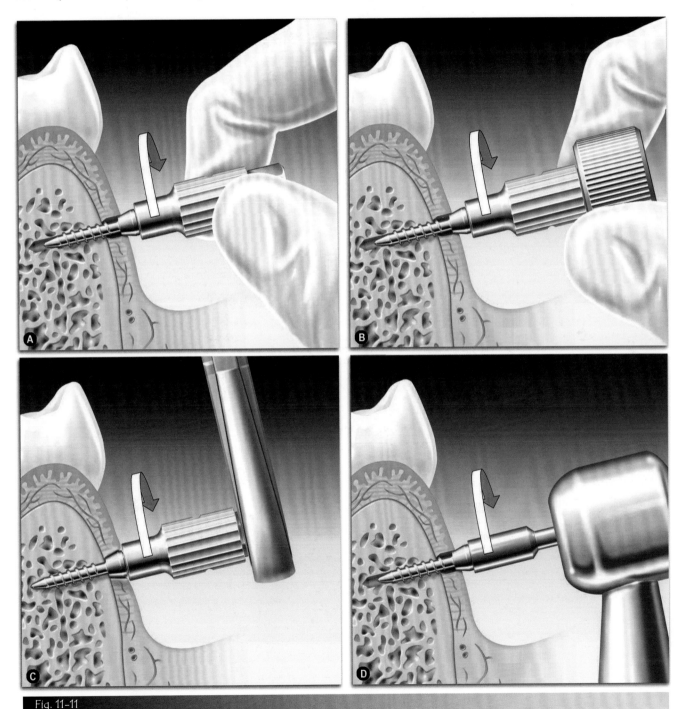

Fig. 11-11

Four different methods of *tomas* pin placement. **A,** Applicator. **B,** Applicator with wheel. **C,** Applicator with torque ratchet. **D,** Machine-driven with driver.

the office for another 10 to 15 minutes. If the pressure and hypersensitivity symptoms do not subside, remove the *tomas* pin and re-place it in another location. However, this has not been necessary to date.

Typically, pin placement and attachment to the orthodontic appliances are performed at the same appointment. The pin is loaded immediately without any healing period. Clinical applications have shown that the *tomas* pin can be loaded with up to 250 g without any problem. After placing the pin, the patient should avoid touching the pin with the fingers, tongue, or other objects. Oral hygiene should be performed as normal without any undue force on the pin with the toothbrush. The first postoperative appointment

is usually scheduled 2 weeks after initial placement. Subsequently, standard orthodontic appointment intervals are implemented.

ORTHODONTIC MECHANICS

The *tomas* pins have changed our conventional orthodontic treatment mechanics concepts and have provided treatment alternatives not previously possible. For example, upper molar distalization can be used to reliably correct Class II malocclusions. Distalization of the entire lower arch for Class III treatment is also possible. In addition, lower molar distalization can be used to resolve anterior crowding in some cases. In these cases, we usually start with posterior segmental

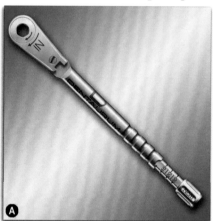
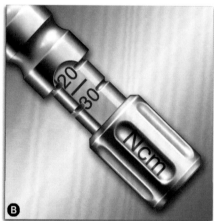
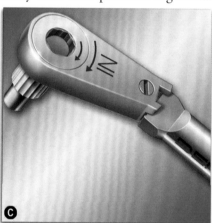

Fig. 11–12

Ratchet use for *tomas* pin placment. **A,** Ratchet wrench. **B,** Torque setting adjusted to 20 N-cm. **C,** Ratchet "breaks" at head upon reaching 20 N-cm.

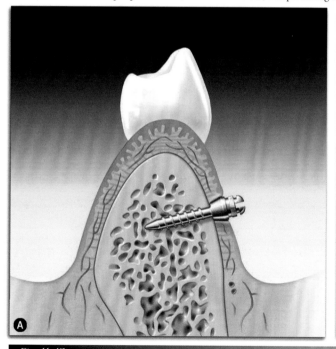
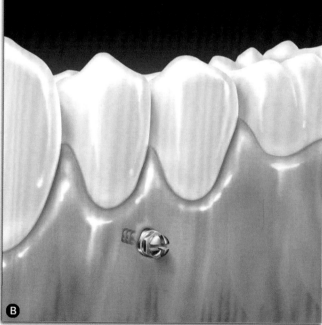

Fig. 11–13

tomas pin after placement. **A,** Cross section through the mandible. **B,** Facial surface showing pin within attached gingiva.

mechanics, which minimizes the duration that anterior brackets are in place. Once a Class I posterior occlusion is achieved, only a short phase of full fixed appliance therapy is necessary.

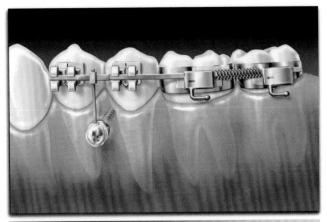

Fig. 11-14

tomas pin connected to orthodontic appliances.

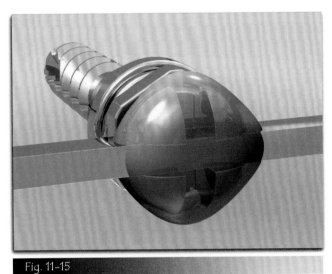

Fig. 11-15

Fixation of the stabilization wire with light-cured composite.

The anchorage system can be direct (Fig. 11-16, *A*) or indirect (Fig. 11-16, *B*). In both situations the wire is fixed to the pin with light-cured composite. When distalizing teeth with open coils, it is important to have enough interbracket distance for the open coil spring. This minimizes activation or wire change appointments during distalization (Figs. 11-17 and 11-18). To prevent open coil spring changes during distalization, a small stop can be crimped to the main wire to reactivate the spring. The rate of molar distalization averages 1.0 to 1.5 mm per month. In most cases, it is difficult to avoid some distal tipping.

To intrude single teeth or upright tipped molars, specific orthodontic mechanics are used. In these cases, as well as in other preprosthetic orthodontic cases, usually only a limited number of brackets, bands, and wires are necessary to solve the problem (Fig. 11-19). This makes treatment more efficient, convenient, and less expensive.

REMOVAL PROCEDURE

Pin removal is much easier than expected. Remove the composite by squeezing the light-cured material gently with a Weingart plier. This shatters the composite, allowing easy removal of the stabilization wire. The applicator and wheel are the standard instruments used to unscrew the *tomas* pin. In our experiences, anesthesia is not required for pin removal in more than 90% of the patients. The small bony and gingival defects remaining upon removal are left uncovered and heal within a few days. To date, no complications have been observed after pin removal.

POTENTIAL COMPLICATIONS

Our evaluation of 158 pins reveals no nerve lesions, blood vessel perforations, contralateral cortex or mucosal perforations, or loss of interdental papilla.

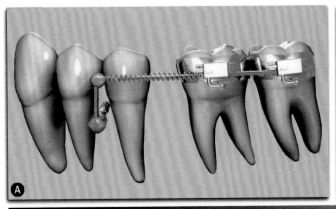
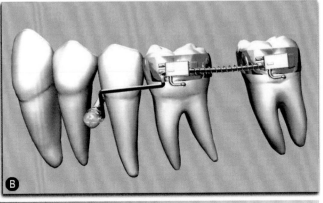

Fig. 11-16

Examples of orthodontic mechanics for the distalization of molars. **A,** Direct anchorage. **B,** Indirect anchorage.

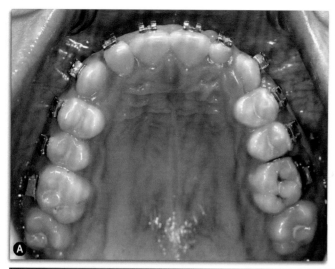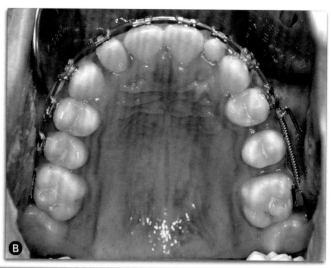

Fig. 11–17

Clinical example for unilateral distalization of teeth to provide enough space to build up an upper right lateral incisor with a veneer. **A,** The pin was placed between second premolar and first molar. **B,** After 4 months, more than enough space was created without side effects anteriorly.

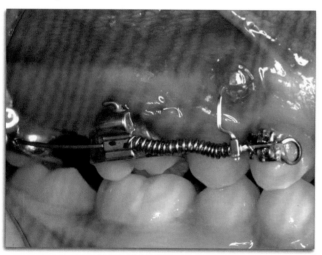

Fig. 11–18

Typical case of a unilateral Class II. One *tomas* pin placed between the premolars is attached to a segmental wire to distalize the posterior segment to a Class I occlusion. The second molar has already been distalized and maintained in its position by a crimpable stop mesial to the tube. Note that there is no bracket on the second premolar to have a longer span for open coil activation.

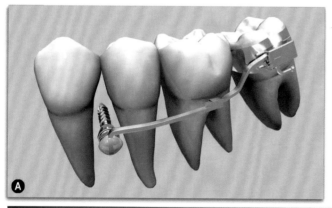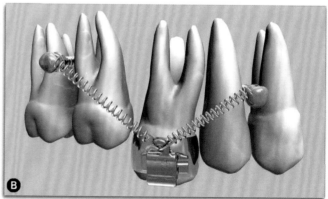

Fig. 11–19

Examples of orthodontic mechanics using limited orthodontic appliances. **A,** Uprighting molars. **B,** Intruding molars.

In addition, no root lesion or root resorption was observed. The rate of pin loss was 6% for the upper jaw and 14.8% for the lower jaw. Patients with a dolichofacial growth pattern showed significantly lower loss rates. The most interesting result was the loss rate when followed over the last 4 years (Fig. 11-20). In the year 2001, the loss rate was 35%; whereas in the year 2004, the loss rate was only 5%. Two reasons explain the increased success rate. First, as our experience increased, our clinical judgment also increased. Second, modifications and improvements were incorporated into the *tomas* system. The main clinical reasons for failure were lack of primary stability, lack of immediate loading, placement close to roots of deciduous teeth, direct anchorage mechanics with long cantilevers, and placement close to frena.

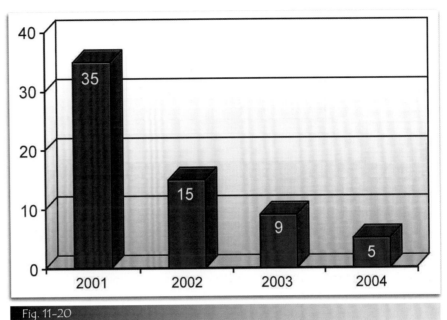

Fig. 11-20

Loss rate of *tomas* pins. From 2001 to 2004, 158 pins were placed.

SUMMARY

The *tomas* pin with a diameter of 1.6 mm and a length of 8 or 10 mm proved suitable for orthodontic anchorage purposes. Larger screws require more bone for placement, minimizing the available sites for placement. tomas pins offer a flexible range of applications, as well as simple insertion and removal, minimum patient stress, and a favorable cost-benefit ratio. The *tomas* tray is organized in a specific layout such that the surgical procedure can be performed efficiently and effectively.

REFERENCES

1. Roberts-Harry D, Sandy J. Orthodontics, IX: anchorage control and distal movement. *Br Dent J.* 196:255-263, 2004.
2. Geron S, Shpack N, Kandos S, Davidovitch M, Vardimon AD. Anchorage loss: a multifactorial response. *Angle Orthod.* 73:730-737, 2003.
3. Papadopoulos MA, Mavropoulos A, Karamouzos, A. Cephalometric changes following simultaneous first and second molar distalization using a non-compliance intraoral appliance. *J Orofac Orthop.* 65:123-136, 2004.
4. Kinzinger GS, Fritz UB, Sander FG, Diedrich PR. Efficiency of a pendulum appliance for molar distalization related to second and third molar eruption stage. *Am J Orthod Dentofacial Orthop.* 125:8-23, 2004.
5. Douglass JB, Killiany DM. Dental implants used as orthodontic anchorage. *J Oral Implantol.* 13:28-38, 1987.
6. Schneider G, Simmons K, Nason R, Felton D. Occlusal rehabilitation using implants for orthodontic anchorage. *J Prosthodont.* 7:232-236, 1998.
7. Roberts WE, Marshall KJ, Mozsary PG. Rigid endosseous implant utilized as anchorage to protract molars and close an atrophic extraction site. *Angle Orthod.* 60:135-152, 1990.
8. Wehrbein H, Merz BR, Diedrich P, Glatzmaier J. The use of palatal implants for orthodontic anchorage: design and clinical application of the orthosystem. *Clin Oral Implants Res.* 7:410-416, 1996.
9. Keles A, Erverdi N, Sezen S. Bodily distalization of molars with absolute anchorage. *Angle Orthod.* 73:471-482, 2003.
10. Block MS, Hoffman DR. A new device for absolute anchorage for orthodontics. *Am J Orthod Dentofacial Orthop.* 107:251-258, 1995.
11. Janssens F, Swennen G, Dujardin T, Glineur R, Malevez C. Use of an onplant as orthodontic anchorage. *Am J Orthod Dentofacial Orthop.* 122:566-570, 2002.
12. Melsen B, Petersen JK, Costa A. Zygoma ligatures: an alternative form of maxillary anchorage. *J Clin Orthod.* 32:154-158, 1998.
13. Sfondrini MF, Cacciafesta V, Sfondrini D. The uprighting of mesially tipped and impacted mandibular second molars: the use of the mandibular ramus as orthodontic anchorage. *Orthodontics.* 1:3-12, 2004.
14. De Clerck H, Cornelis M, Timmerman H. Dental tours de force, IV: the use of a bone anchor for holding upright a tipped molar in the lower jaw. *Ned Tijdschr Tandheelkd.* 111:10-13, 2004.
15. Kim S, Park Y, Chung K. Severe anterior open bite malocclusion with multiple odontoma treated by C-lingual retractor and horseshoe mechanics. *Angle Orthod.* 73:206-212, 2003.
16. Erverdi N, Tosun T, Keles A. A new anchorage site for the treatment of anterior open bite: zygomatic anchorage—case report. *World J Orthod.* 3:147-153, 2002.

17. Park HS, Bae SM, Kyung HM, Sung JH. Micro-implant anchorage for treatment of skeletal Class I bialveolar protrusion. *J Clin Orthod.* 35:417-422, 2001.

18. Costa A, Raffiani M, Melsen B. Miniscrews as orthodoontic anchorage: a preliminary report. *Int J Adult Orthodon Orthognath Surg.* 13:201-209, 1998.

19. Maino BG, Bednar J, Pagin P, Mura P. The spider screw for skeletal anchorage. *J Clin Orthod.* 37:90-97, 2003.

20. Sugawara J, Daimaruya T, Umemori M, et al. Distal movement of mandibular molars in adult patients with the skeletal anchorage system. *Am J Orthodon Dentofacial Orthop.* 125:130-138, 2004.

21. Cheng SJ, Tseng IY, Lee JJ, Kok SH. A prospective study of the risk factors associated with failure of mini-implants used for orthodontic anchorage. *Int J Oral Maxillofac Implants.* 19:100-106, 2004.

CHAPTER

12

The Aarhus Anchorage System

Birte Melsen

Over the past several decades, it has been increasingly difficult to obtain satisfactory patient compliance during orthodontic mechanotherapy. In an attempt to overcome this limitation, orthodontists have developed a wide range of "compliance free" appliances.[1-8] None of these appliances, however, adequately fulfills the requirements of absolute anchorage. For this purpose, only ankylosed teeth, dilacerated teeth, and implants (see Chapter 1 for classification) can provide absolute anchorage and not be mobilized by orthodontic forces.[9]

One of the first skeletal anchorage systems designed specifically for orthodontics was the skeletal fixation wire inserted in the zygoma. Melsen and colleagues[10] chose the zygoma as an alternate anchorage site because mutilated adult dentitions usually do not have enough teeth present to offer the required anchorage with which to adequately move the remaining teeth. The zygoma fixation wires were used as anchorage for retraction and intrusion of flared and supererupted incisors in patients with insufficient posterior anchorage (Fig. 12-1). More recently Sfondrini and colleagues[11] used a similar technique in the ascending ramus region to deimpact a mesioangular impacted second molar.

The surgical procedure for placement of the zygoma wire was performed under local anesthesia. A 1-cm long incision was made on the superior aspect of the infrazygomatic crest, and a horizontal bony canal was drilled through the bone. A double 0.012-inch stainless steel wire was then pulled through the canal and twisted at the anterior aspect of the infrazygomatic crest. Once the incision was closed with sutures, the fixation wire was bent and adapted such that the correct point of force application was established. Next, a 50-g closed coil spring was applied from the fixation wire to the anterior teeth. Although the infrazygomatic crest bone quality generally provided sufficient anchorage for tooth movement,[12] about 20% of the wires came loose before treatment was terminated. One possible explanation was that the bony hole was too close to the surface and the wire "worked" its way through the thin layer of bone. Apart from these cases, tooth movement was well controlled by the fixation wires. Tooth movement was usually complete after 3 to 6 months, and the wires were cut and removed under local anesthesia. In spite of the failures, the zygoma fixation wires provided an inexpensive and simple anchorage approach for use where posterior teeth could not serve as anchorage.

Recently, fixation wires have been replaced by miniplate implants (MPIs) in the infrazygomatic crest area, and the indications have widened to include open bite closure via intrusion of molars.[13-17] In addition, miniscrew implants (MSIs), a modification of osteosynthesis screws, have been introduced for orthodontic anchorage, for which the applications appear promising.

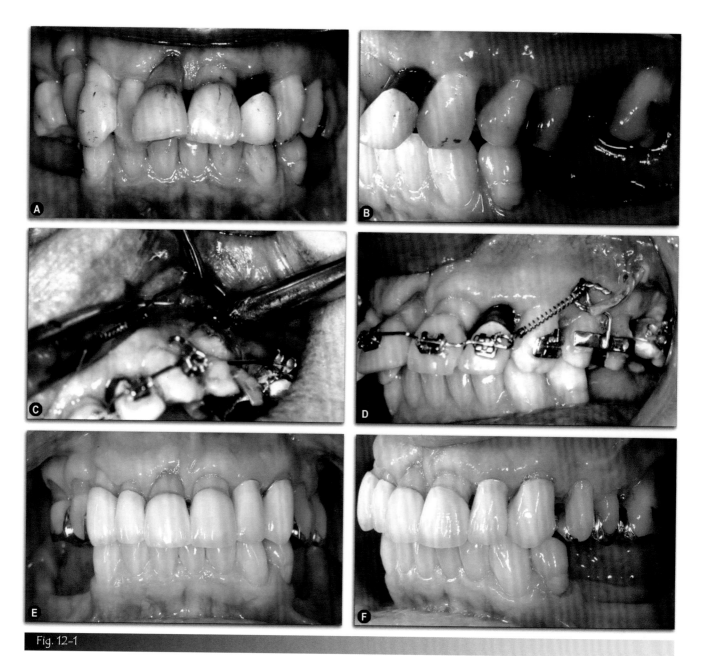

Fig. 12-1

Patient with insufficient posterior dental anchorage treated with zygoma fixation wires for anchorage. **A,** Pretreatment anterior photograph. **B,** Pretreatment left buccal photograph. Note lack of posterior teeth for anchorage. **C,** Insertion of zygomatic fixation wire. **D,** Buccal photograph of zygoma fixation wire as anchorage. **E,** Posttreatment anterior photograph. **F,** Posttreatment left buccal photograph. *(continued)*

THE AARHUS ANCHORAGE SYSTEM

Two types of implant systems are used for increasing anchorage: osseointegrated and nonosseointegrated. The surface of implants designed for osseointegration is treated to increase its roughness, thereby enhancing integration. This category includes the palatal implant,[18-20] the retromolar implant,[21-23] and the traditional dental implant.[5] However, the surface of nonintegrated implants is polished to decrease the potential for integration. This category includes cortically stabilized MSIs, miniplate implants, and fixation wire implants (see Chapter 1). These implants are much more versatile in that they can be inserted in edentulous areas, in interradicular areas, and in sites away from teeth such as the infrazygomatic crest, the hard palate, the retromolar area, and the symphysis.

For MSIs, there is a large variation with respect to material, size, and design. Most MSIs are produced from titanium-vanadium alloys, the same material used for dental and orthopedic implants. Some of the MSIs, however, are produced from resorbable materials, porcelain, and Vitalium.[24] The Leone Mini Orthodontic Implant System (Leone SpA, Firenze, Italy) is produced from stainless steel. The Aarhus

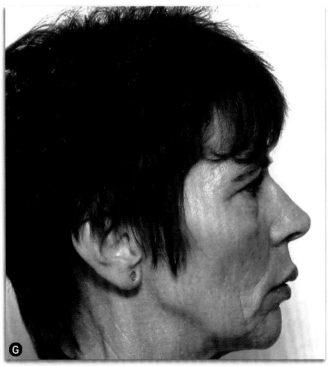

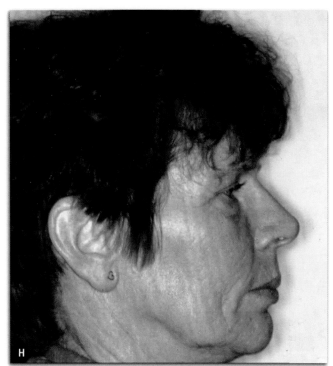

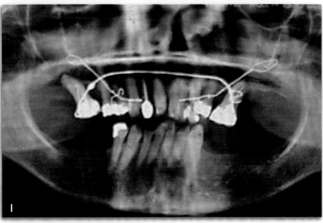

Fig. 12-1 (continued)

G, Pretreatment lateral profile photograph. **H,** Posttreatment lateral profile photograph. **I,** Panoramic radiograph showing zygomatic fixation wires. **J,** Cephalometric superimposition demonstrating maxillary incisor intrusion with retraction.

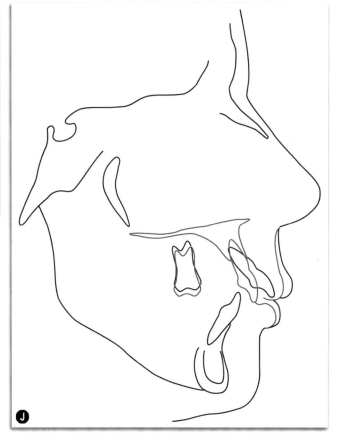

Anchorage System® (Medicon Instrumente, Tuttlingen, Germany) is produced from titanium-vanadium.

Although the biocompatibility of titanium alloys are well known, to date there have been no published reports related to any of the available MSIs on the market. Therefore, our group compared the biocompatibility of the Aarhus MSIs with a well-known sample (Leibinger surgical screw, Stryker Leibinger GmbH & Co. KG, Freiburg, Germany). Extracts were made according to ISO 10993-5.[25] The extraction medium was Dulbecco's Modified Eagles

Media without serum. The miniscrews were placed in sterile, inert, closed containers in accordance with ISO 10992-12,[26] and the extraction was performed at 37° C for 48 hours. Cultures of human oral fibroblasts were established from explants of human dental pulp

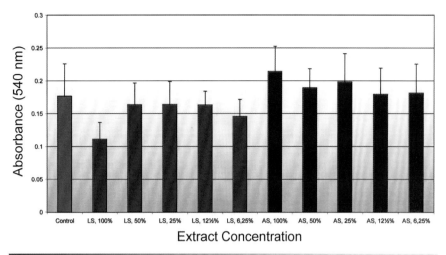

Fig. 12-2

Biocompatibility of the Aarhus Anchorage System. Two different samples, LS (Leibinger screw) and AS (Aarhus miniscrew) were tested relative to control medium.

The MTT-assay was performed per Mossman's procedure,[28] and the experiment was performed in duplicate. The absorbance readings are shown in Fig. 12-2. For each group the mean and standard error of the mean were calculated. Statistical analysis was performed by One Way ANOVA. Apart from a significant difference between LS 100% and controls ($p < 0.05$), no statistically significant differences were found between controls and the remaining exposure groups, which indicates that the Aarhus miniscrews are biocompatible.

Most MSIs are available in varying lengths between 5 and 12 mm with diameters ranging from 1 to 2.5 mm. A small diameter (1 to 1.4 mm) facilitates placement between roots.[29] This small diameter, however, reduces the mechanical properties of the miniscrew[30] and increases the risk of generating high local strains in the bone during loading, possibly causing loosening or fracture of the MSI (Fig. 12-3). Because of the increase risk of fracture with smaller diameters, the Aarhus anchorage system is available in two diameters, 1.5 mm and 2.0 mm. The Aarhus miniscrews are self-drilling (no pilot hole is required), and self-tapping (the miniscrew cuts its own threads during placement) and therefore rarely require an incision or a pilot hole (Fig. 12-4).

tissue and were propagated according to Arenholt-Bindslev and Bleeg's procedure.[27] At confluence, the primary cultures were dissociated enzymatically and were seeded into 96-well plates at a density of 25,000 cells per well. Two days after seeding, the cells were exposed for 24 hours to freshly made extracts (graded dilutions in Modified Eagles Media; 5 wells per dilution, with 10 wells serving as controls). All wells were supplemented with 10% fetal calf serum during the exposure. Cytotoxicity of the MSIs was evaluated by determining the mitochondrial function of the hepatocytes using the tetrazolium dye 3-[4,5-dimethylthiazol-2-yl]-2,5-diphenyltetrazolium bromide (MTT) following exposure to the compound.

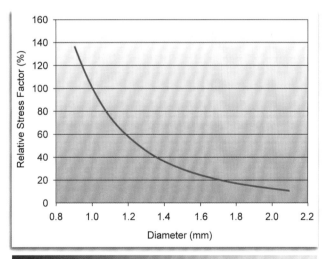

Fig. 12-3

Relative stress factor of bending/torsional stress for a miniscrew subjected to a constant bending/torsional moment relative to the diameter of the screw (set to 100% for a 1.0-mm diameter).

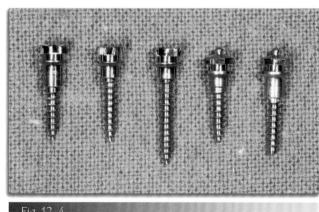

Fig. 12-4

The Aarhus Anchorage System is self-drilling and is available with two different heads, one resembling a bracket with two perpendicular slots and one with a button that can be used for attachment of coil springs or elastics. Multiple threaded body and transmucosal lengths are available. The diameter of the Aarhus miniscrews is either 1.5 or 2.0 mm.

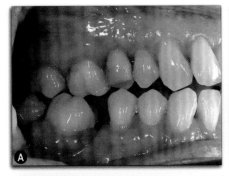
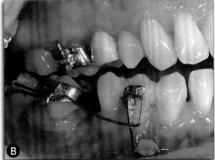
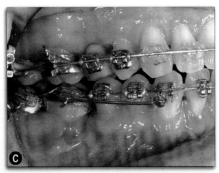

Fig. 12-5

Aarhus Anchorage System used for indirect anchorage to upright, intrude, and mesially displace mandibular right second and third molars. **A,** Pretreatment right buccal photograph. **B,** Progress right buccal photograph of initial miniscrew placement. **C,** Progress right buccal photograph at completion of miniscrew use. **D,** Pretreatment periapical radiograph of tipped molars. **E,** Progress periapical radiograph at completion of miniscrew use.

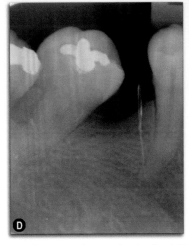
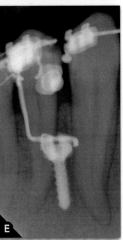

Initially, Costa and colleagues[31] designed the head of the miniscrew such that the abutment head had the shape of a bracket. This allowed the miniscrew to be connected to the appliances via a rectangular wire, thereby providing indirect anchorage from the miniscrew (Fig. 12-5). The first miniscrews were made by Citeza Surgical (San Lazzaro di Savena, Italy) and used an Allen wrench recessed hole in the center of the screw for placement. After the orthodontic loading period, however, the bone density had increased considerably such that several of the miniscrews fractured upon removal as a result of the high stress generated by unscrewing. To minize the risk of fracture upon removal, the design was changed so that the screwdriver seated around the circumference of the bracket head instead of in the center of the screw.

TREATMENT PLANNING

During treatment planning, the final treatment goal should be defined and the tooth movements described in detail. This is best done by combining the tracing of the lateral head film with an occlusogram (Fig. 12-6). Based on this three-dimensional visual treatment objective, it is possible to identify where absolute anchorage is needed, as well as the miniscrew insertion site for either direct or indirect anchorage (see Chapter 1 for a description of anchorage types). The type and direction of tooth movement should be planned carefully before the MSI is placed.[32] Based of the line of action of the force, one then can decide whether the MSI can serve as direct or indirect anchorage. In the case of indirect anchorage, the

tooth or teeth to which the MSIs will be consolidated can also be chosen. By considering the force system carefully before treatment, the potential side effects can be minimized or eliminated altogether.

PRESURGICAL ORTHODONTICS

Based on the treatment plan, orthodontic treatment can be divided into several phases. The miniscrew will likely serve as anchorage for only one or two of these phases. Therefore, there is no need to place the miniscrews before they are needed. Another concern is a mandibular functional shift that makes it difficult to determine the exact nature and direction of tooth movement. In this case, it is important to determine the position of the mandible before placing miniscrews for orthodontic anchorage (Fig. 12-7).

SURGICAL PROCEDURE

Based on the desired line of action of the force, the MSI placement position is determined on a panoramic radiograph or, when necessary, on a periapical radiograph. In radicular alveolar bone areas, a template can be used as guideline for the insertion (Fig. 12-8). Based on skull studies by Melsen and Costa,[33] possible insertion sites in the maxilla include the tuberosity area, the sub–anterior nasal spine, the hard palate, the infrazygomatic crest, and the alveolar process where

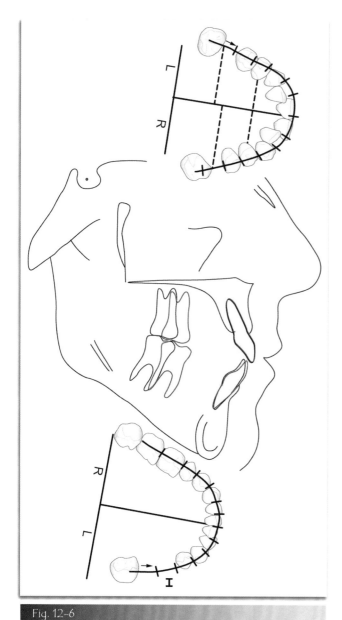

Fig. 12-6

Three dimensional visual treatment objective for determining miniscrew placement and desired tooth movement.

teeth are either absent or the interradicular bone allows adequate space (Fig. 12-9, *A* to *C*). Mandibular sites include the retromolar area, the alveolar process, and the symphyseal region (Fig. 12-9, *D* to *F*). In the alveolar process, primary stability may be enhanced if the threaded body is inserted bicortically (Fig. 12-10). It is crucial, however, that the screw does not perforate the lingual cortex. This can be avoided by measuring the thickness of the alveolar process and subtracting the mucosal thickness before choosing the appropriate length of miniscrew. Additional control is achieved by limiting local anesthesia to the buccal mucosa only. In this case, the patient will experience sensitivity at the slightest contact of the lingual periosteum, and

miniscrew placement should stop.

Because the Aarhus miniscrew is self-drilling, an incision or pilot hole rarely is required. The mucosa should be cleaned with chlorhexidine before miniscrew placement. During placement, the mucosa should be held tight with the thumb and index finger, and the MSI should be screwed directly into the bone. When 2.0-mm screws are used, or in cases with a very thick and dense cortex (mandibular symphysis or retromolar area), a pilot hole can be placed with a slow-speed handpiece. The pilot drill, which should be water cooled and should have the same length as the miniscrew, should have a diameter of about 0.2 mm less than the miniscrew (Fig. 12-11).

The thickness of the mucosa is an important factor in determining the length of the miniscrew for two main reasons. First, the mucosal thickness alters the center of rotation of the miniscrew because the mucosal thickness causes the miniscrew head to be either closer or further away from the surface of the bone. Second, thicker mucosa may require a longer transmucosal collar in order to minimize soft tissue trauma from orthodontic mechanics (Fig. 12-12).[34] Whenever possible, MSIs should be inserted through attached gingiva to minimize local irritation (Fig. 12-12, *C*). In some cases, local irritation cannot be avoided. This is particularly the case in the symphyseal region. The lack of keratinized gingiva and the activity of the mentalis muscle may result in the generation of granulation tissue around the screw. If oral hygiene is maintained, granulation rarely leads to loss of the implant or to infection (Fig. 12-13, *A*). An alternative would be to allow the MSI to be mostly covered by soft tissue with only a ligature penetrating the mucosa (Fig. 12-13, *B*).

ORTHODONTIC MECHANICS

Based on animal experiments, the Aarhus miniscrews can be loaded immediately if the force is controlled.[35] Loading is performed initially with 50-g NiTi closed coil springs because these provide a more consistent force than elastics. As the bone density increases over time with orthodontic loading, the force can be increased. The mechanics applied should be carefully considered before inserting the miniscrews. The line of action should be as perpendicular to the long axis of the screw as possible. Moments that generate torsion around the screw increase the possibility of screw loosening and failure (Fig. 12-14). It is also important to place the miniscrews so that they will not interfere with the planned tooth movement.

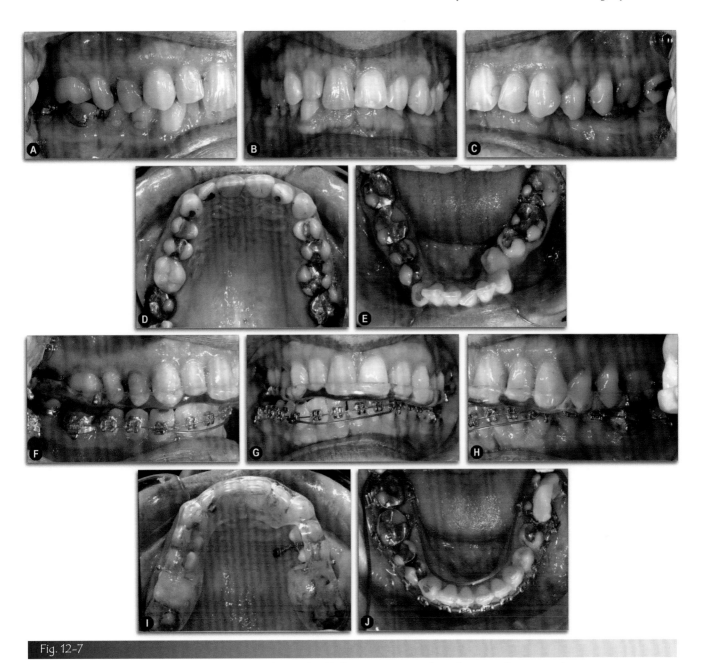

Fig. 12-7

Patient with mandibular functional shift that had to be stabilized before treatment in order to determine the exact tooth movements necessary. **A,** Pretreatment right buccal photograph. **B,** Pretreatment anterior photograph. **C,** Pretreatment left buccal photograph. Note bilateral buccal crossbite and supererupted premolars. **D,** Pretreatment maxillary occlusal photograph. **E,** Pretreatment mandibular occlusal photograph. Note collapse of left buccal segment and crowding. **F,** Progress right buccal photograph. Note maxillary flat plane splint to open bite and allow leveling and alignment of the mandibular arch. **G,** Progress anterior photograph. **H,** Progress left buccal photograph. **I,** Progress maxillary occlusal photograph. Note miniscrew in palate with closed coil spring to lingually displace and intrude left buccal segment. **J,** Progress mandibular occlusal photograph. *(continued)*

REMOVAL PROCEDURE

MSI removal is usually uneventful and can frequently be done without local anesthesia. In cases in which the miniscrew is covered by mucosa, an incision is necessary in order to gain access to the miniscrew; therefore, local anesthesia is required. In rare cases, bone density and bone-to-miniscrew contact is high enough that miniscrew removal might be difficult (Table 12-1). For these cases, two solutions have been suggested: (1) Attempt to loosen the miniscrew and then dismiss the patient for 4 to 7 days. During the interim the microfractures in the bone will have begun to remodel, making miniscrew removal easier at the second attempt. (2) Use a trephine to remove the bone around the circumference of the miniscrew.

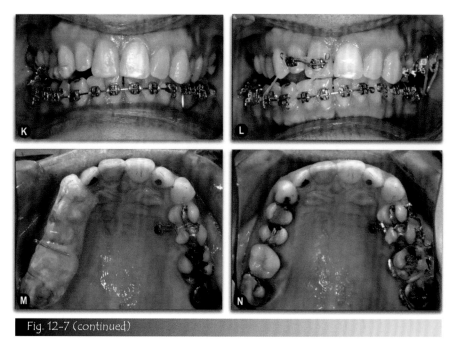

Fig. 12-7 (continued)

K, Progress anterior photograph. Note splint removed on left side. **L,** Progress anterior photograph. Note intermaxillary elastics to closed bite and correct crossbite. **M,** Progress maxillary occlusal photograph. **N,** Progress maxillary occlusal photograph.

POTENTIAL COMPLICATIONS

Primary stability is crucial for the maintenance of the miniscrew as anchorage. Failure rates between 10% and 25% have been reported.[36,37] In a prospective study, Cheng and colleagues[36] found that the anatomic location and the periimplant soft tissue were important factors for determining miniscrew prognosis. This finding also is corroborated by an ongoing study at the Orthodontic Department in Aarhus, where MSIs inserted through mobile mucosa had a higher failure rate than MSIs inserted through attached gingiva. According to Miyawaki and colleagues,[37] factors such as small miniscrew diameter, high mandibular plane angle, and

periimplant inflammation are also considered risk factors. This finding is also confirmed by an ongoing study at the Orthodontic Department in Aarhus. According to these studies, increasing the diameter of the miniscrew from 1.0 to 1.5 mm reduces the maximal stress of the miniscrew by up to 300%. If a miniscrew is mobile at the completion of the insertion procedure, a new miniscrew should be placed. Because of the ensuing remodeling associated with the miniscrew hole, the new miniscrew should either be placed a minimum of 5 mm away from the original site or placement should be postponed until healing of the bony defect has occurred (a minimum of 6 weeks later).

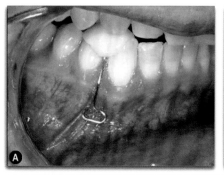
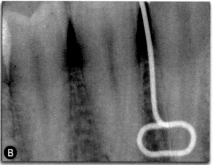
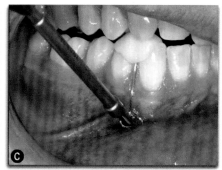

Fig. 12-8

Acrylic radiographic stent for miniscrew placement. **A,** The orthodontic wire emerges from the acrylic and is bent to the approximate site. **B,** The radiograph reveals that the insertion site should be at the distal aspect of the ellipse. **C,** Insertion of the miniscrew.

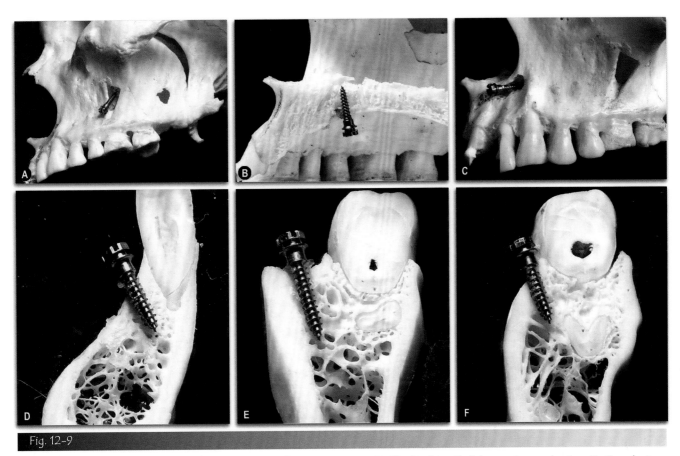

Fig. 12-9

Potential extraalveolar miniscrew insertion sites. **A,** Infrazygomatic crest. **B,** Hard palate. **C,** Sub–anterior nasal spine. **D,** Symphysis. **E,** External oblique ridge. **F,** Retromolar area.

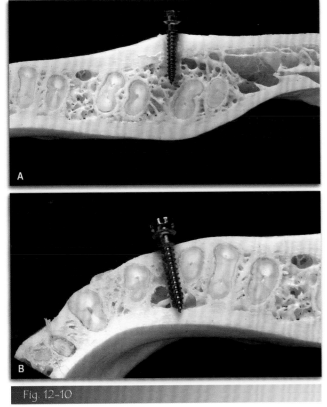

Fig. 12-10

Intraalveolar miniscrew placement. **A,** Monocortical stabilization. **B,** Bicortical stabilization.

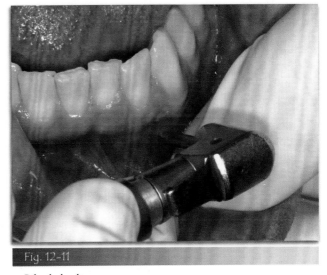

Fig. 12-11

Pilot hole placement.

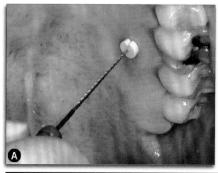
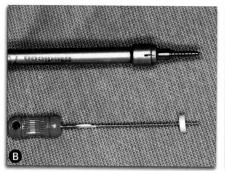
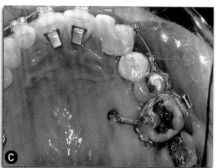

Fig. 12–12

Mucosal thickness measurement. **A,** Endodontic file with rubber stop is inserted through mucosa until contacting bone. **B,** The height of the transmucosal collar should correspond to the soft tissue measurement from the endodontic file. **C,** Miniscrew implant in place.

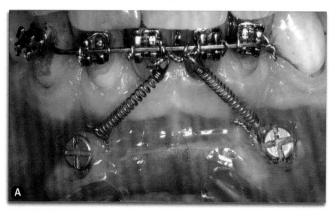
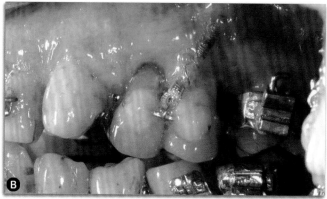

Fig. 12–13

Miniscrew implant position relative to mucosa. **A,** Miniscrew in mobile mucosa in the symphysis. Note that mobility of the mucosa caused granulation tissue development around miniscrew but did not require treatment or analgesics. **B,** Miniscrew covered by mobile mucosa in maxillary vestibule. Note that this situation was well tolerated by patient.

SUMMARY

The interest in skeletal anchorage has increased dramatically over the past decade. This is predominantly the result of the increased number of patients seeking interdisciplinary dental treatment and the lack of patient compliance during orthodontic mechanotherapy. Although traditional dental implants can be used for anchorage, they are too site-specific to have broad application. MSIs, however, are smaller, more cost-effective, and useful in many anatomic sites, and they can be loaded immediately. Moreover, MSIs can be placed by orthodontists. The Aarhus Anchorage System is one such MSI system that can be used for both direct and indirect anchorage. Two different abutment heads are available—one with a bracket-shaped head having two 0.022 × 0.028-inch slots and the other with a button on the head to which a ligature or a coil spring can be added.

ACKNOWLEDGMENTS

The research was supported in part by Medicon Instrumente, Tuttlingen, Germany; AAO Foundation, St. Louis, Missouri; and the Aarhus University Research Foundation, Aarhus, Denmark.

REFERENCES

1. Ghosh J, Nanda RS. Evaluation of an intraoral maxillary molar distalization technique. *Am J Orthod Dentofacial Orthop.* 110(6):639-646, 1996.

2. Keles A, Sayinsu K. A new approach in maxillary molar distalization: intraoral bodily molar distalizer. *Am J Orthod Dentofacial Orthop.* 117(1):39-48, 2000.

3. Kinzinger G, Gross U, Diedrich P. Fixed lingual arch appliance for compliance-free unilateral molar distalization in the mandible: three case studies. *J Orofac Orthop.* 61(6):440-450, 2000.

4. Ngantung V, Nanda RS, Bowman SJ. Posttreatment evaluation of the distal jet appliance. *Am J Orthod Dentofacial Orthop.* 120(2):178-185, 2001.

5. Bolla E, Muratore F, Carano A, Bowman SJ. Evaluation of maxillary molar distalization with the distal jet: a comparison with other contemporary methods. *Angle Orthod.* 72(5):481-494, 2002.

6. Champagne M. The NiTi Distalizer: a non-compliance maxillary molar distalizer. *Int J Orthod Milwaukee.* 13(3):21-24, 2002.

7. Burkhardt DR, McNamara JA Jr, Baccetti T. Maxillary molar distalization or mandibular enhancement: a cephalometric comparison of comprehensive orthodontic treatment including the pendulum and the Herbst appliances. *Am J Orthod Dentofacial Orthop.* 123(2):108-116, 2003.

8. Taner TU, Yukay F, Pehlivanoglu M, Cakirer B. A comparative analysis of maxillary tooth movement produced by cervical headgear and pend-x appliance. *Angle Orthod.* 73(6):686-691, 2003.

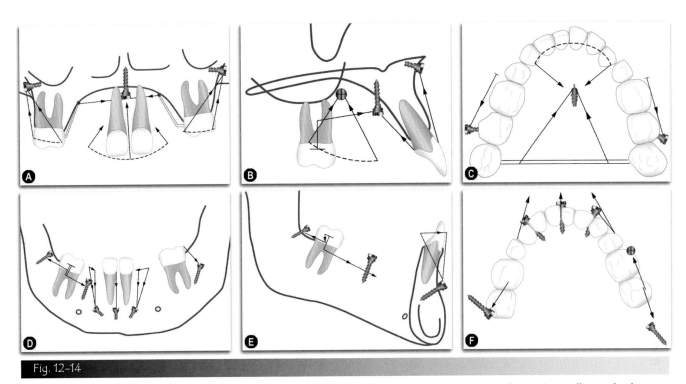

Fig. 12-14

Various force directions possible with miniscrew anchorage. **A,** Maxillary anterior view. **B,** Maxillary lateral view. **C,** Maxillary occlusal view. **D,** Mandibular anterior view. **E,** Mandibular lateral view. **F,** Mandibular occlusal view.

Table 12-1.	Bone-to-Miniscrew Contact and Relative Bone Volume at 4, 12 and 24 Weeks after Loading with 50 g Perpendicular to the Long Axis of the Miniscrew Implant			
Time (Weeks)	Bone to MSI Contact (%)		Bone Density (%) within 1 mm of MSI	
	X	SD	X	SD
4	21.8	14.4	10.6	9.8
12	64.0	13.6	42.5	16.4
24	79.5	17.5	66.3	20.9

MSI, Miniscrew implant.

9. Rozencweig G, Rozencweig S. [Use of implants and ankylosed teeth in orthodontics: review of the literature]. *J Parodontol.* 8(2):179-184, 1989.

10. Melsen B, Petersen JK, Costa A. Zygoma ligatures: an alternative form of maxillary anchorage. *J Clin Orthod.* 32(3):154-158, 1998.

11. Sfondrini MF, Cacciafesta V, Sfondrini D. The uprighting of mesially tipped and impacted mandibular second molars: the use of the mandibular ramus as orthodontic anchorage. *Orthodontics* 1(1):3-12, 2004.

12. Cattaneo PM, Dalstra M, Melsen B. The transfer of occlusal forces through the maxillary molars: a finite element study. *Am J Orthod Dentofacial Orthop.* 123(4):367-373, 2003.

13. Daimaruya T, Nagasaka H, Umemori M, et al. The influences of molar intrusion on the inferior alveolar neurovascular bundle and root using the skeletal anchorage system in dogs. *Angle Orthod.* 71(1):60-70, 2001.

14. Sherwood KH, Burch J, Thompson W. Intrusion of supererupted molars with titanium miniplate anchorage. *Angle Orthod.* 73(5):597-601, 2003.

15. Sugawara J, Baik UB, Umemori M, et al. Treatment and posttreatment dentoalveolar changes following intrusion of mandibular molars with application of a skeletal anchorage system (SAS) for open bite correction. *Int J Adult Orthodon Orthognath Surg.* 17(4):243-253, 2002.

16. Park YC, Lee SY, Kim DH, Jee SH. Intrusion of posterior teeth using mini-screw implants. *Am J Orthod Dentofacial Orthop.* 123(6):690-694, 2003.

17. Erverdi N, Keles A, Nanda R. The use of skeletal anchorage in open bite treatment: a cephalometric evaluation. *Angle Orthod.* 74(3):381-390, 2004.

18. Turley PK, Shapiro PA, Moffett BC. The loading of bioglass-coated aluminium oxide implants to produce sutural expansion of the maxillary complex in the pigtail monkey *(Macaca nemestrina). Arch Oral Biol.* 25(7):459-469, 1980.

19. Wehrbein H, Merz BR, Diedrich P, Glatzmaier J. The use of palatal implants for orthodontic anchorage: design and clinical application of the orthosystem. *Clin Oral Implants Res.* 7(4):410-416, 1996.

20. Wehrbein H, Merz BR, Diedrich P. Palatal bone support for orthodontic implant anchorage: a clinical and radiological study. *Eur J Orthod.* 21(1):65-70, 1999.

21. Roberts WE, Helm FR, Marshall KJ, Gongloff RK. Rigid endosseous implants for orthodontic and orthopedic anchorage. *Angle Orthod.* 59(4):247-256, 1989.

22. Roberts WE, Marshall KJ, Mozsary PG. Rigid endosseous implant utilized as anchorage to protract molars and close an atrophic extraction site. *Angle Orthod.* 60(2):135-152, 1990.

23. Liebenberg WH. The use of endosseous implant for anchorage during the orthodontic movement of a molar using an upright abutment. *J Dent Assoc S Afr.* 51(3):125-129, 1996.

24. Favero L, Brollo P, Bressan E. Orthodontic anchorage with specific fixtures: related study analysis. *Am J Orthod Dentofacial Orthop.* 122(1):84-94, 2002.

25. *ISO 10993-5. Biological Evaluation of Medical Devices—Part 5: Tests for in Vitro Cytotoxicity.* Geneva, Switzerland: International Organization for Standardization, 1999.

26. *ISO 10993-12. Biological Evaluation of Medical Devices—Part 12: Sample Preparation and Reference Materials.* Geneva, Switzerland: International Organization for Standardization, 1996.

27. Arenholt-Bindslev D, Bleeg H. Characterization of two types of human oral fibroblasts with a potential application to cellular toxicity studies: tooth pulp fibroblasts and buccal mucosa fibroblasts. *Int Endod J.* 23:84-91, 1990.

28. Mossman T. Rapid colorimetric assay for cellular growth and survival: application to proliferation and cytotoxicity assays. *J Immunol Methods.* 65:55-63, 1983.

29. Kyung HM, Park HS, Bae SM, et al. Development of orthodontic micro-implants for intraoral anchorage. *J Clin Orthod.* 37(6):321-328, 2003.

30. Dalstra M, Cattaneo PM, Melsen B. Load transfer of miniscrews for orthodontic anchorage. *Orthodontics.* 1(1):53-62, 2004.

31. Costa A, Raffaini M, Melsen B. Miniscrews as orthodontic anchorage: a preliminary report. *Int J Adult Orthodon Orthognath Surg.* 13(3):201-209, 1998.

32. Fiorelli G, Melsen B. *Biomechanics in Orthodontics* [book on CD-ROM; Rel. 2.1]. Arezzo, Italy: Libra Ortodonzia Ed, 2000.

33. Melsen B, Costa A. Immediate loading of implants used for orthodontic anchorage. *Clin Orthod Res.* 3(1):23-28, 2000.

34. Costa A, Pasta G, Bergamaschi G. Intraoral hard and soft tissue depths for temporary anchorage devices. *Semin Orthod.* 11(1):10-15, 2005.

35. Melsen B, Dalstra M. Bone response to loading of miniscrew implants. In: Cope JB, ed. *OrthoTADs: The Clinical Guide and Atlas.* Dallas, Texas: Under Dog Media, LP, 2007:35-45.

36. Cheng SJ, Tseng IY, Lee JJ, Kok SH. A prospective study of the risk factors associated with failure of mini-implants used for orthodontic anchorage. *Int J Oral Maxillofac Implants.* 19(1):100-106, 2004.

37. Miyawaki S, Koyama I, Inoue M, et al. Factors associated with the stability of titanium screws placed in the posterior region for orthodontic anchorage. *Am J Orthod Dentofacial Orthop.* 124(4):373-378, 2003.

The AbsoAnchor

Hyo-Sang Park, Hee-Moon Kyung

Many attempts have been made to use dental implants as orthodontic anchorage. Although dental implants provide absolute anchorage, they require a substantial amount of bone for placement in the edentulous alveolar ridge. More recently, applications with miniaturized dental implants have been used in the hard palate[1] and the retromolar area.[2] These applications have not experienced widespread use, however, because of anatomic limitations, increased costs of the implants, and the extended healing time before force application.

The first reported experimental application of a temporary anchorage device appeared in 1945.[3] However, the miniscrew implants (MSIs) failed within 18 to 35 days of placement. Little interest ensued thereafter until the first clinical report in 1983 by Creekmore and Eklund,[4] who used an MSI placed below the anterior nasal spine to intrude the upper incisors. Since that initial clinical report, several authors[5,6] have used MSIs for orthodontic anchorage applications. These reports interested our group to begin evaluating the use of MSIs. In 1999, the first author reported the use of microimplants to retract the upper incisors, only to find that the entire upper dental arch was distalized.[7] Thereafter, many clinical and experimental reports related to temporary anchorage devices have appeared in the literature.

THE ABSOANCHOR

Although not universally accepted, the term *microimplant* will be defined in this chapter as having a diameter of 1.2 to 1.5 mm and a length of 5 to 12 mm (Fig. 13-1).[8] Moreover, we refer to the use of microimplants for orthodontic anchorage as microimplant anchorage (MIA). The microimplant diameter and length can be chosen for the specific case being treated. For instance, moderate-length microimplants (1.2 to 1.3 mm in diameter, 7 to 8 mm in length) are used most commonly in the

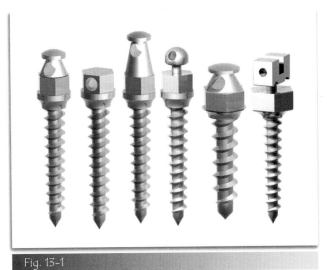

Fig. 13-1

The Absoanchor microimplant system.

facial maxillary alveolar bone. Longer microimplants (10 to 12 mm in length) are usually used in the maxillary palatal alveolar bone, where extra microimplant length compensates for the thick palatal mucosa, which is usually 2 to 5 mm thick. The extra length also ensures that the same length of the microimplant is located within the palatal bone as in other locations. For the mandible, shorter microimplants (5 to 6 mm in length) are commonly used. The Absoanchor® microimplant system (Dentos Co., Daegu, Korea) has two different screw designs, self-tapping and self-drilling. The self-tapping microimplant requires pilot hole drilling before insertion of the microimplant, whereas the self-drilling or drill-free screw does not require pilot hole drilling before insertion (see Chapter 1 for complete description of screw designs).

TREATMENT PLANNING

Force application to the microimplant is principally by the direct method (see Chapter 1 for definitions). The information that is required to establish a treatment plan for MIA is as follows. First, the direction of tooth movement is determined. Next, the line of force required to achieve the desired tooth movement is determined. Finally, the position of the microimplant to achieve the desired line of force is determined. For simplification, two different applications are presented: (1) en masse retraction or protraction of the entire dental arch and (2) minor tooth movement for correcting specific orthodontic problems.

En Masse Tooth Movement

To evaluate the profile, either the E-line[9] or the true vertical line[10] can be used. We prefer the E-line to measure the pretreatment lip protrusion. The line is drawn from the nasal tip to the soft tissue chin (Fig. 13-2, A) and is used to help determine the soft tissue goals because lip position changes during treatment. In this step, growth changes of the upper and lower lips, nose, and chin should be considered in growing patients because growth may drastically affect the profile in some cases.[11,12] In nongrowing patients, the effects of aging on the soft tissue should be considered, because an increase in philtrum height and a decrease in incisor display at rest commonly occur with normal aging.[13] For instance, the upper incisors should usually be positioned to display more than 2 mm at rest in order to minimize the aging effects on the smile line by drooping of the upper lip.

After the soft tissue goals are established, the vertical and horizontal position of the upper incisor can be determined by estimating the ratio of soft tissue movement relative to anterior tooth movement (Fig. 13-2, B). The inclination of the upper incisors should also be decided during this step. In patients with thick lips, the incisors should be positioned further posteriorly than in patients with thin lips.[14] In cases with lip strain, only small lip changes can be expected with incisor retraction. The lower incisor position is then established to create an ideal overjet and overbite relationship with the upper incisor (Fig. 13-2, C). Next, the predicted incisor movement is transferred to an occlusogram. The position of the upper and lower incisors are drawn onto the upper and lower occlusograms, respectively. The remaining posterior teeth are then aligned sequentially from the front to the back. After all teeth are aligned, the amount of distal or mesial movement of posterior teeth is calculated (Fig. 13-2, D).

If the amount of posterior tooth movement is less than 2 mm of distalization, premolar extraction is not considered. If the amount is between 2 and 4 mm, then the extraction decision is made based on the patient's skeletal pattern. If the amount is greater than 4 mm, then premolar extraction is necessary. If so, the premolars are "extracted" on the occlusogram, and the remaining posterior teeth are aligned to close the extraction space without changing the predetermined incisor position (Fig. 13-2, E). When choosing nonextraction treatment, evaluate the maxillary tuberosity and mandibular retromolar area to determine whether ample space is present for distal molar movement. If third molars are present, they should be extracted before distal molar movement.

After the extraction decision is made, the cephalogram is used to determine the force direction and point of force to achieve the desired anterior tooth movement. Once the direction of force and point of force application are decided, the position of microimplant is chosen (Fig. 13-2, F). The best site for a microimplant anteroposteriorly is the alveolar bone between second premolar and first molar. To achieve bodily retraction of the upper incisors in premolar extraction cases, the occlusogingival position of the microimplant should be 8 to 10 mm apical to the arch wire.[15,16] In nonextraction treatment, the occlusogingival position of microimplant should be 6 to 7 mm apical to the arch wire.[17,18]

When treating high-angle patients, maintenance of the vertical position of the upper and lower posterior teeth or actual achievement of intrusion of the posterior teeth is desirable and has the added benefit of allowing autorotation of the mandible.[15,16,19-21] In some cases, however, this may cause a posterior open bite. To correct this problem, the upper incisor should be retracted less than the originally planned amount. Alternatively, the lower incisor can be retracted and intruded. When managing a low-angle patient, nonextraction treatment may be a better option. By group distal movement of the anterior and posterior teeth with the microimplant, the treatment time will be reduced.[17,18]

Minor Tooth Movement

First, the direction of tooth movement is determined. Next, the line of force required to achieve the desired tooth movement is determined. Finally, the position of the microimplant to achieve the desired line of force is determined. This should be done in both the anteroposterior and occlusogingival dimensions. An additional step that might be necessary is the prediction of unwanted tooth rotation or tipping, which might require the design of auxiliary appliances to prevent such undesirable side effects, such as a lingual arch to prevent facial tipping during intrusion from a facially placed microimplant.

PRESURGICAL ORTHODONTICS

Considering the size of the microimplant, there is rarely a need for presurgical orthodontics. The microimplant is usually small enough to be placed in any area in the mouth, including in the facial and lingual/palatal alveolar bone between roots, in the hard palate, and in the retromolar area. The only possible need for presurgical orthodontics would be when space is

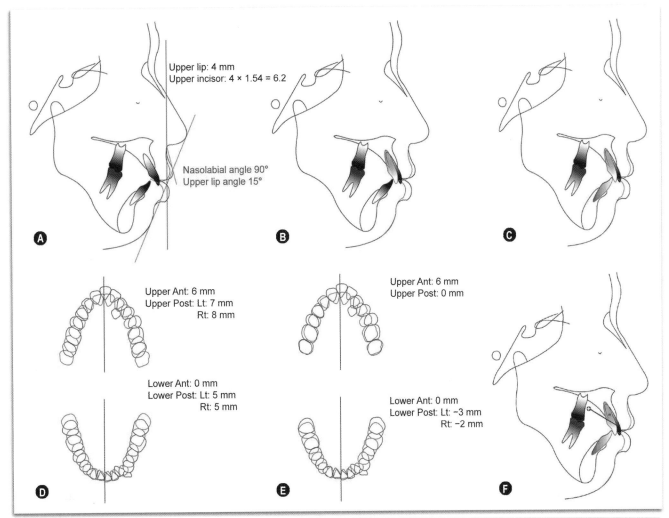

Fig. 13-2

Treatment planning for en masse tooth movement with microimplant anchorage (MIA) sliding mechanics. **A,** Soft tissue profile is used to determine treatment goals. **B,** Final upper incisor position *(red)* is determined. **C,** Final lower incisor position *(red)* is determined. **D,** Final upper incisor position is transferred to occlusogram to determine amount of posterior tooth movement required. **E,** Upper premolars are "extracted," and posterior teeth are aligned into extraction space. **F,** Line of force and microimplant position are determined.

inadequate to place the microimplants between roots. In this case, orthodontically diverging the roots prior to microimplant placement may be necessary.

SURGICAL PROCEDURE

Surgical procedures are slightly different depending on the type of microimplant chosen and the type of soft tissue overlying the intended site. The self-tapping microimplant requires all of the following procedures.[19,22] The self-drilling microimplant does not require a pilot hole before placement. For placement of the microimplant into attached gingiva or palatal masticatory mucosa, no incision is required. The following details all steps required for a self-tapping microimplant in mobile mucosa. Appropriate steps should be deleted for a self-drilling microimplant in keratinized gingiva.

1. Perform local anesthetic infiltration.

2. Place a twisted brass wire between the maxillary first molar and the second premolar to serve as a guide for making the gingival incision and the subsequent pilot hole (Fig. 13-3, A).

3. Make a small vertical incision (3 to 4 mm long) on the facial oral mucosa 3 to 4 mm apical to the mucogingival junction (Fig. 13-3, B).

4. Reflect a mucoperiosteal flap with the periosteal elevator (Fig. 13-3, C).

5. Make an indentation with a No. 2 round bur as an entry point and stabilizing channel for the pilot drill (Fig. 13-3, D).

6. Make a pilot hole with the pilot drill (Fig. 13-3, E).

7. Place the appropriate size of microimplant with the manual screw driver (Fig. 13-3, F).

Two or three periapical radiographs may be used to assess the space between the roots for microimplants. The brass wire acts as a guide for microimplant placement between the tooth roots (Fig. 13-3, G and H). One third of a 2% lidocaine carpule is sufficient to anesthetize the soft tissue and alveolar bone. Profound anesthesia is not indicated because it will interfere with the patient's root sensitivity to a misplaced pilot drill and eliminate the patient's ability to sense tooth root contact.

The authors use approximately 600 rpm for pilot hole drilling. The entire procedure is done under sterile saline irrigation. It is important to not apply heavy forces while creating the pilot hole because this generates heat that can cause bone necrosis, which may decrease microimplant stability and success. Pilot hole drilling in the mobile mucosa may cause twisting of the soft tissue around the drill and tearing of the soft tissue; therefore, it is important to ensure that the reflected flap is held away from the pilot drill. The maxillary microimplants are placed at 30 to 40 degrees to the long axis of the posterior teeth (Fig. 13-4, A). The mandibular microimplants are placed at 10 to 20 degrees to the long axis of the posterior teeth (Fig. 13-4, B). Such angulation allows the use of longer microimplants, which increases stability without the risk of root injury.

The incision and flap reflection is omitted when placing microimplants in attached gingiva or palatal masticatory mucosa (Fig. 13-5, A). The self-drilling microimplant does not require a pilot hole (Fig. 13-5, B and C). This approach, however, is only applicable to the upper arch, particularly in the anterior tooth area where the cortical bone is thinner. Because the mandibular arch has thicker cortical bone, the pilot hole should equal the length of the microimplant. In the maxillary arch, which has thinner and weaker cortical bone,[23] the length of the pilot hole should be less than the length of the selected microimplant. For patients who have unusually thin and weak cortical bone, pilot holes should not exceed one half the length of the microimplant. The pilot drill should be slightly smaller in diameter than that of the microimplant, usually three fourths the size of the microimplant. Because of the quality and quantity of the bone, longer microimplants (8 mm) are used in the maxilla and shorter microimplants (6 mm) are used in the mandible. When inserting microimplants with the manual screwdriver, slow gentle rotational movement increases the success rate and decreases the risk of breaking the small titanium microimplants.

Microimplant placement is easily evaluated after insertion with two or three periapical radiographs. By changing the angulation, a determination can be made as to whether the microimplant touches the roots. Only one radiograph has to demonstrate clearance between the microimplant and root in order to ensure that no contact has been made (Fig. 13-6).

ORTHODONTIC MECHANICS

Orthodontic mechanics is also presented in two parts: (1) en masse retraction or protraction of the entire dental arch and (2) minor tooth movement for correcting specific orthodontic problems.

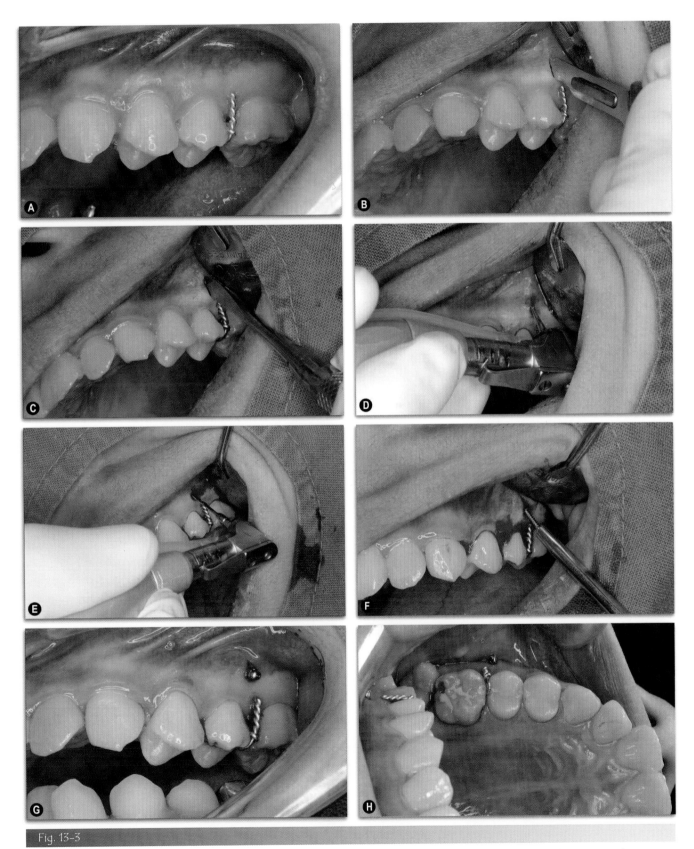

Fig. 13-3

Complete microimplant surgical placement procedure. **A,** Brass wire used as guide for vertical incision and periosteal flap. **B,** Vertical incision. **C,** Periosteal elevator for flap elevation. **D,** No. 2 round bur preparing entry point for pilot drill. **E,** Pilot hole placement. Note the angle of the pilot drill. **F,** Microimplant placement with manual screwdriver. **G,** Buccal photograph of final microimplant position. **H,** Occlusal photograph of final microimplant position.

En Masse Tooth Movement

Most orthodontic mechanics of MIA involve direct force application from the microimplant to the teeth. Detailed procedures in both extraction and nonextraction cases have been described in previous clinical reports.[15-21] Sliding MIA retraction mechanics are usually used with microimplants in extraction treatment for retraction of the upper six anterior teeth (Fig. 13-7, *A*).[15,16,19-21] A nickel titanium closed coil spring (NiTi CCS) force of 150 to 200 g was applied from the upper microimplants between the second premolars and first molars to anterior hooks soldered on the arch wire between the canines and lateral incisors. By using a force passing near to the center of resistance of the six anterior teeth, the anterior teeth tended to be bodily retracted with slight intrusion. An additional intrusion force can be applied from the microimplants in the upper arch to the upper posterior teeth to control the vertical dimension. The purpose of the lower microimplant is purely for vertical control of the lower posterior teeth, which tend to extrude and

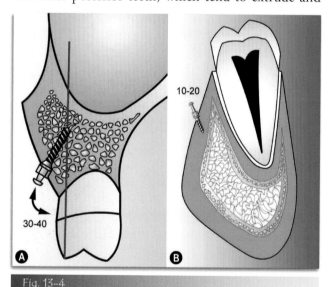

Fig. 13-4

Microimplant angulation. **A,** Maxillary. **B,** Mandibular.

tip mesially during space closure in high-angle cases. The lower microimplant in extraction cases is optional. (See MSI Case Report 8 for more detailed information.) For extraction cases undergoing lingual orthodontic treatment, the microimplant should be placed higher in palatal bone between the maxillary first and second molars[24] or in facial alveolar bone between the second premolar and first molar.[19]

In nonextraction cases with MIA sliding mechanics (Fig. 13-7, *B*),[17,18] two maxillary and two mandibular microimplants are needed. The maxillary microimplants are placed in the facial alveolar bone between second premolars and first molars with facial appliances, or in the palatal alveolar bone between the first and second molars with lingual appliances. The mandibular microimplants are placed in the retromolar area, the alveolar bone distofacial to the second molars, or the alveolar bone between the first and second molars. The distalizing force for the posterior teeth is applied from the microimplant to the canines so that all posterior teeth are distalized simultaneously. If there is crowding of the anterior teeth, it can be resolved by moving the posterior teeth distally and then aligning the anterior teeth in the newly created space without flaring the incisors.

Minor Tooth Movement

During upper molar intrusion (Fig. 13-8), a transpalatal bar is necessary to prevent facial or lingual tipping of the upper molars.[25] In this case, the supererupted upper molars were intruded by placing a microimplant in the palate and attaching an elastic force from the microimplant to the hook soldered on the transpalatal arch.

A mesially tipped lower second molar can be efficiently uprighted with a single microimplant placed distal to the tooth in the retromolar area (Fig. 13-9).[26] Or just as effectively, a mesially tipped third molar can be uprighted by joining two microimplants mesial to

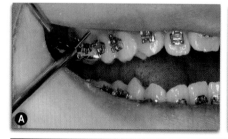
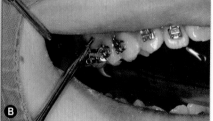
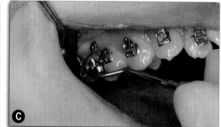

Fig. 13-5

Modified microimplant surgical placement procedure. **A,** Initial self-drilling microimplant placement without a pilot hole or an incision in attached gingiva. **B,** Self-drilling microimplant placement half finished. **C,** Final position of self-drilling microimplant.

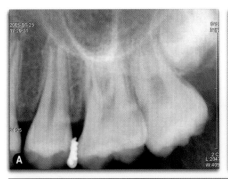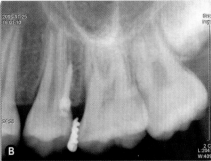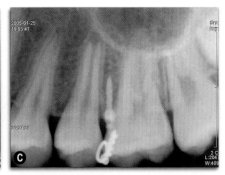

Fig. 13-6

Periapical radiographs used to assess space for microimplants. **A,** Pretreatment periapical radiograph. **B,** Periapical radiograph after microimplant placement. Note overlap with tooth root. **C,** Periapical radiograph after microimplant placement. Note clearance between the microimplant and tooth roots.

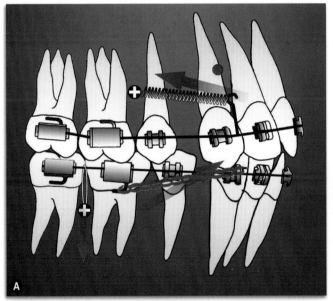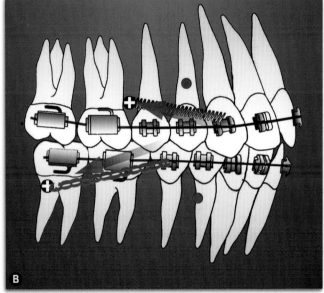

Fig. 13-7

Biomechanics for microimplant anchorage (MIA) sliding mechanics. **A,** Extraction treatment. **B,** Nonextraction treatment.

the tooth (Fig. 13-10). In this case, a bracket was attached to the joined microimplants and the tipped molar and then was uprighted with up to a 400-g force with a section of arch wire. The edentulous alveolar ridge is a good site for placement of microimplants. When comparing the two methods, two joined microimplants have better stability and anchorage value, and the edentulous ridge is more accessible, but at twice the cost.

When uprighting lingually tipped lower molars, one microimplant can be placed just facial to the tipped molar (Fig. 13-11).[27] Because the cortical bone on the lower posterior teeth is approximately 3 mm thick,[23,28] a 6-mm long microimplant can be placed at 10 to 20 degrees without penetrating the marrow space. Moreover, there is more than 6 mm of space between outer surface of the facial bone and the lower second molar roots at a level 5 to 7 mm apical to the alveolar crest. Therefore, the potential for tooth root contact is minimal.

REMOVAL PROCEDURE

The microimplant removal procedure is simple and noninvasive. Without anesthesia, the screwdriver is aligned over the microimplant and screwed in the opposite direction as it was for placement (Fig. 13-12). If the microimplant is covered by soft tissue, local anesthesia, incision, and flap reflection may be required.

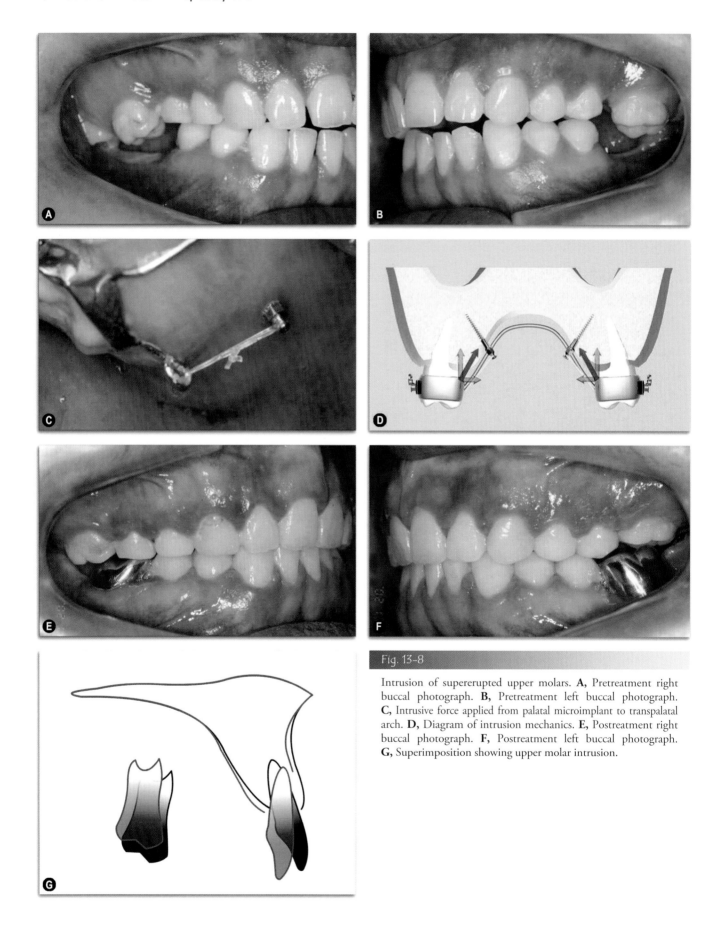

Fig. 13-8

Intrusion of supererupted upper molars. **A,** Pretreatment right buccal photograph. **B,** Pretreatment left buccal photograph. **C,** Intrusive force applied from palatal microimplant to transpalatal arch. **D,** Diagram of intrusion mechanics. **E,** Postreatment right buccal photograph. **F,** Postreatment left buccal photograph. **G,** Superimposition showing upper molar intrusion.

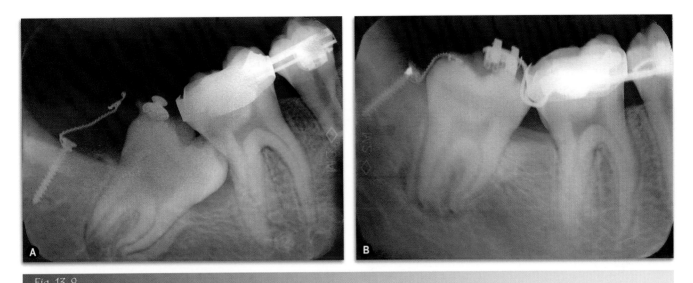

Fig. 13-9

Uprighting of mesioangularly impacted lower molar. **A,** Pretreatment periapical radiograph. **B,** Posttreatment periapical radiograph.

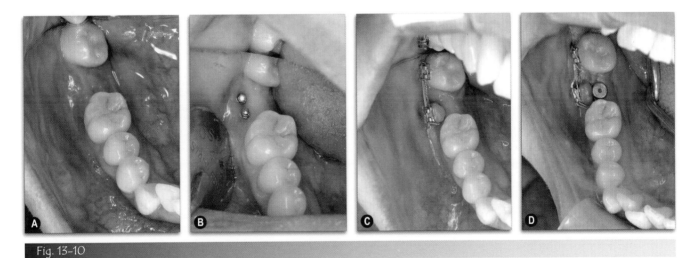

Fig. 13-10

Uprighting of mesiolingually tipped lower molar. **A,** Pretreatment lower occlusal photograph. **B,** Progress lower occlusal photograph showing two microimplants joined together by composite bonding. **C,** Progress lower occlusal photograph showing sectional arch wire attachment. **D,** Progress lower occlusal photograph after molar uprighting.

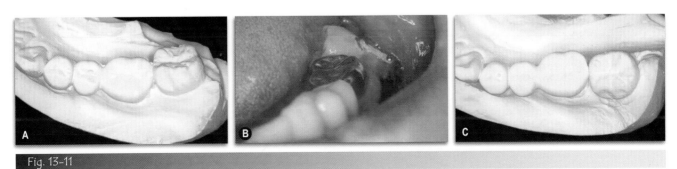

Fig. 13-11

Uprighting of lingually tipped lower molar. **A,** Pretreatment lower occlusal model. **B,** Anterior photograph showing single point force application from microimplant to button. **C,** Posttreatment lower occlusal model.

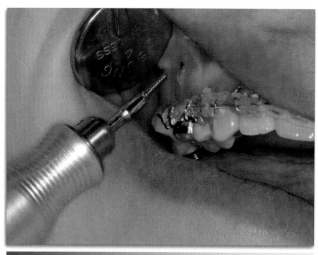

Fig. 13–12

Removal of microimplant with manual screwdriver.

POTENTIAL COMPLICATIONS

The most serious potential complication iis not being able to use the microimplant for the entire treatment duration. The success rate of the microimplants for orthodontic anchorage has been reported at 93.3%[29] and 91.6%,[30] respectively, during 15 months of force application. The risk factors associated with failure of the microimplants were inflammation around the microimplant head, microimplants placed in the mandible, and microimplants placed on the patient's right side, which may have been due to patient handedness or to operator handedness.

SUMMARY

The microimplant is small enough to be placed in most any bony location within the oral cavity, which may expand the clinical application of microimplants to many orthodontic problems. The placement and removal procedures are simple, the microimplants are relatively inexpensive, and they provide absolute anchorage for movement of the entire dentition, individual teeth, or the entire occlusal plane.

ACKNOWLEDGMENTS

This research was supported in part by Dentos Co., Daegu, Korea.

REFERENCES

1. Wehrbein H, Feifel H, Diedrich P. Palatal implant anchorage reinforcement of posterior teeth: a prospective study. *Am J Orthod Dentofacial Orthop.* 116:678-686, 1999.
2. Roberts WE, Nelson CL, Goodacre CJ. Rigid implant anchorage to close a mandibular first molar extraction site. *J Clin Orthod.* 28:693-704, 1994.
3. Gainsforth BL, Higley LB. A study of orthodontic anchorage possibilities in basal bone. *Am J Orthod Oral Surg.* 31:406-417, 1945.
4. Creekmore TD, Eklund MK. The possibility of skeletal anchorage. *J Clin Orthod.* 17:266-269, 1983.
5. Kanomi R. Mini-implant for orthodontic anchorage. *J Clin Orthod.* 31:763-767, 1997.
6. Costa A, Raffini M, Melsen B. Miniscrews as orthodontic anchorage: a preliminary report. *Int J Adult Orthodon Orthognath Surg.* 13:201-209, 1998.
7. Park HS. The skeletal cortical anchorage using titanium microscrew implants. *Korean J Orthod.* 29:699-706, 1999.
8. Kyung HM, Park HS, Bae SM, et al. Development of orthodontic micro-implants for intraoral anchorage. *J Clin Orthod.* 37(6):321-328, 2003.
9. Rickets RM. Esthetics, environment and the law of lip relation. *Am J Orthod.* 54:272-289, 1968.
10. Arnett GW, Jelic JS, Kim J, et al. Soft tissue cephalometric analysis: diagnosis and treatment planning of dentofacial deformity. *Am J Orthod Dentofacial Orthop.* 116:239-253, 1999.
11. Nanda RS, Meng H, Kapilla S, et al. Growth changes in the soft tissue facial profile. *Angle Orthod.* 60:177-190, 1990.
12. Genecov JS, Sinclair PM, Dechow PC. Development of the nose and soft tissue profile. *Angle Orthod.* 60:191-198, 1990.
13. Dickens ST, Sarver DM, Proffit WR. Changes in frontal soft tissue dimensions of the lower face by age and gender. *World J Orthod.* 3:313-320, 2002.
14. Oliver BM. The influence of the lip thickness and strain on upper lip response to incisor retraction. *Am J Orthod.* 82:141-149, 1982.
15. Park HS, Bae SM, Kyung HM, et al. Micro-implant anchorage for treatment of skeletal Class I bialveolar protrusion. *J Clin Orthod.* 35:417-422, 2001.
16. Park HS, Kwon TG. Sliding mechanics with microscrew implant anchorage. *Angle Orthod.* 74:703-710, 2004.
17. Park HS, Kwon TG, Sung JH. Nonextraction treatment with microscrew implant. *Angle Orthod.* 74:539-549, 2004.
18. Park HS, Lee SK, Kwon OW. Group distal movement of teeth with microscrew implants. *Angle Orthod.* 75:510-517, 2005.
19. Park HS. *The use of micro-implant orthodontic anchorage.* Seoul: Nare Publishing Co, 2001.
20. Park HS, Kwon OW. The treatment of openbite with microscrew implants anchorage. *Am J Orthod Dentofacial Orthop.* 126:627-636, 2004.
21. Park HS. A new protocol of sliding mechanics with micro-implant anchorage (MIA). *Korean J Orthod.* 30:677-685, 2000.
22. Park HS, Bae SM, Kyung HM, et al. Simultaneous incisor retraction and distal molar movement with microimplant anchorage. *World J Orthod.* 5:164-171, 2004.
23. Park HS. An anatomical study using CT images for the implantation of micro-implants. *Korean J Orthod.* 32:435-441, 2002.
24. Lee JS, Park HS, Kyung HM. Micro-implant anchorage in lingual orthodontic treatment for a skeletal Class II malocclusion. *J Clin Orthod.* 35:643-647, 2001.
25. Park HS. Intrusion molar con anclaje de microimplantes (MIA, micro-implants anchorage). *Orthodoncia Clinica.* 6:31-36, 2003.
26. Park HS, Kyung HM, Sung JH. A simple method of molar uprighting with micro-implant anchorage. *J Clin Orthod.* 36:592-596, 2002.
27. Park HS, Kwon OW, Sung JH. Uprighting second molars with micro-implant anchorage. *J Clin Orthod.* 38:100-103, 2004.
28. Kruger E, Schilli W. *Mandibular fracture, oral and maxillofacial traumatology.* Vol 2. Chicago; Quintessence Publishing Co, 1986:19-43.
29. Park HS. Clinical study on success rate of microscrew implants for orthodontic anchorage. *Korean J Orthod.* 33:151-156, 2003.
30. Park HS, Jeong SH, Kwon OH. Factors affecting the clinical success of screw implants used as orthodontic anchorage. *Am J Orthod Dentofacial Orthop.* 130(1):18-25, 2006.

CHAPTER

14

The Spider Screw

B. Giuliano Maino, John R. Bednar, Paola Mura

Anchorage control and patient compliance are two of the most critical factors affecting the final outcome of orthodontic treatment. Tooth movement—such as en masse anterior retraction, molar protraction, and intrusion of supererupted teeth—is difficult to achieve without suitable anchorage.[1-3] Molar intrusion is sometimes more difficult to achieve and frequently unpredictable because molars are multirooted with a large root surface area and are located at the terminal aspect of the arch wire, which is less efficient for tooth movement than the intermediate zone of the premolars.[4] It follows that a skeletal-based, as opposed to a dental-based, anchorage system that is independent of patient compliance would be of significant benefit to orthodontists. One such temporary anchorage device is the miniscrew implant (MSI), which is small, easy to place and use, and well accepted by patients and can be loaded immediately.[5-9]

THE SPIDER SCREW SYSTEM

The Spider Screw (HDC Company, Sarcedo, Italy) is a self-tapping, commercially pure titanium MSI that can be loaded immediately with forces in the range of 50 to 250 g.[10-12] Complete osseointegration is neither expected nor desired with this system. The Spider Screw anchorage system can be used to support a variety of orthodontic tooth movements in clinical situations involving mutilated dentitions, poor cooperation, or extraction cases requiring maximum anchorage.

The head of the Spider Screw is designed with internal and external rectangular slots 0.022 × 0.028-inch in size. The Spider Screw also has two round internal vertical slots 0.025-inch in diameter (Fig. 14-1). The extramucosal head of the screw is small enough to avoid soft tissue irritation yet large enough to accommodate orthodontic attachments. The different slots permit a variety of ways in which to connect the MSI to the orthodontic appliances. The internal rectangular slot is used to attach elastic or stainless steel ligatures in a

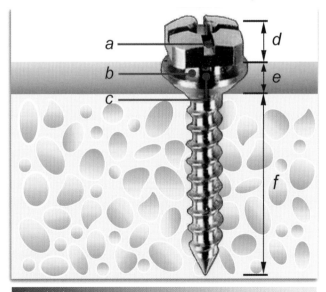

Fig. 14-1

Spider Screw anatomic features. (a) External rectangular slot, (b) internal rectangular slot, (c) internal round slot, (d) abutment head, (e) transmucosal collar, (f) threaded body.

manner that keeps the ties above the soft tissue to prevent soft tissue trauma. The slot size also allows use with the most commonly used orthodontic wires. The external rectangular slot is used mostly for placement of the MSI into bone and for attachment of rectangular arch wires. The vertical slot is used to ligate closed coil springs to the head of the MSI.

This system is available in either 1.5- or 2.0-mm diameters. The 1.5-mm diameter MSI comes in 6-, 8-, or 10-mm lengths, whereas the 2.0-mm diameter MSI comes in 7-, 9-, or 11-mm lengths. Spider Screws are dispensed in prepackaged, sterile, single-use blister packs.

The 1.5-mm diameter Spider Screw is available with either a short or long transmucosal collar (Fig. 14-2). The transmucosal collar length is determined by the depth of the soft tissue, whereas the MSI length is determined by the depth of the hard tissue. The 1.5-mm diameter MSI is indicated for placement in areas with limited space, such as in interradicular bone. The various Spider Screw lengths are placed in the following locations: 6 mm is placed in the anterior region from canine to canine, 8 mm is more adaptable and can be used most anywhere, and 10 mm is placed in the posterolateral region.

The 2.0-mm diameter Spider Screw is available in three different transmucosal collar and abutment head designs to accommodate the soft tissues: *low profile flat, low profile,* and *regular* (Fig. 14-3). These variations provide multiple options to ensure proper adaptation of the soft tissues, thereby minimizing the possibility of inflammation. The low-profile flat screw has a short transmucosal collar and a flat head profile for use in the thin soft tissues in the anterior part of the mouth. The low-profile screw has a longer transmucosal collar and a flat head for use in the thick soft tissues of posterior segments. The regular design has an intermediate length transmucosal collar and a higher profile head and when combined with a resin core can be used as a temporary prosthetic abutment.

TREATMENT PLANNING
Every treatment plan requires careful evaluation of the forces necessary to elicit the desired movements and of the anchorage necessary to support these forces. The most frequently used anchorage systems involving extraoral traction or intraoral elastics are associated with several problems. For example, intraoral elastics cause undesirable effects[3] and necessitate appliance placement in the lower arch even when not required by the treatment objectives. In addition, extraoral traction

or intraoral elastics depend on patient cooperation. Moreover, many adults avoid orthodontic treatment because of esthetic limitations of conventional anchorage. Skeletal anchorage provides a solution to achieve sagittal and vertical movement without cooperation and without compromising the final orthodontic result. Skeletal anchorage also allows appliance placement in one arch or one segment only.

Treatment planning must include a careful choice of Spider Screw size and location, as well as the manner in which the Spider Screw will be used: indirect anchorage, direct anchorage, or prosthetic anchorage. For indirect anchorage, the reactive segment is attached to and stabilized by the MSI, and the reactive segment is used to

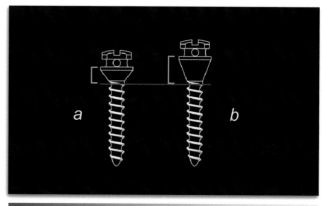

Fig. 14-2

Design characteristics of the 1.5-mm diameter Spider Screw. *(a)* Short transmucosal collar, *(b)* long transmucosal collar. Note that gold bracket indicates transmucosal collar.

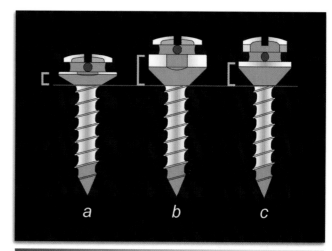

Fig. 14-3

Design characteristics of the 2.0-mm diameter Spider Screw. *(a) Low profile flat* with short transmucosal collar and a flat head profile, *(b) low profile* with longer transmucosal collar and a flat head, *(c) regular* with intermediate-length transmucosal collar and a higher profile head. Note that gold bracket indicates transmucosal collar.

move the active segment. For direct anchorage, the active segment is attached directly to the MSI for tooth movement (see Chapter 1). For prosthetic anchorage, the MSI is placed in the edentulous alveolar ridge and is temporarily restored. The restoration is then used for orthodontic anchorage and is removed afterward. The placement location dictates the ability to control retraction, protraction, extrusion, or intrusion of teeth. The placement of the Spider Screw requires a location that has sufficient bone depth to accommodate the MSI length and at least 2.5 mm of bone width to protect the local anatomic structures.[6,10-12] Typical insertion sites include the maxillary tuberosity, the mandibular retromolar area, edentulous ridges, interradicular sites, the palatal vault, and the alveolar processes above the root apices in the anterior region.

For example, a patient presented with an upper dental midline discrepancy to the right side and an interincisal diastema (Fig. 14-4, *A* to *D*). The treatment plan was designed to close the diastema while reopening space for the missing maxillary left first molar to achieve a bilateral Class I canine relationship. Skeletal

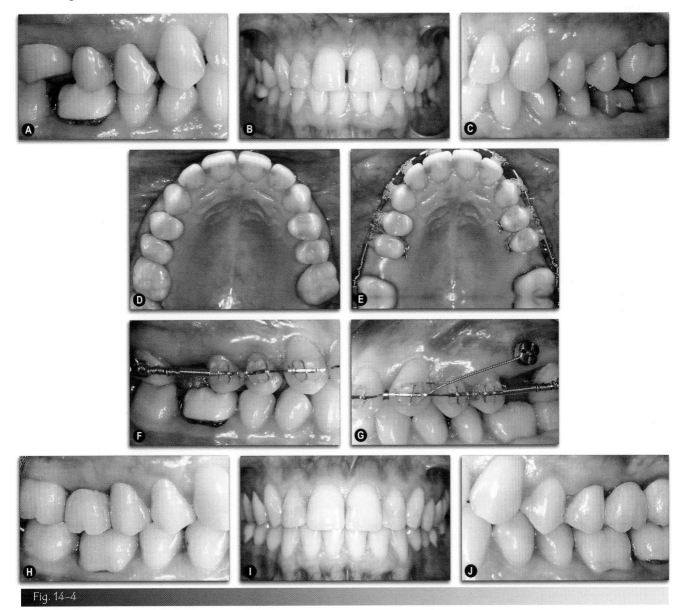

Fig. 14-4

Spider Screw indirect anchorage to distalize maxillary left second molar for replacement of missing first molar. **A,** Pretreatment right buccal photograph. Note Class III canine relationship. **B,** Pretreatment anterior photograph. **C,** Pretreatment left buccal photograph. Note Class I canine relationship. **D,** Pretreatment maxillary occlusal photograph. **E,** Progress maxillary occlusal photograph after molar distalization. **F,** Progress right buccal photograph. Note that reciprocal space opening was used. **G,** Progress left buccal photograph. Note that the Spider Screw was ligated to the canine, which provided indirect anchorage to distalize the second molar. **H,** Posttreatment right buccal photograph. **I,** Posttreatment anterior photograph. **J,** Posttreatment left buccal photograph.

anchorage became the option of choice because the patient rejected extraoral traction and mandibular appliances. Treatment proceeded as follows (Fig. 14-4, *E* to *G*). The maxillary right third molar was extracted, and anchorage was provided by placement of a Spider Screw (2.0-mm diameter, 9 mm long) in the residual space between the maxillary left second premolar and left second molar. The Spider Screw was used as indirect anchorage in this case. A 0.012-inch metal ligature extending from the Spider Screw to the maxillary left canine resisted forward movement of the canine from the compressed open coil spring. On the patient's right side, a compressed open coil spring was used to distalize the first molar while the reactive force corrected the Class III premolar and canine relationship and shifted the maxillary midline as the diastema closed (Fig. 14-4, *H* to *J*).

Miniscrews can be incorporated into treatment planning when it is difficult to achieve the desired results with traditional anchorage. Miniscrews are particularly useful in adult cases when there are compromised periodontal conditions or partially edentulous arches. Miniscrews are also useful for molar intrusion because intrusion of supererupted molars can create undesirable effects in open bite cases.[4] Another patient presented with a malocclusion characterized by supereruption of the maxillary left second premolar, first molar, and second molar toward the edentulous ridge in the mandibular left quadrant (Fig. 14-5, *A*). The supereruption created an esthetic problem and precluded the possibility of prosthetic treatment in the mandibular left quadrant. Anchorage for intrusion in the maxillary left quadrant was provided by two Spider Screws. One (1.5-mm diameter, 10 mm long) was placed in the interradicular bone between the maxillary left first and second premolars, and a second (2.0-mm diameter, 11 mm long) was inserted distal to the maxillary left second molar. The segmental orthodontic appliance

consisted of brackets with a sectional 0.016 × 0.022-inch arch wire. Two 150-g closed coil springs were attached directly from the Spider Screws to the appliance to initiate intrusion (Fig. 14-5, *B*). In the final 2 months of treatment, a bracket was placed on the maxillary left second premolar for intrusion using an elastic from the mesial Spider Screw. Appliance placement was limited to three teeth in the maxillary left quadrant to achieve the desired results (Fig. 14-5, *C*). Routine home care and periodic professional hygiene with scaling and root planing were performed during orthodontic treatment.[13-15]

Another use of MSIs is in patients with multiple missing teeth in whom adequate anchorage is not available. In these cases, Spider Screws can be used to create temporary prosthetic anchorage. For example, a patient presented with a missing maxillary central incisors and a semiankylotic maxillary right lateral incisor resulting from facial trauma (Fig. 14-6, *A*). Traditional orthodontic treatment was initiated; however, the maxillary right canine and lateral incisor further intruded (Fig. 14-6, *B*). The decision was then made to use skeletal anchorage. Two Spider Screws (2.0-mm diameter, 11 mm long, regular head) were placed in the central incisor positions (Fig. 14-6, *C* and *D*) and were built up with a resin core to create a temporary prosthetic abutment usable for orthodontic treatment. The MSIs were used to extrude the right lateral incisor, avoid intrusion of the adjacent teeth, and temporarily replace the central incisors for esthetics (Fig. 14-6, *E*). After luxation of the right lateral incisor, the Spider Screws were used to facilitate the completion of orthodontic treatment without side effects (Fig. 14-6, *F*). Upon completion of orthodontic treatment, the temporary crowns attached to the Spider Screws were left in place until definitive dental implants and final restorations were placed.

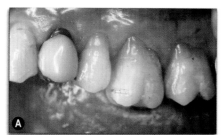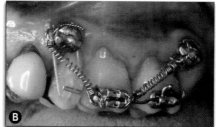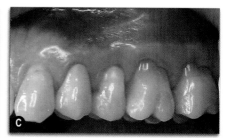

Fig. 14-5

Spider Screw direct anchorage to intrude supererupted maxillary posterior teeth. **A,** Pretreatment left buccal photograph. **B,** Progress left buccal photograph. Note Spider Screws were used directly to intrude molars using closed coil springs. **C,** Posttreatment left buccal photograph.

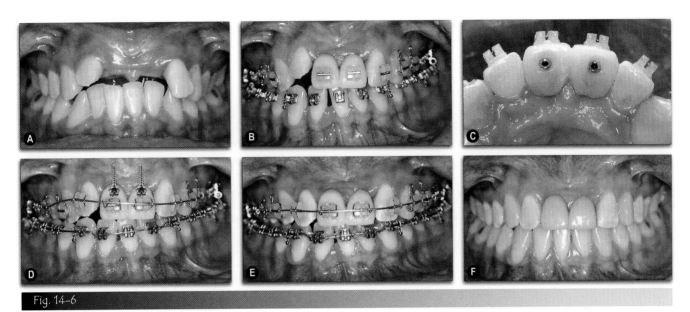

Fig. 14-6

Spider Screw prosthetic anchorage to replace missing central incisors and extrude semiankylotic lateral incisor. **A,** Pretreatment anterior photograph. **B,** Progress anterior photograph after side effects occurred. Spider Screws were then placed in the missing incisor positions. **C,** Progress anterior occlusal photograph with Spider Screws in place. **D,** Progress anterior photograph during initial leveling. **E,** Progress anterior photograph during detailing phase. **F,** Posttreatment anterior photograph.

PRESURGICAL ORTHODONTICS

Although TAD placement usually does not require presurgical orthodontics, it may be necessary to diverge roots orthodontically in order to create adequate space for interradicular placement in some cases. For example, in select cases with Class II malocclusions, the maxillary first molars are distalized into super Class I positions before miniscrews are placed mesial to the first molars. The MSIs are then used as anchorage for retraction of the remaining teeth.

SURGICAL PROCEDURE

The surgical armamentarium for Spider Screw insertion includes a slow-speed contraangle handpiece, a pilot drill (1.2 mm for 1.5-mm diameter screw, 1.5 mm for 2.0-mm diameter screw) with depth stops according to screw length, a contraangle adapter, and a hand screwdriver. Every effort must be made to avoid contact with local anatomic structures. When it is necessary to insert the MSIs close to anatomic structures, such as the tooth roots, the maxillary sinus, or neurovascular structures, a surgical template fabricated from orthodontic wire and acrylic resin should be used to precisely locate the insertion point in the bone to avoid adjacent structures.[10-12] The acrylic fits over the occlusal surfaces of the teeth near the surgical site. The wire is embedded in the acrylic and is bent so that it corresponds to the point of screw placement (Fig. 14-7, *A*). Long cone radiographs are taken to visualize the surgical template relative to the

adjacent anatomic structures (Fig. 14-7, *B*). To obtain additional information in the vertical plane, notches are cut into the wire at selected heights. These notches are then visible on the radiographs and can be used to determine the insertion site. Once the insertion site has been determined, the surgical site is prepared while keeping the surgical template in place during the entire procedure.

First, the intraoral tissues are cleaned with 0.2% chlorhexidine, and then the region is anesthetized with local anesthetic. For the 2-mm screw the contraangle handpiece is used to create a 1.5-mm diameter pilot hole (Fig. 14-8, *A*). A slow-speed of 60 to 100 rpm is maintained to *feel* the transition from cortical to medullary bone and to minimize bone overheating. Sterile saline solution is used to cool the site. No incision is required in keratinized gingiva. However, a small 5-mm incision can be made, if necessary, in mobile mucosa before placing the pilot hole. Once the pilot hole has been prepared, the selected screw is removed from its sterilized package with the contraangle adapter and is inserted into the pilot hole at approximately 20 to 30 rpm (Fig. 14-8, *B*).

When the MSI is placed adjacent to tooth roots, we suggest using a small quantity of local anesthetic to anesthetize the soft tissue and bone only. This leaves the periodontal ligament and tooth root sensitive and minimizes the possibility of contacting the tooth root with the pilot hole or screw. Because the screw is

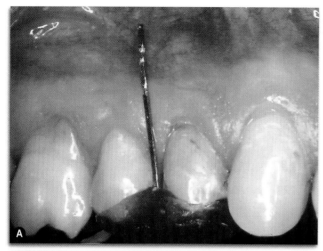

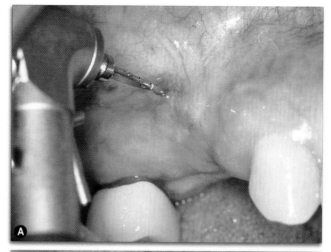

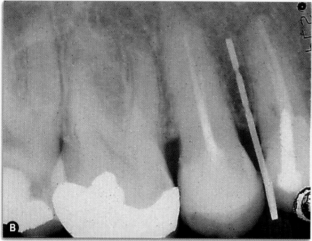

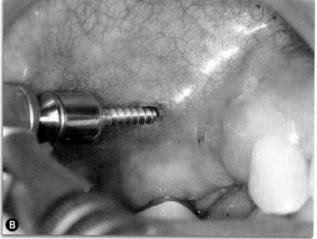

Fig. 14-7

Surgical template. **A,** Acrylic adapted over teeth with wire bent to anticipated MSI site. **B,** Periapical radiograph confirming MSI position.

Fig. 14-8

Spider Screw placement protocol. **A,** Pilot hole preparation with 1.5-mm drill. **B,** Spider Screw (2.0-mm diameter) insertion with slow-speed contraangle handpiece.

maintained only by mechanical retention, it should be placed perpendicular to the direction of the applied forces. If it appears that bone support is inadequate, it is advisable to use a longer screw to reach the opposite cortical plate, thereby providing bicortical stabilization. If a screw is inserted in bone of poor quality, it should be loaded immediately to promote mechanical stability. If the screw has minor mobility, light forces applied immediately[7] often cause a slight inclination of the MSI in bone and favor better stabilization. The final placement is achieved with a hand screwdriver until the collar of the screw reaches its ideal position in the surrounding tissue.

Immediately after MSI placement, an antiinflammatory is prescribed and a 0.2% chlorhexidine rinse is advised for the next 7 days. Subsequently, the patient is instructed to follow routine hygiene procedures; the same around the MSI as around the teeth. It should be

recalled that osseointegration is neither expected nor desired for this anchorage system. Although some studies have reported a degree of osseointegration with immediately loaded MSIs, we have found no difficulty in removing the Spider Screws to date.[16,17]

ORTHODONTIC MECHANICS

The Spider Screw is connected to the teeth by force modules or ligatures attached to the orthodontic screw head. When spring forces are placed on the Spider Screw, it is best to secure them with a metal ligature attached to the vertical slot in order to avoid accidental detachment. The internal rectangular slot also helps to maintain elastic and ligature ties away from the soft tissues and avoids trauma to them. Forces applied to the miniscrew can vary from 50 g up to 200 g and occasionally 300 g, depending on the quantity of bone and the desired orthodontic movements.[4,10-12] In sites of less

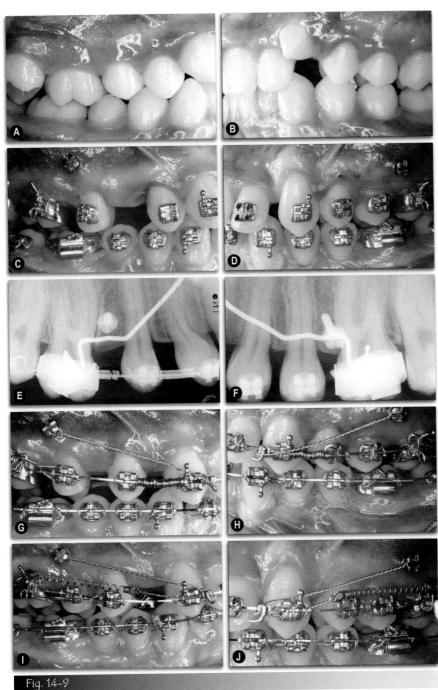

Fig. 14-9

Indirect anchorage to distalize the buccal segments in a Class II malocclusion. **A,** Pretreatment right buccal photograph. **B,** Pretreatment left buccal photograph. **C,** Progress right buccal photograph after maxillary first molar distalization. **D,** Progress left buccal photograph after maxillary first molar distalization. **E,** Right bitewing radiograph after maxillary first molar distalization. **F,** Left bitewing radiograph after maxillary first molar distalization. **G,** Progress right buccal photograph. Note right canine was ligated to Spider Screw to distalize first premolar. **H,** Progress left buccal photograph. Note left canine was ligated to Spider Screw to distalize first and second premolars. **I,** Progress right buccal photograph. Note right canine was directly retracted with Spider Screw via closed coil spring. **J,** Progress left buccal photograph. Note left canine was directly retracted with Spider Screw via closed coil spring.

bone quality, the force applied should be decreased as necessary.

Miniscrew implant anchorage can be indirect, direct, or via prosthetics. In Class II noncooperative patients, indirect anchorage is generally used. For example, in a Class II patient (Fig. 14-9), two Spider Screws (1.5-mm diameter, 9 mm long) can be inserted mesial to the maxillary first molars after distalization of the molars to a Class I relationship (Fig. 14-9, *C* to *F*). In this case the Spider Screws are used to retract the teeth anteriorly into the created space. An 0.016 × 0.022-inch rectangular wire with stops mesial to the first molars and hooks mesial to the canines was inserted. Indirect anchorage mechanics were used to retract the premolars and canines. On the right side, a metal ligature was placed from the MSI to the canine, and a 150-g open coil spring was placed between the first and second premolars in order to distalize the second premolar (Fig. 14-9, *G* and *I*). On the left side a metal ligature was placed to the hook, and a 150-g open coil spring was extended from the molar to the canine (Fig. 14-9, *H* and *J*).

Spider Screws also offer reliable direct anchorage for retraction of groups of teeth or individual teeth (Fig. 14-10). To retract and simultaneously intrude teeth, MSIs should be located above the occlusal plane. In that position, power arms are inserted into the vertical slots of the brackets. This moves the point of force application closer to the center of resistance and makes possible pure translation or bodily movement of the teeth and minimizes the intrusive component of the orthodontic force.

Biomechanically, the vertical MSI position should be determined relative to the occlusal plane and depends on the type of tooth movement desired. For

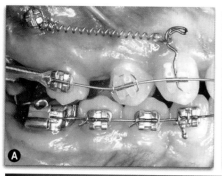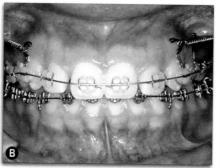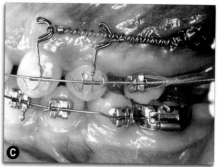

Fig. 14-10

Direct anchorage to retract anterior teeth en masse. **A,** Progress right buccal photograph. **B,** Progress anterior photograph. **C,** Progress left buccal photograph. Note closed coil springs are attached directly from Spider Screw to power arm through canine bracket.

intrusion and retraction, the MSIs should be placed as high in the vestibule as possible (Figs. 14-11 and 14-12). When only retraction is the main objective, the MSIs should be placed closer to the occlusal surface of the teeth. When intrusion cannot be tolerated, the MSIs should be used indirectly. In this type of case, the canine is ligated directly to the MSI, and then the first molar is used to attach a horizontal force to retract the incisors directly (Fig. 14-13).

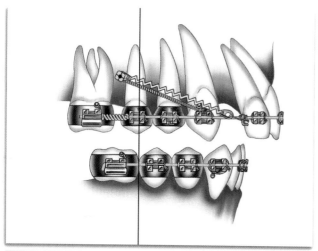

Fig. 14-11

Diagram illustrating direct anchorage mechanics for simultaneous intrusion and retraction of anterior teeth using Spider Screw system.

Facial inclination of the clinical crowns tends to occur with molar intrusion. Control can be achieved by torquing arch wires or with transpalatal bars. Alternatively, crown control can be maintained by the placement of a palatal miniscrew and the application of palatal and facial forces simultaneously (Fig. 14-14). Precise intrusion occurs quickly when using proper forces (Fig. 14-15). It is important, however, to prevent inflammation, eliminate pockets, and establish a sound periodontal environment before intrusion is attempted. Good home care, professional cleaning, and scaling and root planing are necessary during treatment.[13-15]

The regular Spider Screw can be used in edentulous areas both as anchorage and as a provisional prosthesis simultaneously (Fig. 14-16, *A*). To fabricate the temporary abutment, a prefabricated resin core is secured to the head of the regular Spider Screw by a small screw. The resin core is then shaped into a tooth form and is cemented in place (Fig. 14-16, *B*).[10-12] For example, in a Class II malocclusion with a missing upper right second premolar and first molar, a temporary four-unit bridge extended from the maxillary right first premolar to the maxillary right second molar. The maxillary right lateral incisor was rotated, and a carious lesion was present on its distal surface (Fig. 14-17, *A* and *D*). The treatment plan was to create a

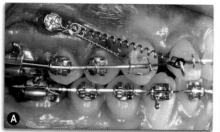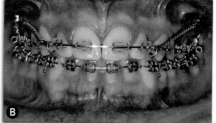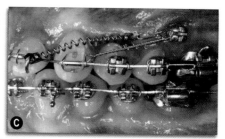

Fig. 14-12

Direct anchorage for simultaneous intrusion and retraction of anterior teeth using Spider Screw system. **A,** Progress right buccal photograph. **B,** Progress anterior photograph. **C,** Progress left buccal photograph.

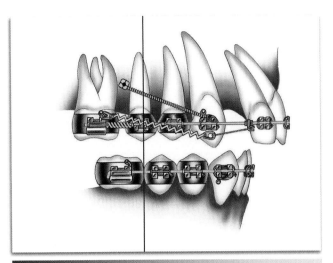

Fig. 14-13

Diagram illustrating indirect anchorage mechanics for retraction without intrusion of anterior teeth using Spider Screw system.

Class I canine relationship by retracting the upper right canine and then rotating the lateral incisor so that it could be restored properly. The bridge was removed, and a Spider Screw (2.0-mm diameter, 11 mm long) was inserted into the edentulous ridge in the second premolar position where it served as an abutment for a three-unit temporary bridge in the maxillary right quadrant (Fig. 14-17, *G* to *J*). Brackets were placed on the maxillary teeth, and a segmental 0.016 × 0.022-inch stainless steel wire was inserted. The maxillary right first premolar and canine were retracted by 150-g elastic forces applied on the buccal and palatal surfaces (Fig. 14-17, *B* and *E*). The maxillary right lateral incisor was then rotated into proper alignment. At the completion of orthodontic treatment, the Spider Screw was removed and the final prosthetic reconstruction was placed (Fig. 14-17, *C* and *F*).

REMOVAL PROCEDURE

Spider Screw anchorage does not depend on osseointegration. One study has demonstrated that 2-mm diameter implants placed in beagle dogs and used for intrusion had less than 25% osseointegration.[9] The forces applied were similar to those used in clinical practice, and the screws were easily removed. In clinical practice the screws are also easily removed, indirectly suggesting minimal Spider Screw osseointegration. Other studies also indicate that in spite of the presence of a certain degree of osseointegration, the smooth surface of the screw facilitates easy removal.[17] To remove the miniscrew, simply unscrew it with the appropriate screwdriver. Removal can usually be accomplished without anesthesia, and healing takes place in a few

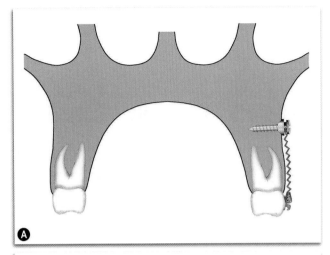

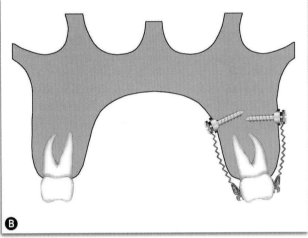

Fig. 14-14

Diagram illustrating torque control with Spider Screws. **A,** Facial tipping would occur during intrusion with a Spider Screw on the facial surface only. **B,** Pure intrusion would occur during intrusion with a Spider Screw on the facial and palatal.

days (Fig. 14-18). A 0.2% chlorhexidine rinse is recommended for the first few days after removal.

POTENTIAL COMPLICATIONS

One possible complication is inflammation of the periimplant tissues, especially in areas of frenum tissue or muscle tissue.[18,19] These problems can be controlled with proper oral hygiene and topical application of a 0.2% chlorhexidine rinse. Sometimes, insertion of the MSI high in the vestibule creates mucosal complications. In these cases, the clinician should attempt to use anchorage mechanics that requires minimal adjustments at the abutment head of the screw. In the event of MSI mobility, it can be replaced with a longer and larger-diameter MSI. If this is not sufficient, another site for placement should be chosen. If, during insertion of the MSI, the periodontal ligament is inadvertently contacted,

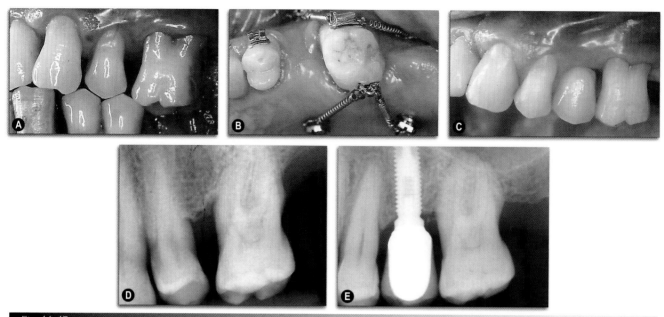

Fig. 14-15

Direct anchorage to intrude and distalize supererupted maxillary second molar into normal position. **A,** Pretreatment left buccal photograph. **B,** Progress left occlusal photograph of Spider Screw mechanics. Note two Spider Screws are used on both the facial and palatal surfaces to control torque and tip. **C,** Posttreatment left buccal photograph. **D,** Pretreatment bitewing radiograph. **E,** Posttreatment bitewing radiograph. Note bone level improvement.

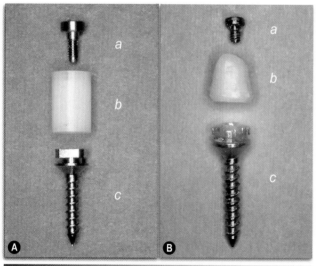

Fig. 14-16

Fabrication of tooth-shaped abutment on Spider Screw. **A,** Original components. *(a)* Long abutment screw, *(b)* untrimmed acrylic abutment, *(c)* Spider Screw *regular.* **B,** Adjusted components. *(a)* Short abutment screw, *(b)* trimmed and adjusted acrylic abutment, *(c)* Spider Screw *regular.*

the patient will show symptoms of pain to percussion or mastication. If a root is contacted during insertion, the patient will develop sensitivity to hot and/or cold. In these cases, the MSI should be removed; antiinflammatory and antibiotic therapy may be initiated.

SUMMARY

The Spider Screw is versatile and can be placed intraorally in any location with sufficient bone and is immediately loadable after placement. The simplicity of surgical insertion makes the Spider Screw a viable anchorage option in the conventional orthodontic practice. Through the use of a surgical guide, it can be placed precisely and dependably in areas of reduced space approximating important anatomic structures. MSIs of 2.0-mm diameter and up to 11 mm long can be used in areas of bone that have reduced quality or quantity. The variety of transmucosal heights and the specifically designed orthodontic head controls tissue trauma and inflammation while simultaneously providing ease of use by the orthodontist.

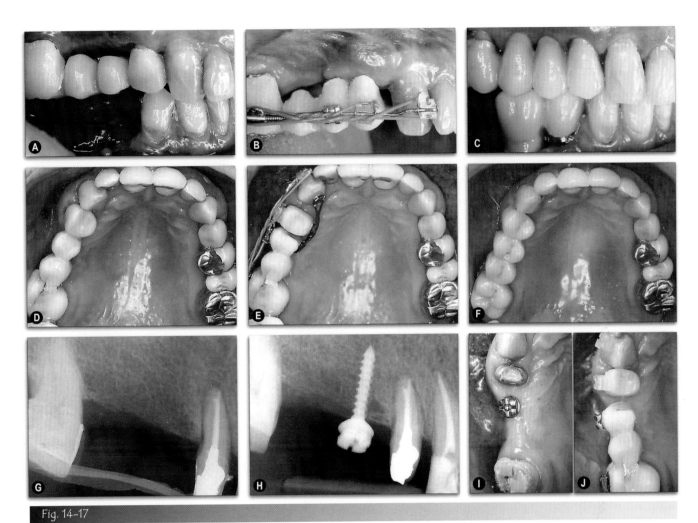

Fig. 14-17

Spider Screw prosthetic anchorage to correct Class II malocclusion with missing maxillary right second premolar and first molar with rotated right lateral incisor. **A,** Pretreatment right buccal photograph. **B,** Progress right buccal photograph. Note that four-unit bridge has been replaced with three-unit bridge attached to Spider Screw mesially. This allows retraction of anterior teeth into the created space. **C,** Posttreatment right buccal photograph. **D,** Pretreatment maxillary occlusal photograph. **E,** Progress maxillary occlusal photograph. Note that canine is being retracted into created space. **F,** Posttreatment maxillary occlusal photograph. **G,** Pretreatment periapical radiograph of four-unit bridge. **H,** Progress periapical radiograph with Spider Screw in place. **I,** Progress maxillary occlusal photograph. Note four-unit bridge has been removed, Spider Screw is placed in the second premolar position. **J,** Progress maxillary occlusal photograph with new three-unit temporary bridge anchored to Spider Screw.

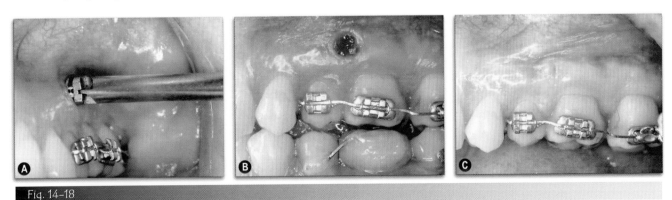

Fig. 14-18

Spider Screw removal procedure. **A,** Spider Screw removal with manual screwdriver. **B,** Left buccal photograph immediately after Spider Screw removal. **C,** Left buccal photograph 7 days after Spider Screw removal. Note healed soft tissue

REFERENCES

1. Weinstein S, Haak DC, Morris LY, et al. One equilibrium theory of tooth position. *Angle Orthod.* 33:1-26, 1963.
2. Pilon JJGM, Kuijpers-Jagtman AM, Maltha JC. Magnitude of orthodontic forces and rate of bodily tooth movement: an experimental study in Beagle dogs. *Am J Orthod Dentofacial Orthop.* 110:16-23, 1996.
3. Fogel MS. A cephalometric assessment of prepared mandibular anchorage. *Am J Orthod.* 43:511-536, 1957.
4. Unemori M, Sugawara J, Mitani H, et al. Skeletal anchorage system for open-bite correction. *Am J Orthod Dentofacial Orthop.* 115:166-174, 1999.
5. Roberts WE, Nelson CL, Goodacre CJ. Rigid implant anchorage to close a mandibular first molar extraction site. *J Clin Orthod.* 27:693-704, 1994.
6. Kanomi R. Mini-implant for orthodontic anchorage. *J Clin Orthod.* 31:763-767, 1997.
7. Melsen B, Verna C: A rational approach to orthodontic anchorage. *Prog Orthod.* 1:11-22, 2000.
8. Higuchi KW, Slack JM. The use of titanium fixtures for intraoral anchorage to facilitate orthodontic tooth movement. *Int J Oral Maxillofac Implants.* 6:388-344, 1991.
9. Ohmae M, Saito S, Morohashi T, et al. A clinical and histological evaluation of titanium mimi-implants as anchors for orthodontic intrusion in the beagle dog. *Am J Orthod Dentofacial Orthop.* 119:489-497, 2001.
10. Maino BG, Bednar J, Pagin P, Mura P. The Spider Screw for skeletal anchorage. *J Clin Orthod.* 37:90-97, 2003.
11. Maino BG, Pagin P, Mura P. Anclaje absoluto de carga immediata. *Revista Espanola De Ortodoncia.* 33:21-30, 2003.
12. Maino BG, Mura P, Bednar J. Miniscrews implants: The Spider Screw Anchorage System. *Semin Orthod.* 11:40-46, 2005.
13. Boyd RL, Leggot PJ, Quinn RS, et al. Periodontal implications of orthodontic treatment in adults with reduced or normal periodontal tissue vs those of adolescents. *Am J Orthod Dentofacial Orthop.* 96:191-199, 1989.
14. Melsen B, Agerbaek N, Markennstam G. Intrusion of incisors in adult patients with marginal bone loss. *Am J Orthod.* 96:232-241, 1989.
15. Melsen B. Limitations in adult orthodontics. In: Melsen B, ed. *Current controversies in orthodontics.* Chicago: Quintessence Publishing Co, 1991.
16. Costa A, Raffaini M, Melsen B. Miniscrews as orthodontic anchorage: a preliminary report. *Int J Adult Orthod.* 32:154-158, 1998.
17. Costa A, Dalstra M, Melsen B. L'Aarhus Anchorage System. *Ortognatodonzia Italiana.* 9:487-496, 2000.
18. Young-Chel Park, Seung-Yeon Lee, Kim DH, Jee SH. Intrusion of posterior teeth using mini-screw implants. *Am J Orthod Dentofacial Orthop.* 123:690-694, 2003.
19. Miyakawa S, Koyama I, Inoue M, et al. Factors associated with the stability of titanium screws placed in the posterior region for orthodontic anchorage. *Am J Orthod Dentofacial Orthop.* 124:373-378, 2003.

CHAPTER

15

The LOMAS System

Eric J. W. Liou, James C. Y. Lin

THE LOMAS SYSTEM

An ideal orthodontic miniscrew should be applicable to all orthodontic anchorage requirements, capable of withstanding the forces applied without the risk of fracture, loadable during the entire treatment period, and easily used in all mechanics situations. In addition, the miniscrew should be compatible with the standard orthodontic edgewise appliance, which requires it to function like a bracket, a tube, and a hook so that arch wires, elastics, and coil springs can be attached.

The Lin/Liou Orthodontic Mini Anchor System (LOMAS, Mondeal Medical System Gmbh,

Tuttlingen, Germany)[1,2] was developed to fulfill the ideal criteria (Fig. 15-1). The LOMAS miniscrew is a self-drilling and self-tapping orthodontic miniscrew that can be used for direct osseous orthodontic anchorage within the dental arches interradicularly and in non–tooth-bearing areas. The LOMAS miniscrew implant (MSI) is made of titanium alloy, which provides increased tensile and compressive strength for the self-drilling and heavy orthodontic forces.[3] The anatomic design of the LOMAS miniscrew consists of a threaded body, a transmucosal collar or platform, and an abutment head (Fig. 15-2).

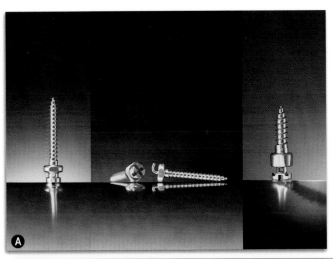
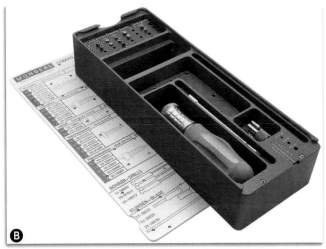

Fig. 15-1

Lin/Liou Orthodontic Mini Anchor System (LOMAS). **A,** Three different head designs. **B,** Surgical kit.

Threaded Body

The threaded body has a sharp cutting tip for self-drilling, a tapered shape for self-tapping, and deeper thread depth for better mechanical retention and decreased failure.[4] The LOMAS miniscrew comes in three lengths (7, 9, and 11 mm) and three diameters (1.5, 2.0, and 2.3 mm) for different locations within the oral cavity (Table 15-1). The 1.5-mm diameter LOMAS miniscrew is designed for use in interdental areas. The 7-mm length is used anteriorly and 9-mm length posteriorly. The force level should not exceed 200 g. The 2.0-mm diameter LOMAS miniscrew is designed for use in non–tooth-bearing areas (Fig. 15-3), such as the infrazygomatic crest of the maxilla or the mandibular external oblique ridge (buccal shelf). In the infrazygomatic crest the 9- or 11-mm lengths are used, whereas in the external oblique ridge the 7- or 9-mm lengths are used. The force level can be as high as 400 to 600 g. The 2.3-mm diameter LOMAS miniscrew is the emergency MSI in case the 2.0-mm diameter LOMAS miniscrew fails. The miniscrew should be placed only in a non–tooth-bearing area or edentulous alveolar ridge. The force level can be higher than 600 g.

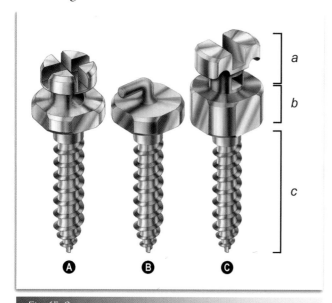

Fig. 15-2

Anatomy of LOMAS miniscrews. **A,** Standard head. **B,** Hook head. **C,** Quattro head. Abutment head *(a),* transmucosal collar *(b),* and threaded body *(c).*

Transmucosal Collar

The transmucosal collar or platform is the component that lies between the threaded body and the abutment head and abuts against the outer cortical bone. The collar emerges through the soft tissue, and its thickness elevates the abutment head to prevent soft tissue impingement from elastics or coil springs. The collar comes in two thicknesses: the *flat* platform is 1 mm tall (Fig. 15-2, *A* and *B*), and the *regular* platform is 2 mm tall (Fig. 15-2, *C*) for the different MSI sites (Table 15-1). The 1.5-mm diameter miniscrew has the flat platform for use in interdental areas. The 2.0- and 2.3-mm diameter miniscrews have the regular platform for use in non–tooth-bearing areas.

Abutment Head

Three different abutment heads are available: the *standard,* the *hook,* and the *Quattro* (Fig. 15-2). All are compatible with the traditional orthodontic edgewise appliance. The *standard* miniscrew has an 0.022 × 0.028-inch bracket slot and an 0.8-mm round auxiliary tube. The bracket slot is for placement of orthodontic arch wires; the round auxiliary tube is for the ligation of elastics, ligature wires, or coil springs or for the insertion of an auxiliary arch wire. The *hook* miniscrew has an inverted L-shaped hook for easy application of elastics or coil springs (Fig. 15-4, *A*). The Quattro miniscrew has an 0.018 × 0.025-inch or 0.022 × 0.028-inch Lewis-type bracket for arch wire placement. The Quattro miniscrew also has a rectangular auxiliary tube for insertion of an auxiliary rectangular arch wire (Fig. 15-4, *B*). The bracket wings have undercuts for ligation of arch wires with elastic or stainless steel ligatures or for attachment of elastics.

TREATMENT PLANNING

The incorporation of miniscrews as osseous anchorage has greatly broadened the spectrum of orthodontic treatment.[5] This does not mean, however, that miniscrews should be used routinely in every case and without regard for sound diagnosis and treatment planning. When using miniscrews, one should consider certain guidelines. Because anchorage is no longer an issue, treatment should be planned as though patient

Table 15-1.		LOMAS Miniscrew Implant (MSI) Dimensions and Locations		
Diameter (mm)	Platform (mm)	Length (mm)	MSI Sites	Loading Force (g)
1.5	1.0	7, 9, 11	Interdental areas	<200
2.0	2.0	7, 9, 11	Non–tooth-bearing areas	<400-600
2.3	2.0	7, 9, 11	Emergency	<600-800

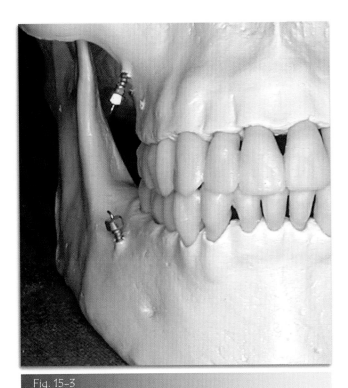

Fig. 15-3

Placement location of LOMAS miniscrews in maxillary infrazygomatic crest and mandibular external oblique ridge.

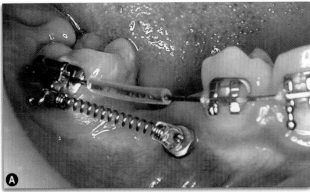

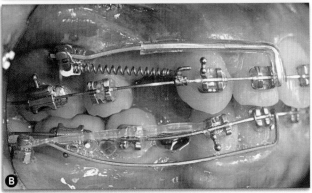

Fig. 15-4

LOMAS attachment mechanics. **A,** LOMAS hook miniscrew allows direct attachment of NiTi closed coil springs. **B,** LOMAS Quattro miniscrew allows attachment of lever arms, elastic modules, and NiTi closed coil springs.

compliance were perfect or as if the case were being set up for jaw surgery. However, the planned tooth movement still should be within the boundaries of the biologic system.

The length and width of the alveolar ridge limits the possible tooth movements regardless of what is possible with miniscrew anchorage. For distalization or retraction of maxillary teeth, the boundaries are the palatal cortical plate and the posterior wall of the maxillary tuberosity. For distalization or retraction of mandibular teeth, the boundaries are the lingual cortical plate of the alveolar ridge and the ascending ramus. For maxillary intrusion, the boundaries are the floors of the nasal cavity and maxillary sinus.

Although interdental implant sites are easier to access, they are indicated only when teeth adjacent to the miniscrew are not to be moved mesiodistally. For example, the placement of a 1.5-mm LOMAS miniscrew between the maxillary posterior teeth in a Class II case would be contraindicated if the teeth are planned to be distalized (Fig. 15-5, *A*).

The selected interdental site should be wider than 5.5 mm mesiodistally. This is based on the fact that an orthodontic miniscrew might migrate in bone and contact the tooth roots under heavy orthodontic forces. At least a 2-mm zone of clearance should be maintained

between the miniscrew and the tooth roots to prevent the possibility of tooth root damage during surgical miniscrew placement or orthodontic tooth movement.[6,7] Therefore, when a 1.5-mm diameter LOMAS miniscrew is used, the interseptal bone width should be at least 5.5 mm (2.0 mm + 1.5 mm + 2.0 mm; Fig. 15-6).

The apical third of the interseptal bone is always wider mesiodistally than the middle or gingival third. The LOMAS miniscrew should be placed as close to the apical third as possible. The most frequent site in the maxilla and mandible is the apical third of the interseptal bone between the first molar and second premolar where the width is usually wider than 5.5 mm.

The non–tooth-bearing areas are universal MSI sites regardless of whether the posterior teeth are planned to be moved mesiodistally. For example, a 2.0-mm LOMAS miniscrew can be inserted into the infrazygomatic crest for en masse retraction of the entire maxillary dentition in a Class II nonextraction case or for maxillary anterior retraction in a Class II extraction case (Fig. 15-5, *B*).

The most frequent non–tooth-bearing MSI sites for the LOMAS miniscrews are the infrazygomatic crest

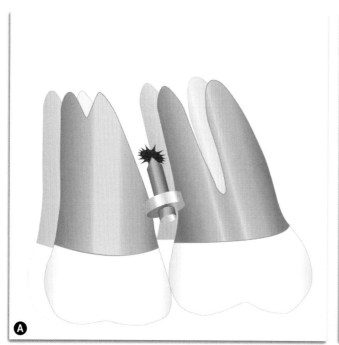
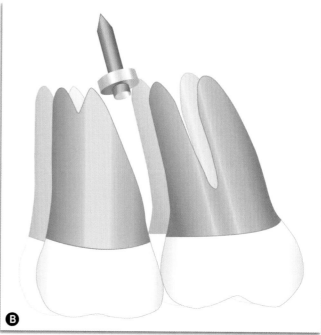

Fig. 15-5

Diagnostic decision for interradicular LOMAS miniscrew placement. **A,** When moving teeth mesiodistal, there is an increased risk of moving the teeth into the miniscrew when it is placed interradicularly. **B,** When moving teeth mesiodistal, there is little risk of moving the teeth into the miniscrew when placed in the infrazygomatic crest.

and the external oblique ridge and can be used as anchorage sites for canine retraction, anterior retraction, anterior en masse retraction, and posterior intrusion.[8-14] The paramedian hard palate, sub–anterior nasal spine region, maxillary tuberosity, mandibular symphysis, and retromolar area are also feasible sites for LOMAS miniscrews anchorage.[2]

PRESURGICAL ORTHODONTICS

When interdental miniscrew placement sites are planned, presurgical orthodontics are required to align the dentition and tooth roots to at least a 0.016 × 0.022-inch stainless steel arch wire and to maximize the amount of interradicular bone in the apical third to at least 5.5 mm. When the apical third of the planned miniscrew placement site is less than 5.5 mm after initial alignment, the miniscrew placement site should be moved to a non–tooth-bearing area so that treatment proceeds without delay. Treatment time is delayed too much when the tooth roots are diverged orthodontically before MSI placement and are again made parallel after MSI removal.

Unlike interdental MSI sites, presurgical orthodontics are not necessary when the non–tooth-bearing areas are the intended miniscrew sites. The chance of tooth root contact during placement or tooth movement is almost

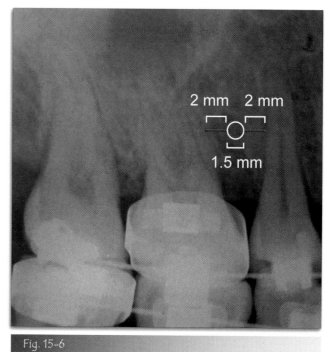

Fig. 15-6

Space requirements for a 1.5-mm diameter LOMAS miniscrew is at least 5.5 mm of interseptal bone to prevent potential tooth root contact.

zero if the miniscrews are placed appropriately. Orthodontic tooth movement can be performed before, during, or after the dentition is aligned.

SURGICAL PROCEDURE

The placement protocol for LOMAS miniscrews is referred to as the *bone density–guided insertion technique* because it is based on the bone density of the MSI site.[2]

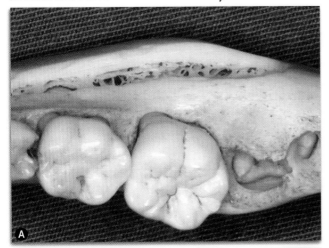

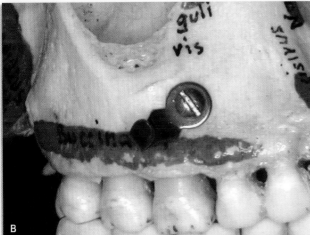

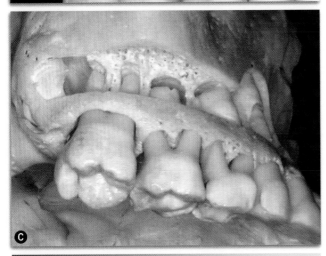

Fig. 15-7

Common sites for different bone density within the oral cavity. **A,** D1 bone is found in the mandibular external oblique ridge. **B,** D2 bone is found in the maxillary infrazygomatic crest. **C,** D3 bone is sometimes found in the infrazygomatic crest and D4 bone is found in interradicular bone.

The bone quality is classified into four types according to its Misch bone density category.[15] Density type D1 is dense cortical bone as seen in the external oblique ridge (Fig. 15-7, *A*). D2 is porous cortical and coarse trabecular bone as seen in the infrazygomatic crest (Fig. 15-7, *B*) and interseptal bone of the mandibular posterior teeth. D3 is porous cortical and fine trabecular bone as seen in the infrazygomatic crest and the interseptal bone of maxillary and mandibular posterior teeth (Fig. 15-7, *C*). D4 is thin cortical bone with fine trabecular bone as seen in the interseptal bone of the maxillary and mandibular anterior teeth.

General Guidelines for Bone Density–Guided Insertion Technique

General guidelines for bone density–guided insertion technique are as follows:

1. Standard photographs, radiographs, and computed tomographic (CT) images should be acquired of the prospective miniscrew site before the surgical procedure.
2. The LOMAS miniscrews should remain in place the shortest duration possible to achieve the desired treatment result. Therefore, the best time for LOMAS miniscrew placement is immediately before use.
3. All surgical procedures should be performed under local infiltration anesthesia; block anesthesia is not necessary.
4. The Misch bone density is established using Hounsfield

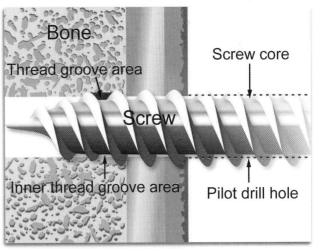

Fig. 15-8

Anatomy of threaded body and its relationship to the pilot hole, which should be 75% smaller than the threaded body diameter.

Table 15-2.	CT Values of Bone Density
Misch Bone Density	Hounsfield Units
D1	>1250
D2	850-1250
D3	350-850
D4	150-350

CT, Computed tomography.

units from the CT images[16] (Table 15-2).

5. When CT images are not available, bone density can be established by pressing a No. 15 surgical blade firmly into the cortical bone at the MSI site. If the blade cuts and makes an indention in the cortical bone surface, the bone density is D3 or D4; otherwise, the bone density is D1 or D2.

6. In D1 and D2 bone (infrazygomatic crest and external oblique ridge), a pilot hole at approximately 75% of the MSI size is drilled in the cortical bone (Fig. 15-8).[17] The drill speed should be limited to 500 to 800 rpm under sterile saline irrigation to prevent bone necrosis from overheating.[18,19]

7. In D3 and D4 bone (maxillary and mandibular interseptal bone), no pilot hole is required; the LOMAS miniscrew is placed directly with the LOMAS screwdriver.[2]

8. The emergence of the LOMAS miniscrew should be in attached gingiva or at the mucogingival junction. MSI emergence in mobile mucosa frequently causes soft tissue irritation.[20]

9. The LOMAS miniscrews can either be loaded immediately or after 2 weeks of soft tissue healing.[4]

10. Neither antibiotics nor analgesics are required postoperatively. However, a 2% chlorhexidine mouth rinse is prescribed, and the patient is instructed to brush the LOMAS miniscrews gently after each meal as with normal orthodontic appliances.

Specific Guidelines for Bone Density–Guided Insertion Technique

Specific guidelines for bone density–guided insertion technique are as follows based on insertion site.

Interdental Sites

The interdental sites lie between the roots of the maxillary and mandibular teeth. Guidelines are as follows:

1. A vertical bitewing radiograph is taken of the planned interdental site. The insertion site is approximated by drawing a line along the occlusal plane and bisecting that line through the interproximal contact (Fig. 15-9, A).

2. The site is defined by moving from the occlusal plane along the interproximal contact line to the most coronal point that has a mesiodistal width of greater than 5.5 mm (I-point).

3. The angle of the bisecting line and the distance of the I-point from the occlusal plane is measured on the radiograph.

4. The angle between the occlusal plane and the interproximal contact line and the I-point are transferred to the patient by using a periodontal probe to penetrate through the attached gingiva or mucosa (Fig. 15-9, B).

5. A 1.5-mm diameter and 9-mm long LOMAS miniscrew is used for posterior teeth, and a 1.5-mm diameter and 7-mm long LOMAS miniscrew is used for anterior teeth (Fig. 15-9, C).

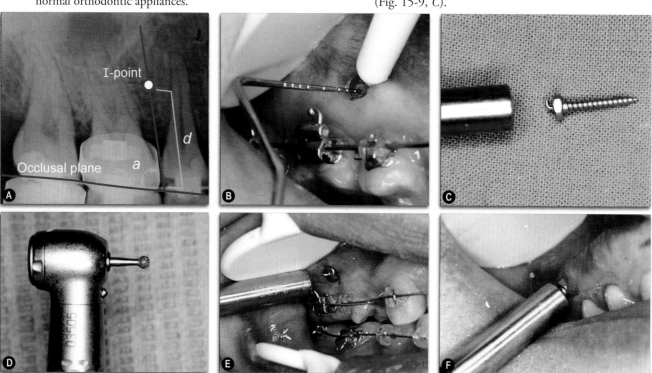

Fig. 15-9

Radiographic evaluation and surgical placement of the interradicular LOMAS miniscrew. **A,** Vertical bitewing radiograph is used to determine miniscrew position. **B,** Periodontal probe is used to transfer measurement to interproximal site. **C,** Appropriate LOMAS miniscrew is chosen. **D,** A No. 2 round diamond in a high-speed handpiece is used to remove the attached gingiva and periosteum. **E,** The LOMAS miniscrew is placed at a right angle at the I-point. **F,** The LOMAS miniscrew is placed at a 30- to 40-degree angle if the I-point is high in the vestibule.

6. When the I-point is located in attached gingiva, use a No. 2 round diamond in a high-speed handpiece to remove the attached gingiva and periosteum (Fig. 15-9, *D*). Place the selected LOMAS miniscrew at a right angle at the I-point with the LOMAS screwdriver (Fig. 15-9, *E*).

7. When the I-point is located in mobile mucosa, make a new I-point slightly below the mucogingival junction, remove the overlying attached gingiva and periosteum, and place the LOMAS miniscrew into the new I-point at a 30- to 40-degree angle relative to the occlusal plane toward the real I-point (Fig. 15-9, *F*).

8. The site and LOMAS miniscrew are irrigated thoroughly with saline.

9. Postoperative radiographs are taken.

10. The LOMAS miniscrew is loaded immediately.

Infrazygomatic Crest

The infrazygomatic crest is a bony ridge running along the curvature between the alveolar process and zygomatic process of the maxilla (Figs. 15-3 and 15-7, *B*). The thickness of the infrazygomatic crest ranges from 5.5 to 8.8 mm in adults.[21] In younger individuals, the infrazygomatic crest lies between the maxillary second premolar and first molar; in adults it lies above the maxillary first molar. Guidelines are as follows:

1. The thickness of the infrazygomatic crest and floor of the maxillary sinus is evaluated on the posteroanterior cephalometric and panoramic radiographs (Fig. 15-10, *A* and *B*) or on CT images if available.

2. A 2.0-mm diameter and 9-mm long LOMAS miniscrew is used for a thinner infrazygomatic crest

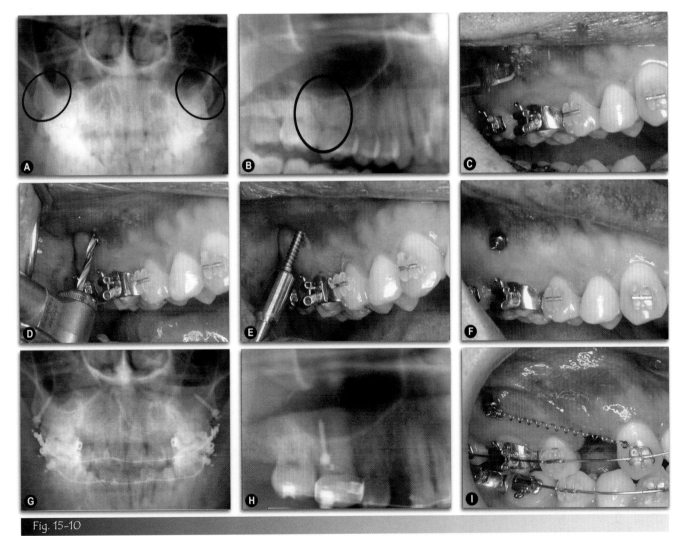

Fig. 15-10

LOMAS placement in infrazygomatic crest. **A,** Pretreatment posteroanterior cephalometric radiograph to evaluate infrazygomatic crest thickness and floor of the maxillary sinus. **B,** Pretreatment panoramic radiograph to evaluate infrazygomatic crest thickness and floor of the maxillary sinus. **C,** Vertical incision with a No. 15 surgical blade at the mucogingival junction above the maxillary first molar. **D,** Pilot hole prepared at 60 to 75 degrees and 13 to 15 mm above occlusal plane. **E,** LOMAS miniscrew is screwed into the infrazygomatic crest. **F,** Final position of LOMAS miniscrew. **G,** Position of miniscrew on posteroanterior cephalometric radiograph. **H,** Position of miniscrew on panoramic radiograph. **I,** Direct loading of miniscrew with NiTi closed coil spring.

and a low maxillary sinus floor. A 2.0-mm diameter and 11-mm long LOMAS miniscrew is used for a thicker infrazygomatic crest and a high maxillary sinus floor.

3. A 2-mm vertical incision is made with a No. 15 surgical blade at the mucogingival junction above the maxillary first molar (Fig. 15-10, C). A periosteal elevator is used to raise a mucogingival flap and expose the cortical bone.

4. The bone density is established using the No. 15 surgical blade as previously described.

5. When the bone density is D2, a 1.5-mm pilot hole is prepared at 60 to 75 degrees and 13 to 15 mm above the occlusal plane (Fig. 15-10, D).[21] The selected LOMAS miniscrew is screwed into the infrazygomatic crest with the LOMAS screwdriver (Fig. 15-10, E and F).

6. When the bone density is D3, the selected LOMAS miniscrew is screwed directly into the infrazygomatic crest without a pilot hole.

7. The site and LOMAS miniscrew are irrigated thoroughly with saline.

8. Postoperative radiographs are taken (Fig. 15-10, G and H).

9. The LOMAS miniscrew is loaded immediately (Fig. 15-10, I).

Mandibular External Oblique Ridge

The external oblique ridge is a pillar of cortical bone running from the ascending ramus down to the lateral extent of the mandibular body at the molar region (Figs. 15-3 and 15-7, A). The anteroinferior extent of the external oblique ridge is usually lateral to and distal to the first molar (Fig. 15-11). Therefore, when a LOMAS miniscrew is placed in the external oblique ridge, it is always placed between the first and second molars. Guidelines are as follows:

1. The anteroinferior extent of the external oblique ridge is determined on the panoramic and posteroanterior cephalometric radiographs (Fig. 15-12, A and B) or on the CT images when they are available.

2. A 2-mm vertical incision is made with a No. 15 surgical blade at the mucogingival junction between the first and second molars. A periosteal elevator is used to raise a mucogingival flap and expose the cortical bone (Fig. 15-12, C).

3. A 1.5-mm pilot hole is prepared at 30 to 40 degrees to the facial surface of the first molar, which is also at a right angle relative to the surface of the external oblique ridge (Fig. 15-12, D).

4. A 2.0-mm diameter and 7- or 9-mm long LOMAS miniscrew is selected.

5. The selected LOMAS miniscrew is screwed into the external oblique ridge with the LOMAS screwdriver (Fig. 15-12, E and F).

6. The site and LOMAS miniscrew are irrigated thoroughly with saline.

7. Postoperative radiographs are taken (Fig. 15-12, G and H).

8. The LOMAS miniscrew is loaded immediately (Fig. 15-12, I).

ORTHODONTIC MECHANICS

LOMAS mechanics are designed around the concept of *one LOMAS miniscrew at one site for multiple purposes,* such as retraction or protraction, intrusion or extrusion of anterior and/or posterior teeth, in either extraction or nonextraction cases. The combination of LOMAS miniscrews and the following auxiliary appliances provide the ability to treat various malocclusions:

1. Crimpable hooks or power arms (Fig. 15-13) can be attached on the arch wire distal to the canines for en masse retraction or at any other site for different purposes.

2. Nickel titanium closed coil springs (NiTi CCSs; Fig. 15-13) are attached from the LOMAS miniscrews to the crimpable hooks for en masse retraction, or from the LOMAS miniscrews to the hooks on the second molars for the protraction, or directly to the arch wire for intrusion of anterior or posterior teeth.

3. CNA transpalatal arch (32CNA-TPA) and CNA lingual holding arch (32CNA-LHA) are made of 0.032-inch beta NiTi wire (CNA, Ortho Organizer, Carlsbad, California) and are built with mesial angulation and buccal root torque. They are inserted into weldable/bondable lingual sheaths for active control of intermolar width, molar rotation, and torque during retraction or protraction.

4. CNA lever arms are made of 0.017 × 0.025-inch beta-NiTi wire (CNA). They are used to intrude or extrude anterior teeth (Fig. 15-14)

Although the LOMAS miniscrews can be used for individual tooth intrusion or extrusion, retraction or protraction, or correction of a posterior crossbite, the following LOMAS mechanics pertain primarily to complete extraction and nonextraction treatment.

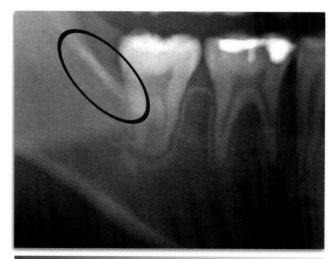

Fig. 15-11

The external oblique ridge runs from the ascending ramus down to the mandibular body, where it ends distolateral to the mandibular first molar.

LOMAS Extraction Mechanics

LOMAS extraction mechanics are as follows:

1-1. En masse retraction of anterior teeth (Fig. 15-13)

These mechanics are indicated for correction of Class I bimaxillary dentoalveolar protrusion, Class II division 1 maxillary dentoalveolar protrusion, or Class III mandibular dentoalveolar protrusion cases that do not require anterior intrusion. The LOMAS miniscrews can be placed in the maxillary and/or mandibular interdental bone between the first molars and second premolars or in the infrazygomatic crest and/or the external oblique ridge. The main arch wire should be 0.016 × 0.022-inch or thicker stainless steel with anterior lingual root torque to prevent lingual tipping of the anterior teeth and distal tipping of the posterior teeth during retraction. Crimpable hooks are attached on the arch wire distal to the canines. Bilateral medium-force NiTi CCSs are attached diagonally from the LOMAS miniscrews to the crimpable hooks for en masse retraction. A 32CNA-TPA or 32CNA-LHA with mesial angulation and lingual crown torque is inserted into the lingual sheaths on the molars for control of intermolar width, molar rotation, and torque during en masse retraction.

1-2. En masse retraction and intrusion of anterior teeth (Fig. 15-14)

These mechanics are almost identical to the preceding mechanics (1-1), except that CNA lever arms are added for intrusion. The mechanics are indicated for

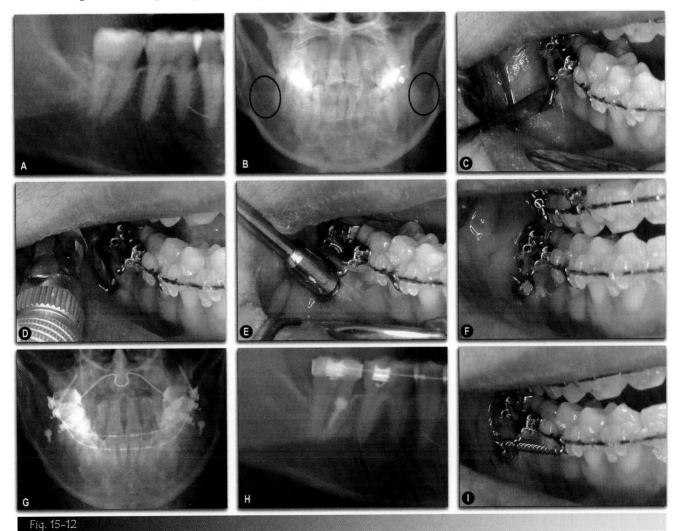

Fig. 15-12

LOMAS placement in external oblique ridge. **A,** Pretreatment panoramic radiograph to evaluate external oblique ridge. **B,** Pretreatment posteroanterior cephalometric radiograph to evaluate external oblique ridge. **C,** After the vertical incision, a periosteal elevator is used to reflect the soft tissue at the mucogingival junction between the first and second molars. **D,** Pilot hole prepared at 30 to 40 degrees to the facial surface of the first molar. **E,** LOMAS miniscrew is screwed into the external oblique ridge. **F,** Final position of LOMAS miniscrew. **G,** Position of miniscrew on posteroanterior cephalometric radiograph. **H,** Position of miniscrew on panoramic radiograph. **I,** Direct loading of miniscrew with NiTi closed coil spring.

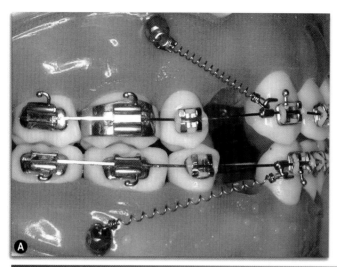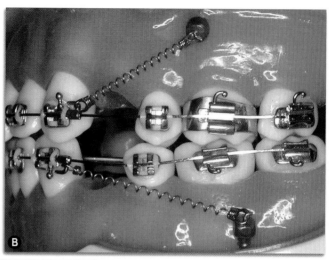

Fig. 15-13

Extraction mechanics 1-1 for en masse retraction of anterior teeth. **A,** Right buccal photograph. **B,** Left buccal photograph.

correction of Class I bimaxillary dentoalveolar protrusion, Class II division 1 maxillary dentoalveolar protrusion, or Class III mandibular dentoalveolar protrusion cases that require anterior retraction and intrusion. The CNA lever arms are inserted into the auxiliary tubes on the molars and are hooked over the arch wire between the canines and lateral incisors for en masse intrusion of the anterior teeth. Alternatively, the CNA lever arms can be inserted into the auxiliary rectangular tube of the LOMAS Quattro screws, if used.

2-1. En masse retraction of anterior teeth and posterior tooth intrusion (Fig. 15-15)

These mechanics are indicated for correction of high-angle Class I bimaxillary dentoalveolar protrusion or Class II division 1 maxillary dentoalveolar protrusion

with an anterior open bite requiring anterior retraction/posterior intrusion for mandibular counterclockwise rotation. For maximal counterclockwise rotation, both the maxillary and mandibular posterior teeth should be intruded. When the appropriate amount of overbite has been obtained or the gummy smile has been eliminated, the mechanics are switched to extraction mechanics 2-2 (Fig. 15-16). The LOMAS miniscrews can be placed in the maxillary and/or mandibular interdental bone between the first molars and second premolars, or in the infrazygomatic crest and/or the external oblique ridge. The main arch wire should be 0.016 × 0.022-inch or thicker stainless steel with anterior lingual root torque to prevent lingual tipping of the anterior teeth. Crimpable hooks are attached on the arch wire distal to the canines. Bilateral medium-

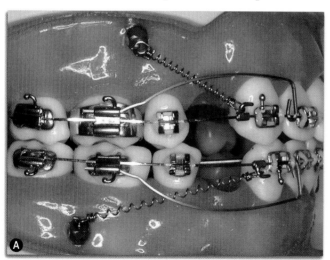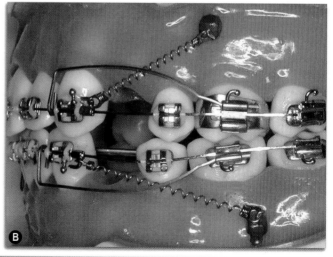

Fig. 15-14

Extraction mechanics 1-2 for en masse retraction and intrusion of anterior teeth. **A,** Right buccal photograph. **B,** Left buccal photograph.

force NiTi CCSs are attached diagonally from the LOMAS miniscrews to the crimpable hooks for en masse retraction. Bilateral medium-force NiTi CCSs are also attached vertically to the arch wire for posterior intrusion. A 32CNA-TPA or 32CNA-LHA with mesial angulation and lingual crown torque is inserted into the lingual sheaths on the molars.

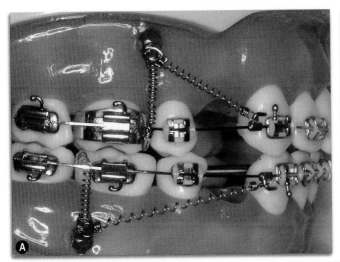
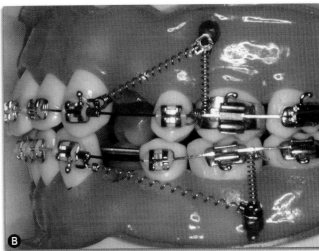

Fig. 15-15

Extraction mechanics 2-1 for en masse retraction of anterior teeth and posterior tooth intrusion. **A,** Right buccal photograph. **B,** Left buccal photograph.

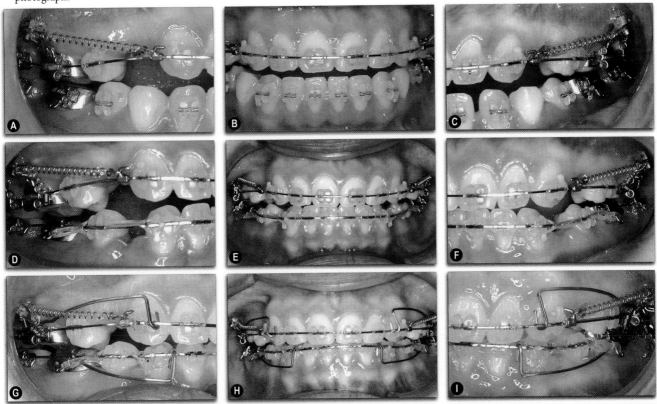

Fig. 15-16

Transition of different extraction mechanics during open bite treatment. **A,** Right buccal photograph of extraction mechanics 1-1. **B,** Anterior photograph of extraction mechanics 1-1. **C,** Left buccal photograph of extraction mechanics 1-1. **D,** Right buccal photograph of extraction mechanics 2-1. **E,** Anterior photograph of extraction mechanics 2-1. **F,** Left buccal photograph of extraction mechanics 2-1. **G,** Right buccal photograph of extraction mechanics 2-2. **H,** Anterior photograph of extraction mechanics 2-2. **I,** Left buccal photograph of extraction mechanics 2-2.

2-2. En masse retraction and intrusion of anterior teeth and posterior tooth intrusion (Fig. 15-17)

These mechanics are almost identical to the preceding mechanics (2-1), except that CNA lever arms are added for intrusion. These mechanics are indicated for correction of high-angle Class I bimaxillary dentoalveolar protrusion or Class II division 1 maxillary dentoalveolar protrusion with a gummy smile and anterior open bite that requires anterior retraction and intrusion and posterior intrusion for mandibular counterclockwise rotation. For maximal counterclockwise rotation, both the maxillary and mandibular posterior teeth should be intruded.

3-1. En masse retraction of anterior teeth and intrusion with posterior tooth distalization (Fig. 15-18)

These mechanics are indicated for anterior retraction of more than 7 mm and posterior distalization and intrusion for counterclockwise mandibular rotation, such as in high-angle Class I bimaxillary dentoalveolar protrusion or Class II division 1 maxillary dentoalveolar protrusion with anterior open bite. The treatment results of these mechanics are similar to those with orthognathic surgery.[22] For maximal counterclockwise rotation, both the maxillary and mandibular posterior teeth should be intruded. When the appropriate amount of overbite has been obtained or the gummy smile has been eliminated, the mechanics are switched to extraction mechanics 3-2 (Fig. 15-19). The LOMAS

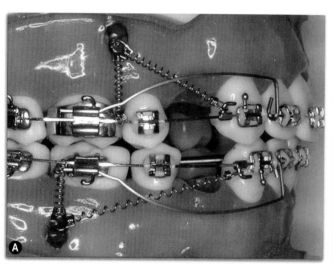
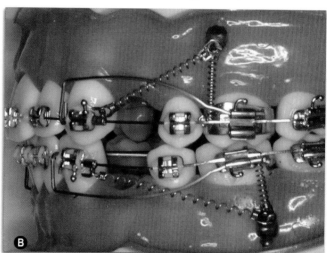

Fig. 15–17

Extraction mechanics 2-2 for en masse retraction and intrusion of anterior teeth and posterior tooth intrusion. **A,** Right buccal photograph. **B,** Left buccal photograph.

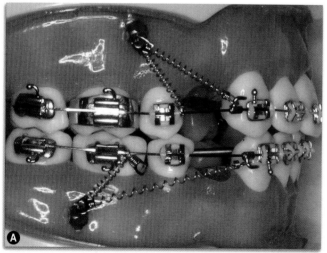
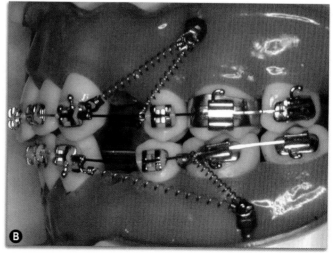

Fig. 15–18

Extraction mechanics 3-1 for en masse retraction of anterior teeth and intrusion with posterior tooth distalization. **A,** Right buccal photograph. **B,** Left buccal photograph.

miniscrews should be placed only in the infrazygomatic crest or the external oblique ridge. The interdental sites are contraindicated. The main arch wire should be 0.016 × 0.022-inch or thicker stainless steel with anterior lingual root torque to prevent lingual tipping of the anterior teeth. Crimpable hooks are attached on the arch wire distal to the canines. Bilateral medium-force NiTi CCSs are attached diagonally from the LOMAS miniscrews to the crimpable hooks for en masse retraction. Bilateral medium-force NiTi CCSs are also attached diagonally to the arch wire just mesial to the second premolar brackets for posterior distalization and intrusion. A 32CNA-TPA or 32CNA-LHA with mesial angulation and lingual crown torque is inserted into the lingual sheaths on the molars.

3-2. En masse retraction and intrusion of anterior teeth and intrusion with posterior tooth distalization (Fig. 15-19)

These mechanics are almost identical to the preceding mechanics (3-1), except that CNA lever arms are added for intrusion. These mechanics are indicated for anterior intrusion and retraction of more than 7 mm and posterior distalization and intrusion for counterclockwise mandibular rotation, such as in high-angle Class I bimaxillary dentoalveolar protrusion or Class II division 1 maxillary dentoalveolar protrusion with a gummy smile. The treatment results of these mechanics are similar to those with orthognathic surgery.[22] For maximal counterclockwise rotation, both the maxillary and mandibular posterior teeth should be intruded.

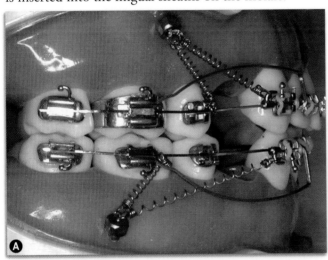
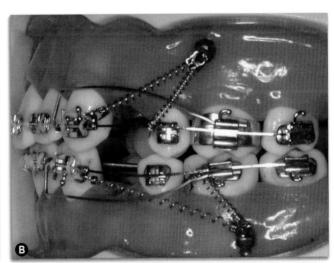

Fig. 15-19

Extraction mechanics 3-2 for en masse retraction and intrusion of anterior teeth and intrusion with posterior tooth distalization. **A,** Right buccal photograph. **B,** Left buccal photograph.

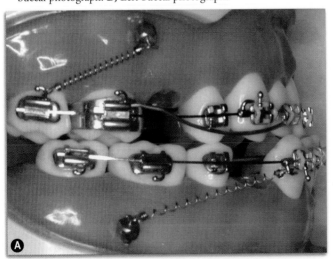
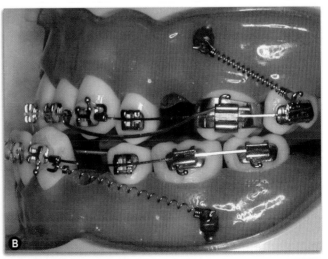

Fig. 15-20

Extraction mechanics 4 for en masse protraction of the maxillary posterior teeth, extrusion of maxillary anterior teeth, and en masse retraction of mandibular anterior teeth. **A,** Right buccal photograph. **B,** Left buccal photograph.

4. En masse protraction of the maxillary posterior teeth, extrusion of maxillary anterior teeth, and en masse retraction of mandibular anterior teeth (Fig. 15-20)

These mechanics are indicated for correction of a mild skeletal Class III with an anterior crossbite. The maxillary second and mandibular first premolars are extracted and the maxillary dentition is extruded, resulting in downward tilting of the maxillary occlusal plane and clockwise mandibular rotation. The LOMAS miniscrews should be placed only in the infrazygomatic crest or external oblique ridge. The maxillary arch wire should be 0.016 × 0.022-inch or thicker stainless steel with anterior facial root torque to prevent facial tipping of the anterior teeth. The mandibular arch wire should be 0.016 × 0.022-inch or thicker stainless steel with anterior lingual root torque. Bilateral heavy-force NiTi CCSs are attached from the LOMAS miniscrews to the hooks of the maxillary second molars for en masse protraction. Bilateral heavy-force NiTi CCSs are also attached diagonally to the arch wire distal to the canines for en masse anterior retraction. A 32CNA-TPA with mesial angulation and lingual crown torque is inserted into the lingual sheaths on the molars. Extrusion CNA lever arms are inserted into the auxiliary rectangular tube in the LOMAS Quattro miniscrews and are hooked over the arch wire between the maxillary canines and lateral incisors for anterior extrusion.

LOMAS Nonextraction Mechanics

LOMAS nonextraction mechanics are as follows:

1-1. En masse distalization of the entire dentition (Fig. 15-21)

These mechanics are indicated for correction of Class I or Class II cases with anterior crowding and/or mild dentoalveolar protrusion where premolar extraction is undesirable. The LOMAS miniscrews should be placed in the infrazygomatic crest and/or the external oblique ridge. The third molars should be extracted if present. The main arch wire should be 0.016 × 0.022-inch or thicker stainless steel with anterior lingual root torque to prevent lingual tipping of the anterior teeth and distal tipping of the posterior teeth during retraction. Crimpable hooks are attached on the arch wire distal to the canines. Bilateral heavy-force NiTi CCSs are attached from the LOMAS miniscrews to the crimpable hooks for en masse retraction. A 32CNA-TPA or 32CNA-LHA with mesial angulation and lingual crown torque is inserted into the lingual sheaths on the molars for control of intermolar width, molar rotation, and torque during en masse retraction.

1-2. En masse distalization of the entire dentition with anterior tooth en masse intrusion and retraction (Fig. 15-22)

These mechanics are almost identical to the preceding mechanics (1-1), except that CNA lever arms are added for intrusion. The mechanics are indicated for correction of Class I or Class II cases with anterior crowding and/or mild dentoalveolar protrusion or Class II division 2 cases that require anterior and posterior distalization without premolar extraction. The CNA lever arms are inserted into the auxiliary tubes on the molars and are hooked over the arch wire between the canines and lateral incisors for en masse intrusion of the anterior teeth. Alternatively, the CNA lever arms could be inserted into the auxiliary rectangular tube of the LOMAS Quattro screws, if used.

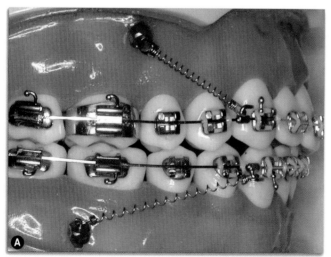 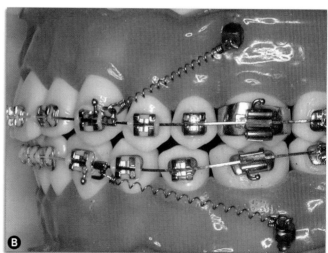

Fig. 15-21

Nonextraction mechanics 1-1 for en masse distalization of the entire dentition. **A,** Right buccal photograph. **B,** Left buccal photograph.

3-1. En masse distalization of the entire dentition with posterior tooth intrusion (Fig. 15-23)

There are no nonextraction mechanics 2-1 because the results are the same as for 3-1. These mechanics are indicated for high-angle Class I or Class II cases with anterior crowding and/or mild dentoalveolar protrusion and anterior open bite in which distalization of the entire dentition with posterior intrusion is required for mandibular counterclockwise rotation. For maximal counterclockwise rotation, both the maxillary and mandibular posterior teeth should be intruded. When the appropriate amount of overbite has been obtained or the gummy smile has been eliminated, the mechanics are switched to nonextraction mechanics 3-2 (Fig. 15-24). The LOMAS miniscrews should be placed only in the infrazygomatic crest or external oblique ridge. The interdental sites are contraindicated. The third molars should be extracted if present. The main arch wire should be 0.016 × 0.022-inch or thicker stainless steel with anterior lingual root torque to prevent lingual tipping of the anterior teeth. Crimpable hooks are attached on the arch wire distal to the canines. Bilateral heavy-force NiTi CCSs are attached diagonally from the LOMAS miniscrews to the crimpable hooks for en masse distalization. Bilateral medium-force NiTi CCSs are attached diagonally from the LOMAS miniscrews to the arch wire just mesial to the second premolar brackets for posterior distalization and intrusion. A 32CNA-TPA or 32CNA-LHA with mesial angulation and lingual crown torque is inserted into the lingual sheaths on the molars.

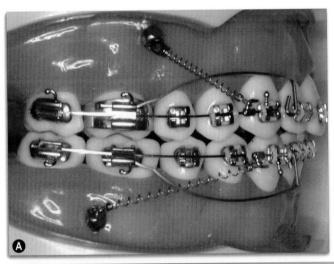 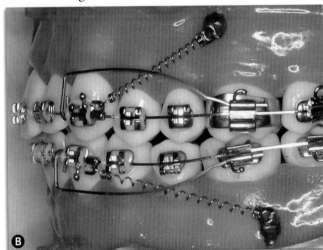

Fig. 15-22

Nonextraction mechanics 1-2 for en masse distalization of the entire dentition with anterior tooth en masse intrusion and retraction. **A,** Right buccal photograph. **B,** Left buccal photograph.

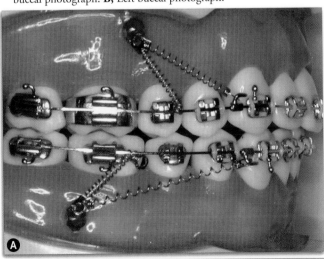 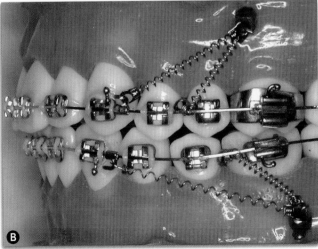

Fig. 15-23

Nonextraction mechanics 3-1 for en masse distalization of the entire dentition with posterior tooth intrusion. **A,** Right buccal photograph. **B,** Left buccal photograph.

3-2. En masse intrusion and distalization of the entire dentition (Fig. 15-25)

These mechanics are almost identical to extraction mechanics (2-1), except that CNA lever arms are added for intrusion. The mechanics are indicated for high-angle Class I or Class II cases with anterior crowding and/or mild dentoalveolar protrusion and a gummy smile in which retraction and intrusion of the entire dentition is required for mandibular counterclockwise rotation. For maximal counterclockwise rotation, both the maxillary and mandibular posterior teeth should be intruded.

4. En masse distalization of the mandibular dentition with en masse protraction and extrusion of the maxillary dentition (Fig. 15-26)

These mechanics are indicated for correction of a mild skeletal Class III with an anterior crossbite. Protraction and extrusion of the maxillary dentition results in downward tilting of the maxillary occlusal plane and clockwise mandibular rotation. The LOMAS miniscrews should be placed in the infrazygomatic crest and the external oblique ridge. The interdental miniscrew sites are contraindicated. The maxillary arch wire should be 0.016 × 0.022-inch or thicker

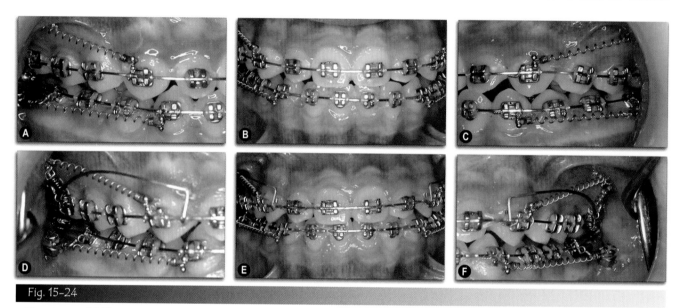

Fig. 15-24

Transition of different nonextraction mechanics during Class I mild bimaxillary protrusion treatment. **A,** Right buccal photograph of nonextraction mechanics 1-1. **B,** Anterior photograph of nonextraction mechanics 1-1. **C,** Left buccal photograph of nonextraction mechanics 1-1. **D,** Right buccal photograph of extraction mechanics 3-2. **E,** Anterior photograph of extraction mechanics 3-2. **F,** Left buccal photograph of extraction mechanics 3-2.

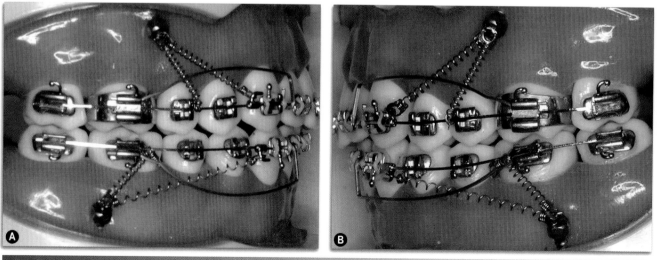

Fig. 15-25

Nonextraction mechanics 3-2 for en masse intrusion and distalization of the entire dentition. **A,** Right buccal photograph. **B,** Left buccal photograph.

stainless steel with anterior facial root torque to prevent facial tipping of the anterior teeth. The mandibular arch wire should be 0.016 × 0.022-inch or thicker stainless steel with anterior lingual root torque. Bilateral heavy-force NiTi CCSs are attached from the LOMAS miniscrews to the hooks of the maxillary second molars for en masse protraction. Bilateral heavy-force NiTi CCSs are also attached diagonally to the arch wire distal to the mandibular canines for en masse distalization. A 32CNA-TPA with mesial angulation and lingual crown torque is inserted into the lingual sheaths on the molars. Extrusion CNA lever arms are inserted into the auxiliary rectangular tube in the LOMAS Quattro miniscrews and are hooked over the arch wire between the maxillary canines and lateral incisors for anterior extrusion.

REMOVAL PROCEDURE

The LOMAS miniscrews can be removed whenever they are no longer needed or when the orthodontic appliances are removed at the end of the treatment (Fig. 15-27). It may be safest to leave them in place until the end of treatment just in case their use is required at a later point in treatment. No incision or flap is required, and the wound heals within a week. First, a small amount of local infiltration anesthesia may be injected around the LOMAS miniscrew. The LOMAS miniscrew is unscrewed with the LOMAS screwdriver. Povidone-iodine (Betadine) is applied around the wound for disinfection, and then 2% chlorhexidine is prescribed for 7 days postoperatively.

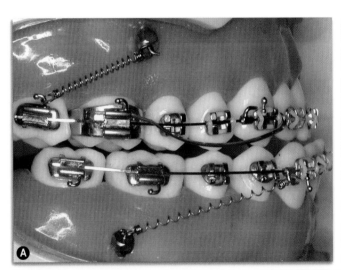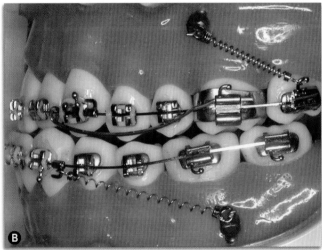

Fig. 15-26

Nonextraction mechanics 4 for en masse distalization of the mandibular dentition with en masse protraction and extrusion of the maxillary dentition. **A,** Right buccal photograph. **B,** Left buccal photograph.

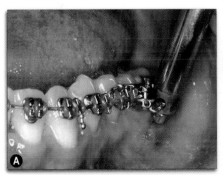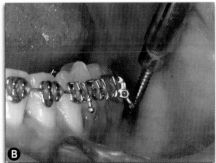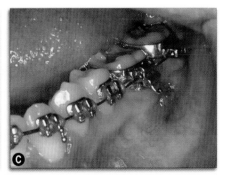

Fig. 15-27

LOMAS miniscrew removal procedure. **A,** Seat screwdriver head on LOMAS miniscrew. **B,** Unscrew LOMAS miniscrew. **C,** Wound usually heals within a week.

POTENTIAL COMPLICATIONS

A clinical review of our 59 patients reveals that the 120-week success rate of LOMAS miniscrews was 91.1%; failure was therefore 8.9%.[4] Miniscrew loosening occurred mostly in the earlier cases and was within the first 20 weeks after miniscrew placement, suggesting that the learning curve of miniscrew placement plays a role in success and failure.

For a loosened miniscrew, the miniscrew should be removed and the wound allowed to heal for at least a month before the replacement. Seating a loose miniscrew deeper into bone does not overcome its failure and may increase the potential for infection by pushing bacteria into the miniscrew site.

SUMMARY

The Lin/Liou Orthodontic Mini Anchor System is a self-drilling and self-tapping orthodontic miniscrew. By using the bone density–guided insertion technique, the LOMAS miniscrew can be placed in interdental and non–tooth-bearing areas. To avoid tooth root injury, miniscrews can be placed in interdental areas when the teeth will not be moved mesiodistally. In contrast, the infrazygomatic crests and the external oblique ridges are universal miniscrew sites regardless of whether the teeth will be moved mesiodistally. The LOMAS miniscrew is compatible with the traditional edgewise appliance system. The miniscrew is made with a hook, rectangular auxiliary tube, and a bracket so that it is universally adaptable to any type of tooth movement. Although miniscrews broaden the spectrum of orthodontic treatment, they should not be used as a mainstream treatment option, but rather as a treatment adjunct.

REFERENCES

1. Lin JC, Liou EJ, Liaw JL. The application of a new osseous miniscrew for orthodontic anchorage. *J Taiwan Assoc Orthod.* 14:33-38, 2002.
2. Lin JC, Liou EJ. A new bone screw for orthodontic anchorage. *J Clin Orthod.* 37:676-681, 2003.
3. Misch CE. A scientific rationale for dental implant design. In: Misch CE, ed. *Contemporary Implant Dentistry.* 2nd ed. St Louis: Mosby, 1999.
4. Yang LI, Liou EJ. Clinical evaluation on the factors related to orthodontic miniscrew failure. Paper presented at: 3rd Asia Implant Orthodontics Conference; Dec 4 to 6, 2004; Taipei, Taiwan.
5. Favero L, Brollo P, Bressan E. Orthodontic anchorage with specific fixtures: related study analysis. *Am J Orthod Dentofacial Orthop.* 122:84-94, 2002.
6. Liou EJ, Pai BC, DDS, Lin JC. Do miniscrews remain stationary under orthodontic force? *Am J Orthod Dentofacial Orthop.* 126:42-47, 2004.
7. Wang YC, Liou EJ. The stability of self-drilling miniscrews throughout orthodontic loading. Paper presented at: 3rd Asia Implant Orthodontics Conference; Dec 4-6, 2004; Taipei, Taiwan.
8. Melsen B, Peterson JK, Costa A. Zygoma ligatures: an alternative form of maxillary anchorage. *J Clin Orthod.* 32:154-158, 1998.
9. Costa A, Raffainl M, Melsen B. Miniscrews as orthodontic anchorage: a preliminary report. *Int J Adult Orthodon Orthognath Surg.* 13:201-209, 1998.
10. Umemori M, Sugawara J, Mitani H, et al. Skeletal anchorage system for open-bite correction. *Am J Orthod Dentofacial Orthop.* 115:166-174, 1999.
11. Melsen B, Costa A. Immediate loading of implants used for orthodontic anchorage. *Clin Orthod Res.* 3:23-28, 2000.
12. Clerck H, Geerinckx V, Siciliano S. The zygoma anchorage system. *J Clin Orthod.* 36:455-459, 2002.
13. Chung KR, Kim YS, Linton Lee J, Lee YJ. The miniplate with skeletal anchorage system. *J Clin Orthod.* 36:407, 2002.
14. Kuroda S, Katayama A, Takano-Yamamoto T. Severe anterior open-bite case treated using titanium screw anchorage. *Angle Orthod.* 74:558-567, 2004.
15. Misch CE. Bone character: second vital implant criterion. *Dent Today.* 7(5):39-40, 1998.
16. Misch CE, Kircos LT. Diagnostic imaging and techniques. In: Misch CE, editor, *Contemporary Implant Dentistry.* 2nd ed. St Louis; Mosby, 1999.
17. Heidemann W, Gerlach KL, Grobel KH, Kollner HG. Influence of different pilot sizes on torque measurements and pullout analysis of osteosynthesis screws. *J Craniomaxillofac Surg.* 26:50-55, 1998.
18. Matthews J, Hirsch C. Temperature measured in human cortical bone when drilling. *J Bone Joint Surg Am.* 45:297-308, 1972.
19. Misch CE. Density of bone: effect on surgical approach and healing. In: Misch CE, ed. *Contemporary Implant Dentistry.* 2nd ed. St Louis; Mosby, 1999.
20. Cheng SJ, Tseng IY, Lee JJ, Kok SH. A prospective study of the risk factors associated with failure of mini-implants used for orthodontic anchorage. *Int J Oral Maxillofac Implants.* 19:100-106, 2004.
21. Chen PH, Liou EJ. CT-image study on the thickness of infrazygomatic crest of maxilla and its implications for implant orthodontics. Paper presented at: 3rd Asia Implant Orthodontics Conference; Dec 4-6, 2004; Taipei, Taiwan.
22. Liou EJ. Orthognathic-like miniscrew orthodontics. Paper presented at: 3rd Asia Implant Orthodontics Conference; Dec 4-6, 2004; Taipei, Taiwan.

The MiniScrew Anchorage System

Aldo Carano, Stefano Velo

THE MINISCREW ANCHORAGE SYSTEM

The miniscrew anchorage system (MAS) is a miniscrew implant (MSI) system manufactured from type 5 titanium alloy. The miniscrews are conical and are available in three different sizes (Fig. 16-1, *A*).[1] The type A miniscrew is 1.3 mm in diameter at the transmucosal collar and tapers to 1.1 mm at the apex. The type B miniscrew is 1.5 mm in diameter at the transmucosal collar and tapers to 1.3 mm at the apex. Type A and B miniscrews are 11 mm long. The type C miniscrew is 1.5 mm in diameter at the transmucosal collar and tapers to 1.3 mm at the apex but is only 9 mm long.

The abutment head of the miniscrew is composed of two spheres. The superior sphere is 2.2 mm in diameter, whereas the inferior sphere is 2.0 mm in diameter. The spheres are connected by a narrower-diameter neck that is used for attachment of elastics, power chains, or closed coil springs. The superior sphere has an 0.6-mm diameter hole oriented perpendicular to the long axis of the miniscrew for insertion of ligature wire or auxiliaries, such as *monkey hooks*. An internal hexagonally shaped recess is also oriented parallel to the long axis of the miniscrew for insertion of the screwdriver (Fig. 16-1, *B*)

Two pilot hole drills are available depending on the diameter of the MAS (Fig. 16-2). The 1.3-mm MAS uses the smaller pilot hole drill, which is tapered from 0.9 mm at the tip to 1.1 mm at the base. The 1.5-mm

MAS uses the larger pilot hole drill, which is tapered from 1.1 mm at the tip to 1.25 mm at the base. The discrepancy between the diameters of the pilot hole drill and the miniscrew is one of the main factors influencing torsional moment during MSI placement. In vitro tests suggest that the torsional moment occurring during MSI placement increases when the pilot hole drill diameter is decreased, that is, the pilot hole itself is smaller. Therefore, the difference in pilot hole drill diameter and miniscrew diameter is 0.3 mm for the MAS.

The MAS is self-tapping and has small a diameter (1.3 to 1.5 mm), which makes placement in tight spaces easier. However, this small diameter might lead to increased miniscrew fracture in thicker and denser bone upon either placement or removal. Therefore, experiments were carried out to test the mechanical strength of the MAS during torsion and flexure. In torsion, the 1.5-mm diameter MAS fractured at a level of 48.7 N, and the 1.3-mm diameter MAS fractured at a level of 37.4 N. In flexure, the 1.5-mm diameter MAS yielded at 120.4 N, and the 1.3-mm diameter MAS yielded at 63.7 N. All of these values increased substantially by thickening the transmucosal collar (Fig. 16-3).

Miniscrew implant shape and thread form are also important.[2] A symmetric thread form is preferred to an asymmetric thread form (Fig. 16-4), and a cylindrical shape is preferred to a conical shape. A conical shape, however, is preferable in sites where limited space is available, such as in interradicular bone, because a smaller screw apex decreases the risk of tooth root contact. For this reason, the MAS miniscrews were designed with a conical shape.

TREATMENT PLANNING

Skeletal anchorage is indicated in cases in which absolute anchorage is necessary or in which traditional intraoral or extraoral anchorage systems are insufficient to achieve ideal treatment results. When MSI anchorage is planned as a part of orthodontic treatment, four primary factors should be considered: the required tooth movements, the anticipated biomechanics, the correct MSI placement locations, and the benefits for the patient (decreased treatment duration, better results, decreased costs). For instance, if teeth are missing and are to be restored, one realistic alternative to an MSI would be a traditional dental implant that could be used for orthodontic anchorage and then prosthetically restored after orthodontics.

Recently, miniaturized dental implants were developed specifically for placement in the hard palate. These palatal implants can be used as anchorage for space closure, intrusion, anterior retraction, of even maxillary molar distalization.[3,4] More recently, miniplate implants were developed and have been used for molar intrusion.[5,6] Although these orthodontic implants provide alternative anchorage to traditional anchorage, they are limited in application. The surgical protocol for placement is more invasive, and a second procedure is required for removal. These implants are frequently placed by a surgeon, which increases the costs. The palatal implant, in particular is limited only to placement in the palate. Moreover, a cost-benefit ratio remains to be documented for comparing palatal implants for molar distalization, miniplate implants for molar intrusion, or traditional orthodontic mechanics.[7,8]

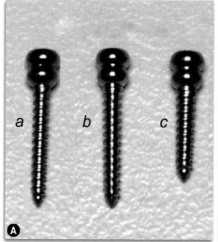
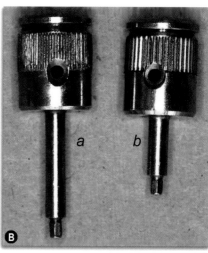

Fig. 16-1

The miniscrew anchorage system (MAS). **A,** Type A MAS *(a)* is 11 mm long and tapered from 1.3 to 1.1 mm. Type B MAS *(b)* is 11 mm long and tapered from 1.5 to 1.3 mm. Type C MAS *(c)* is 9 mm long and tapered from 1.5 to 1.3. **B,** Screwdrivers for MAS placement. Long *(a)* and short *(b)* are available for different intraoral locations.

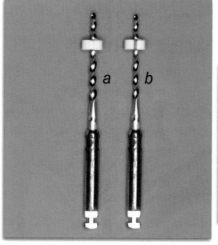

Fig. 16-2

Pilot hole drills. Drill *(a)* for larger diameter MAS is tapered from 1.25 to 1.1 mm. Drill *(b)* for smaller diameter MAS is tapered from 1.1 to 0.9 mm.

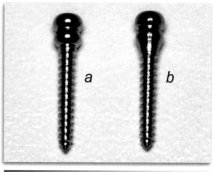

Fig. 16-3

Comparison of MAS generations. First generation *(a)*. Second generation *(b)*. Note that second-generation neck is thicker to minimize the potential of breakage during placement or removal.

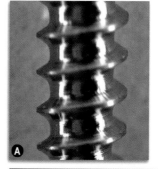
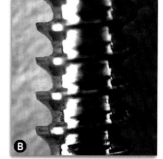

Fig. 16-4

Miniscrew implant designs. **A,** A symmetric thread form. **B,** An asymmetric thread form.

Alternatively, MSIs have been used extensively in the last few years as an alternative method for achieving absolute orthodontic anchorage.[9-14] The major benefits of MSIs include small size, decreased costs, easy placement and removal, and simplicity of use.

When evaluating the exact site for MSI placement, it is important to relate the interradicular space available to the miniscrew diameter and shape, as well as to the bony dimension required between the miniscrew and the tooth root, in order to minimize root contact and ensure periodontal health. Currently, the majority of the available miniscrews have a diameter ranging from 1.2 to 2 mm. Conical miniscrews have a smaller diameter at the apex that gradually increases to the transmucosal collar. Because of this smaller diameter at the apical half of conical miniscrews, the MAS miniscrew is beneficial in narrower interradicular spaces where the available space is less than 3 to 4 mm.

Proper placement and use of MSI anchorage depends on two primary factors: safe placement location and ideal mechanical vectors. Both factors are interrelated and are affected by the other. In a recent study, our group evaluated the intraoral hard and soft tissues of 50 maxillae and mandibles to determine possible placement locations for MSI placement location.[15] Briefly, the patient's ages ranged from 20 and 40 years, and all had completely dentate arches. Three-dimensional cone beam computed tomography images were captured with a NewTom cone beam computed tomography machine (DVT9000). The maxillary alveolar ridge was evaluated on both the facial and palatal surface, whereas the mandibular alveolar ridge was evaluated on the facial surface only. For each region, four horizontal slices were evaluated relative to the alveolar crest, 2, 5, 8, and 11 mm apical to the crest on both the mesial and distal aspects of each tooth.

The results demonstrate that several sites are more applicable for MSI placement than others. In general, less space is available in a mesiodistal direction, but faciopalatal depth was always greater than 7 mm. To date, no scientific data are available quantifying the amount of bone necessary to adequately stabilize a miniscrew yet prevent encroachment of the periodontal ligament (PDL). However, when considering that the PDL is approximately 0.25 mm wide,[16] one can assume that a minimum clearance of 1 mm of alveolar bone between the miniscrew and PDL would be sufficient to maintain MSI stability and provide periodontal health.

Combining this information with measurements of the interradicular spaces and of known miniscrew

diameters, safe zones for miniscrew insertion can be identified (Fig. 16-5). Based on this study, it appears that relatively *safe zones* in the maxilla for MSI placement in order of most to least safe are as follows:

1. Facially and palatally between the canine and lateral incisor
2. Facially and palatally between the first molar and second premolar at a level of 2 to 8 mm from the alveolar crest
3. Facially and palatally between the first and second molar at a level of 2 to 8 mm from the alveolar crest

Unsafe zones in the maxilla for MSI placement are as follows:

1. The maxillary tuberosity, especially if the third molars are unerupted
2. The interradicular spaces greater than 8 mm apical to the alveolar crest in the maxillary molar and premolar area because of maxillary sinus proximity

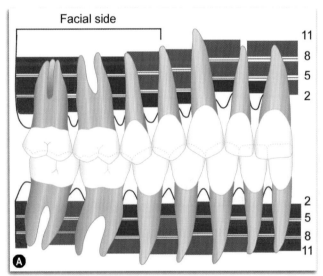

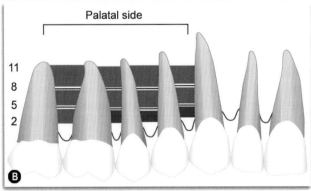

Fig. 16-5

Map of safe zones for miniscrew placement based on cone beam computed tomography data. **A,** Facial surface of maxilla and mandible. **B,** Palatal surface of maxilla. Note green areas are safe zones for miniscrews with a diameter of 1.3 mm. Blue areas are intermediate zones, where 1.3 diameter miniscrews sometimes can be placed safely. Red areas are not suitable for miniscrew placement.

Relatively *safe zones* in the mandible for MSI placement in order of most to least safe are as follows:

1. The interradicular space between the first and second molars
2. The interradicular space between the first and second premolars
3. The interradicular space between the first molar and second premolar at a level of 11 mm apical to the alveolar crest
4. The interradicular space between the canine and first premolar at a level of 11 mm apical to the alveolar crest

The *safe zone map* (Fig. 16-5) indicates that green areas, which have a mesiodistal dimension of greater than 3.1 mm, are safe zones for miniscrews with a diameter of 1.3 mm. Miniscrews with a 1.5-mm diameter would be considered safe if the mesiodistal bone dimension were at least 3.5 mm. Considering this, miniscrew diameters of 2 mm or greater may not be safe in posterior maxillary interradicular spaces. Blue areas represent intermediate zones where only 1.3-mm diameter miniscrews may be safely placed after accurate treatment planning using panoramic or periapical radiographs and good surgical skill. Red areas are not suitable for miniscrew placement.

If the angulation of the miniscrew is oriented perpendicular to the long axis of the teeth, there is a greater chance of tooth root contact than with an oblique angulation. Therefore, the MAS miniscrews are oriented at 30 to 40 degrees relative to the long axis of the teeth (Fig. 16-6). This also allows the use of a longer miniscrew. The combination of these parameters—that is, using a conical miniscrew, angling the miniscrew on placement, and understanding the local bony dimensions—greatly reduces the risk of tooth root contact.

Ideal mechanical vectors are achieved by first understanding the desired tooth movement. Once tooth movement has been determined, the location and angulation of the miniscrew should be determined based on bone width and thickness and the force vectors applied to the miniscrew and the teeth of the active segment. For instance, a miniscrew placed at the level of the mucogingival junction generates a mostly horizontal force vector, whereas a miniscrew placed more apically generates a horizontal and intrusive force vector (Fig. 16-7). In some instances, however, the ideal MSI position is not possible because of local anatomic constraints. In these cases, the orthodontist must be creative in designing alternative miniscrew positions, orthodontic attachment points, or mechanical systems necessary to obtain an ideal result.

Anterior Retraction

In cases with premolar extraction, the MAS can be used to retract the anterior teeth without anchorage loss of the posterior teeth. Depending on the desired tooth movement, the miniscrew should be placed at the mucogingival junction for translation and more apical for intrusion and translation. The miniscrew is usually placed between the first molar and second premolar roots, which generally provides ample space for safe miniscrew placement. Extraction spaces may also be used for MSI placement, but only after sufficient time has passed for healing of the extraction site (3 to 6 months). Caution should be used in the mandible

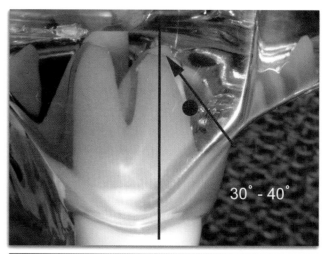
Fig. 16-6

Ideal MAS placement orientation is 30 to 40 degrees relative to the long axis of the tooth.

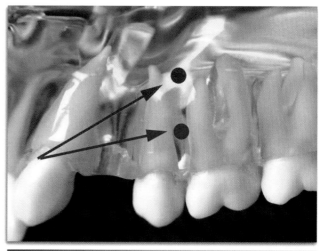
Fig. 16-7

MAS force vector orientation. For a horizontal force *(blue arrow)*, the miniscrew should be placed at the level of the mucogingival junction *(blue circle)*. For a horizontal and intrusive force *(red arrow)*, the miniscrew should be placed more apically *(red circle)*.

when placing a miniscrew between the premolars in order to avoid the mental nerve.

Incisor Intrusion

In deep bite cases with excessive gingival display, placement of miniscrews allows rapid intrusion of maxillary anterior teeth without bite-opening auxiliaries. Miniscrews can usually be placed between the maxillary lateral incisors and canines.

Unilateral Occlusal Plane Intrusion

Canted occlusal plane correction is often considered impossible with traditional orthodontic mechanics. Using miniscrew anchorage, however, this treatment goal is much more attainable. To achieve unilateral intrusion of a canted occlusal plane, miniscrews are placed between the maxillary lateral incisor and canine or between the canine and first premolar (depending on alveolar bone space) on the side that is inferiorly positioned (Fig. 16-8). In the mandible, the miniscrew is usually placed between the lateral incisor and canine.

Dental Midline Correction

Significant dental midline deviation is also difficult to treat ideally with traditional orthodontic mechanics. MSI anchorage makes midline correction much simpler. In these cases, the miniscrew can be placed either on the facial or on the palatal with the abutment head at the level of the gingival margin. This position places the line of action of the force more occlusally with a horizontal vector.

Molar Intrusion

The MAS is a reliable system for intruding supererupted molars. However, because of space

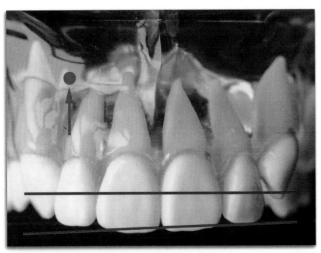

Fig. 16-8

MAS placement position (*green circle*) for correcting a canted occlusal plane.

limitations between the molar roots and access in the posterior part of the mouth, the miniscrews usually have to be angled considerably to prevent tooth root contact. Also, because the tooth to be intruded is moving toward the miniscrew, there is an increased risk of moving the tooth into the miniscrew. Moreover, multiple screws are often necessary to handle the increased forces used for intrusion. For these reasons, MAS use is limited to cases with simple intrusion of one or two molars. In open bite cases, in which bilateral intrusion of both posterior segments is required, miniscrews are not the ideal solution and alternative approaches should be explored.[8]

Molar Distalization

Previous studies of molar distalization using conventional anchorage have demonstrated variable amounts of anterior anchorage loss.[7] Skeletal anchorage, however, may decrease or eliminate anterior anchorage loss. The palatal implant placed in the palate is a good source of skeletal anchorage; however, this implant requires an invasive surgical procedure for both placement and removal. The MAS in combination with the Distal Jet[1] (American Orthodontics, Sheboygan, Wisconsin) may provide a less invasive alternative to the anchorage loss so common during molar distalization. In these cases, the miniscrew is placed in the maxillary alveolar process, between the palatal roots of the first and second premolar. This mechanical system limits or prevents mesial movement of the anterior teeth during molar distalization (Fig. 16-9).

Molar Protraction

Molar protraction is often required to close extraction sites or edentulous spaces. Molar protraction is not easily achieved and often causes problems such as anterior anchorage loss and molar dumping. These problems can be avoided by placing a miniscrew mesial to the space to be closed and at a level vertically such that the protraction force passes through the center of resistance of the molars.

Intermaxillary Anchorage

The MAS can be used as intermaxillary anchorage in either Class II or Class III cases. For Class II treatment that requires maxillary arch distalization, the miniscrew is placed between roots of the mandibular first molar and second premolars, erring toward the first molar root (Fig. 16-10). This miniscrew position may also prevent mesial movement of the first molar if it does move forward and contacts the MSI. Whether this is

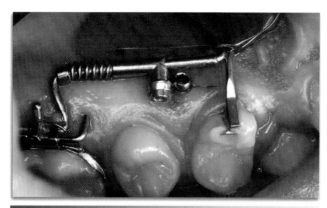

Fig. 16-9

MAS placed between the first and second premolar palatal roots. The Distal Jet abuts against the MAS to prevent anterior anchorage loss during molar distalization.

clinically acceptable and does not cause damage to the tooth root needs to be evaluated first in animal experiments. The mechanics can be established either directly or indirectly. For direct anchorage, the elastic force is attached directly from the mandibular MAS to the maxillary lateral incisor. For indirect anchorage,

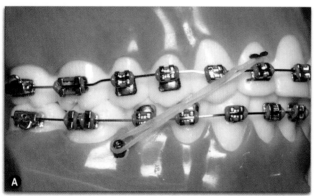

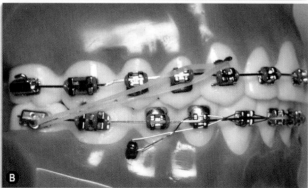

Fig. 16-10

Miniscrew location for Class II intermaxillary elastics. **A,** For direct anchorage, the elastic force is attached directly from the mandibular MAS to the maxillary lateral incisor. **B,** For indirect anchorage, the elastic force is attached from the mandibular second molar to the maxillary lateral incisor. The mandibular arch is stabilized by indirect ligation to the MAS.

the elastic force is attached from the mandibular second molar to the maxillary canine with the MAS ligated to the mandibular first premolar to prevent incisor proclination. Although possible, it is more difficult to place the miniscrew between the first and second molar because access and interradicular space is considerably decreased.

For Class III treatment that requires maxillary arch advancement, the miniscrew is placed between the mandibular canine and first premolar roots to anchor Class III elastics. When the mandibular arch requires distalization, the miniscrew can be placed either between the maxillary first and second molars or between the first molar and the second premolars to anchor Class III elastics.

PRESURGICAL ORTHODONTICS

Because of the small size of the MAS, presurgical orthodontics is rarely required. However, in some circumstances, presurgical orthodontics may prove beneficial before placing the miniscrews.

Anterior Retraction

For anterior retraction, both arches must be leveled and aligned before extractions take place. After a short healing period, the miniscrews are placed and retraction begins in rectangular stainless steel arch wires.

Incisor Intrusion

Numerous techniques have been suggested to intrude upper and lower incisors without anchorage loss. The standard MAS technique consists of bonding acrylic bite plates to the palatal surfaces of the maxillary central and sometimes lateral incisors without the use of miniscrews.[17] In very severe deep bite cases, however, in which maximum intrusion of the maxillary incisors is desired, miniscrews are inserted to add a vertical force and minimize posterior extrusion. The miniscrews are placed after leveling and aligning so that the interradicular space at the placement site is maximum. To avoid maxillary incisor proclination during intrusion, the arch wire should be 0.017 × 0.025-inch (0.022-inch slot) and cinched back.

Unilateral Occlusal Plane Intrusion

When vertical asymmetry correction is required, leveling and alignment should precede the placement of miniscrews. To prevent maxillary incisor flaring during intrusion, a cinched back 0.017 × 0.025-inch arch wire (0.022-inch slot) should be used.

Dental Midline Correction

For dental midline correction, a full-sized rectangular wire should be used in both arches to obtain a proper asymmetric force.

Molar Intrusion

Miniscrews should be used for molar intrusion in patients with supererupted molars in whom only one or two molars need to be intruded and in whom the placement location is easily accessible. In open bite cases, where bilateral intrusion of both posterior segments is required, the screws are not the ideal solution, and alternative methods are available.[8]

If an individual molar is to be intruded, the molar should be excluded from the initial leveling and alignment. After leveling, the miniscrew is placed and intrusion is initiated. If two molars are to be intruded together, then these teeth are included in the initial leveling and alignment, with the miniscrew being used simultaneously for intrusion.

Molar Distalization

Molar distalization is best achieved using the MAS-supported Distal Jet, which places the force approximately at the center of resistance and provides a more translatory force. To decrease anterior anchorage loss, the Distal Jet should be used independent of fixed edgewise appliances. After distalization, the edgewise appliance is placed to retract the anterior teeth.

Molar Protraction

Molar protraction is not easily achieved, even if with miniscrew anchorage. Complete leveling and alignment is necessary before protraction is begun. Insufficient leveling before protraction allows molar tipping rather than bodily movement.

Intermaxillary Anchorage

When using miniscrews for attachment of intermaxillary elastics, leveling and alignment should be performed first, followed by engagement of full-sized rectangular arch wires before miniscrew placement. Although miniscrews prevent anchorage loss in an arch, they do not prevent adverse effects in the opposite arch. Therefore, in Class II cases in which intermaxillary elastics are worn from a miniscrew in the mandibular arch, acrylic bite plates are bonded to the cingulum of the maxillary incisors to prevent bite deepening during incisor retraction.

SURGICAL PROCEDURE

Before the MAS surgical procedure, the miniscrew placement site is determined using a periapical radiograph and a surgical guide (Fig. 16-11). First, local anesthesia is performed with mepivacaine (Fig. 16-12, A). Next, the miniscrews site is prepared using the appropriate-size pilot hole drill through the gingival tissue and the cortical bone. The angulation of the pilot hole drill should be the same as that of the final miniscrew position (Fig. 16-12, B). A rubber endodontic stopper is placed on the pilot hole drill to establish the depth to which the pilot hole extends into bone. The depth is only 2 to 3 mm and usually does not extend into medullary bone because the miniscrew is self-tapping. After pilot hole preparation, the MAS is placed with a manual screwdriver (Fig. 16-12, C). If the pilot hole does extend into medullary bone, however, it is critical that the depth of the pilot hole be at least 2 mm shorter than the miniscrew length.

The preferable vertical level of insertion is at the mucogingival junction with an angulation of 30 to 40 degrees relative to the long axis of the tooth. If,

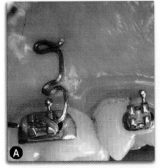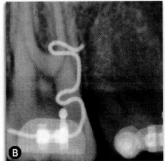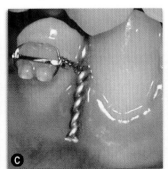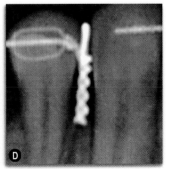

Fig. 16-11

Determination of MAS insertion point. **A,** Orthodontic wire bent and adjusted to approximate insertion point. **B,** Periapical radiograph showing insertion point. Note that wire can be bent and adjusted until appropriate position is achieved. **C,** Brass wire around interproximal contact bent and adjusted to approximate insertion point. **D,** Periapical radiograph showing insertion point. Note that wire can be bent and adjusted until appropriate position is achieved.

however, the miniscrew is placed higher in the maxilla, it should be placed more perpendicular to the long axis of the tooth to prevent perforation of the maxillary sinus. When properly placed, the abutment head of the MAS emerges from the soft tissue, and the desired force can be applied immediately (Fig. 16-12, *D*). If the mucosa is compressed by the force modules attached to the miniscrews, auxiliaries can be attached to move the force module attachment point away from the miniscrew head. For example, monkey hooks[18] have been used for this purpose. Once MSI primary stability has been established, an orthodontic force of 50 to 250 g can be applied immediately. Neither antibiotics nor analgesics are required postoperatively.

Careful attention is required during MSI insertion to prevent injuries to vessels, nerves, or tooth roots. Presurgical and postsurgical radiographs (panoramic or periapical) with metallic markers attached to vacuum-formed stents can assist in miniscrew site localization. If, upon placement, a miniscrew contacts a tooth root, the miniscrew can either be moved to a different location altogether or the angulation can be changed slightly, which is often sufficient to eliminate miniscrew-root contact.

ORTHODONTIC MECHANICS

The MAS can be used as either direct or indirect anchorage (see Chapter 1 for description). Direct anchorage consists of applying the force directly from the miniscrew to the active segment to be moved. If mechanical factors do not allow direct attachment, the miniscrew can be used as indirect anchorage. For indirect anchorage, the miniscrew is ligated or bonded (via an orthodontic wire) to the teeth of the reactive segment, which is then used indirectly to move the teeth

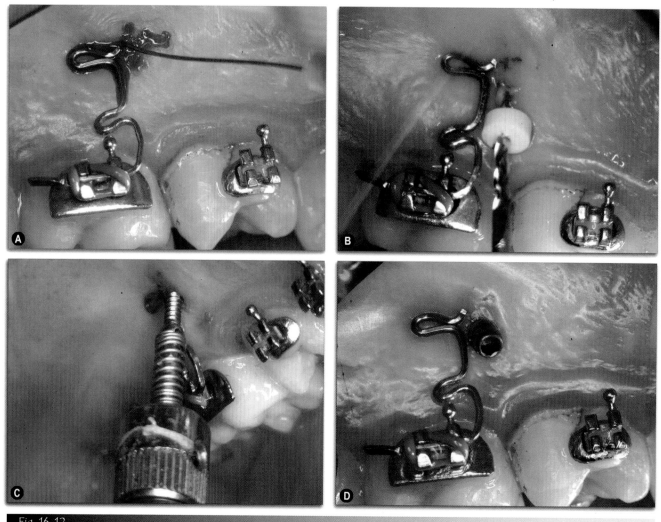

Fig. 16-12

MAS insertion sequence. **A,** Injection of local anesthetic. **B,** Preparation of pilot hole with rubber endodontic stopper to prevent overinsertion of drill. **C,** Placement of MAS using screwdriver. **D,** Final position of MAS.

of the active segment (Fig. 16-13). Indirect anchorage is rarely necessary with the MAS, however, because the small size of the miniscrew allows placement in the exact site necessary for direct force application.

Anterior Retraction

When closing premolar extraction sites, the miniscrew is usually placed either between first molar and second premolar roots or, after the extraction site has healed, in the new bone of the extraction site. Vertically, the abutment head is located at the mucogingival junction and sometimes even more apically depending on whether pure translation or translation with intrusion is desired, respectively.

The distalizing force is delivered by elastic power chain and is replaced monthly. The force should not be more than 250 g per MAS. Forces higher than about 400 g increase the risk of miniscrew mobility and subsequent failure. Closed coil springs are not used because they are less hygienic and more uncomfortable for the patient. As a rule, en masse retraction is used (Fig. 16-14). The power chains are attached from the miniscrew to the bracket directly or through a power arm crimped on the arch wire (Fig. 16-15). When the force is applied directly to the bracket, an intrusive component is present during retraction. However, when the force is applied to a power arm crimped on the arch wire, the force is almost purely horizontal and through the center of resistance; therefore, no intrusive component is present. In some cases, direct attachment of the power chain to the miniscrew head causes soft

tissue impingement. In these cases, an auxiliary such as the monkey hook (Fig. 16-16) can be used to keep the power chain away from the soft tissue.

Incisor Intrusion

For maxillary incisor intrusion, the MAS is usually placed between the maxillary lateral incisor and canine. Power chains are stretched from the bracket or the arch wire to monkey hooks attached to the miniscrew head to prevent soft tissue impingement.

Unilateral Occlusal Plane Intrusion

To treat a canted occlusal plane, the MAS is used unilaterally for an asymmetric effect. The intrusive force is applied through a power chain from the miniscrew to the tooth segment to be intruded, thereby levelling the occlusal plane (Fig. 16-17).

Dental Midline Correction

The MAS is useful for midline correction. If both a vertical and a horizontal force vector is desired, the asymmetric force is applied directly to the brackets. If however, only a horizontal force vector is desired without a vertical force vector, the asymmetric force is applied to a power arm crimped on the arch wire.

Molar Intrusion

If molar intrusion is desired, a single miniscrew on the facial surface is usually sufficient for intruding one or two molars. Because the force is applied facial to the center of resistance, facial crown tipping occurs if the teeth are not constrained with a transpalatal arch. Alternatively, lingual crown torque can be bent into the arch wire.

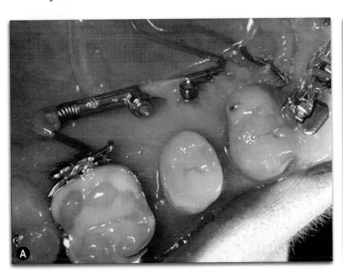 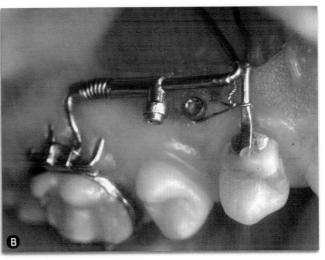

Fig. 16-13

Distal Jet anchorage mechanics. **A,** Direct anchorage where the NiTi open coil spring exerts a mesial force to the miniscrew via a composite stop that contacts the lock on the Distal Jet. **B,** Indirect anchorage where the NiTi open coil spring exerts a mesial force to the Nance button attached to the first premolar, which is ligated indirectly to the miniscrew to prevent forward movement of the premolar.

Although several authors have used miniscrews in the molar region for posterior dental intrusion in skeletal open bite cases, this is not a ideal treatment option. First, the facial interradicular spaces between maxillary first and second molars are generally insufficient for miniscrew stability. Second, surgical access to this posterior region, both on the facial and on the palatal, is limited. Third, the miniscrew must generally be placed very apical for intrusion, and if the MSI is located higher than about 8 mm above the alveolar crest, perforation of the maxillary sinus becomes more probable.

Miniplate implants have also been proposed for molar intrusion.[5,6] The miniplates are generally placed apical to the tooth roots, and considerable force can be applied without risking miniplate failure; however, this technique is more invasive and requires an incision and flap for miniplate placement and removal, and long-term stability is questionable.

Molar Distalization

Miniscrews provide additional anchorage to the Distal Jet molar distalizing appliance, which has traditionally used the acrylic Nance button component as anchorage. The MAS minimizes or even eliminates anterior tooth proclination during molar distalization. The MAS is usually placed in the interradicular bone between the maxillary first and second premolars (Fig. 16-18, *A*). Because the open coil spring exerts a mesial force on the activation lock, composite is bonded between

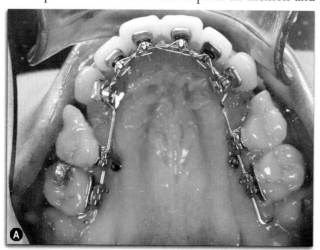
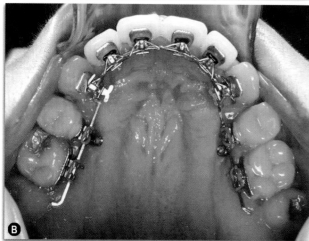

Fig. 16–14

En masse retraction after premolar extraction using lingual orthodontic appliances. **A,** Maxillary occlusal photograph before retraction. Note MAS placed between second premolars and first molars to retract anterior teeth. **B,** Maxillary occlusal photograph after retraction.

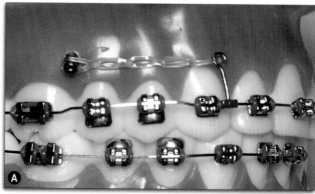
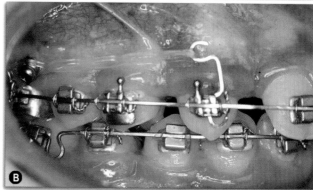
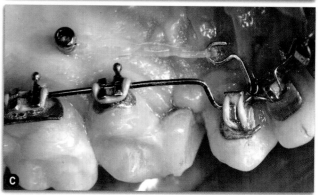

Fig. 16–15

Force application using power arm. **A,** Power arm crimped onto arch wire. **B,** Power arm inserted into vertical bracket slot with facial mechanics. **C,** Power arm inserted into vertical bracket slot with palatal mechanics.

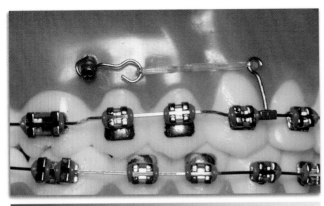

Fig. 16-16

Monkey hook used to move point of force application away from MAS to prevent gingival impingement of power chain.

the miniscrew head to prevent anchorage loss. After molar distalization, the Distal Jet is transformed into a retainer for anterior retraction, and brackets are bonded to the teeth. After anterior retraction is finished, the Distal Jet is removed and final detailing and finishing is initiated. Alternatively, the MAS can be removed after molar distalization and replaced mesial to the distalized molar to prevent mesial molar drift as the anterior teeth are being retracted (Fig. 16-18, B).

Molar Protraction

When protracting molars, it is important to place the MAS at a level that effectively locates the force level mesial to and through the center of resistance of the molar. This prevents molar dumping during protraction and enhances translation.

Intermaxillary Anchorage

Orthodontic mechanics for miniscrew anchorage with intermaxillary elastics do not require specific considerations.

REMOVAL PROCEDURE

Once tooth movement with miniscrew anchorage is complete and the miniscrews are no longer needed,

they are easily removed with a manual screwdriver (Fig. 16-19). Generally, local anesthesia is not necessary. The soft tissues heal within 7 to 14 days, and new bone fills the site within 6 to 12 weeks. If MAS osseointegration has occurred, a minor surgical procedure is necessary for miniscrew removal. Briefly, local anesthesia is performed with mepivacaine, and then the bone around the miniscrew is removed with a round bur in a slow-speed handpiece. The screwdriver is then used to produce a gentle torsional movement around the long axis of the miniscrew to fracture the bone-miniscrew contact.

POTENTIAL COMPLICATIONS

Two types of complication are possible with the MAS, as with any other miniscrew system: miniscrew failure and damage of local anatomic structures. Miniscrew failure can be subcategorized as loss of miniscrew stability and miniscrew breakage. If the miniscrew pilot hole has been adequately prepared, the MAS should be easily inserted and should be immediately stable. If the cutting threads of the MAS strip the bone, primary stability could be compromised. In such a case, the MAS should be moved to another location. Other factors that decrease primary stability include poor bone quality or density, improper pilot hole drilling, and excessive pilot hole depth. After insertion, the miniscrew must be absolutely stable. Otherwise, another site should be prepared.

Miniscrew breakage can occur as a result of excessive forces applied during miniscrew insertion or removal, particularly if partial osseointegration has occurred. Originally, MAS breakage was attributed to the decreased neck diameter. In the second generation, however, the neck diameter was increased and breakage has not been an issue. In addition, the screwdriver length was shortened so that it could only be held by the operator's fingertips, which decreased the torsional

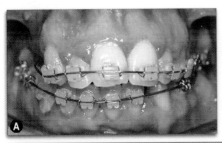
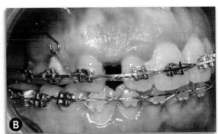
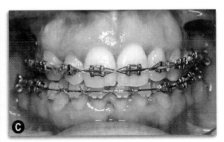

Fig. 16-17

Correction of occlusal plane cant. **A,** Anterior photograph of occlusal plane cant after initial leveling. **B,** Right buccal photograph of MAS mechanics. Note that MAS is placed high in the vestibule between the premolars and a monkey hook is used to move point of attachment of power chain closer to the canine bracket. **C,** Anterior photograph of occlusal plane after cant correction.

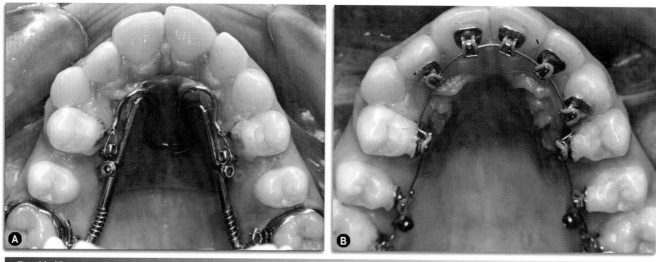

Fig. 16-18

Molar distalization with the MAS-anchored Distal Jet as indirect anchorage. **A,** Maxillary occlusal photograph after molar distalization. **B,** Maxillary occlusal photograph during premolar and anterior retraction. Note that MAS was moved from its initial position distal to the first premolar to distal to the second premolar to prevent contact of the first premolar root with the MAS.

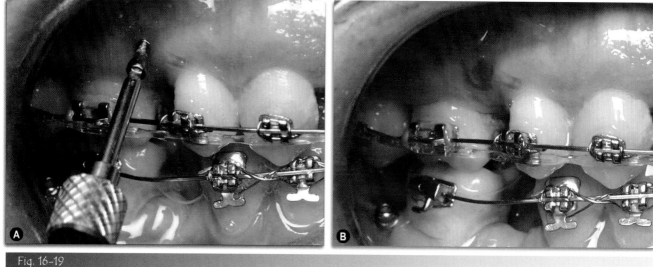

Fig. 16-19

MAS removal. **A,** Screwdriver used to remove MAS. **B,** Condition of miniscrew site after removal. Note that the removal procedure is generally done without local anesthesia and that the soft tissue usually heals within 7 to 10 days after removal.

force that could be generated, thereby minimizing miniscrew breakage.

Special attention is required during miniscrew placement to prevent injuries to local anatomic structures such as vessels, nerves, or tooth roots. Preplacement and postplacement radiographs with orthodontic wires bent and adjusted to the planned miniscrew site are helpful in this regard. In addition, the pilot hole should perforate the cortical bone only

to a depth of no more than 2 to 3 mm. Finally, anesthetic technique is critical. Local anesthesia should not be profound enough to anesthetize the PDL or tooth. Only the soft tissues and bone should be anesthetized. In this way, the patient will feel the miniscrew approaching the tooth root, and the MAS can be directed away from the tooth before contact is made. If, however, tooth root contact is made, endodontic treatment may be required (Fig. 16-20).

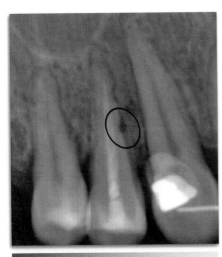

Fig. 16-20

Tooth root contact during miniscrew pilot hole preparation required endodontic treatment. Note radiograph taken at follow-up 2 years after endodontic treatment

SUMMARY

Orthodontic treatment results have often been compromised by orthodontists' lack of control over anchorage and inadequate patient compliance. The introduction of temporary anchorage devices overcomes these limitations. The MAS is one such device. The MAS is composed of three different sizes of titanium miniscrews that are broadly applicable in many different case types and can be placed in many sites within the oral cavity.

ACKNOWLEDGMENTS

The authors would like to thank Dr. Carolina Mannarini for her help in the preparation of this manuscript.

REFERENCES

1. Carano A, Velo S, Leone P, Siciliani G. Clinical applications of the miniscrew anchorage system. *J Clin Orthod.* 39(1):9-24, 2005.

2. Carano A, Lonardo P, Velo S, Incorvati C. Mechanical properties of three different commercially available miniscrews for skeletal anchorage. *Prog Orthod.* 6(1):82-97, 2005.

3. Block MS, Hoffman DR. A new device for absolute anchorage for orthodontics. *Am J Orthod Dentofacial Orthop.* 107:251-258, 1995.

4. Mura P, Maino BJ, Paoletto E. Midplant: l'ancoraggio assoluto in ortodonzia. *Ortodonzia Tecnica Marzo* 3:7-11, 2000.

5. Umemori M, Sugawara J. Skeletal anchorage system for open bite correction. *Am J Orthod. Dentofacial Orthop.* 115:166-174, 1999.

6. Ohmae M, Saito S, Mormhashi T, et al. A clinical and histological evaluation of titanium mini-implants as anchors for orthodontic intrusion in the beagle dog. *Am J Orthod Dentofacial Orthop.* 119:489-497, 2001.

7. Bolla E, Muratore F, Carano A, Bowman J. Evaluation of maxillary molar distalization with the Distal Jet: a comparison with other contemporary methods. *Angle Orthod.* 72(5):481-494, 2002.

8. Carano A, Machata B. Non compliance orthodontics: rapid molar intrusion, *J Clin Orthod.* 36(3):137-142, 2002.

9. Creekmore T, Eklund MK. The possibility of skeletal anchorage. *J Clin Orthod.* 17(4):266-269, 1983.

10. Kanomi R. Mini-implant for orthodontic anchorage. *J Clin Orthod.* 31:763-767, 1997.

11. Park HS. The skeletal cortical anchorage using titanium miniscrew implants. *Korean J Orthod.* 29:699-706, 1999.

12. Costa A, Raffainl M, Melsen B. Miniscrews as orthodontic anchorage: a preliminary report. *Int J Adult Orthodon Orthognath Surg.* 3:201-209, 1998.

13. Deguchi T, Takano-Yamamoto T, Kanomi R, et al. The use of small titanium screws for orthodontic anchorage. *J Dent Res.* 82(5):377-381, 2003.

14. Kyung HM, Park HS, Bae SM, et al: Development of orthodontic micro-implants for intraoral anchorage. *J Clin Orthod.* 37:321-328, 2003.

15. Poggio PM, Incorvati C, Velo S, Carano A. "Safe zones": a guide for miniscrew positioning in the maxillary and mandibular arch. *Angle Orthod.* 76(2):191-197, 2005.

16. Lindhe J, editor: *Textbook of Clinical Periodontology.* Copenhagen, Denmark: Munksgaard, 1984.

17. Carano A, Ciocia C, Farronato G. Use of lingual brackets for deep bite corrections. *J Clin Orthod.* 35:449-450, 2001.

18. Carano A, Bowman SJ. The monkey hook: an auxiliary for impacted, rotated, and displaced teeth. *J Clin Orthod.* 36:375-378, 2002.

The C-Implant

Kyu-Rhim Chung, Seong-Hun Kim, Yoon-Ah Kook

Recently, orthodontic temporary anchorage devices (OrthoTADs) have increased in popularity. These intraosseous anchorage devices enable clinicians to move teeth easily and rapidly without extraoral appliances. However, the conventional one-component designs are used only as anchorage reinforcement (see Chapters 9 to 16).[1-7] The C-orthodontic mini-implant (C-implant®, Cimplant Co., Seoul, Korea), however, was designed to be an independent orthodontic appliance capable of accommodating an arch wire for anterior retraction. The unique design of the screw component increases mechanical retention and osseointegration because of the surface treatment of the implant. The C-implant therefore represents the third generation of implant orthodontics. The conventional prosthetic implant used for orthodontic anchorage was the first generation, and miniscrew implants (MSIs) and miniplate implants (MPIs) used along with conventional orthodontic treatment are the second generation.

THE C-IMPLANT

The C-implant (Fig. 17-1) is a unique titanium device that provides stability through mechanical retention and osseointegration (Fig. 17-2).[8-10] The C-implant has two parts, a head component and a screw component. The screw-shaped component is 1.8 mm in diameter and is available in lengths of 8.5, 9.5, or 10.5 mm. The entire surface, except for the coronal 2 mm (transmucosal collar), is sandblasted, large grit, and acid etched (SLA)

for optimal osseointegration. The head component is 2.5 mm in diameter with a 0.032-inch diameter hole and a neck length of 5.35, 6.35, or 7.35 mm. Each implant comes packaged in a sterile vial and blister pack.

Screw Component

In contrast to conventional MSIs, the screw maintains a constant diameter throughout its length, tapering only slightly at the apex (Fig. 17-3).[1-2] The C-implant is placed in a self-tapping procedure. Because of the width of the apex, the C-implant does not tend to damage the root surface during placement. If the

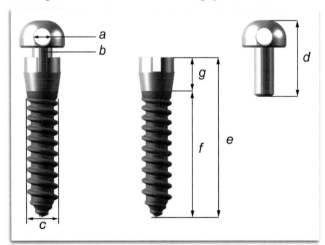

Schematic drawing of the C-implant. *(a)* A 0.032-inch diameter hole for arch wire, *(b)* neck, *(c)* 1.8-mm diameter screw, *(d)* head component, *(e)* screw component, *(f)* SLA surface, *(g)* 2-mm long polished transmucosal collar.

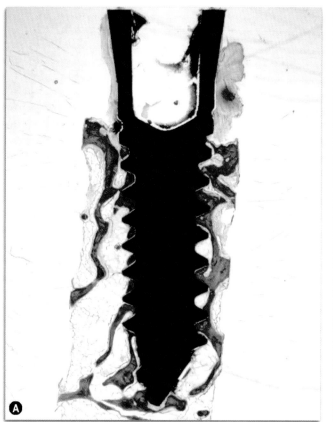
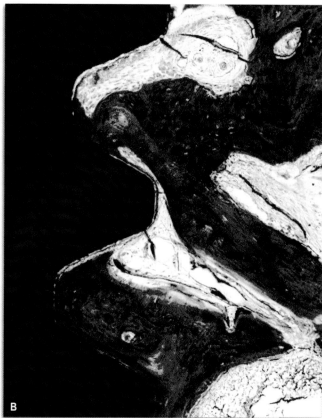

Fig. 17-2

Histologic view of C-implant removed from human alveolus. **A,** 5× magnification. **B,** 100× magnification.

apex of the implant does come in contact with a root surface, the screw cannot perforate the root. At this point, the clinician should discontinue placement and choose another site. The coronal 2 mm of the screw component (transmucosal collar) is polished for soft tissue contact. The entire screw length apical to the transmucosal collar is SLA treated, which maximizes the bone-to-implant contact surface area (Fig. 17-4). Lee and Chung[11] demonstrated that there was no difference between immediately loaded or delayed-loaded C-implants. Their evaluation criteria included osseointegration and bone healing at the implant site upon implant removal.

Head Component

The titanium head is connected to the screw by tapping the neck of the head into an internal hole in the screw with a mallet. This procedure provides mechanical retention without cement or bonding material. The connection between the head and the screw is strong enough to control torque and three-dimensional tooth movement while resisting rotational forces. The two-component design allows placement of the screw

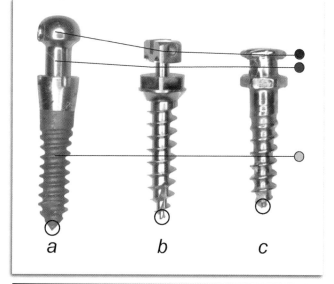

Fig. 17-3

Miniscrew implants. *(a)* C-implant two-component design. The head *(maroon)* is separated from the body *(gold)* by the neck *(blue)*. Note the long span of neck, the polished of the transmucosal collar, and that the SLA surface differs from other systems. *(b)* and *(c)* One-component systems.

component only, thereby preventing undue forces to the neck of the head. This eliminates any potential for

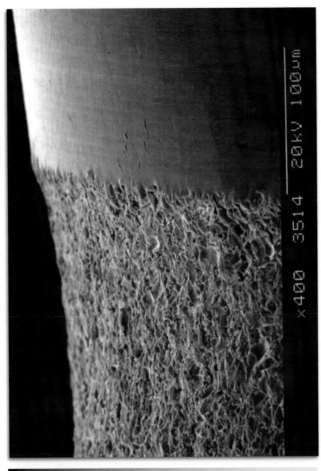

Fig. 17-4

Scanning electron micrograph of C-implant. Note the SLA surface treatment *(bottom)* and polished transmucosal collar *(top)*.

fracture that may occur with other systems. The longer span between the head and the screw components prevents gingival irritation during retraction and also makes it possible to apply multidirectional forces. The clinician can choose the most appropriate length of the neck based on anatomic variation of each patient.

Two-Component Advantage

The force applied from the screwdriver tip to the screw itself differs from most one-component systems. Usually the screwdriver tip fits into the head of one-component screws, potentially applying too much force to the neck during placement or removal. As a result, the neck may fracture in some systems.[12] The C-implant, in contrast, applies a force only to the screw and not to the head, thereby eliminating this potential problem. In addition, the C-implant is less tapered, so it distributes forces more evenly along the length of the screw, reducing the risk of fracturing during placement and removal (Fig. 17-5).

TREATMENT PLANNING

The C-implant is an independent appliance that can be used for anchorage without using the posterior teeth and without changing the posterior occlusion. This biocreative therapy™ is appropriate for cases that require no loss of posterior anchorage, such as in patients who have an ideally intercuspated posterior occlusion in combination with anterior protrusion and crowding. The C-implant can also be used in cases with inadequate posterior anchorage caused by severe dental caries, advanced periodontal disease, or missing teeth. Similar to other MSIs, the C-implant can also function efficiently as an auxiliary for the distalization or intrusion of posterior teeth or for attaching intermaxillary elastics for retraction of anterior teeth or protraction of posterior teeth.

This MSI can be placed in just about any site in alveolar bone because of its small diameter, but the ideal position for anterior retraction without altering the posterior occlusion is between the second premolar and the first molar. If, however, the interradicular space is too small or the alveolar bone is inadequate because of pneumatization of the maxillary sinus, another site should be chosen. The next best choice is between the first and second molars. The placement of C-implants in adolescents should be performed only after eruption of the second premolar.

PRESURGICAL ORTHODONTICS

The C-implant can be applied without banding or bonding, which saves time and allows immediate loading. In patients who have systemic diseases such as diabetes, osteoporosis, osteopenia, or hyperparathyroidism and in those who are smokers or patients undergoing head and neck radiation therapy, Gapski and colleagues[13] strongly suggest following the standard two-stage implant protocol or even using longer periods of healing. In the two-stage protocol, the implant is placed in stage 1 and is uncovered/loaded in stage 2, usually several months later when osseointegration has occurred. Because diseases that directly affect bone metabolism may influence implant healing significantly, C-implants placed in these patients preferably should not be loaded until osseointegration is complete.

SURGICAL PROCEDURE

For en masse retraction, C-implants are usually placed in the interradicular spaces between the second premolar and first molar or the first and second molars, using either an open or a closed technique. The surgical kit for C-implant placement includes the C-implant in a sterile package, a 1.5-mm diameter pilot hole drill, a screw holder, a screwdriver, mosquito hemostats, a dental mirror handle, and a mallet (Fig. 17-6). Before the surgical procedure, the patient should rinse for 3 minutes with 0.2% chlorhexidine.

Stage 1: Screw Placement
Perform stage 1 of implantation as follows (Fig. 17-7):

1. Administer infiltration anesthesia (2% lidocaine with

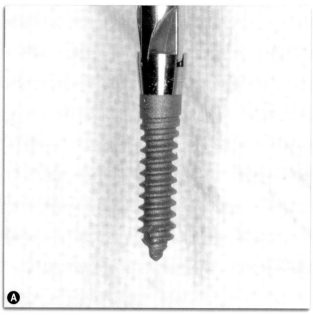

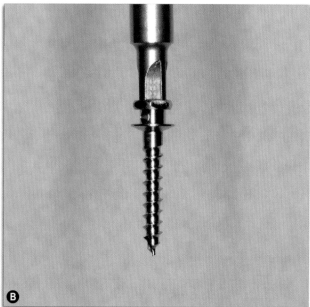

Fig. 17-5

Screwdriver adaptation. **A,** The screwdriver tip of the C-implant fits directly into the screw. **B,** The screwdriver tip of a one-component system fits into the head of the screw, potentially weakening the screw by overloading the neck with a hole in it.

1:100,000 epinephrine) at the mucogingival junction and into the surgical area.
2. Scrub the implant site with H_2O_2 and air dry.
3. Determine the C-implant position based on evaluation of the periapical radiograph and intraoral anatomy. Mark the estimated root position by indenting the keratinized gingiva with an explorer.
4. Use a No. 15 blade to make an incision only if the attached gingiva is insufficient and the implant site is surrounded by mucosa. (Fig. 17-8 demonstrates the open method.)
5. Use a slow-speed handpiece (500 rpm, 40 N-cm) with copious isotonic saline irrigation to place a 1.5-mm pilot hole through the cortical bone. Only the cortex should be perforated, not the cancellous bone. Bleeding is a sign of penetration by the drill through the cortical bone and into the cancellous bone.
6. Remove the color-coded cap from the sterile package and place the screwdriver tip into the screw (Fig. 17-9).
7. Screw the C-implant clockwise into the pilot hole until the top of C-implant body is level with the gingival surface and the soft tissue collar penetrates the soft tissue.

Stage 2: Head Connection
Stage 2 can be done either during the same appointment as stage 1 or weeks to months later after osseointegration has occurred. Perform stage 2 of implantation as follows (Fig. 17-10):

1. Hold the head with a mosquito hemostat and insert the neck into the screw.
2. Insert the tip of an explorer into the hole in the head and rotate the head until the hole is parallel to the occlusal plane.
3. Connect the head to the screw by placing the shaft of a dental mirror between the mallet and the head. Lightly tap with a small mallet 1 to 2 times to seat the head into the screw.
4. Immediately apply orthodontic force to stable implants in dense bone. Verify the stability of the C-implant 4 weeks postoperatively.

Image Transfer System and Surgical Template
Inaccurate placement of MSIs adjacent to tooth roots, particularly when the adjacent teeth are being moved, may damage a root. This damage may occur not only during placement but also if the MSI lies in the path of a moving tooth, which potentially could lead to pressure-induced necrosis or root resorption. Considering this, the use of an accurately fabricated surgical template may provide a tool for ideal placement of MSIs. Our group has recently developed the x-ray Image Transfer System to aid in the transfer of dental anatomy (crown and root location) from a periapical radiograph to a dental model (Fig. 17-11).

The components necessary for Image Transfer System implementation are a standard periapical radiograph,

Fig. 17-6

C-implant surgical kit: two C-implants, 1.5-mm diameter pilot hole drills with the screw holder, a screwdriver, mosquito hemostats, a dental mirror handle, and a mallet.

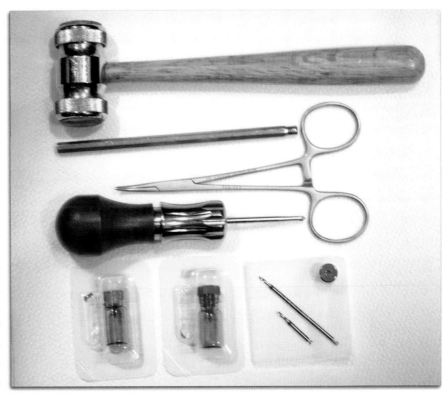

photographic emulsion, a dental model, a film projector, and a film development set. First, expose a periapical radiograph taken with the parallel exposure technique in the planned implant site, including the entire crowns and roots of the adjacent teeth. Second, take an impression of the dentition, including the vestibule, and pour it in dental stone. If applicable, remove all orthodontic attachments from the model. Third, paint the model with a silver halide photographic emulsion (Liquid Light VC; Rockland Colloid

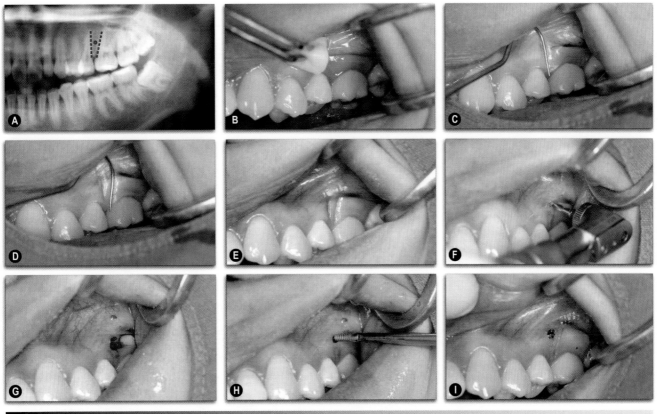

Fig. 17-7

Stage 1 implant procedure: closed method. **A,** Determine implant location using panoramic radiograph. **B,** After local anesthesia, scrub the implant site with H_2O_2 and air dry. **C,** Mark the distal root position on the keratinized gingiva with an explorer. **D,** Mark the mesial root position on the keratinized gingiva with an explorer. **E,** Resultant gingival indentation shows estimated root positions. **F,** Drill pilot hole using slow-speed handpiece at 500 rpm under saline irrigation. **G,** Resulting pilot hole. **H,** Screw the C-implant clockwise into the pilot hole. **I,** The top of the soft tissue collar should be level with the gingival surface.

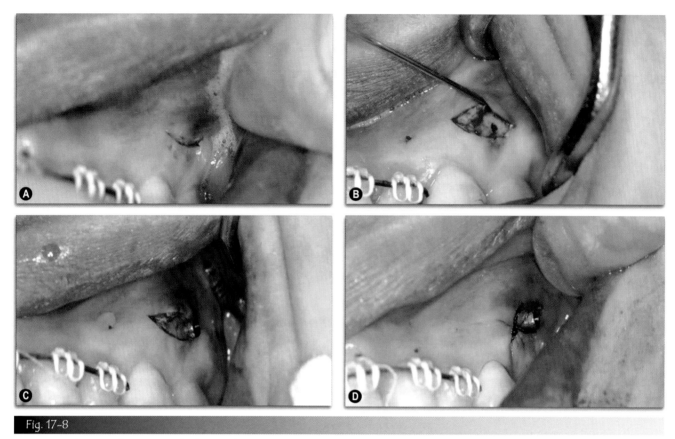

Fig. 17-8

Stage 1 implant procedure: open method. **A,** Semilunar incision at implant site. **B,** Flap reflection. **C,** Screw in place;. **D,** Single-suture closure.

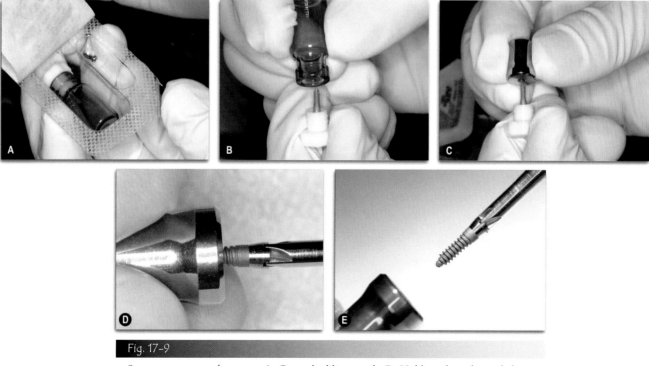

Fig. 17-9

Screw component placement. **A,** Open the blister pack. **B,** Holding the color-coded cap inferiorly, remove the cap and the implant. **C,** Place the apex of the implant in the screw holder. **D,** Insert the screwdriver tip into the screw. **E,** The screw is ready to be placed.

Co., Piermont, New York). Because this is a light-sensitive product, this and subsequent steps must be carried out in a darkroom. Allow the model to dry,

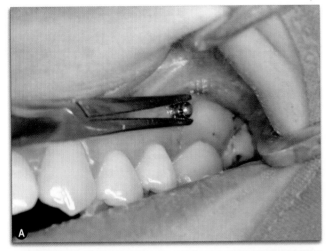

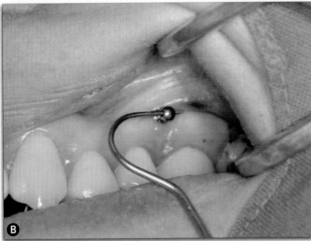

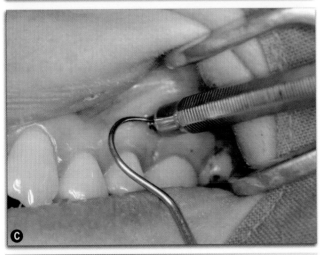

Fig. 17-10

Head component placement. **A,** Hold the head with mosquito hemostats. **B,** Insert explorer into hole to orient parallel to occlusal plane, and stabilize. **C,** Place a dental mirror handle onto the head and lightly tap the head into the screw with a small mallet.

which takes about 60 minutes. Fourth, project the periapical radiographic image onto the model using a safe light filter over the projector. It is important to line the image up exactly with the crowns so that the root anatomy is lined up accurately on the model. After exactly matching the image to the model anatomy, remove the safe filter and expose the emulsion-coated model for about 6 seconds. Fifth, process and develop the exposed model in a procedure similar to that for photographic film. The resulting image on the model is opposite that of the radiograph—the crowns and roots are black, and the bone is white. Sixth, fabricate a surgical stent using cold-cure acrylic on the image-transferred model. After polymerization, trim the surgical stent and drill the pilot hole.

The benefits of the Image Transfer System system include cost-effectiveness and decreased radiation compared with computed tomography or the multiple exposures required when ideally placing a wire guide. During surgery, the surgical stent provides a more accurate and safe placement of the screw. Moreover, the stent is placed not only for the pilot hole but also for MSI placement and is easily removed afterward.

ORTHODONTIC MECHANICS

Using the C-implant, several different traditional clinical mechanics situations are possible. These situations include tip-back mechanics (Fig. 17-12), multiloop edgewise arch wire (MEAW) mechanics (Fig. 17-13), or en masse distalization of the entire upper dentition by applying closed coil springs to only two upper C-implants (Fig. 17-14). In addition, the C-implant can be used as an anchor for a closed coil spring to protract posterior teeth (Fig. 17-15) or an open coil spring to upright molars (Fig. 17-16).

The C-implant can also be used as an independent orthodontic appliance during en masse retraction of anterior teeth without posterior bonding or banding (Fig. 17-17). En masse movement is performed using an 0.016 × 0.022-inch blue Elgiloy arch wire (Elgiloy Specialty Metals, Elgin, Illinois) as the initial wire. Usually, 3/16-inch, 3.5-oz elastics are used for canine retraction, while at the same time the incisors are retracted using 1/4-inch, 3.5-oz elastics attached to soldered hooks between the canines and lateral incisors (Fig. 17-18). After retraction, traditional fixed appliances, clear aligners, or tooth positioners can be used for final detailing.

For intermaxillary fixation during orthognathic surgery, C-implants are usually placed in the

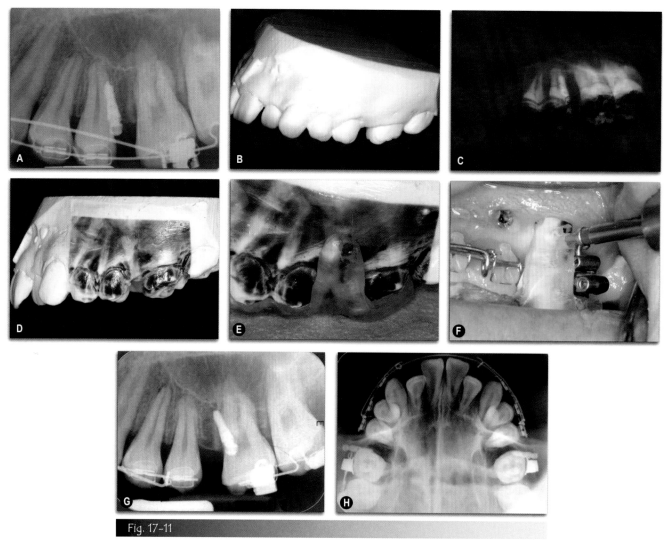

Fig. 17–11

Image Transfer System and surgical stent for molar distalization. **A,** Initial periapical radiograph. Note that this C-implant had been used to distalize the molars and is being removed and re-placed in another location for retraction of the anterior teeth. **B,** Emulsion-coated model. **C,** X-ray image projected onto model. **D,** Final image-transferred model. Note faint red line demarcating mesial of molar root and faint red circle indicating implant location. **E,** Surgical stent on model. **F,** Surgical stent used for pilot hole drill. **G,** Final periapical radiograph of new implant location. **H,** Final occlusal radiograph of new implant location.

interradicular spaces between the canines and first premolars (Fig. 17-19).[14] The intermaxillary fixation C-implants can be used as anchorage for postoperative orthodontic treatment and for outpatient intermaxillary traction as needed.

REMOVAL PROCEDURE

Apply topical anesthetic to the implant site (Fig. 17-20). Remove the head from the screw by inserting the tip of an explorer or using Howe pliers to pull the head laterally away from the screw. Then remove the screw by rotating the screwdriver counterclockwise. If the screw resists removal, heavy wire pliers can be placed slightly

subgingivally to grab around the circumference of the transmucosal collar for rotation and removal. This may traumatize the soft tissue slightly, but the tissue will heal within 7 to 10 days.

POTENTIAL COMPLICATIONS

Although complications are possible, they are rare. Mobility 1 to 3 weeks after screw placement indicates implant failure. The failed C-implant should be removed but can be re-placed in the same patient. The procedure for re-placement is as follows: (1) separate the head from the screw and clean the surface with water irrigation, and (2) sandblast the screw surface, autoclave it, and re-place it using the standard surgical procedure outlined previously.

Another possible problem that may allow loosening of the C-implant is contact with the periodontal ligament. Loosening would occur because of incomplete or inadequate bone volume around the circumference of the screw. If a second site is not available in this situation, a C-tube® (KLS Martin LP, Jacksonville, Florida; see Chapter 20) can be substituted for the C-implant to achieve the same results.

SUMMARY

The two-component C-implant provides several practical advantages over other MSIs in certain circumstances. One such advantage is in retraction of anterior teeth without posterior bonding or banding. This is possible by passing the distal extent of the arch wire through the hole in the head to allow sliding of the arch wire during retraction.

The surface treatment increases the possibility of osseointegration, which may be a benefit in cases requiring heavier orthodontic and orthopedic forces. The nontapering design of the screw allows forces to be distributed more evenly along the length of the screw, thereby decreasing the risk of fracture during placement or removal. Finally, the C-implant causes less soft tissue irritation because the neck length moves the head away from the soft tissue.

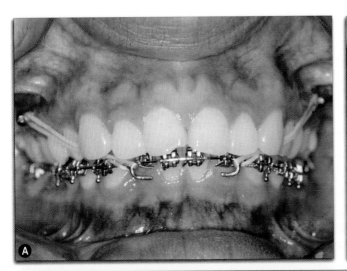
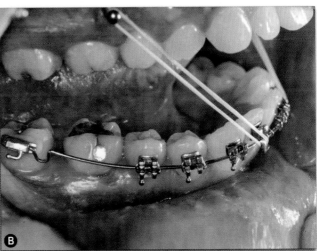

Fig. 17-12

C-implant used as hooks for Class III intermaxillary elastics for Tweed tip-back mechanics. **A,** Anterior photograph. **B,** Buccal photograph.

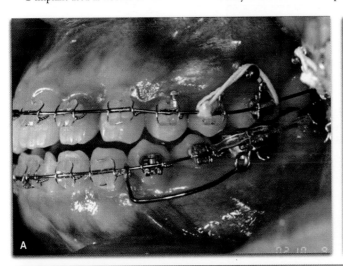
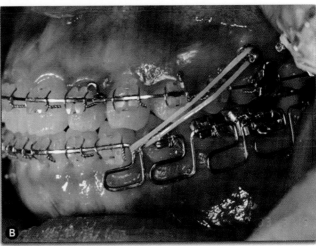

Fig. 17-13

Upper molar intrusion and multiloop edgewise arch wire mechanics. **A,** Buccal photograph of intrusion. **B,** Buccal photograph of multiloop edgewise arch wire mechanics.

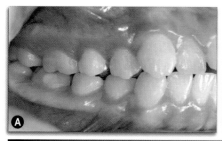 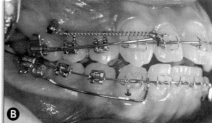 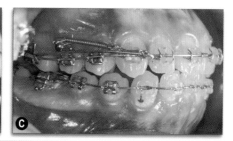

Fig. 17–14

Upper arch distalization after second molar extraction in Class II malocclusion. **A,** Initial buccal photograph. **B,** Progress buccal photograph using 0.018 × 0.025-inch stainless steel sliding jigs and NiTi closed coil springs. **C,** Final buccal photograph.

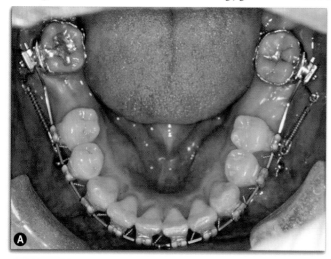 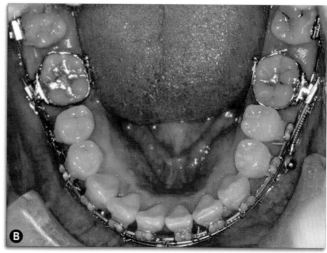

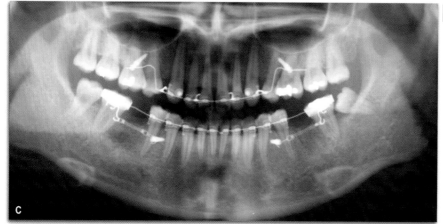

Fig. 17–15

Protraction of posterior teeth using a NiTi closed coil spring from the C-implant to auxiliary hooks on the lower second molars. **A,** Occlusal photograph before protraction. **B,** Occlusal photograph 8 months later. **C,** Panoramic radiograph before protraction. **D,** Panoramic radiograph 8 months later.

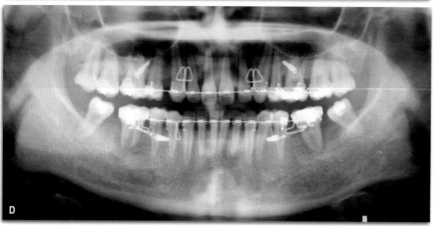

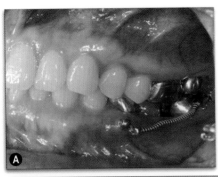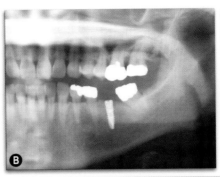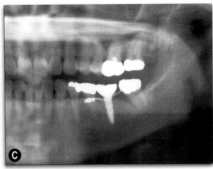

Fig. 17-16

Molar uprighting. **A,** Buccal photograph. **B,** Panoramic radiograph before uprighting. **C,** Panoramic radiograph after uprighting. Note the angle between the implant and tipped molar long axes changed 15 degrees.

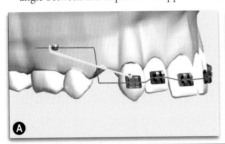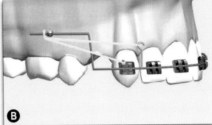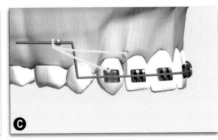

Fig. 17-17

C-orthodontic treatment mechanics using C-implant as a substitute for posterior anchorage teeth during en masse retraction of upper anterior dentition. **A,** 0.016 × 0.022-inch blue Elgiloy is used as initial arch wire for leveling and alignment with ³/₁₆-inch, 3.5-oz elastics used for canine retraction. **B,** Soldered hooks and ¼-inch, 3.5-oz elastics are added for en masse retraction of upper anterior teeth. **C,** Final position of anterior teeth.

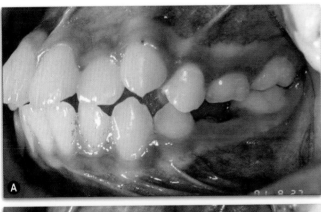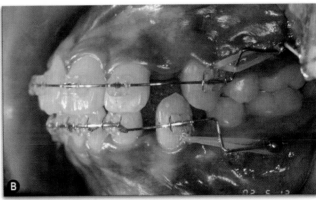

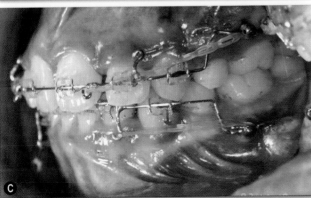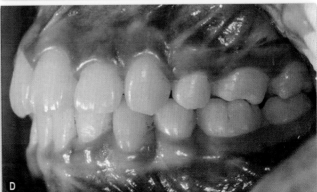

Fig. 17-18

En masse retraction of six anterior teeth in adolescent patient. **A,** Initial buccal photograph; **B,** Progress buccal photograph at start of retraction; **C,** Progress buccal photograph at end of retraction; **D,** Final buccal photograph.

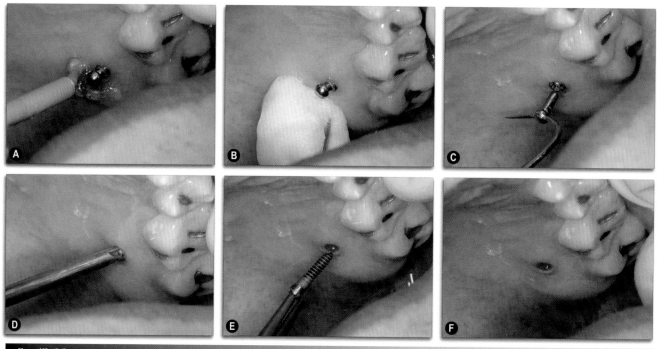

Fig. 17-19

An additional use for the C-implant is for intermaxillary fixation during and after orthognathic surgery.

ACKNOWLEDGMENTS

Supported in part by the Korean Society of Speedy Orthodontics.

REFERENCES

1. Kanomi R. Mini-implant for orthodontic anchorage. *J Clin Orthod.* 31:763-767, 1997.
2. Kyung HM, Park HS, Bae SM, et al. Development of orthodontic micro-implants for intraoral anchorage. *J Clin Orthod.* 37:321-328, 2003.
3. Kyung SH, Hong SG, Park YC. Distalization of maxillary molars with a midpalatal miniscrew. *J Clin Orthod.* 37:22-26, 2003.
4. Maino BG, Bender J, Pagin P, et al. The spider screw for skeletal anchorage. *J Clin Orthod.* 37:90-97, 2003.
5. Costa A, Raffaini M, Melsen B. Microscrews as orthodontic anchorage: a preliminary report. *Int J Adult Orthodon Orthognath Surg.* 13:201-209, 1998.
6. Melsen B, Verna C. A rational approach to orthodontic anchorage. *Prog Orthod.* 1:10-22, 1999.
7. Wehrbein H, Diedrich P. Endosseous titanium implants during and after orthodontic loading an experimental study. *Clin Oral Implants Res.* 4:76-82, 1993.
8. Chung KR, Kim SH, Kook YA. C-orthodontic microimplant. *J Clin Orthod.* 38:478-486, 2004.
9. Chung KR, Kim SH, Kook YA. C-orthodontic microimplant for distalization of mandibular dentition in Class III correction. *Angle Orthod.* 175:119-128, 2005
10. Simon H, Caputo AA. Removal torque of immediately loaded transitional endosseous implants in human subjects. *Int J Oral Maxillofac Implants.* 17:839-845, 2002.
11. Lee SJ, Chung KR. The effect of early loading on the direct bone-to-implant surface contact of the orthodontic osseointegrated titanium implant. *Korean J Orthod.* 31:173-185, 2001.
12. Lim JW, Kim WS, Kim IK, et al. Three dimensional finite element method for stress distribution on the length and diameter of orthodontic miniscrew and cortical bone thickness. *Korean J Orthod.* 33:11-20, 2003.
13. Gapski R, Wang HL, Mascarenhas P, et al. Critical review of immediate loading. *Clin Oral Implants Res.* 14:515-527, 2003.
14. Jones DC: The intermaxillary screw: a dedicated bicortical bone screw for temporary intermaxillary fixation. *Br J Oral Maxillofac Surg.* 37:115-116, 1999.

Fig. 17-20

Removal procedure. **A,** Topically anesthetize the implant site. **B,** Scrub the implant site with H_2O_2 and air dry. **C,** Insert explorer tip into hole in head and remove the head component. **D,** Insert the screwdriver tip into the screw. **E,** Rotate the screw counterclockwise and remove. **F,** No sutures are necessary.

SECTION 5

MiniScrew Implant Case Reports

MSI Case Reports (Continued)

Introduction to Case Reports

Jason B. Cope

The implementation of any orthodontic treatment regimen requires a fundamental understanding of the indications and contraindications, diagnostic and treatment planning criteria, and the basic biologic and biomechanical tenets governing orthodontic mechanotherapy. With this in mind, the chapters were written to provide the historical background and basic concepts required to implement orthodontic temporary anchorage devices (OrthoTADs) on a clinical level. Theory and clinical technique alone, however, often leave a void of clinical treatment examples. The age-old expression "there is more than one way to skin a cat" certainly applies in clinical orthodontics, in that similar cases may be treated by a multitude of different biomechanical approaches. For example, a Class II maxillary protrusive malocclusion can be treated with TADs either by extracting maxillary premolars with maximum anterior retraction or by distalizing the entire maxillary arch. In light of this, it is important to illustrate the various ways that a single case category may be treated. Therefore, a case report section follows each of the three major TAD sections: miniscrew implants (MSIs), palatal implants (PIs), and miniplate implants (MPIs).

The case reports were designed to provide only the basic diagnostic and treatment information (primarily in tabular form) necessary to understand the case, relying more on photographs, radiographs, and superimpositions for illustration of the case, as well as the mechanics used in OrthoTAD treatment. Considering this editorial decision, it is important for the reader to understand the basic layout, because all case reports are identical for both consistency and direct comparison of one case to another. Only cases that had finished treatment with complete diagnostic records were accepted. These guidelines were created to provide the best possible scenario for case-to-case comparison.

Every case report has a brief summary, three tables, photographs, panoramic radiographs, and a superimposition. For tooth identification, the international tooth identification system (Fédération Dentaire Internationale) was chosen (Fig. CR-1). For all facial profile photographs, the profile always faces the right side of the page. For all panoramic radiographs, the patient's left side appears on the right side of the page, as if the reader is facing the patient. No cephalometric radiographs were included. This was done in the interest of space requirements. Instead, the cephalometric information can be ascertained directly from the cephalometric summary in Table 3 and from the superimposition, which also always faces the right side of the page. For the superimpositions, only the pretreatment (black) and posttreatment (red) tracings were used to prevent confusion from having too many lines.

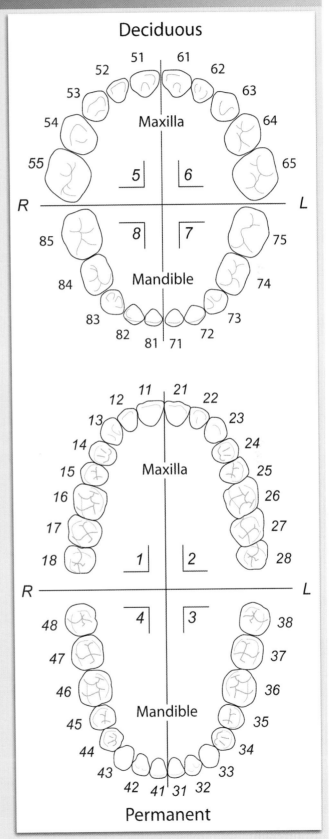

Fig. CR-1. Fédération Dentaire Internationale tooth ID system.

Three tables are used. Table 1 (Diagnosis and Treatment Goals) presents the original diagnosis in the left column, with the final treatment goals for the same values in the right column. These data are categorized based on skeletal, dental, facial soft tissue, periodontium, and other factors. For each item, the author was provided with a specific set of responses from which to choose (Table CR-1). Table 2 (Temporary Anchorage Device Summary) presents the pertinent data for the TAD(s) used: date of placement, loading, unloading, and removal; location of placement; and forces/mechanics used. *Direct* anchorage is the term

used when the TAD is attached directly to the teeth of the active segment for tooth movement. *Indirect* anchorage is the term used when the TAD is attached to and reinforces the teeth of the reactive segment, which is directly used to move the teeth of the active segment. Table 3 (Cephalometric Summary) presents the specific cephalometric values for pretreatment, pre-TAD placement, TAD removal, and posttreatment. At a minimum, the pretreatment and posttreatment values had to be available for the case to be acceptable. This information also was categorized based on skeletal, dental,

Table CR-1.	Diagnosis and Treatment Goals Responses Possible
SKELETAL	
Anteroposterior	Class I, Class II, Class III
Vertical	Normal, deep bite, open bite
Transverse	Normal, bilateral crossbite, bilateral buccal crossbite (Brody bite), bilateral constriction, right crossbite, left crossbite
DENTAL	
Right molar	Class I, End-on Class II, Class II, End-on Class III, Class III
Right canine	Class I, End-on Class II, Class II, End-on Class III, Class III
Left molar	Class I, End-on Class II, Class II, End-on Class III, Class III
Left canine	Class I, End-on Class II, Class II, End-on Class III, Class III
Upper right	X mm crowding or spacing
Upper left	X mm crowding or spacing
Lower right	X mm crowding or spacing
Lower left	X mm crowding or spacing
Missing teeth	Insert tooth numbers
Restore teeth	Insert tooth numbers
Overjet	X mm (positive or negative)
Overbite	X mm (positive or negative)
Upper ML	X mm to right or left of facial midline
Lower ML	X mm to right or left of facial midline
SOFT TISSUE	
Profile	Convex, concave, straight, full
Lips	Competent or incompetent
PERIODONTIUM	
Inadequate KT/TT	Insert tooth numbers
Gingival recession	Insert tooth numbers
Bone loss	Insert tooth numbers
OTHER	Insert other factors not listed above

KT/TT, Keratinized tissue/thin tissue; *ML,* midline.

and facial soft tissues. Because a variety of cephalometric values are in use, a succinct standardized list was designed (Fig. CR-2).

The summary of each case has four specific written responses:

1. Treatment plan: How were the treatment goals to be achieved?
2. Treatment progress: How did treatment progress? (This was used only if progress was different from that planned.)
3. Treatment results: What were the results achieved? (This was used only if the results were different from that planned.)

4. Complications: What problem occurred unexpectedly that was not anticipated? How was it corrected? How could it be prevented? (This was used only if complications occurred.)

It should be apparent that only the treatment plan summary was mandatory. The other three were used only if necessary.

Finally, in each major TAD section, similar cases are grouped together. For example, retraction cases appear together, distalization cases appear together, and intrusion cases appear together. This was done in an attempt to facilitate case comparison.

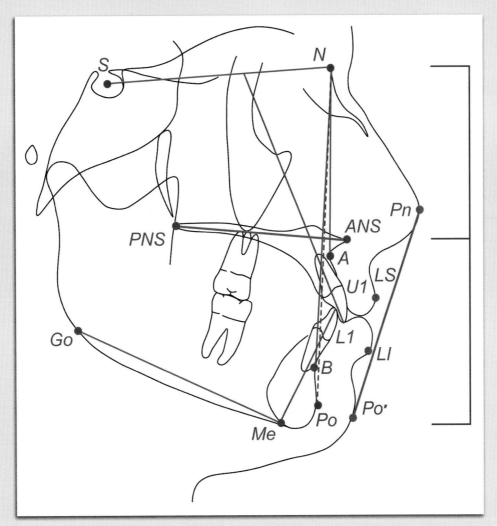

Fig. CR-2. Lateral cephalometric landmarks and measurements. *A*, A point; *ANS*, anterior nasal spine; *B*, B point; *Go*, gonion; *L1*, lower central incisor; *LI*, labrale inferius; *LS*, labrale superius; *Me*, menton; *N*, nasion; *Pn*, pronasale; *PNS*, posterior nasal spine; *Po*, pogonion; *Po'*, soft tissue pogonion; *S*, sella; *U1*, upper central incisor.

CR-MSI

Nonextraction Treatment for Resolution of Anterior Crowding

Kyu-Rhim Chung

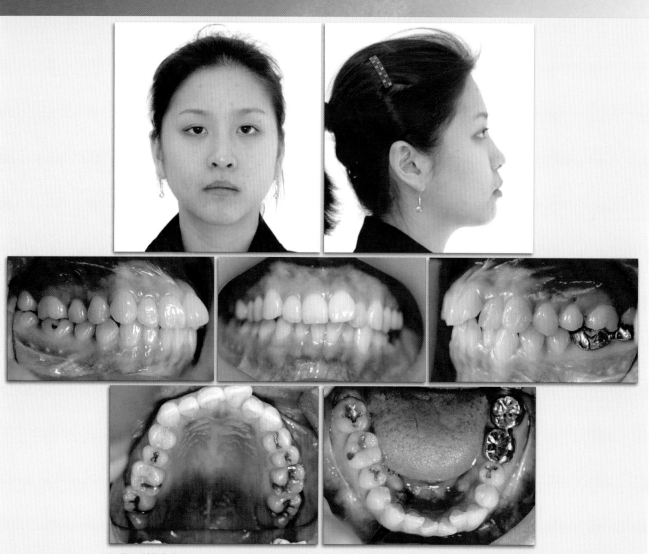

Fig. MSI 1-1. Pretreatment photographs.

Because of the patient's desire to avoid premolar extraction, the treatment plan was to use upper C-implants (Cimplant Co., Seoul, Korea) to resolve the anterior crowding. The strategy was to use the implants in the upper arch to directly distalize the entire upper arch so as to resolve the upper crowding without allowing the anterior teeth to move forward. In the lower arch, tip back mechanics would be used for distalizing the lower dentition while using the upper implants for Class III elastics wear to prevent the lower anterior teeth from moving forward.

The lower arch was distalized using an 0.018-inch NiTi arch wire with an 0.019 × 0.025-inch stainless steel sliding jig to the second molars. Class III elastics ($5/16$ inch, 3.5 oz) were worn from the upper C-implant to the lower sliding jig. Afterward, 0.019 × 0.025-inch stainless steel uprighting sectional arch wires were added for tipping back of the lower first molars. Elastics (³/₁₆ inch, 3.5 oz) were worn from the C-implant to the upper second premolars and first molars for intrusion during leveling of upper second molars while in an 0.016 × 0.022-inch stainless steel arch wire that bypassed the anterior teeth. After leveling, power chain was applied from the C-implant to the upper canines for group distal movement and decrowding of the upper dentition. The only problem encountered was a lack of compliance in wearing intramaxillary Class I elastics for group distal movement of upper dentition. Therefore, the force was changed from elastics to power chain in the latter part of treatment.

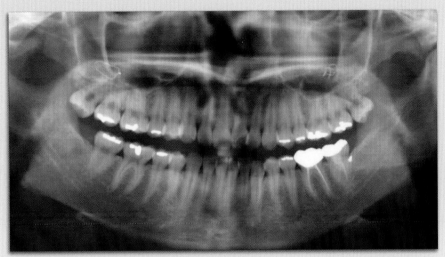

Fig. MSI 1–2. Pretreatment panoramic radiograph.

Table MSI 1–1.	Diagnosis and Treatment Goals	
	Diagnosis	Treatment Goals
SKELETAL		
Anteroposterior	Class II	Class II
Vertical	Normal	Normal
Transverse	Normal	Normal
DENTAL		
Right molar	End-on Class II	Class I
Right canine	Class II	Class I
Left molar	Class I	Class I
Left canine	End-on Class II	Class I
Upper right	3 mm crowding	None
Upper left	2 mm crowding	None
Lower right	2 mm crowding	None
Lower left	2 mm crowding	None
Missing teeth	No. 38, 48	No. 18, 28, 38, 48
Restore teeth	N/A	N/A
Overjet	3 mm	3 mm
Overbite	1.5 mm	2 mm
Upper ML	1 mm left of facial ML	0 mm to facial ML
Lower ML	0 mm to facial ML	0 mm to facial ML
SOFT TISSUE		
Profile	Convex	Straight
Lips	Incompetent	Competent
PERIODONTIUM		
Inadequate KT/TT	None	None
Gingival recession	None	None
Bone loss	None	None

KT/TT, Keratinized tissue/thin tissue; *ML,* midline; *N/A,* not applicable.

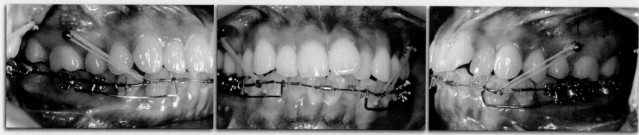

Fig. MSI 1-3. Initial temporary anchorage device (TAD) photographs.

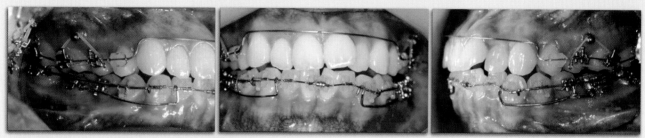

Fig. MSI 1-4. First progress TAD photographs.

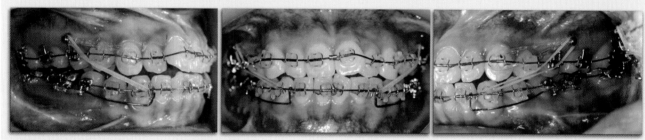

Fig. MSI 1-5. Second progress TAD photographs.

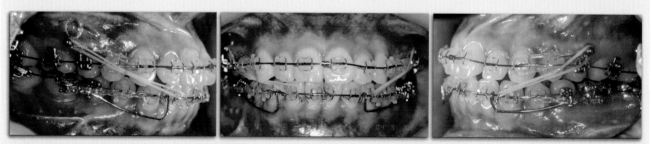

Fig. MSI 1-6. Third progress TAD photographs.

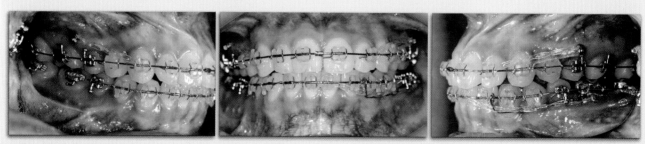

Fig. MSI 1-7. Final TAD photographs.

Table MSI 1–2.	Temporary Anchorage Device Summary	
Procedure	Data	
Appliances placed	14 Apr 2004	
TAD placed	7 Apr 2004	7 Apr 2004
Location of TAD	Distofacial No. 15	Distofacial No. 25
Type of TAD	MSI	MSI
TAD loaded	14 Apr 2004	14 Apr 2004
Healing duration	7 days	7 days
Force in grams	250-500	250-500
Mechanics used	Direct	Direct
TAD unloaded	10 Mar 2005	10 Mar 2005
TAD loading duration	11 months	11 months
TAD removed	23 Mar 2005	23 Mar 2005
Appliances removed	22 Mar 2005	
Treatment duration	11 months	

TAD, Temporary anchorage device; *MSI*, miniscrew implant.

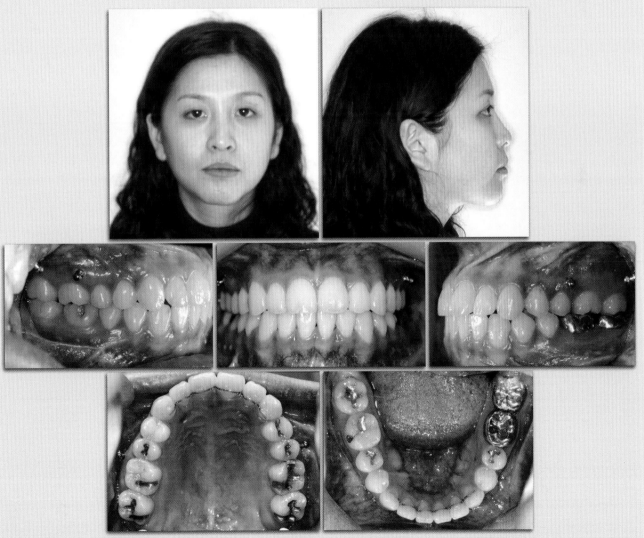

Fig. MSI 1–8. Posttreatment photographs.

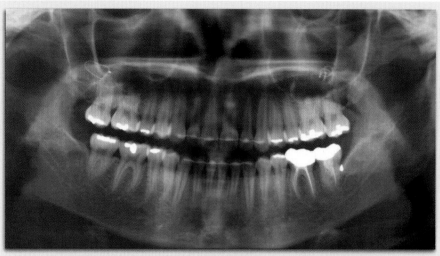

Fig. MSI 1–9. Posttreatment panoramic radiograph.

Table MSI 1-3.	Cephalometric Summary	
	Pretreatment	Posttreatment
SKELETAL		
SNA (degrees)	86.0	85.5
SNB (degrees)	82.0	81.0
ANB (degrees)	4.0	4.5
SN-ANS/PNS (degrees)	12.0	12.5
SN-GoMe (degrees)	29.5	29.0
N-ANS (mm)	55.0	54.0
ANS-Me (mm)	64.0	63.0
DENTAL		
U1-SN (degrees)	115.0	106.0
L1-GoMe (degrees)	102.0	98.0
U1-APo (mm)	9.5	7.5
L1-APo (mm)	4.0	4.0
SOFT TISSUE		
LS-PnPo' (mm)	1.5	1.0
LI-PnPo' (mm)	3.5	2.5

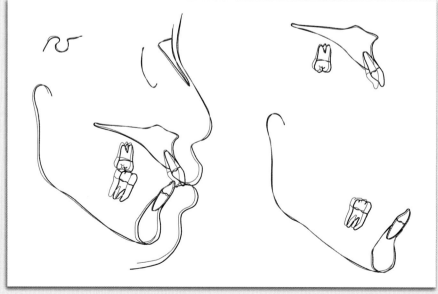

Fig. MSI 1–10. Cephalometric superimposition.

CR-MSI 2

Distalization of the Lower Arch to Create a Nonextraction Surgical Class II Case

Siegrid Brix, Axel Bumann

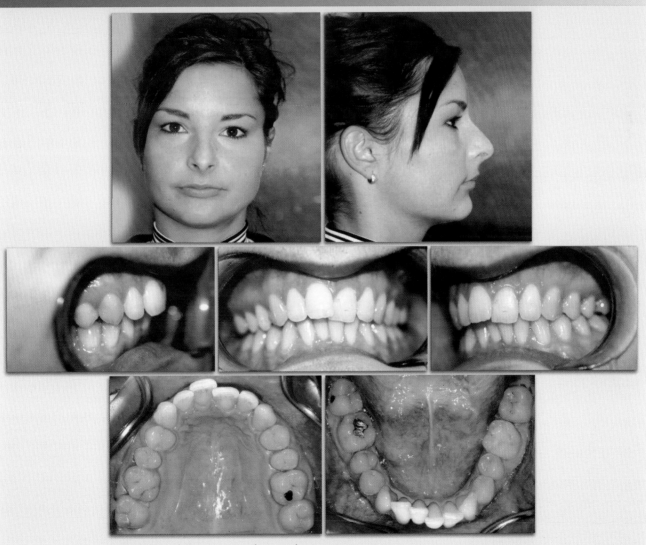

Fig. MSI 2-1. Pretreatment photographs.

The aim of treatment was to resolve lower anterior crowding without extraction in a Class II surgical case. The plan was to use *tomas*® pins (Dentaurum, Inc., Newtown, Pennsylvania) to distalize the lower arch, thereby increasing the dental Class II relationship from a half to a full step. The mandible would then be advanced surgically to a normal skeletal relationship.

Before orthodontic treatment, the patient was treated with an occlusal splint to eliminate myogenic pain. Following pain resolution, the *tomas* pins were used to distalize the lower second molars individually. Next, the first molars were distalized, followed by the second premolars. The remainder of the lower arch was then bonded to resolve the anterior crowding by distalization into the created space. The upper ach was bonded, leveled, and aligned, followed by surgical mandibular advancement to achieve a normal occlusion.

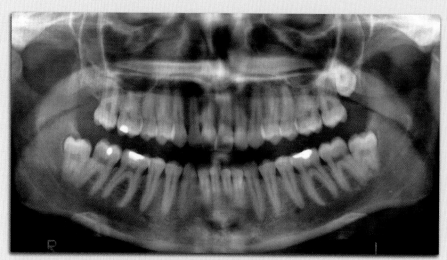

Fig. MSI 2–2. Pretreatment panoramic radiograph.

Table MSI 2-1.	Diagnosis and Treatment Goals	
	Diagnosis	Treatment Goals
SKELETAL		
Anteroposterior	Class II	Class I
Vertical	Normal	Normal
Transverse	Normal	Normal
DENTAL		
Right molar	End-on Class II	Class I
Right canine	End-on Class II	Class I
Left molar	End-on Class II	Class I
Left canine	End-on Class II	Class I
Upper right	3 mm crowding	None
Upper left	1 mm crowding	None
Lower right	3 mm crowding	None
Lower left	3 mm crowding	None
Missing teeth	No. 18	No. 18, 38, 48
Restore teeth	N/A	N/A
Overjet	7 mm	2 mm
Overbite	2 mm	2 mm
Upper ML	1 mm right of facial ML	0 mm to facial ML
Lower ML	2 mm right of facial ML	0 mm to facial ML
SOFT TISSUE		
Profile	Convex	Straight
Lips	Competent	Competent
PERIODONTIUM		
Inadequate KT/TT	None	None
Gingival recession	Lingual No. 31, 32, 43	Maintain
Bone loss	None	None

KT/TT, Keratinized tissue/thin tissue; *ML,* midline; *N/A,* not applicable.

Table MSI 2-2.	Temporary Anchorage Device Summary	
Procedure	Data	
Appliances placed	5 Jun 2001	
TAD placed	30 Apr 2002	
Location of TAD	Distofacial No. 34	Distofacial No. 44
Type of TAD	MSI	MSI
TAD loaded	30 Apr 2002	30 Apr 2002
Healing duration	0 days	0 days
Force in grams	150-180	150-180
Mechanics used	Direct and indirect	Direct and indirect
TAD unloaded	11 Mar 2003	11 Mar 2003
TAD loading duration	11 months	11 months
TAD removed	24 Mar 2003	24 Mar 2003
Appliances removed	6 Jul 2004	
Treatment duration	37 months	

TAD, Temporary anchorage device; *MSI,* miniscrew implant.

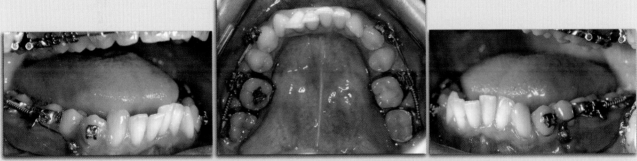

Fig. MSI 2-3. Initial temporary anchorage device (TAD) photographs.

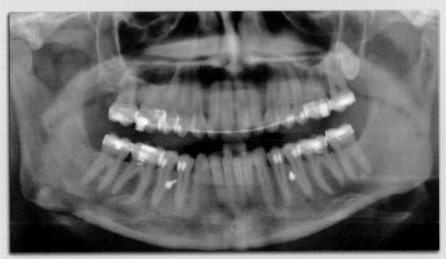

Fig. MSI 2-4. Initial TAD panoramic radiograph.

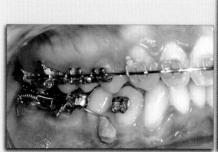 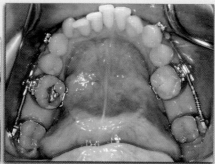 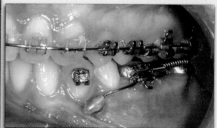

Fig. MSI 2-5. First progress TAD photographs.

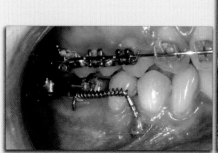 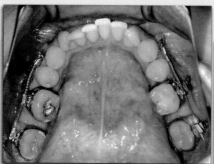 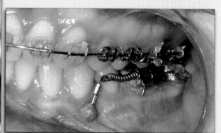

Fig. MSI 2-6. Second progress TAD photographs.

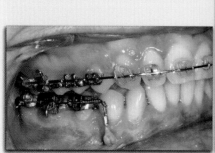 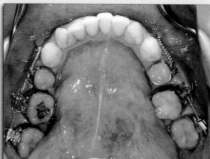 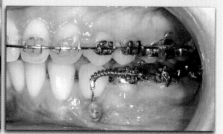

Fig. MSI 2-7. Third progress TAD photographs.

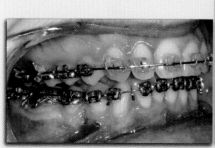 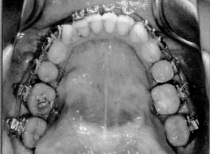 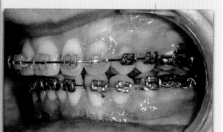

Fig. MSI 2-8. Final TAD photographs.

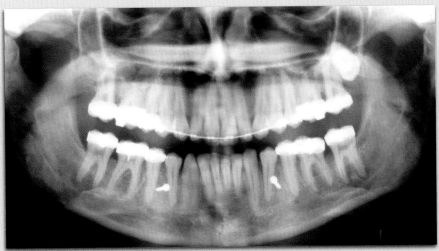

Fig. MSI 2-9. Final TAD panoramic radiograph.

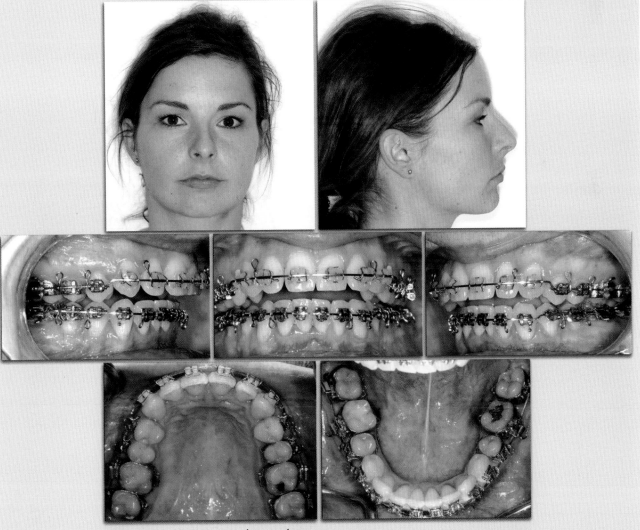

Fig. MSI 2-10. Presurgery photographs.

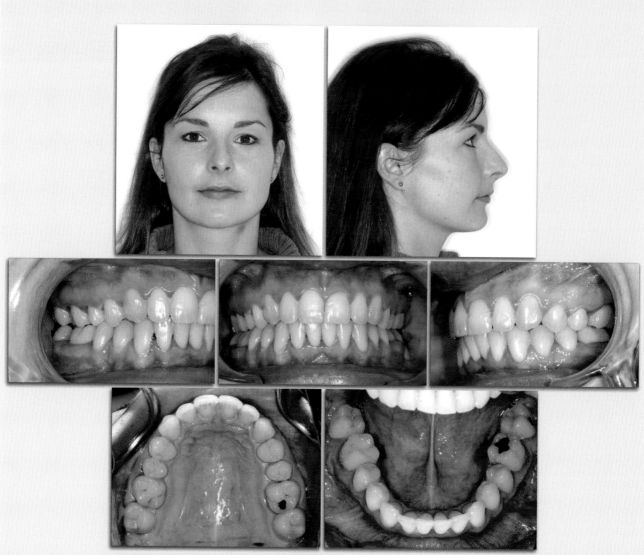

Fig. MSI 2–11. Posttreatment photographs.

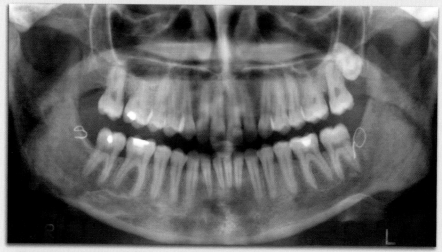

Fig. MSI 2–12. Posttreatment panoramic radiograph.

Table MSI 2-3.	Cephalometric Summary	
	Pretreatment	Posttreatment
SKELETAL		
SNA (degrees)	76.2	76.2
SNB (degrees)	72.1	74.1
ANB (degrees)	4.1	2.1
SN-ANS/PNS (degrees)	12.0	12.0
SN-GoMe (degrees)	35.4	35.0
N-ANS (mm)	60.5	62.2
ANS-Me (mm)	63.5	65.5
DENTAL		
U1-SN (degrees)	92.6	92.8
L1-GoMe (degrees)	106.2	102.1
U1-APo (mm)	5.0	4.3
L1-APo (mm)	1.0	2.5
SOFT TISSUE		
LS-PnPo' (mm)	–5.0	–5.0
LI-PnPo' (mm)	–7.0	–6.0

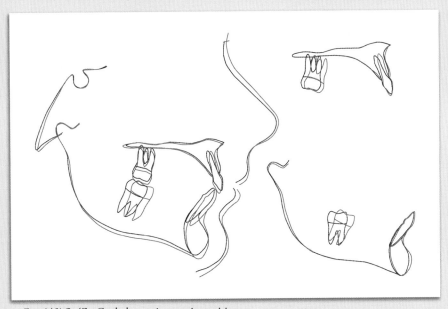

Fig. MSI 2-13. Cephalometric superimposition.

CR-MSI

Nonsurgical Treatment of a Class III Skeletal Pattern by Lower Arch Distalization

Isao Koyama

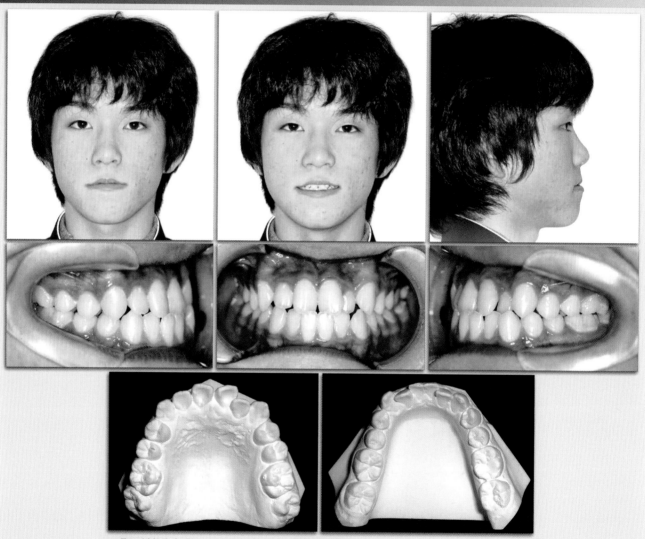

Fig. MSI 3-1. Pretreatment photographs.

The treatment plan was to use lower miniscrew implants (MSIs) to distalize the entire lower arch in order to eliminate the need for premolar extraction or orthognathic surgery. To accomplish the goals, the lower third molars were extracted. Next, the lower arch was distalized indirectly.

The MSIs were ligated directly to the premolars to prevent forward premolar movement. Then an open coil spring was placed between the premolars and the molars to distalize the molars. Finally, the premolars were retracted, followed by the anterior teeth.

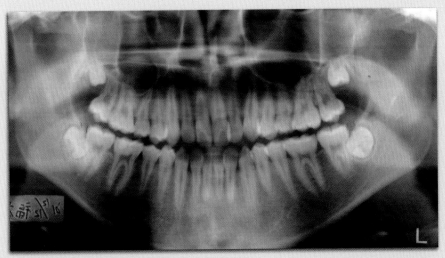

Fig. MSI 3-2. Pretreatment panoramic radiograph.

Table MSI 3-1.	Diagnosis and Treatment Goals	
	Diagnosis	Treatment Goals
SKELETAL		
Anteroposterior	Class III	Class III
Vertical	Normal	Normal
Transverse	Normal	Normal
DENTAL		
Right molar	Class III	Class I
Right canine	Class III	Class I
Left molar	Class III	Class I
Left canine	Class III	Class I
Upper right	0 mm crowding	None
Upper left	2 mm crowding	None
Lower right	1 mm crowding	None
Lower left	1 mm crowding	None
Missing teeth	None	No. 38, 48
Restore teeth	N/A	N/A
Overjet	–0.5 mm	2 mm
Overbite	1 mm	2 mm
Upper ML	0 mm to facial ML	0 mm to facial ML
Lower ML	0 mm to facial ML	0 mm to facial ML
SOFT TISSUE		
Profile	Concave	Straight
Lips	Competent	Competent
PERIODONTIUM		
Inadequate KT/TT	None	None
Gingival recession	No. 31, 32, 41, 42	Maintain
Bone loss	None	None

KT/TT, Keratinized tissue/thin tissue; *ML,* midline; *N/A,* not applicable.

| Table MSI 3-2. | Temporary Anchorage Device Summary | |
Procedure	Data	
Appliances placed	1 Jun 2002	
TAD placed	15 Jul 2002	
Location of TAD	Distofacial No. 35	Distofacial No. 45
Type of TAD	MSI	MSI
TAD loaded	8 Nov 2002	8 Nov 2002
Healing duration	112 days	112 days
Force in grams	200	200
Mechanics used	Indirect	Indirect
TAD unloaded	14 Apr 2004	14 Apr 2004
TAD loading duration	20 months	20 months
TAD removed	7 Mar 2005	7 Mar 2005
Appliances removed	7 Mar 2005	
Treatment duration	33 months	

TAD, Temporary anchorage device; *MSI*, miniscrew implant.

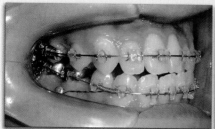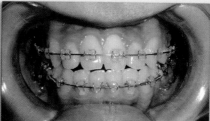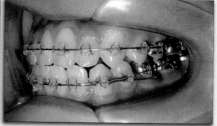

Fig. MSI 3-3. Initial temporary anchorage device (TAD) photographs.

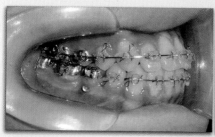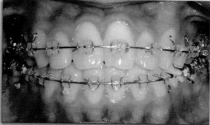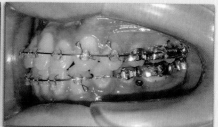

Fig. MSI 3-4. Final TAD photographs.

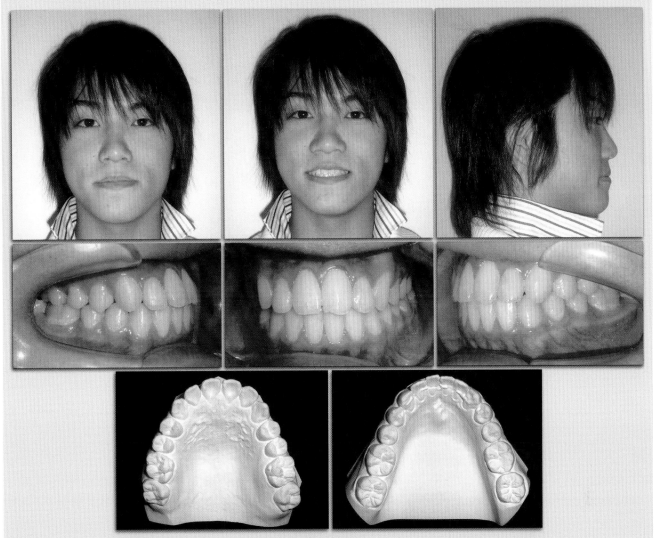

Fig. MSI 3-5. Posttreatment photographs.

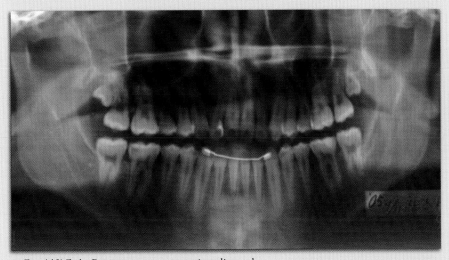

Fig. MSI 3-6. Posttreatment panoramic radiograph.

Table MSI 3-3.	Cephalometric Summary	
	Pretreatment	Posttreatment
SKELETAL		
SNA (degrees)	81.0	83.0
SNB (degrees)	84.0	83.0
ANB (degrees)	–3.0	0.0
SN-ANS/PNS (degrees)	6.5	11.0
SN-GoMe (degrees)	36.0	37.0
N-ANS (mm)	60.0	59.0
ANS-Me (mm)	59.0	58.0
DENTAL		
U1-SN (degrees)	107.0	115.0
L1-GoMe (degrees)	80.0	90.0
U1-APo (mm)	8.0	9.0
L1-APo (mm)	9.0	6.0
SOFT TISSUE		
LS-PnPo′ (mm)	–2.0	–3.5
LI-PnPo′ (mm)	2.0	1.0

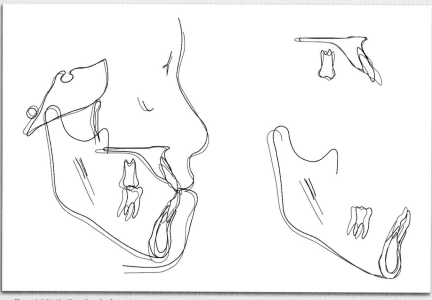

Fig. MSI 3-7. Cephalometric superimposition.

CR-MSI

Bidentoalveolar Protrusion Treated with Premolar Extraction and Maximum Retraction

James C.Y. Lin, Johnny J.L. Liao, Eric J.W. Liou

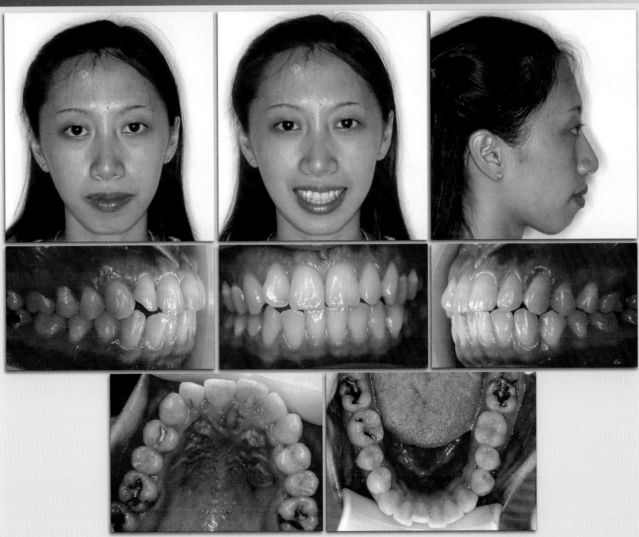

Fig. MSI 4-1. Pretreatment photographs.

Based on the patient's desire to eliminate her dental and soft tissue protrusion, the treatment plan was to extract all four first premolars, followed by maximum anterior retraction using the Lin/Liou Orthodontic Mini Anchor System (LOMAS; Mondeal Medical Systems Gmbh, Tuttlingen, Germany). After extraction, the anterior teeth were retracted en masse directly from the miniscrew implants with no posterior anchorage loss.

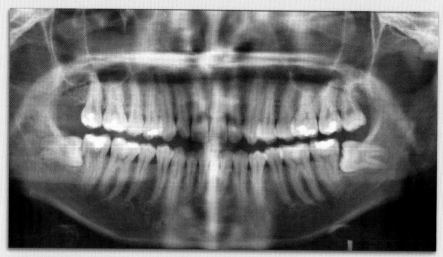

Fig. MSI 4–2. Pretreatment panoramic radiograph.

Table MSI 4-1.	Diagnosis and Treatment Goals	
	Diagnosis	Treatment Goals
SKELETAL		
Anteroposterior	Class II	Class I
Vertical	Normal	Normal
Transverse	Normal	Normal
DENTAL		
Right molar	Class I	Class I
Right canine	Class I	Class I
Left molar	Class I	Class I
Left canine	Class I	Class I
Upper right	2 mm crowding	None
Upper left	1 mm crowding	None
Lower right	1 mm crowding	None
Lower left	1 mm crowding	None
Missing teeth	No. 18	No. 14, 18, 24, 34, 44, 28
Restore teeth	N/A	N/A
Overjet	1 mm	1 mm
Overbite	0 mm	1 mm
Upper ML	0 mm to facial ML	0 mm to facial ML
Lower ML	0 mm to facial ML	0 mm to facial ML
SOFT TISSUE		
Profile	Convex	Straight
Lips	Incompetent	Competent
PERIODONTIUM		
Inadequate KT/TT	None	None
Gingival recession	None	None
Bone loss	None	None

KT/TT, Keratinized tissue/thin tissue; *ML,* midline; *N/A,* not applicable.

| Table MSI 4–2. | | Temporary Anchorage Device Summary | | |
Procedure		Data		
Appliances placed	7 Jun 1995			
TAD placed	26 Dec 1995	26 Dec 1995	26 Dec 1995	26 Dec 1995
Location of TAD	Distofacial No. 15	Distofacial No. 25	Distofacial No. 36	Distofacial No. 46
Type of TAD	MSI	MSI	MSI	MSI
TAD loaded	26 Dec 1995	26 Dec 1995	26 Dec 1995	26 Dec 1995
Healing duration	0 days	0 days	2 weeks	2 weeks
Force in grams	250	250	250	250
Mechanics used	Direct	Direct	Direct	Direct
TAD unloaded	30 Apr 1997	30 Apr 1997	30 Apr 1997	30 Apr 1997
TAD loading duration	16 months	16 months	16 months	16 months
TAD removed	30 Apr 1997	30 Apr 1997	30 Apr 1997	30 Apr 1997
Appliances removed	8 Jul 1997			
Treatment duration	25 months			

TAD, Temporary anchorage device; *MSI*, miniscrew implant.

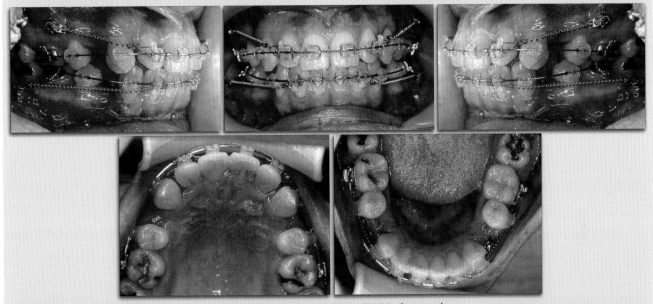

Fig. MSI 4-3. Initial temporary anchorage device (TAD) photographs.

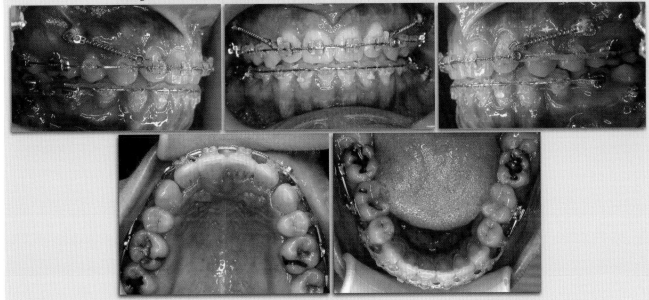

Fig. MSI 4-4. Final TAD photographs.

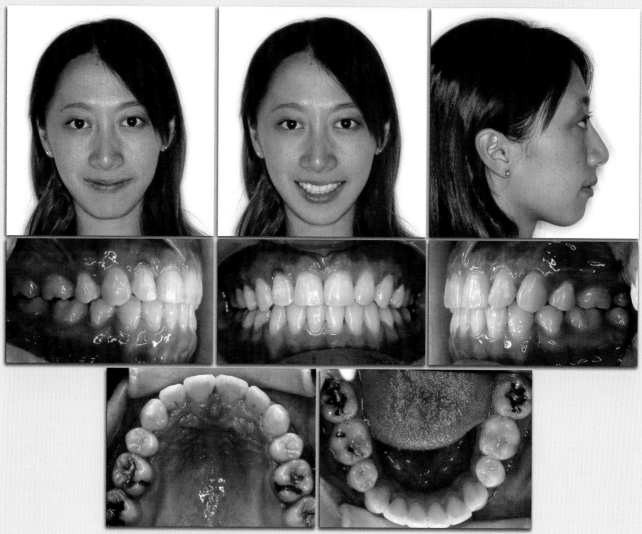

Fig. MSI 4-5. Posttreatment photographs.

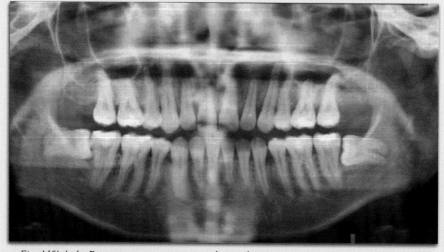

Fig. MSI 4-6. Posttreatment panoramic radiograph.

Table MSI 4–3.	Cephalometric Summary	
	Pretreatment	Posttreatment
SKELETAL		
SNA (degrees)	78.5	76.0
SNB (degrees)	72.0	71.0
ANB (degrees)	6.5	5.0
SN-ANS/PNS (degrees)	18.0	15.0
SN-GoMe (degrees)	44.0	47.5
N-ANS (mm)	57.0	58.5
ANS-Me (mm)	66.0	66.5
DENTAL		
U1-SN (degrees)	104.0	87.5
L1-GoMe (degrees)	106.0	88.0
U1-APo (mm)	11.0	6.0
L1-APo (mm)	8.5	2.5
SOFT TISSUE		
LS-PnPo′ (mm)	3.0	–1.0
LI-PnPo′ (mm)	7.0	1.5

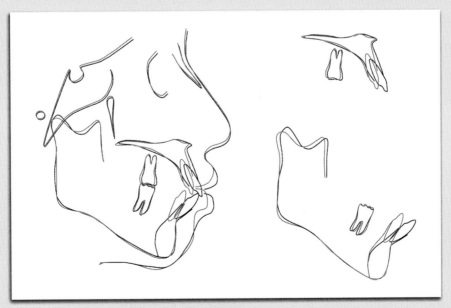

Fig. MSI 4-7. Cephalometric superimposition.

5
CR-MSI

Maximum Anchorage in Lingual Orthodontic Premolar Extraction Treatment of Bidentoalveolar Protrusion

Masayoshi Kawakami

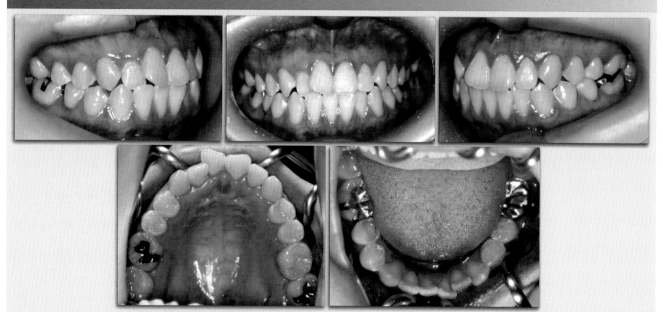

Fig. MSI 5-1. Pretreatment photographs.

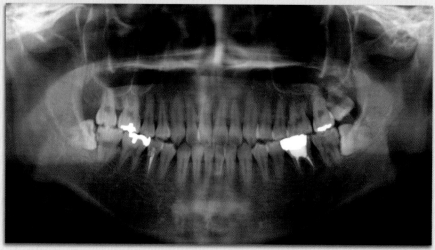

Fig. MSI 5-2. Pretreatment panoramic radiograph.

Because of the patient's refusal to wear facial appliances or use headgear, the treatment plan was to extract four premolars, followed by maximum anterior retraction with lingual appliances. Four miniscrew implants (MSIs) were placed distal to the first molars. Indirect anchorage was used by ligating the first molars to the MSIs. The molars were then used to retract the anterior teeth en masse.

All photos herein reprinted from Kawakami M, Miyawaki S, Noguchi H, Kirita T LI. Screw-type implants used as anchorage for lingual orthodontic mechanics: A case of bimaxillary protrusion with second premolar extraction. *Angle Orthod.* 74:716-719, 2004, with permission from The Angle Orthodontist.

Table MSI 5-1.	Diagnosis and Treatment Goals	
	Diagnosis	Treatment Goals
SKELETAL		
Anteroposterior	Class I	Class I
Vertical	Open bite	Normal
Transverse	Normal	Normal
DENTAL		
Right molar	Class III	Class I
Right canine	Class I	Class I
Left molar	Class I	Class I
Left canine	Class I	Class I
Upper right	3 mm crowding	None
Upper left	1 mm crowding	None
Lower right	0 mm crowding	None
Lower left	2 mm crowding	None
Missing teeth	No. 18	No. 15, 18, 25, 28, 35, 38, 45, 48
Restore teeth	N/A	N/A
Overjet	2 mm	3 mm
Overbite	0 mm	3 mm
Upper ML	1 mm right of facial ML	0 mm to facial ML
Lower ML	1 mm left of facial ML	0 mm to facial ML
SOFT TISSUE		
Profile	Convex	Straight
Lips	Incompetent	Competent
PERIODONTIUM		
Inadequate KT/TT	None	None
Gingival recession	None	None
Bone loss	None	None

KT/TT, Keratinized tissue/thin tissue; *ML,* midline; *N/A,* not applicable.

Table MSI 5-2.	Temporary Anchorage Device Summary			
Procedure	Data			
Appliances placed	14 Sep 1999			
TAD placed	14 Jul 1999	14 Jul 1999	14 Jul 1999	14 Jul 1999
Location of TAD	Distofacial No. 16	Distofacial No. 26	Distofacial No. 36	Distofacial No. 46
Type of TAD	MSI	MSI	MSI	MSI
TAD loaded	14 Sep 1999	14 Sep 1999	14 Sep 1999	14 Sep 1999
Healing duration	56 days	56 days	56 days	56 days
Force in grams	50-100	50-100	50-100	50-100
Mechanics used	Indirect	Indirect	Indirect	Indirect
TAD unloaded	16 May 2001	16 May 2001	16 May 2001	16 May 2001
TAD loading duration	20 months	18 months	20 months	20 months
TAD removed	13 Jul 2001	16 May 2001	13 Jul 2001	13 Jul 2001
Appliances removed	26 Dec 2001			
Treatment duration	27 months			

TAD, Temporary anchorage device; *MSI,* miniscrew implant.

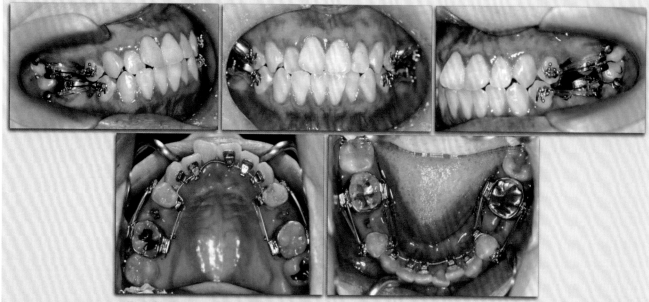

Fig. MSI 5-3. Initial temporary anchorage device (TAD) photographs.

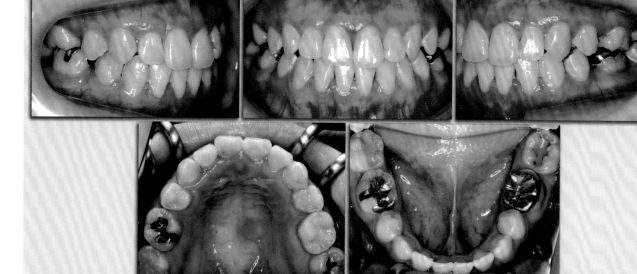

Fig. MSI 5-4. Posttreatment photographs.

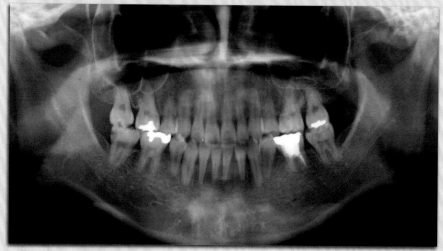

Fig. MSI 5-5. Posttreatment panoramic radiograph.

Table MSI 5-3.	Cephalometric Summary		
	Pretreatment	Posttreatment	1 Year Posttreatment
SKELETAL			
SNA (degrees)	79.8	78.8	78.3
SNB (degrees)	78.3	77.6	77.3
ANB (degrees)	1.5	1.4	1.0
SN-ANS/PNS (degrees)	8.7	8.8	9.3
SN-GoMe (degrees)	37.6	37.0	37.0
N-ANS (mm)	57.5	58.1	58.7
ANS-Me (mm)	75.5	75.3	75.6
DENTAL			
U1-SN (degrees)	118.1	110.7	112.3
L1-GoMe (degrees)	98.6	90.6	84.2
U1-APo (mm)	10.2	7.2	8.0
L1-APo (mm)	8.5	5.9	5.2
SOFT TISSUE			
LS-PnPo' (mm)	1.5	0.0	–1.0
LI-PnPo' (mm)	5.5	3.0	2.0

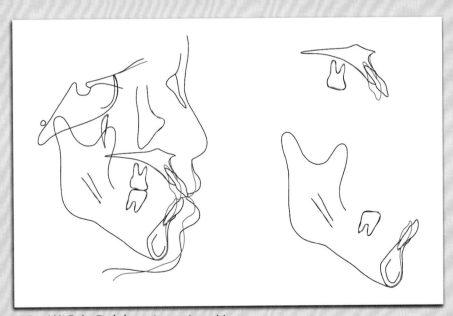

Fig. MSI 5-6. Cephalometric superimposition.

CR–MSI

Treatment of Bidentoalveolar Protrusion with Premolar Extraction and Maximum Anchorage

Isao Koyama

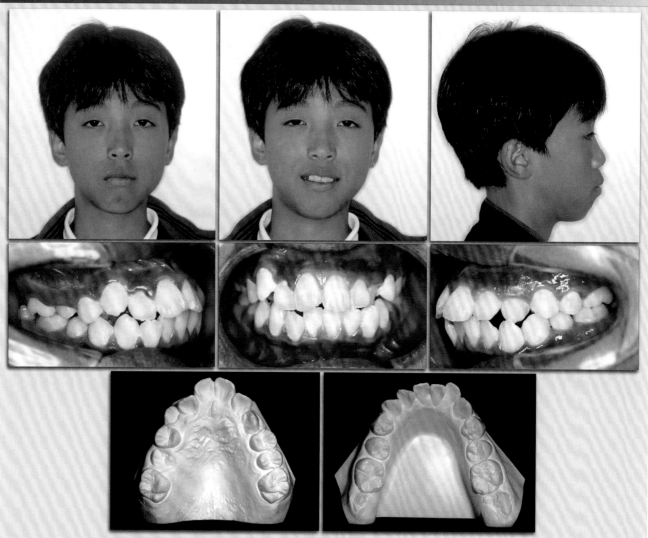

Fig. MSI 6-1. Pretreatment photographs.

The treatment plan was to extract the first premolars in order to retract the anterior teeth maximally and improve the procumbent lips and convex profile. En masse retraction of the anterior teeth was accomplished by attachment directly from the miniscrew implants to the anterior teeth.

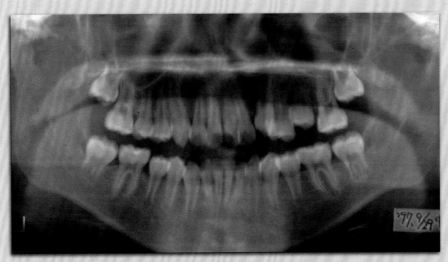

Fig. MSI 6-2. Pretreatment panoramic radiograph.

Table MSI 6-1.	Diagnosis and Treatment Goals	
	Diagnosis	Treatment Goals
SKELETAL		
Anteroposterior	Class I	Class I
Vertical	Normal	Normal
Transverse	Normal	Normal
DENTAL		
Right molar	Class I	Class I
Right canine	Class I	Class I
Left molar	Class I	Class I
Left canine	Class I	Class I
Upper right	1 mm crowding	None
Upper left	0 mm crowding	None
Lower right	1 mm crowding	None
Lower left	1 mm crowding	None
Missing teeth	None	No. 14, 24, 34, 44
Restore teeth	N/A	N/A
Overjet	5.5 mm	2 mm
Overbite	2 mm	2 mm
Upper ML	0 mm to facial ML	0 mm to facial ML
Lower ML	0 mm to facial ML	0 mm to facial ML
SOFT TISSUE		
Profile	Convex	Straight
Lips	Incompetent	Competent
PERIODONTIUM		
Inadequate KT/TT	None	None
Gingival recession	None	None
Bone loss	None	None

KT/TT, Keratinized tissue/thin tissue; *ML,* midline; *N/A,* not applicable.

Table MSI 6-2.	Temporary Anchorage Device Summary			
Procedure	Data			
Appliances placed	19 Jan 1998			
TAD placed	14 Nov 1997	14 Nov 1997	14 Nov 1997	14 Nov 1997
Location of TAD	Mesiofacial No. 15	Mesiofacial No. 25	Mesiofacial No. 35	Mesiofacial No. 45
Type of TAD	MSI	MSI	MSI	MSI
TAD loaded	2 Mar 1998	2 Mar 1998	2 Mar 1998	2 Mar 1998
Healing duration	56 days	56 days	56 days	56 days
Force in grams	200	200	200	200
Mechanics used	Direct	Direct	Direct	Direct
TAD unloaded	26 Jul 1999	26 Jul 1999	26 Jul 1999	26 Jul 1999
TAD loading duration	15 months	15 months	15 months	15 months
TAD removed	26 Jul 1999	26 Jul 1999	26 Jul 1999	26 Jul 1999
Appliances removed	22 May 2000			
Treatment duration	28 months			

TAD, Temporary anchorage device; *MSI*, miniscrew implant.

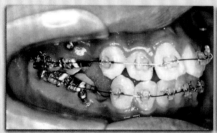 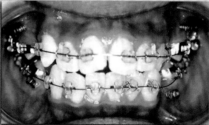 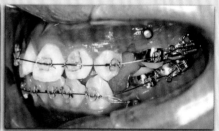

Fig. MSI 6-3. Initial temporary anchorage device (TAD) photographs.

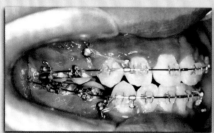 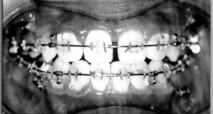 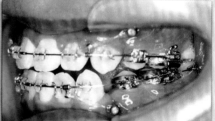

Fig. MSI 6-4. Progress TAD photographs.

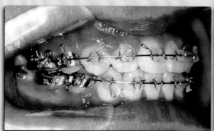 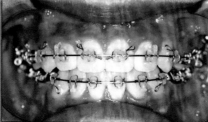 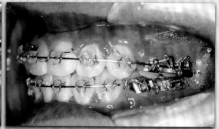

Fig. MSI 6-5. Final TAD photographs.

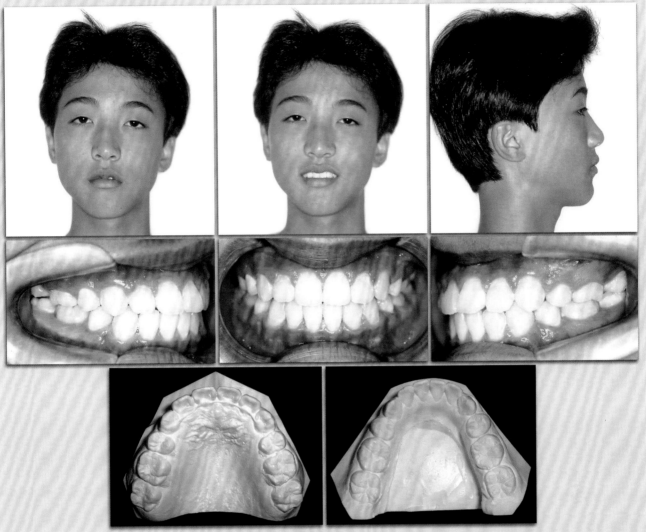

Fig. MSI 6-6. Posttreatment photographs.

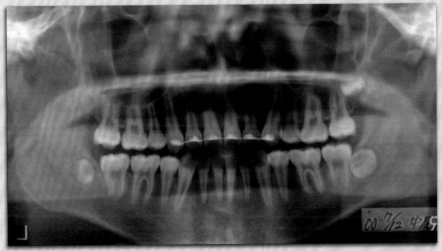

Fig. MSI 6-7. Posttreatment panoramic radiograph.

Table MSI 6–3.	Cephalometric Summary	
	Pretreatment	Posttreatment
SKELETAL		
SNA (degrees)	85.0	85.0
SNB (degrees)	80.0	83.5
ANB (degrees)	5.0	1.5
SN-ANS/PNS (degrees)	6.0	5.0
SN-GoMe (degrees)	36.0	32.0
N-ANS (mm)	57.0	61.0
ANS-Me (mm)	56.0	60.0
DENTAL		
U1-SN (degrees)	121.0	117.0
L1-GoMe (degrees)	97.0	89.0
U1-APo (mm)	15.0	6.0
L1-APo (mm)	8.0	3.0
SOFT TISSUE		
LS-PnPo′ (mm)	7.0	–2.0
LI-PnPo′ (mm)	10.0	1.0

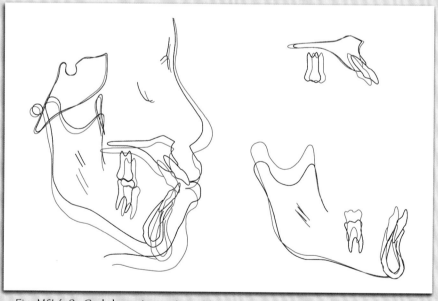

Fig. MSI 6–8. Cephalometric superimposition.

7

Upper Premolar Extraction and Anterior Retraction without Upper Posterior Appliances

Kyu-Rhim Chung, Seong-Hun Kim

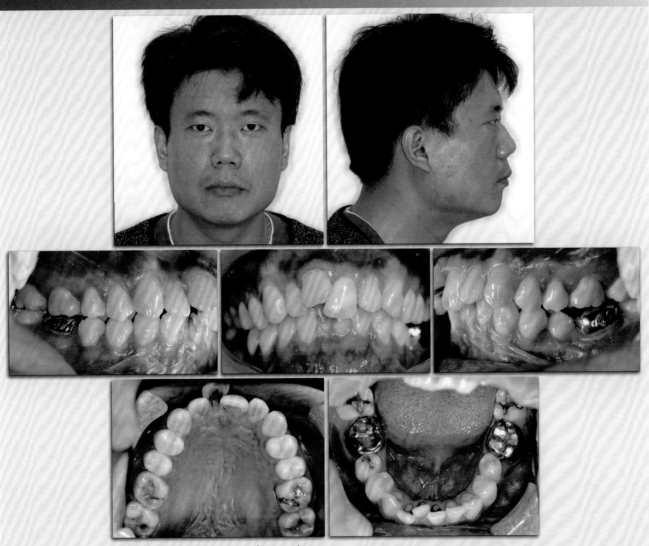

Fig. MSI 7-1. Pretreatment photographs.

The patient presented with poor oral hygiene, several faulty restorations with recurrent decay, and a lower anterior tooth size discrepancy. The treatment strategy was to extract the upper first premolars and correct the Class II canine relationship by retracting the upper anterior teeth. To do this, C-implants (Cimplant Co., Seoul, Korea) were placed in the upper arch for upper anterior intrusion and retraction by sliding mechanics on an 0.016 × 0.022-inch blue Elgiloy arch wire (Elgiloy Specialty Metals, Elgin, Illinois). The lower anterior excess tooth mass was resolved by interproximal enamel reduction. Toward the end of treatment, the upper canines were slightly upright. Therefore, an 0.017 × 0.022-inch stainless steel arch wire with T-loops was used to control the canine angulation.

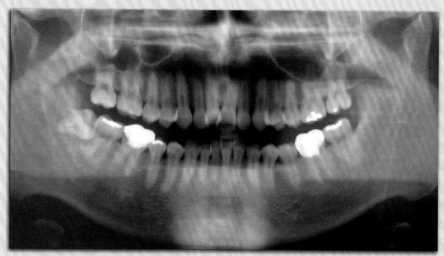

Fig. MSI 7–2. Pretreatment panoramic radiograph.

Table MSI 7-1.	Diagnosis and Treatment Goals	
	Diagnosis	Treatment Goals
SKELETAL		
Anteroposterior	Class II	Class II
Vertical	Normal	Normal
Transverse	Normal	Normal
DENTAL		
Right molar	Class II	Class II
Right canine	Class II	Class I
Left molar	Class II	Class II
Left canine	Class II	Class I
Upper right	5 mm crowding	None
Upper left	2.5 mm crowding	None
Lower right	2 mm crowding	None
Lower left	1.5 mm crowding	None
Missing teeth	No. 18, 28, 38	No. 14, 18, 24, 28, 38
Restore teeth	N/A	No. 16, 17
Overjet	5.5 mm	2 mm
Overbite	3 mm	2 mm
Upper ML	1 mm right of facial ML	0 mm to facial ML
Lower ML	1 mm left of facial ML	0 mm to facial ML
SOFT TISSUE		
Profile	Convex	Straight
Lips	Incompetent	Competent
PERIODONTIUM		
Inadequate KT/TT	No. 31, 41, 43	Maintain
Gingival recession	No. 34, 35, 44, 45	Maintain
Bone loss	None	None
OTHER	Lower anterior excess tooth mass of 1.5 mm	

KT/TT, Keratinized tissue/thin tissue; *ML,* midline; *N/A,* not applicable.

Table MSI 7-2.	Temporary Anchorage Device Summary	
Procedure	Data	
Appliances placed	8 Mar 2003	
TAD placed	2 Mar 2003	2 Mar 2003
Location of TAD	Distofacial No. 15	Distofacial No. 25
Type of TAD	MSI	MSI
TAD loaded	8 Mar 2003	8 Mar 2003
Healing duration	7 days	7 days
Force in grams	200-500	200-500
Mechanics used	Direct	Direct
TAD unloaded	4 Nov 2004	4 Nov 2004
TAD loading duration	20 months	20 months
TAD removed	9 Nov 2004	9 Nov 2004
Appliances removed	8 Nov 2004	
Treatment duration	20 months	

TAD, Temporary anchorage device; *MSI*, miniscrew implant.

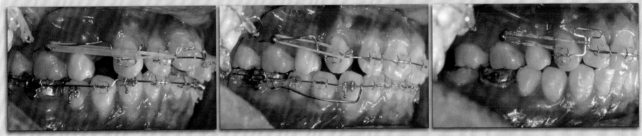

Fig. MSI 7-3. Initial *(left)*, progress *(center)*, and final *(right)* temporary anchorage device (TAD) buccal photographs.

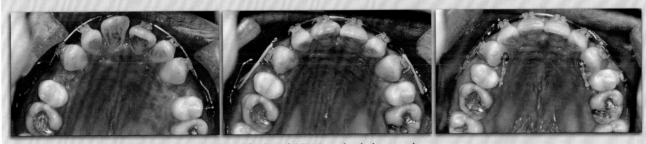

Fig. MSI 7-4. Initial *(left)*, progress *(center)*, and final *(right)* TAD occlusal photographs.

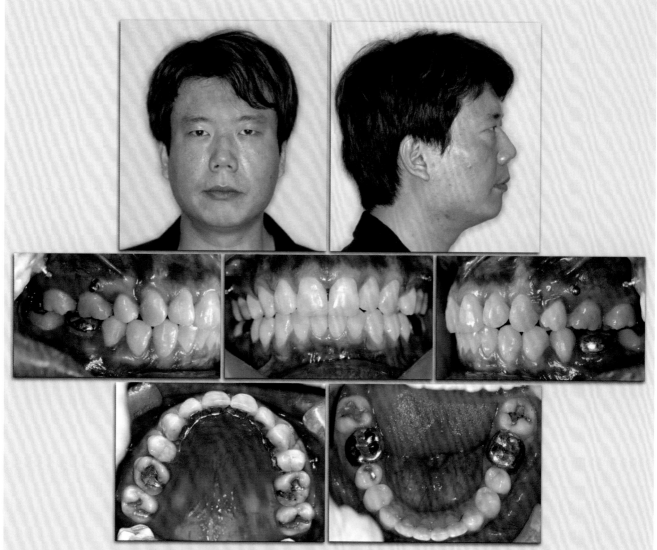

Fig. MSI 7-5. Posttreatment photographs.

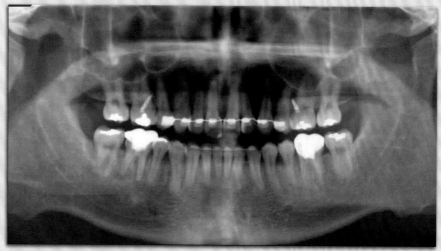

Fig. MSI 7-6. Posttreatment panoramic radiograph.

Table MSI 7-3.	Cephalometric Summary	
	Pretreatment	Posttreatment
SKELETAL		
SNA (degrees)	81.0	80.0
SNB (degrees)	76.5	76.0
ANB (degrees)	4.5	4.0
SN-ANS/PNS (degrees)	9.0	8.5
SN-GoMe (degrees)	25.0	26.0
N-ANS (mm)	61.0	62.0
ANS-Me (mm)	81.0	81.0
DENTAL		
U1-SN (degrees)	113.0	92.0
L1-GoMe (degrees)	103.0	106.0
U1-APo (mm)	12.5	8.0
L1-APo (mm)	4.0	4.0
SOFT TISSUE		
LS-PnPo′ (mm)	5.0	1.5
LI-PnPo′ (mm)	3.0	1.5

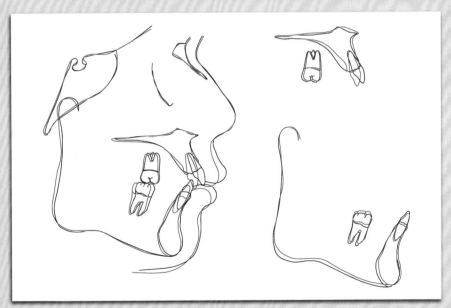

Fig. MSI 7-7. Cephalometric superimposition.

Treatment of Class II Bialveolar Protrusion with Maximum Retraction

Hyo-Sang Park

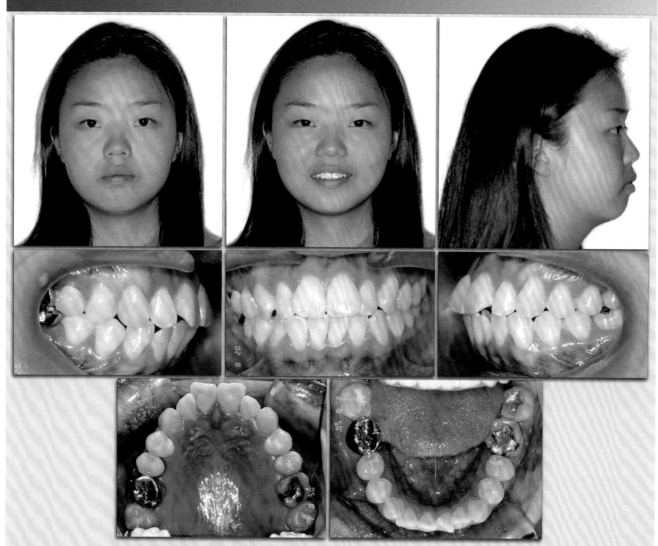

Fig. MSI 8-1. Pretreatment photographs.

Because of significant bialveolar protrusion and lip protrusion, the treatment plan was to extract four first premolars to improve the facial profile. Instead of retracting the canines followed later by the incisors, microscrew implants were to be placed between the second premolars and first molars in order to allow for en masse retraction of all six anterior teeth. The microscrew implants were positioned to prevent soft tissue impingement of mechanics around the canine eminence and such that the line of force passed through the center of resistance of the anterior segment.

A straight facial profile was obtained with good intercuspation. The cephalometric superimposition demonstrates that the upper anterior teeth were retracted with intrusion and that the upper posterior teeth showed no anchorage loss. The upper and lower lips were retracted along with the retraction of the anterior teeth, resulting in improvement of the facial profile.

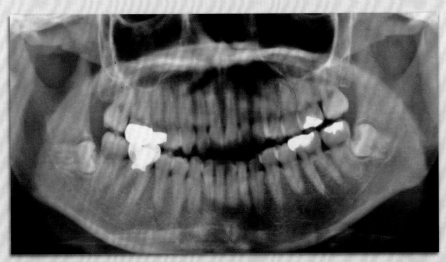

Fig. MSI 8-2. Pretreatment panoramic radiograph.

Table MSI 8-1.	Diagnosis and Treatment Goals	
	Diagnosis	Treatment Goals
SKELETAL		
Anteroposterior	Class I	Class I
Vertical	Normal	Normal
Transverse	Normal	Normal
DENTAL		
Right molar	Class I	Class I
Right canine	Class I	Class I
Left molar	Class I	Class I
Left canine	Class I	Class I
Upper right	0.5 mm crowding	None
Upper left	0.5 mm crowding	None
Lower right	0 mm crowding	None
Lower left	1 mm crowding	None
Missing teeth	No. 18, 28	No. 14, 18, 24, 28, 34, 38, 44, 48
Restore teeth	N/A	N/A
Overjet	3.5 mm	2 mm
Overbite	1.5 mm	2 mm
Upper ML	0 mm to facial ML	0 mm to facial ML
Lower ML	1 mm left of facial ML	0 mm to facial ML
SOFT TISSUE		
Profile	Convex	Straight
Lips	Incompetent	Competent
PERIODONTIUM		
Inadequate KT/TT	None	None
Gingival recession	None	None
Bone loss	None	None

KT/TT, Keratinized tissue/thin tissue; *ML,* midline; *N/A,* not applicable.

Table MSI 8-2.	Temporary Anchorage Device Summary	
Procedure	Data	
Appliances placed	11 Oct 2002	
TAD placed	31 May 2003	31 May 2003
Location of TAD	Distofacial No. 15	Distofacial No. 25
Type of TAD	MSI	MSI
TAD loaded	28 Jun 2003	28 Jun 2003
Healing duration	28 days	28 days
Force in grams	200	200
Mechanics used	Direct	Direct
TAD unloaded	20 Mar 2004	11 Aug 2004
TAD loading duration	9 months	14 months
TAD removed	11 Aug 2004	
Appliances removed	11 Aug 2004	
Treatment duration	22 months	

TAD, Temporary anchorage device; *MSI*, miniscrew implant.

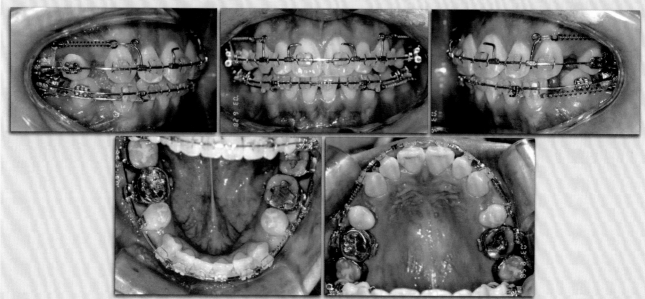

Fig. MSI 8-3. Initial temporary anchorage device (TAD) photographs.

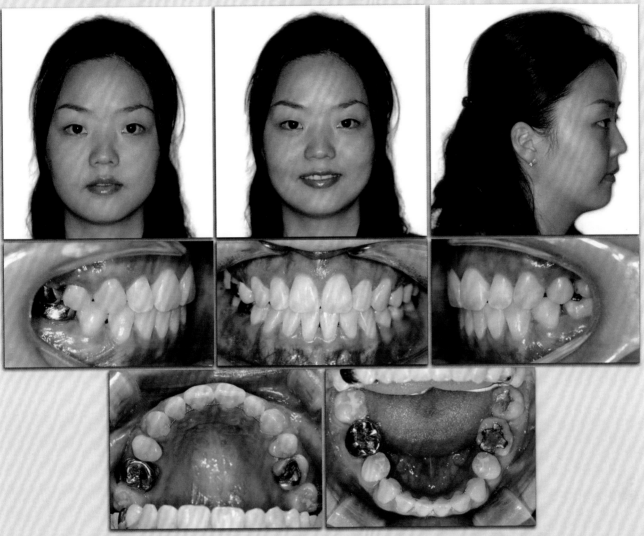

Fig. MSI 8-4. Posttreatment photographs.

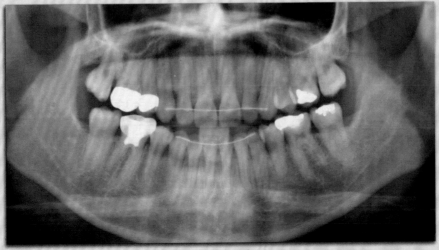

Fig. MSI 8-5. Posttreatment panoramic radiograph.

Table MSI 8-3.	Cephalometric Summary	
	Pretreatment	Posttreatment
SKELETAL		
SNA (degrees)	77.7	77.7
SNB (degrees)	73.7	73.2
ANB (degrees)	4.0	4.5
SN-ANS/PNS (degrees)	13.1	13.1
SN-GoMe (degrees)	38.4	38.9
N-ANS (mm)	52.1	52.1
ANS-Me (mm)	69.0	70.0
DENTAL		
U1-SN (degrees)	145.2	121.2
L1-GoMe (degrees)	99.9	88.9
U1-APo (mm)	12.0	3.5
L1-APo (mm)	6.5	1.0
SOFT TISSUE		
LS-PnPo' (mm)	3.5	–0.5
LI-PnPo' (mm)	6.5	–1.0

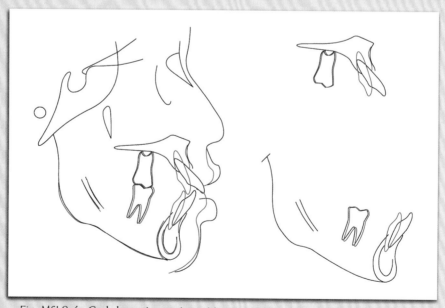

Fig. MSI 8-6. Cephalometric superimposition.

CR–MSI

En Masse Retraction of Anterior Teeth in a Bidentoalveolar Protrusion Case

Seong-Hun Kim, Kyu-Rhim Chung, Yoon-Ah Kook

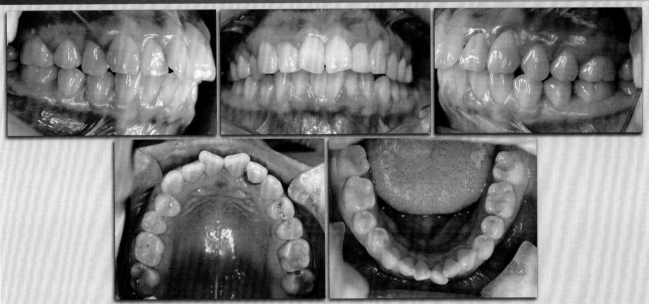

Fig. MSI 9-1. Pretreatment photographs.

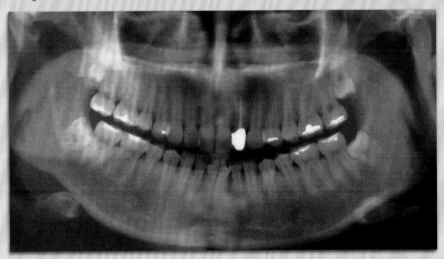

Fig. MSI 9-2. Pretreatment panoramic radiograph.

The treatment plan was to extract the upper first and lower second premolars for crowding resolution. Upper C-implants (Cimplant Co., Seoul, Korea) were used for maximum retraction of the upper anterior teeth, with only moderate anchorage required in the lower arch. No appliances were used on the upper posterior teeth for anterior retraction because the C-implants were used for sliding mechanics. Two 0.019 × 0.025-inch stainless steel uprighting springs were used for simultaneous lower anterior intrusion and molar uprighting.

Table MSI 9-1.	Diagnosis and Treatment Goals	
	Diagnosis	Treatment Goals
SKELETAL		
Anteroposterior	Class II	Class II
Vertical	Normal	Normal
Transverse	Normal	Normal
DENTAL		
Right molar	Class II	Class I
Right canine	Class II	Class I
Left molar	Class II	Class I
Left canine	Class II	Class I
Upper right	4 mm crowding	None
Upper left	2 mm crowding	None
Lower right	3 mm crowding	None
Lower left	3 mm crowding	None
Missing teeth	None	No. 14, 24, 35, 45
Restore teeth	N/A	N/A
Overjet	5 mm	2 mm
Overbite	2 mm	2 mm
Upper ML	0 mm to facial ML	0 mm to facial ML
Lower ML	2 mm left of facial ML	0 mm to facial ML
SOFT TISSUE		
Profile	Convex	Straight
Lips	Incompetent	Competent
PERIODONTIUM		
Inadequate KT/TT	None	None
Gingival recession	None	None
Bone loss	None	None
OTHER	No. 18, 28, 38, 48 impacted	

KT/TT, Keratinized tissue/thin tissue; *ML,* midline; *N/A,* not applicable.

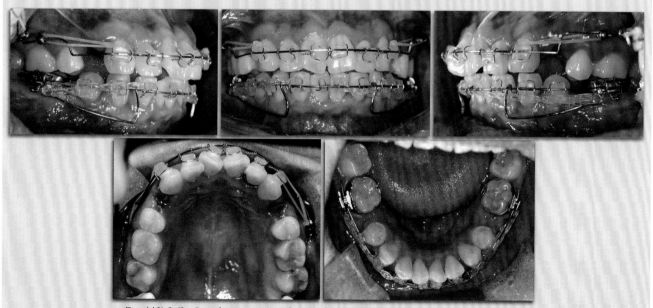

Fig. MSI 9-3.   Initial temporary anchorage device (TAD) photographs.

Table MSI 9–2.	Temporary Anchorage Device Summary	
Procedure	Data	
Appliances placed	10 Apr 2003	
TAD placed	16 Jul 2003	16 Jul 2003
Location of TAD	Distofacial No. 15	Distofacial No. 25
Type of TAD	MSI	MSI
TAD loaded	23 Jul 2003	23 Jul 2003
Healing duration	7 days	7 days
Force in grams	250-400	250-400
Mechanics used	Direct	Direct
TAD unloaded	1 Oct 2004	1 Oct 2004
TAD loading duration	15 months	15 months
TAD removed	8 Oct 2004	8 Oct 2004
Appliances removed	8 Oct 2004	
Treatment duration	18 months	

TAD, Temporary anchorage device; *MSI*, miniscrew implant.

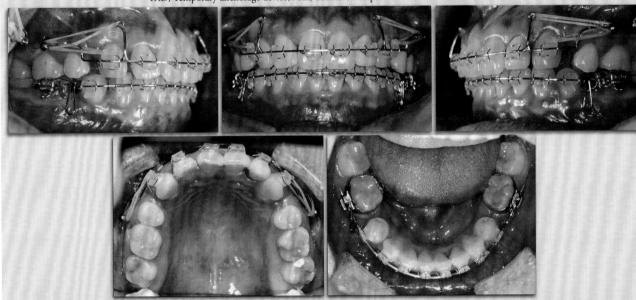

Fig. MSI 9-4.   Progress TAD photographs.

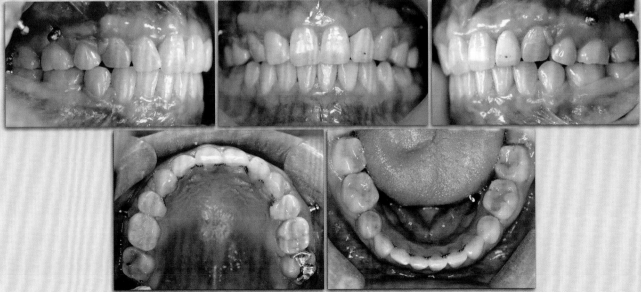

Fig. MSI 9-5.   Posttreatment photographs.

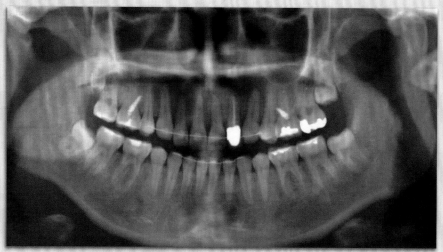

Fig. MSI 9-6. Posttreatment panoramic radiograph.

Table MSI 9-3.	Cephalometric Summary	
	Pretreatment	Posttreatment
SKELETAL		
SNA (degrees)	81.5	81.0
SNB (degrees)	75.0	74.5
ANB (degrees)	6.5	6.5
SN-ANS/PNS (degrees)	11.0	12.0
SN-GoMe (degrees)	36.0	35.5
N-ANS (mm)	63.0	63.0
ANS-Me (mm)	69.0	69.0
DENTAL		
U1-SN (degrees)	108.5	84.0
L1-GoMe (degrees)	110.0	94.0
U1-APo (mm)	10.0	4.0
L1-APo (mm)	6.0.	1.0
SOFT TISSUE		
LS-PnPo' (mm)	2.0	1.0
LI-PnPo' (mm)	3.0	–1.0

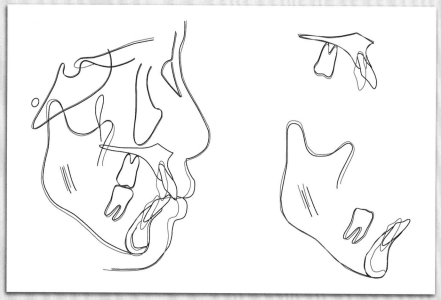

Fig. MSI 9-7. Cephalometric superimposition.

Extraction Treatment of Anterior Crowding

Ryoon-Ki Hong

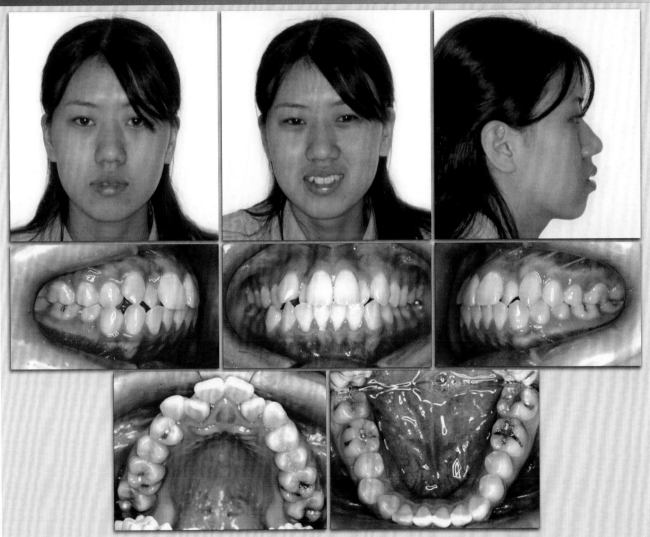

Fig. MSI 10-1. Pretreatment photographs.

The treatment plan was to extract the first premolars and use a miniscrew implant in the upper right quadrant to distalize the buccal segment from a Class II to a Class I relationship. After the Class II molar correction on the upper right, standard mechanics were used to close the extraction spaces by anterior retraction.

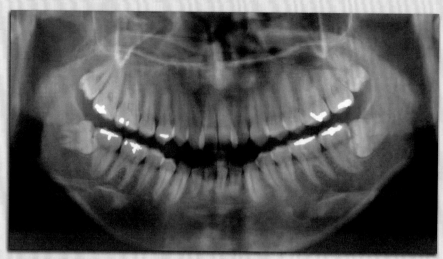

Fig. MSI 10-2. Pretreatment panoramic radiograph.

Table MSI 10-1.	Diagnosis and Treatment Goals	
	Diagnosis	Treatment Goals
SKELETAL		
Anteroposterior	Class I	Class I
Vertical	Normal	Normal
Transverse	Normal	Normal
DENTAL		
Right molar	Class II	Class I
Right canine	Class II	Class I
Left molar	Class I	Class I
Left canine	Class I	Class I
Upper right	5.4 mm crowding	None
Upper left	4.3 mm crowding	None
Lower right	1.2 mm crowding	None
Lower left	0.5 mm crowding	None
Missing teeth	None	No. 14, 18, 24, 28, 34, 38, 44, 48
Restore teeth	N/A	N/A
Overjet	4 mm	3 mm
Overbite	3 mm	2.5 mm
Upper ML	1 mm left of facial ML	0 mm to facial ML
Lower ML	0 mm to facial ML	0 mm to facial ML
SOFT TISSUE		
Profile	Convex	Straight
Lips	Incompetent	Competent
PERIODONTIUM		
Inadequate KT/TT	None	None
Gingival recession	None	None
Bone loss	None	None

KT/TT, Keratinized tissue/thin tissue; *ML,* midline; *N/A,* not applicable.

Table MSI 10-2.	Temporary Anchorage Device Summary
Procedure	**Data**
Appliances placed	31 Mar 2001
TAD placed	1 Sep 2001
Location of TAD	Distofacial No. 15
Type of TAD	MSI
TAD loaded	15 Sep 2001
Healing duration	14 days
Force in grams	150
Mechanics used	Indirect
TAD unloaded	10 Jul 2002
TAD loading duration	10 months
TAD removed	25 Oct 2002
Appliances removed	24 Feb 2003
Treatment duration	23 months

TAD, Temporary anchorage device; *MSI*, miniscrew implant.

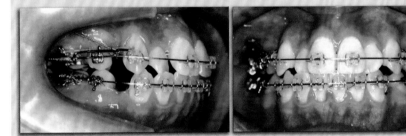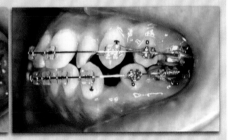

Fig. MSI 10-3.   Initial temporary anchorage device (TAD) photographs.

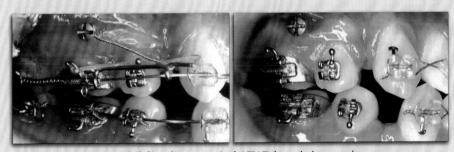

Fig. MSI 10-4.   Initial *(left)* and progress *(right)* TAD buccal photographs.

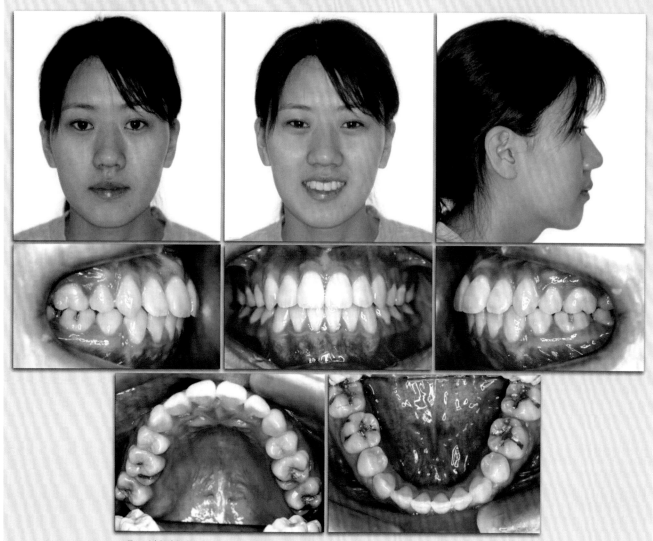

Fig. MSI 10-5. Posttreatment photographs.

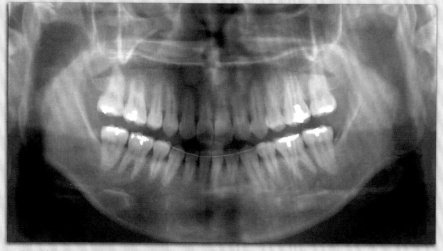

Fig. MSI 10-6. Posttreatment panoramic radiograph.

Table MSI 10–3.	Cephalometric Summary	
	Pretreatment	Posttreatment
SKELETAL		
SNA (degrees)	81.7	81.4
SNB (degrees)	77.2	77.4
ANB (degrees)	4.6	4.0
SN-ANS/PNS (degrees)	10.0	10.0
SN-GoMe (degrees)	42.7	42.7
N-ANS (mm)	59.0	58.9
ANS-Me (mm)	75.2	75.3
DENTAL		
U1-SN (degrees)	110.2	101.8
L1-GoMe (degrees)	96.0	86.1
U1-APo (mm)	11.7	7.7
L1-APo (mm)	7.9	3.8
SOFT TISSUE		
LS-PnPo′ (mm)	2.0	–2.0
LI-PnPo′ (mm)	6.0	0.0

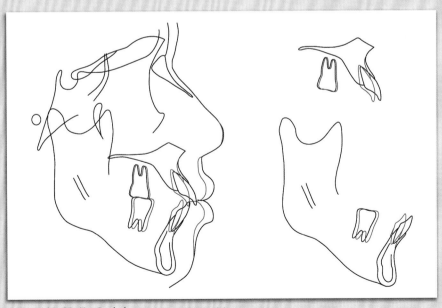

Fig. MSI 10-7. Cephalometric superimposition.

11
CR–MSI

Lingual Orthodontic Treatment of Class I Crowding Following Premolar Extraction

Ryoon-Ki Hong

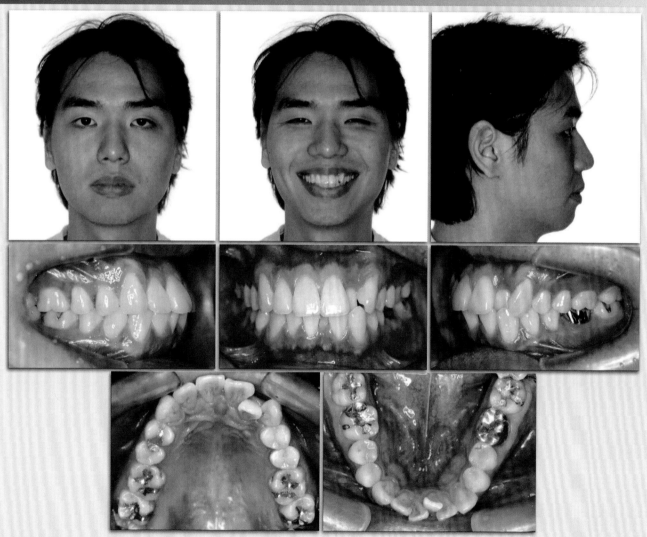

Fig. MSI 11–1. Pretreatment photographs.

The patient had moderate crowding in both arches; however, the anterior teeth were proclined considerably. Therefore the plan was to extract the four first premolars followed by traditional lingual appliance mechanics for space closure in all quadrants except the upper right.

Because of the Class II canine relationship in the upper right, a miniscrew implant (MSI) was placed for retraction of the upper right anterior teeth. Treatment proceeded as planned to achieve an ideal Class I occlusion.

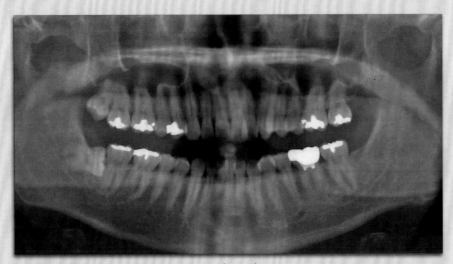

Fig. MSI 11–2. Pretreatment panoramic radiograph.

Table MSI 11–1.	Diagnosis and Treatment Goals	
	Diagnosis	Treatment Goals
SKELETAL		
Anteroposterior	Class I	Class I
Vertical	Normal	Normal
Transverse	Normal	Normal
DENTAL		
Right molar	Class I	Class I
Right canine	Class II	Class I
Left molar	Class I	Class I
Left canine	Class I	Class I
Upper right	0 mm crowding	None
Upper left	3 mm crowding	None
Lower right	1 mm crowding	None
Lower left	2.3 mm crowding	None
Missing teeth	No. 28, 38	No. 14, 18, 24, 28, 34, 38, 44, 48
Restore teeth	N/A	N/A
Overjet	2.5 mm	3 mm
Overbite	1.5 mm	2.5 mm
Upper ML	0 mm to facial ML	0 mm to facial ML
Lower ML	0 mm to facial ML	0 mm to facial ML
SOFT TISSUE		
Profile	Convex	Straight
Lips	Competent	Competent
PERIODONTIUM		
Inadequate KT/TT	None	None
Gingival recession	None	None
Bone loss	None	None
OTHER	Mesiodens apical to No. 11 and 12	

KT/TT, Keratinized tissue/thin tissue; *ML,* midline; *N/A,* not applicable.

Table MSI 11-2.	Temporary Anchorage Device Summary
Procedure	Data
Appliances placed	5 Mar 2002
TAD placed	27 Jun 2003
Location of TAD	Distopalatal No. 16
Type of TAD	MSI
TAD loaded	11 Jul 2003
Healing duration	14 days
Force in grams	200
Mechanics used	Indirect
TAD unloaded	7 Oct 2003
TAD loading duration	3 months
TAD removed	7 Oct 2003
Appliances removed	7 Apr 2004
Treatment duration	25 months

TAD, Temporary anchorage device; *MSI*, miniscrew implant.

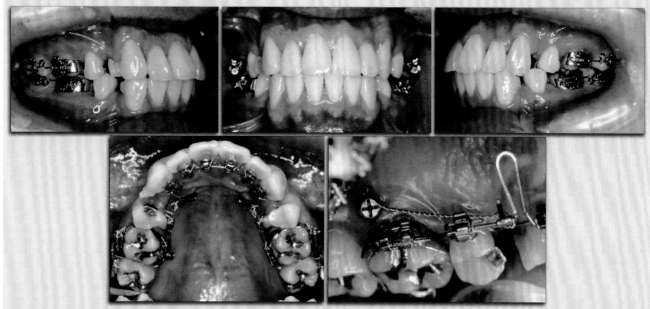

Fig. MSI 11-3.   Initial temporary anchorage device (TAD) photographs.

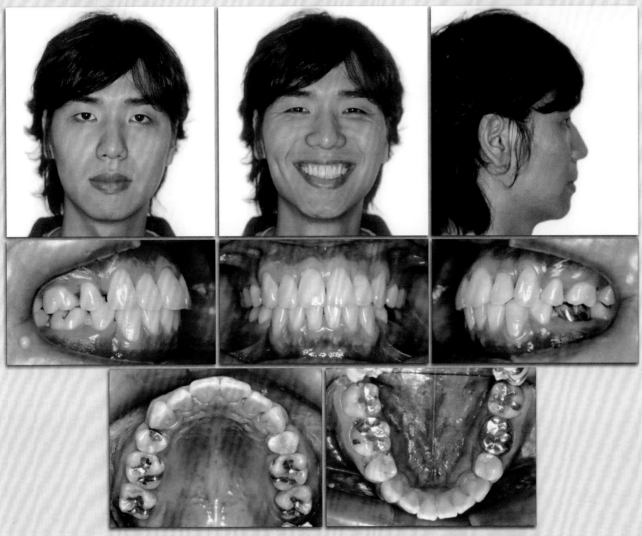

Fig. MSI 11-4. Posttreatment photographs.

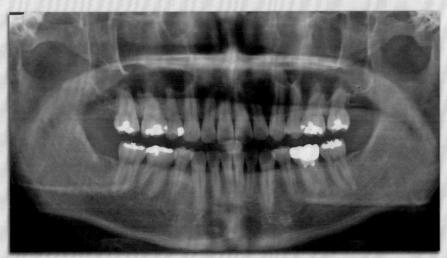

Fig. MSI 11-5. Posttreatment panoramic radiograph.

Table MSI 11-3.	Cephalometric Summary	
	Pretreatment	Posttreatment
SKELETAL		
SNA (degrees)	81.0	80.9
SNB (degrees)	79.7	79.0
ANB (degrees)	1.3	1.9
SN-ANS/PNS (degrees)	7.0	7.0
SN-GoMe (degrees)	27.7	27.0
N-ANS (mm)	60.0	59.4
ANS-Me (mm)	78.1	79.4
DENTAL		
U1-SN (degrees)	115.3	102.5
L1-GoMe (degrees)	109.0	99.4
U1-APo (mm)	13.6	9.3
L1-APo (mm)	10.1	5.7
SOFT TISSUE		
LS-PnPo' (mm)	–0.5	–3.0
LI-PnPo' (mm)	2.5	1.0

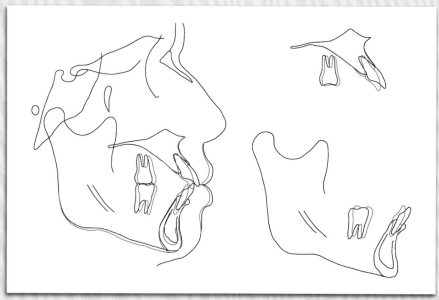

Fig. MSI 11-6. Cephalometric superimposition.

12

Bialveolar Protrusion Treated by First Premolar Extraction and Maximum Retraction

Johnny J.L. Liao, James C.Y. Lin, Eric J.W. Liou

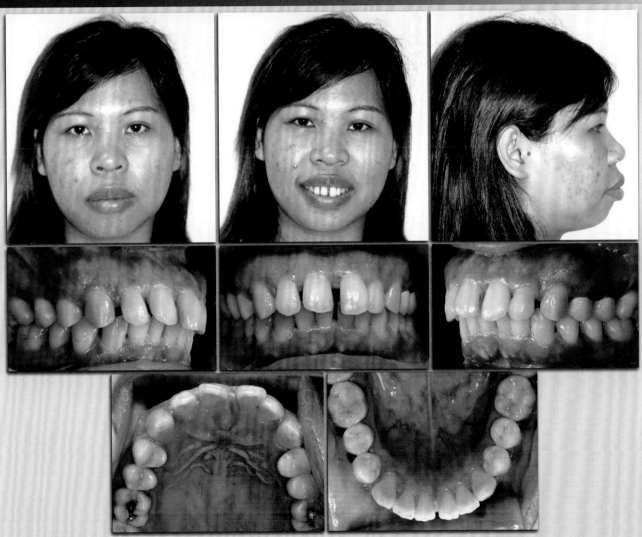

Fig. MSI 12-1. Pretreatment photographs.

The patient had a significant bialveolar protrusion and lip protrusion. The treatment plan was to extract all four first premolars and maximally retract the anterior teeth to decrease the facial convexity using upper miniscrew implants (MSIs).

In spite of the improved facial profile and dental relationship, several problems were encountered during treatment. The MSIs failed twice. The first MSIs were the Micro-Implant Anchorage system (MIA), the second was the Orthodontic Mini Anchor System (OMAS). Both were located in the interradicular area, which suggests that the patient's pretreatment generalized horizontal bone loss may have been a contributing factor. The second OMAS MSIs were placed in the infrazygomatic crest and were larger in diameter (2.0 as opposed to 1.5 mm) where more bone stock was available, with no further sequellae. It also appears that some root resorption occurred on the upper anterior teeth.

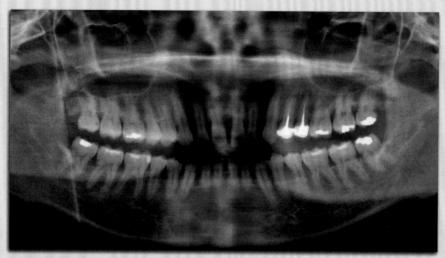

Fig. MSI 12–2. Pretreatment panoramic radiograph.

Table MSI 12–1.	Diagnosis and Treatment Goals	
	Diagnosis	Treatment Goals
SKELETAL		
Anteroposterior	Class II	Class II
Vertical	Normal	Normal
Transverse	Normal	Normal
DENTAL		
Right molar	Class I	Class I
Right canine	Class I	Class I
Left molar	Class I	Class I
Left canine	Class I	Class I
Upper right	2 mm spacing	None
Upper left	2 mm spacing	None
Lower right	1 mm spacing	None
Lower left	1 mm spacing	None
Missing teeth	None	No. 14, 18, 24, 28, 34, 38, 44, 48
Restore teeth	N/A	N/A
Overjet	5 mm	2 mm
Overbite	4 mm	2 mm
Upper ML	0 mm to facial ML	0 mm to facial ML
Lower ML	0 mm to facial ML	0 mm to facial ML
SOFT TISSUE		
Profile	Convex	Full
Lips	Incompetent	Competent
PERIODONTIUM		
Inadequate KT/TT	None	None
Gingival recession	None	None
Bone loss	No. 11, 12, 16, 21, 22, 26	Maintain

KT/TT, Keratinized tissue/thin tissue; *ML,* midline; *N/A,* not applicable.

Table MSI 12-2.	Temporary Anchorage Device Summary			
Procedure	Data			
Appliances placed	8 Sep 2002			
TAD placed	8 Sep 2002	8 Sep 2002	10 Dec 2002	10 Dec 2002
Location of TAD	Mesiofacial No. 16	Mesiofacial No. 26	Zygoma apical No. 16	Zygoma apical No. 16
Type of TAD	MSI	MSI	MSI	MSI
TAD loaded	8 Sep 2002	8 Sep 2002	10 Dec 2002	10 Dec 2002
Healing duration	0 days	0 days	0 days	0 days
Force in grams	150	150	150	150
Mechanics used	Direct	Direct	Direct	Direct
TAD unloaded	10 Dec 2002	10 Dec 2002	1 Oct 2004	1 Oct 2004
TAD loading duration	3 months	3 months	20 months	20 months
TAD removed	10 Dec 2002	10 Dec 2002	1 Oct 2004	1 Oct 2004
Appliances removed	1 Oct 2004			
Treatment duration	25 months			

TAD, Temporary anchorage device; *MSI*, miniscrew implant.

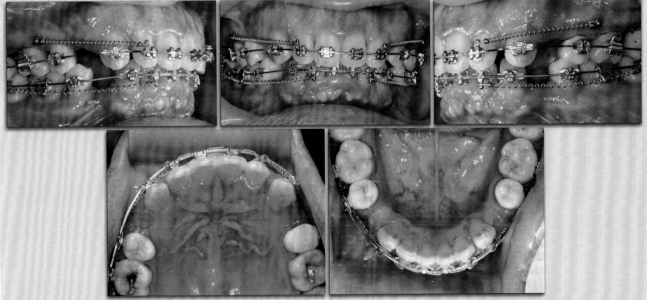

Fig. MSI 12-3.   Initial temporary anchorage device (TAD) photographs.

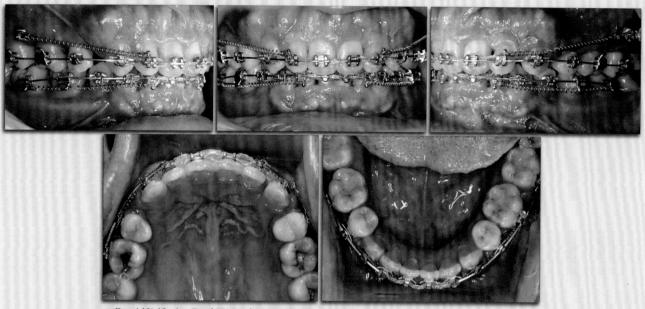

Fig. MSI 12–4.   Final TAD photographs.

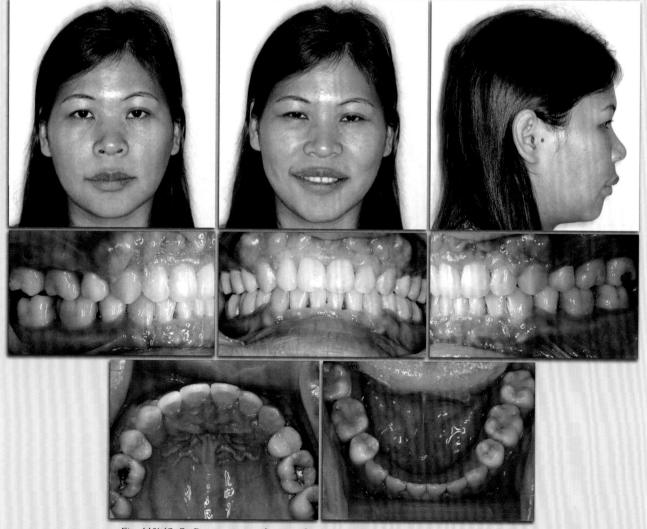

Fig. MSI 12–5.   Posttreatment photographs.

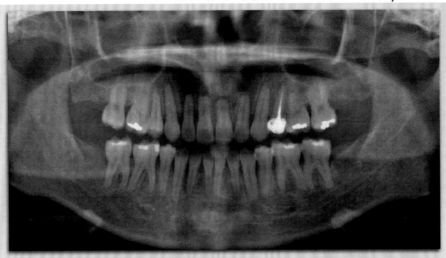

Fig. MSI 12-6. Posttreatment panoramic radiograph.

Table MSI 12-3.	Cephalometric Summary	
	Pretreatment	Posttreatment
SKELETAL		
SNA (degrees)	85.0	80.5
SNB (degrees)	78.5	78.0
ANB (degrees)	6.5	2.5
SN-ANS/PNS (degrees)	9.5	9.5
SN-GoMe (degrees)	38.5	37.0
N-ANS (mm)	47.5	44.0
ANS-Me (mm)	73.0	75.5
DENTAL		
U1-SN (degrees)	112.0	89.0
L1-GoMe (degrees)	114.5	89.5
U1-APo (mm)	18.0	6.5
L1-APo (mm)	13.5	5.0
SOFT TISSUE		
LS-PnPo′ (mm)	6.0	2.0
LI-PnPo′ (mm)	12.0	2.5

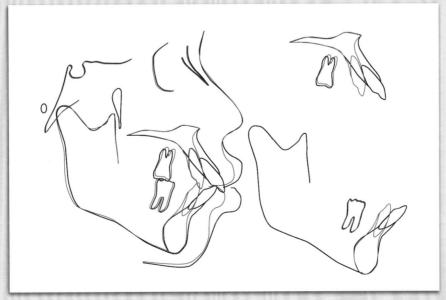

Fig. MSI 12-7. Cephalometric superimposition.

CR-MSI

Adult Class II Subdivision Malocclusion Treated with Extraction of Decayed Maxillary Second Premolars

Eric J.W. Liou, James C.Y. Lin

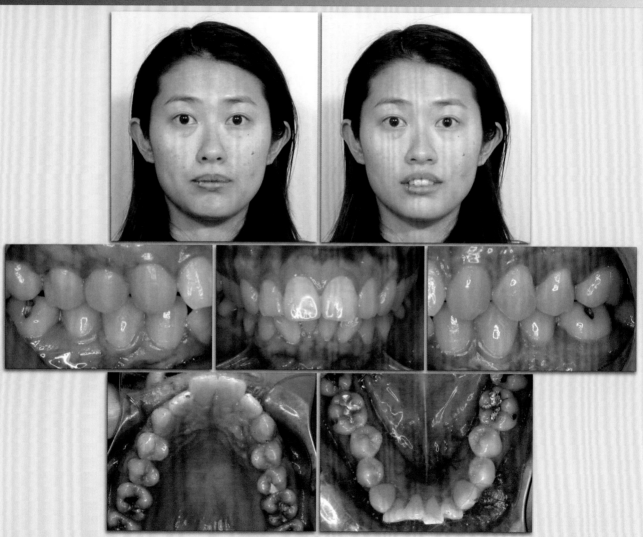

Fig. MSI 13-1. Pretreatment photographs.

The original treatment plan was to restore tooth No. 15 and to extract teeth No. 14, 24, 34, and 44 to resolve the protrusive upper incisors and Class II malocclusion. However, the patient requested that the decayed tooth No. 15 be extracted instead of tooth No. 14. Therefore, the extraction pattern was altered. Miniscrew implants (MSIs) 2.0 mm in diameter by 17 mm long were to be placed in the infrazygomatic crests for en masse retraction and intrusion

of the upper premolars and anterior teeth.

Although the radiographs suggested that the MSIs were placed into the maxillary sinus, there were never any signs or symptoms of sinus infection during treatment. The maxillary sinus remained clear at the end of the treatment, as revealed on the radiographs. The only unexpected complication was palatal tipping of the maxillary incisors after en masses retraction and intrusion. We anticipated that the composite retraction-and-intrusion vector of the NiTi closed coil springs and the titanium-molybdenum alloy (TMA) lever arms would move the maxillary incisors bodily, or at least would not tip palatally too much. To correct this, labial crown torque was placed on the maxillary incisors at the end of treatment. Currently, labial crown torque is placed on the maxillary incisors at the beginning of the en masse retraction and intrusion to prevent palatal tipping.

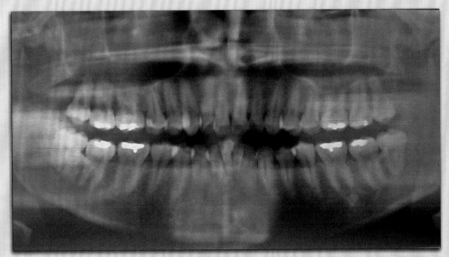

Fig. MSI 13-2. Pretreatment panoramic radiograph.

Table MSI 13-1.	Diagnosis and Treatment Goals	
	Diagnosis	Treatment Goals
SKELETAL		
Anteroposterior	Class I	Class I
Vertical	Normal	Normal
Transverse	Normal	Normal
DENTAL		
Right molar	End-on Class III	Class I
Right canine	End-on Class III	Class I
Left molar	Class I	Class I
Left canine	Class I	Class I
Upper right	1 mm crowding	None
Upper left	1.5 mm crowding	None
Lower right	3 mm crowding	None
Lower left	3 mm crowding	None
Missing teeth	None	No. 15, 25, 34, 44
Restore teeth	N/A	N/A
Overjet	6 mm	2 mm
Overbite	3 mm	2 mm
Upper ML	0.5 mm right of facial ML	0 mm to facial ML
Lower ML	1 mm right of facial ML	0 mm to facial ML
SOFT TISSUE		
Profile	Convex	Straight
Lips	Incompetent	Competent
PERIODONTIUM		
Inadequate KT/TT	None	None
Gingival recession	None	None
Bone loss	None	None
OTHER	Distal decay No. 15	

KT/TT, Keratinized tissue/thin tissue; *ML*, midline; *N/A*, not applicable.

Table MSI 13–2. Procedure	Temporary Anchorage Device Summary Data	
Appliances placed	15 Apr 2002	
TAD placed	10 Jul 2002	
Location of TAD	Zygoma apical No. 16	Zygoma apical No. 26
Type of TAD	MSI	MSI
TAD loaded	24 Jul 2002	24 Jul 2002
Healing duration	14 days	14 days
Force in grams	450	450
Mechanics used	Direct	Direct
TAD unloaded	10 Apr 2003	10 Apr 2003
TAD loading duration	9 months	9 months
TAD removed	17 Oct 2003	17 Oct 2003
Appliances removed	17 Oct 2003	
Treatment duration	18 months	

TAD, Temporary anchorage device; *MSI,* miniscrew implant.

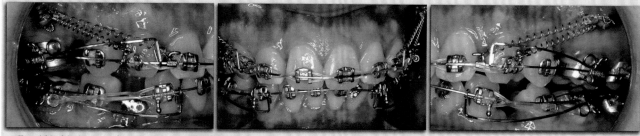

Fig. MSI 13–3.   Initial temporary anchorage device (TAD) photographs.

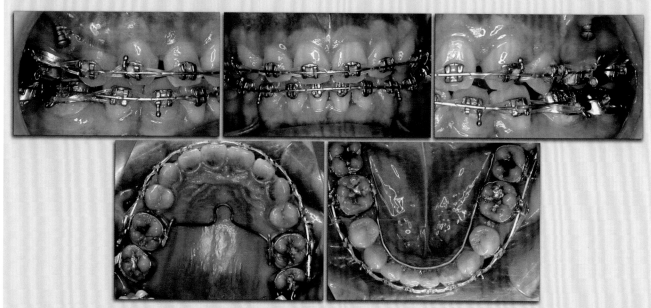

Fig. MSI 13–4.   Final TAD photographs.

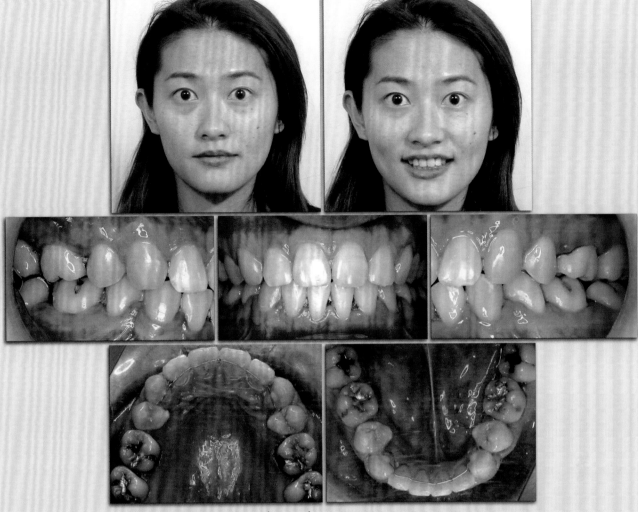

Fig. MSI 13-5. Posttreatment photographs.

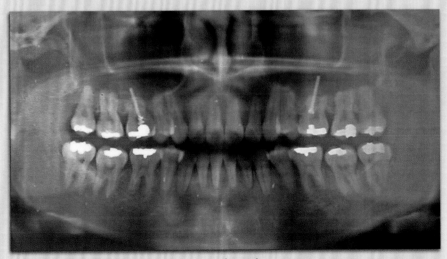

Fig. MSI 13-6. Posttreatment panoramic radiograph.

Table MSI 13-3.	Cephalometric Summary	
	Pretreatment	Posttreatment
SKELETAL		
SNA (degrees)	88.5	85.5
SNB (degrees)	82.5	81.5
ANB (degrees)	6.0	4.0
SN-ANS/PNS (degrees)	9.0	9.0
SN-GoMe (degrees)	31.0	30.0
N-ANS (mm)	60.0	60.0
ANS-Me (mm)	67.0	66.0
DENTAL		
U1-SN (degrees)	122.0	104.0
L1-GoMe (degrees)	101.0	101.0
U1-APo (mm)	11.0	2.5
L1-APo (mm)	2.5	–1.0
SOFT TISSUE		
LS-PnPo′ (mm)	0.5	–5.0
LI-PnPo′ (mm)	1.5	–4.5

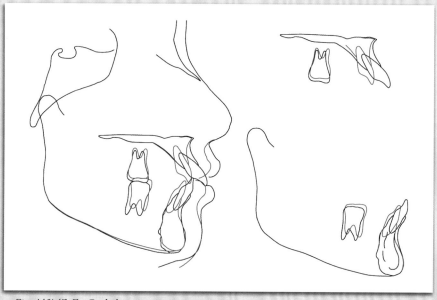

Fig. MSI 13-7. Cephalometric superimposition.

CR–MSI

14

Canted Occlusal Plane and Anterior Open Bite Treatment

Johnny J.L. Liao, James C.Y. Lin, Eric J.W. Liou

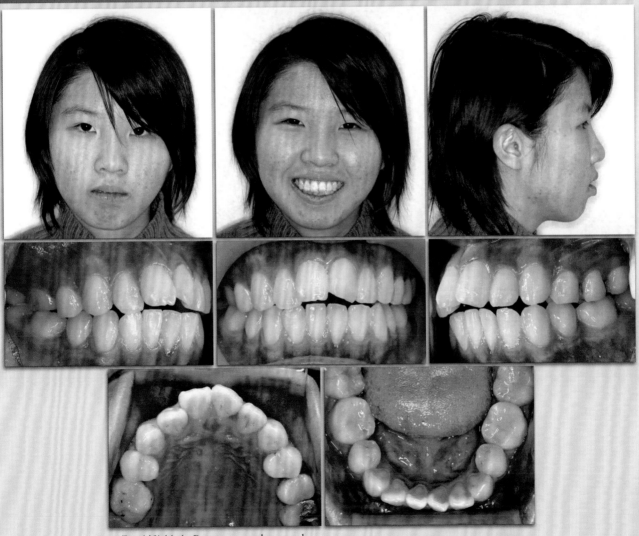

Fig. MSI 14–1. Pretreatment photographs.

The treatment plan was to extract the upper left second premolar in order to correct the left posterior arch asymmetry and to extract all second molars to retract and intrude the posterior teeth and close the open bite. A miniscrew implant (MSI) was to be placed on the upper right for intrusion and occlusal cant correction. After the occlusal cant was corrected bilaterally, MSIs were to be used to retract and intrude the upper arch to achieve a normal overbite and overjet.

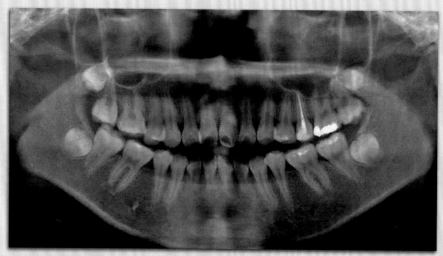

Fig. MSI 14–2. Pretreatment panoramic radiograph.

Table MSI 14–1.	Diagnosis and Treatment Goals	
	Diagnosis	Treatment Goals
SKELETAL		
Anteroposterior	Class II	Class II
Vertical	Open bite	Normal
Transverse	Normal	Normal
DENTAL		
Right molar	End-on Class II	Class I
Right canine	End-on Class II	Class I
Left molar	Class III	Class I
Left canine	End-on Class II	Class I
Upper right	1.5 mm crowding	None
Upper left	0 mm crowding	None
Lower right	1.5 mm crowding	None
Lower left	1.5 mm crowding	None
Missing teeth	No. 14, 34, 44	No. 14, 17, 25, 27, 34, 37, 44, 47
Restore teeth	N/A	N/A
Overjet	4.5 mm	2 mm
Overbite	0 mm	2 mm
Upper ML	0 mm to facial ML	0 mm to facial ML
Lower ML	0 mm to facial ML	0 mm to facial ML
SOFT TISSUE		
Profile	Convex	Full
Lips	Incompetent	Competent
PERIODONTIUM		
Inadequate KT/TT	None	None
Gingival recession	None	None
Bone loss	None	None
OTHER	No. 25 endodontically treated	

KT/TT, Keratinized tissue/thin tissue; *ML,* midline; *N/A,* not applicable.

Table MSI 14-2.	Temporary Anchorage Device Summary	
Procedure	Data	
Appliances placed	28 Aug 2002	
TAD placed	22 Nov 2003	13 Mar 2004
Location of TAD	Distofacial No. 15	Distofacial No. 24
Type of TAD	MSI	MSI
TAD loaded	22 Nov 2003	13 Mar 2004
Healing duration	0 days	0 days
Force in grams	200	100
Mechanics used	Direct	Direct
TAD unloaded	13 Nov 2004	13 Nov 2004
TAD loading duration	12 months	8 months
TAD removed	13 Nov 2004	13 Nov 2004
Appliances removed	13 Nov 2004	
Treatment duration	27 months	

TAD, Temporary anchorage device; *MSI,* miniscrew implant.

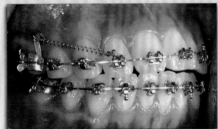 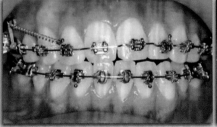 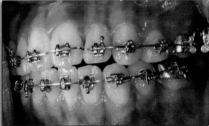

Fig. MSI 14-3. Initial temporary anchorage device (TAD) photographs.

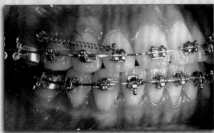 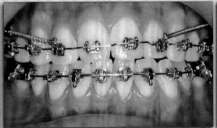 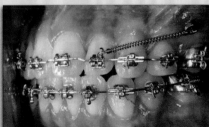

Fig. MSI 14-4. Final TAD photographs.

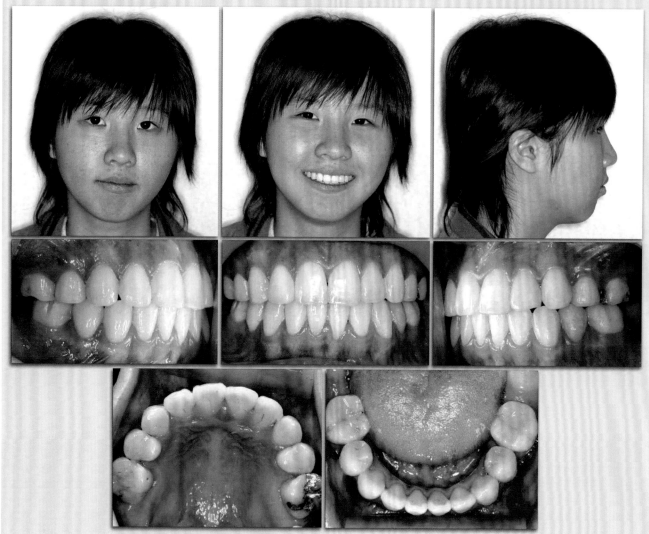

Fig. MSI 14–5. Posttreatment photographs.

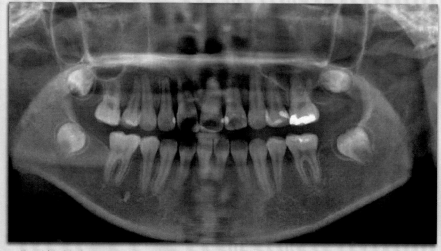

Fig. MSI 14–6. Posttreatment panoramic radiograph.

Table MSI 14-3.	Cephalometric Summary	
	Pretreatment	Posttreatment
SKELETAL		
SNA (degrees)	84.5	82.5
SNB (degrees)	78.5	76.5
ANB (degrees)	6.0	6.0
SN-ANS/PNS (degrees)	6.0	5.0
SN-GoMe (degrees)	42.5	44.0
N-ANS (mm)	48.0	50.5
ANS-Me (mm)	70.0	71.0
DENTAL		
U1-SN (degrees)	116.5	105.5
L1-GoMe (degrees)	94.0	87.5
U1-APo (mm)	10.5	6.5
L1-APo (mm)	5.5	3.0
SOFT TISSUE		
LS-PnPo′ (mm)	1.0	–1.0
LI-PnPo′ (mm)	6.5	2.5

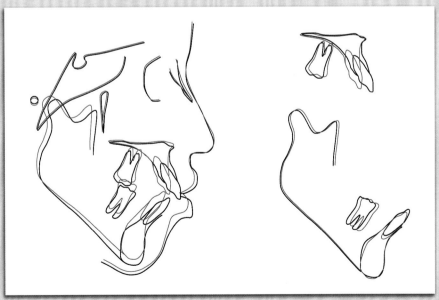

Fig. MSI 14-7. Cephalometric superimposition.

15

En Masse Retraction and Upper Anterior Intrusion in Class I Bialveolar Protrusion

George Anka

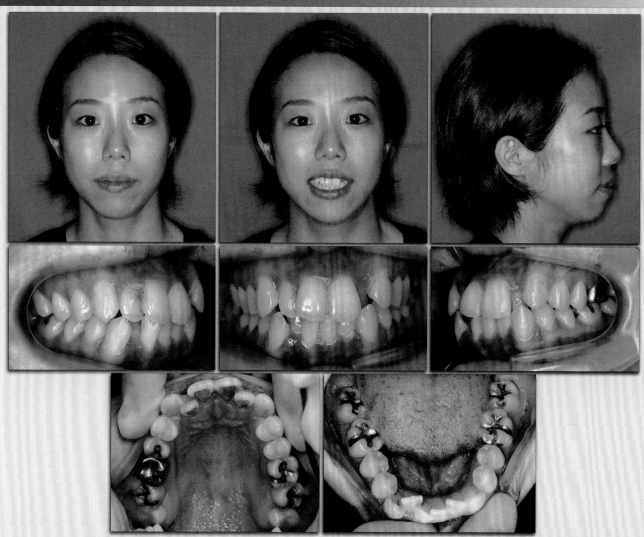

Fig. MSI 15–1. Pretreatment photographs.

The treatment plan was to extract the four first premolars to alleviate the crowding. After the initial alignment was finished, miniscrew implants (MSI) were to be placed to aid in anterior retraction. The MSIs placed in the upper anterior region were used to intrude the upper anterior teeth to minimize the excessive gingival display.

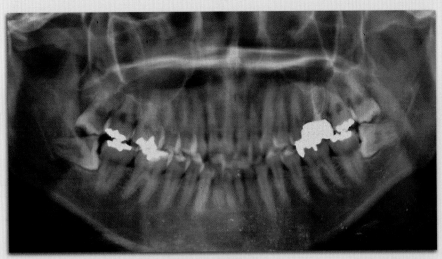

Fig. MSI 15–2. Pretreatment panoramic radiograph.

Table MSI 15–1.	Diagnosis and Treatment Goals	
	Diagnosis	Treatment Goals
SKELETAL		
Anteroposterior	Class I	Class I
Vertical	Normal	Normal
Transverse	Normal	Normal
DENTAL		
Right molar	Class I	Class I
Right canine	Class I	Class I
Left molar	Class I	Class I
Left canine	Class I	Class I
Upper right	7 mm crowding	None
Upper left	6 mm crowding	None
Lower right	5 mm crowding	None
Lower left	4 mm crowding	None
Missing teeth	None	No. 14, 18, 24, 28, 34, 38, 44, 48
Restore teeth	N/A	N/A
Overjet	2 mm	2 mm
Overbite	2 mm	2 mm
Upper ML	2 mm left of facial ML	0 mm to facial ML
Lower ML	0 mm to facial ML	0 mm to facial ML
SOFT TISSUE		
Profile	Full	Straight
Lips	Incompetent	Competent
PERIODONTIUM		
Inadequate KT/TT	No. 31, 33, 41, 43	Maintain
Gingival recession	None	None
Bone loss	None	None
OTHER	Decay in all posterior teeth; No. 38 and 48 impacted; No. 26 endodontically treated.	

KT/TT, Keratinized tissue/thin tissue; *ML,* midline; *N/A,* not applicable.

Table MSI 15-2.	Temporary Anchorage Device Summary					
Procedure	Data					
Appliances placed	13 Jul 2001					
TAD placed	14 Sep 2002	14 Sep 2002	14 Sep 2002	14 Sep 2002	14 Sep 2002	14 Sep 2002
Location of TAD	Mesiofacial No. 16	Mesiofacial No. 26	Mesiofacial No. 12	Mesiofacial No. 22	Mesiofacial No. 36	Mesiofacial No. 46
Type of TAD	MSI	MSI	MSI	MSI	MSI	MSI
TAD loaded	28 Sep 2002	28 Sep 2002	28 Sep 2002	28 Sep 2002	28 Sep 2002	28 Sep 2002
Healing duration	14 days	14 days	14 days	14 days	14 days	14 days
Force in grams	200-300	200-300	200-300	200-300	200-300	200-300
Mechanics used	Direct	Direct	Direct	Direct	Direct	Direct
TAD unloaded	31 Mar 2003	31 Mar 2003	31 Mar 2003	31 Mar 2003	31 Mar 2003	31 Mar 2003
TAD loading duration	6 months	6 months	6 months	6 months	6 months	6 months
TAD removed	15 Dec 2003	15 Dec 2003	15 Dec 2003	15 Dec 2003	15 Dec 2003	15 Dec 2003
Appliances removed	15 Dec 2003					
Treatment duration	29 months					

TAD, Temporary anchorage device; *MSI*, miniscrew implant.

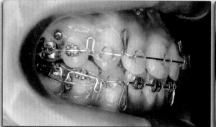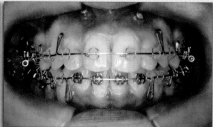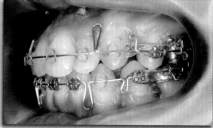

Fig. MSI 15-3. Initial temporary anchorage device (TAD) photographs.

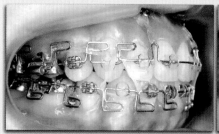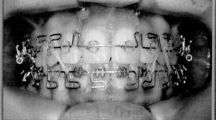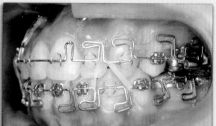

Fig. MSI 15-4. Final TAD photographs.

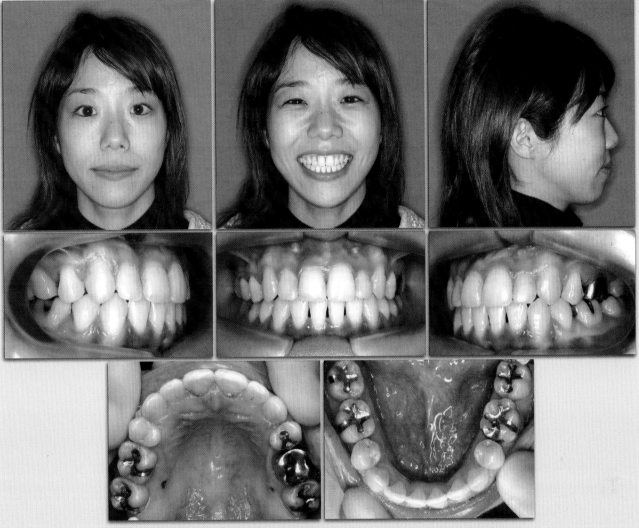

Fig. MSI 15-5. Posttreatment photographs.

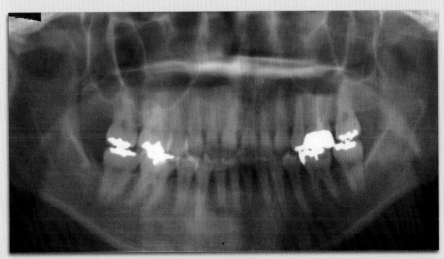

Fig. MSI 16-6. Posttreatment panoramic radiograph.

Table MSI 15-3.	Cephalometric Summary	
	Pretreatment	Posttreatment
SKELETAL		
SNA (degrees)	76.3	76.9
SNB (degrees)	76.6	75.4
ANB (degrees)	−0.2	1.5
SN-ANS/PNS (degrees)	7.3	9.6
SN-GoMe (degrees)	48.0	48.1
N-ANS (mm)	120.2	114.6
ANS-Me (mm)	50.7	62.8
DENTAL		
U1-SN (degrees)	115.5	103.4
L1-GoMe (degrees)	90.0	80.3
U1-APo (mm)	16.8	8.8
L1-APo (mm)	12.6	6.4
SOFT TISSUE		
LS-PnPo′ (mm)	1.7	0.5
LI-PnPo′ (mm)	5.0	2.7

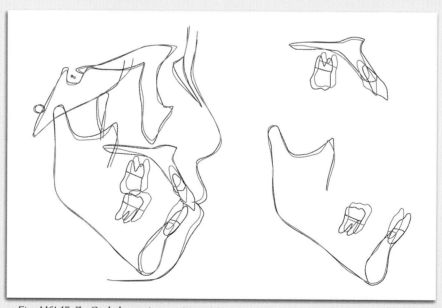

Fig. MSI 15-7. Cephalometric superimposition.

Protraction of Lower Molars to Close Extraction Spaces and Avoid Mandibular Advancement

Jason B. Cope

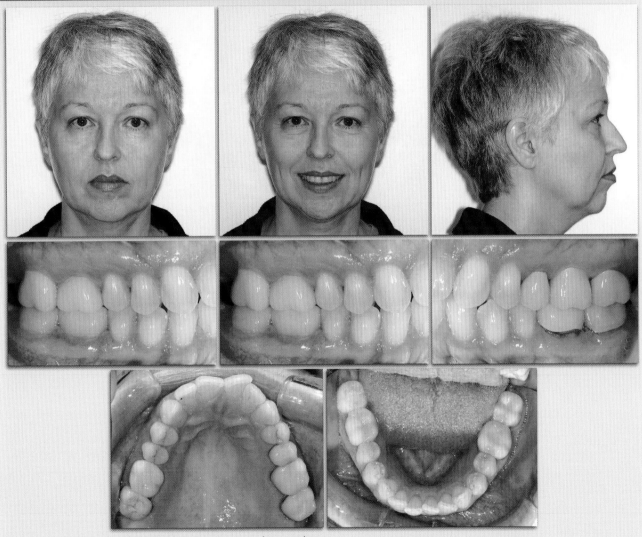

Fig. MSI 16-1. Pretreatment photographs.

The treatment plan originally was to extract upper second premolars and lower first premolars followed by space closure and mandibular advancement. However, the patient declined surgical treatment. The alternative treatment plan was to extract upper first premolars (for anterior retraction) and lower second premolars (for maximum posterior protraction). Ortho Implants (IMTEC Corp., Ardmore, Oklahoma) were to be placed bilaterally between the lower canines and first premolars for protraction.

The soft tissue around the lower right miniscrew implant (MSI) became infected 6 weeks after placement. The infection was treated with 150 mg clindamycin 3 times daily and chlorhexidine rinses twice daily for 8 days without further sequelae. The MSI was not removed or replaced because it was stable. The most probable reason for the infection was inadequate oral hygiene around an MSI that was placed slightly too deep. To prevent this problem, a longer MSI should have been placed so that more of the abutment head was located supramucosally.

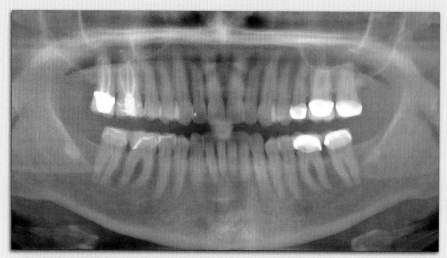

Fig. MSI 16-2. Pretreatment panoramic radiograph.

Table MSI 16-1.	Diagnosis and Treatment Goals	
SKELETAL		
Anteroposterior	Class II	Class II
Vertical	Normal	Normal
Transverse	Normal	Normal
DENTAL		
Right molar	End-on Class II	Class II
Right canine	End-on Class II	Class I
Left molar	End-on Class II	Class II
Left canine	End-on Class II	Class I
Upper right	1 mm crowding	None
Upper left	2 mm crowding	None
Lower right	2 mm crowding	None
Lower left	3 mm crowding	None
Missing teeth	No. 18, 28, 38, 48	No. 14, 18, 24, 28, 35, 38, 45, 48
Restore teeth	N/A	N/A
Overjet	7 mm	2 mm
Overbite	3 mm	3 mm
Upper ML	0 mm to facial ML	0 mm to facial ML
Lower ML	1.5 mm right of facial ML	0 mm to facial ML
SOFT TISSUE		
Profile	Convex	Convex
Lips	Incompetent	Competent
PERIODONTIUM		
Inadequate KT/TT	None	None
Gingival recession	None	None
Bone loss	None	None

KT/TT, Keratinized tissue/thin tissue; ML, midline; N/A, not applicable.

| Table MSI 16-2. | Temporary Anchorage Device Summary | |
Procedure	Data	
Appliances placed	28 May 2003	
TAD placed	11 Feb 2004	11 Feb 2004
Location of TAD	Distofacial No. 33*	Distofacial No. 43
Type of TAD	MSI	MSI
TAD loaded	11 Feb 2004	11 Feb 2004
Healing duration	0 days	0 days
Force in grams	100-150	100-150
Mechanics used	Direct	Direct
TAD unloaded	11 Oct 2004	11 Oct 2004
TAD loading duration	8 months	8 months
TAD removed	11 Oct 2004	11 Oct 2004
Appliances removed	9 Aug 2005	
Treatment duration	27 months	

*No. 33 miniscrew implant (MSI) gingiva was infected on 3/31/2004 and was treated with 150 mg clindamycin 3 times daily and chlorhexidine rinses twice daily for 8 days without sequelae. *TAD*, Temporary anchorage device.

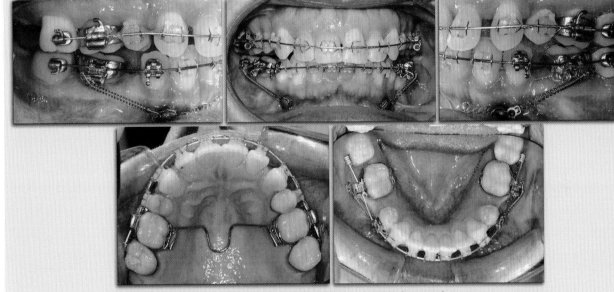

Fig. MSI 16-3. Initial temporary anchorage device (TAD) photographs.

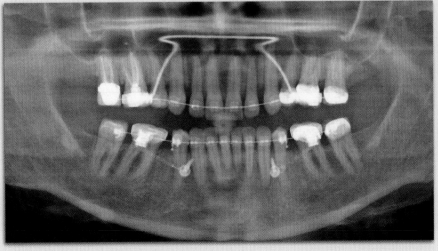

Fig. MSI 16-4. Initial TAD panoramic radiograph.

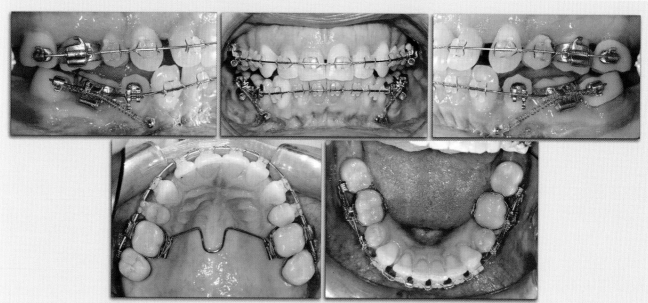

Fig. MSI 16-5. Final TAD photographs.

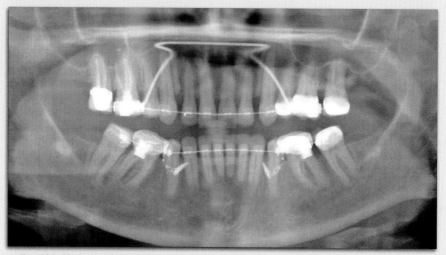

Fig. MSI 16-6. Final TAD panoramic radiograph.

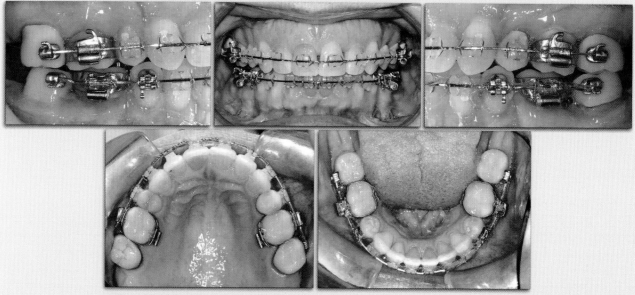

Fig. MSI 16-7. Progress photographs.

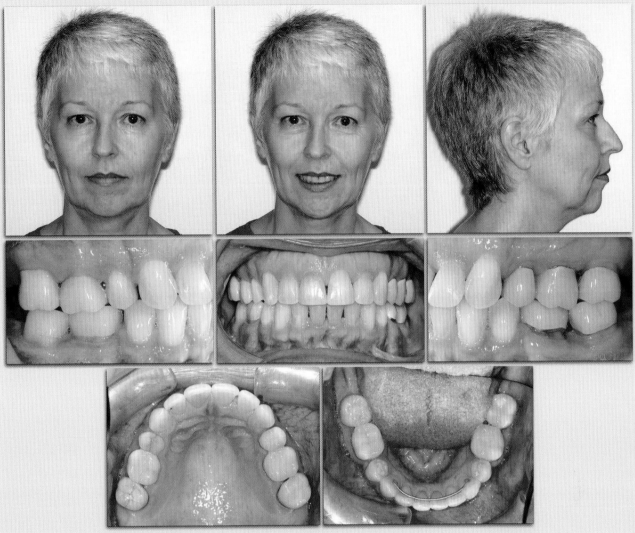

Fig. MSI 16-8. Posttreatment photographs.

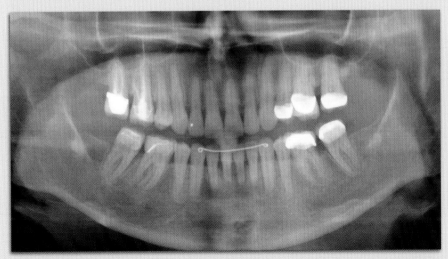

Fig. MSI 16-9. Posttreatment panoramic radiograph.

Table MSI 16-3.	Cephalometric Summary			
	Pretreatment	Pre-TAD	Post-TAD	Posttreatment
SKELETAL				
SNA (degrees)	83.8	83.7	82.9	84.0
SNB (degrees)	77.8	76.8	76.9	78.0
ANB (degrees)	6.0	6.9	6.0	6.0
SN-ANS/PNS (degrees)	4.8	4.9	4.9	4.4
SN-GoMe (degrees)	34.3	36.7	35.9	35.1
N-ANS (mm)	49.3	49.3	48.7	49.5
ANS-Me (mm)	72.7	74.5	73.7	74.8
DENTAL				
U1-SN (degrees)	110.6	98.0	99.8	98.7
L1-GoMe (degrees)	105.4	104.1	104.7	98.7
U1-APo (mm)	13.4	9.3	8.7	7.8
L1-APo (mm)	8.2	5.6	6.4	4.0
SOFT TISSUE				
LS-PnPo′ (mm)	–4.7	–4.0	–4.1	–4.5
LI-PnPo′ (mm)	2.9	3.1	2.7	0.5

TAD, Temporary anchorage device.

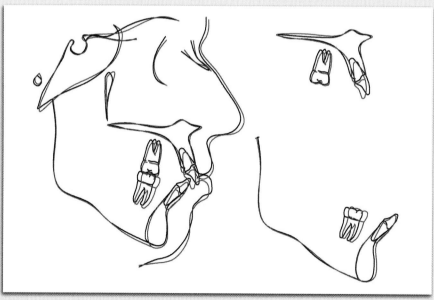

Fig. MSI 16-10. Cephalometric superimposition.

Patient with Multiple Missing Teeth Treated by Space Closure Instead of Restorations

Thomas S. Drechsler, Axel Bumann

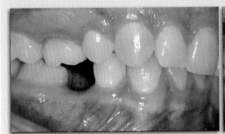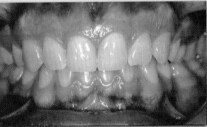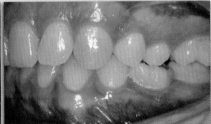

Fig. MSI 17–1. Pretreatment photographs.

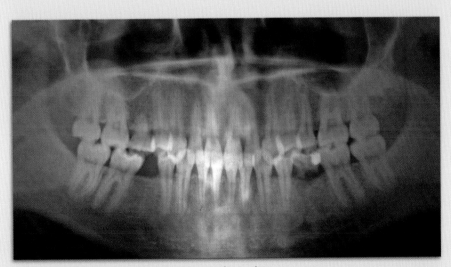

Fig. MSI 17–2. Pretreatment panoramic radiograph.

The patient had congenitally missing upper right and both lower second premolars. The deciduous second molars were retained in the upper right and lower left quadrants and were to be extracted. The *tomas®* pin (Dentaurum, Inc., Newtown, Pennsylvania) was placed distal to teeth No. 14, 34, and 44 to aid in protracting the posterior teeth using sectional arches to close the extraction spaces.

Table MSI 17-1.	Diagnosis and Treatment Goals	
	Diagnosis	Treatment Goals
SKELETAL		
Anteroposterior	Class I	Class I
Vertical	Deep bite	Normal
Transverse	Normal	Normal
DENTAL		
Right molar	Class III	Class I
Right canine	Class II	Class I
Left molar	Class II	Class III
Left canine	Class I	Class I
Upper right	0 mm crowding	None
Upper left	0 mm crowding	None
Lower right	6.5 mm spacing	None
Lower left	1 mm crowding	None
Missing teeth	No. 15, 18, 35, 38, 45, 48	No. 15, 18, 35, 38, 45, 48
Restore teeth	N/A	N/A
Overjet	2 mm	2 mm
Overbite	5.5 mm	5.5 mm
Upper ML	0 mm to facial ML	0 mm to facial ML
Lower ML	1 mm left of facial ML	1 mm left of facial ML
SOFT TISSUE		
Profile	Straight	Straight
Lips	Competent	Competent
PERIODONTIUM		
Inadequate KT/TT	None	None
Gingival recession	None	None
Bone loss	None	None
OTHER	Retained deciduous teeth No. 55 and 75	

KT/TT, Keratinized tissue/thin tissue; ML, midline; N/A, not applicable.

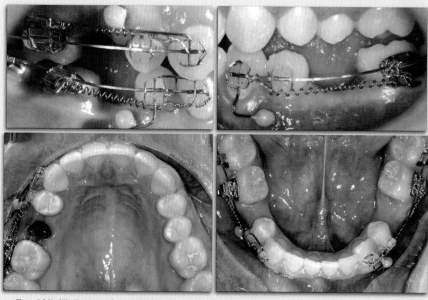

Fig. MSI 17-3. Initial temporary anchorage device (TAD) photographs.

| Table MSI 17-2. | Temporary Anchorage Device Summary | | |
Procedure	Data		
Appliances placed	5 Feb 2001		
TAD placed	5 Feb 2001	5 Feb 2001	5 Feb 2001
Location of TAD	Distofacial No. 14	Distofacial No. 44	Distofacial No. 34
Type of TAD	MSI	MSI	MSI
TAD loaded	5 Feb 2001	5 Feb 2001	5 Feb 2001
Healing duration	0 days	0 days	0 days
Force in grams	150	150	150
Mechanics used	Indirect	Direct and indirect	Direct and indirect
TAD unloaded	17 Oct 2001	16 Jan 2002	16 Jan 2002
TAD loading duration	8 months	11 months	11 months
TAD removed	17 Oct 2001	16 Jan 2002	16 Jan 2002
Appliances removed	16 Jan 2002		
Treatment duration	11 months		

TAD, Temporary anchorage device; *MSI*, miniscrew implant.

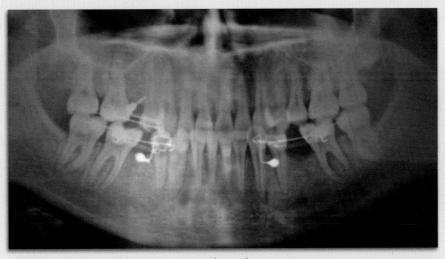

Fig. MSI 17-4. Initial TAD panoramic radiograph.

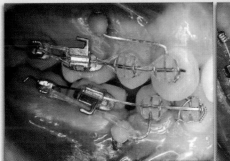
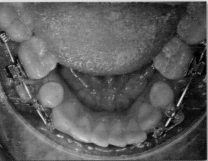
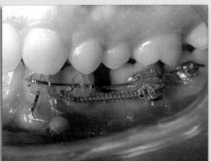

Fig. MSI 17-5. Progress TAD photographs.

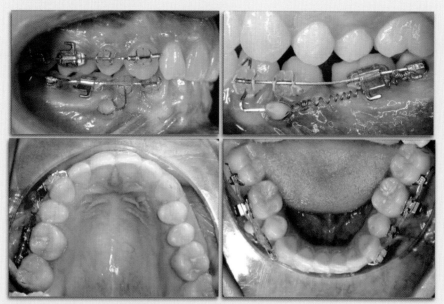

Fig. MSI 17–6. Final TAD photographs.

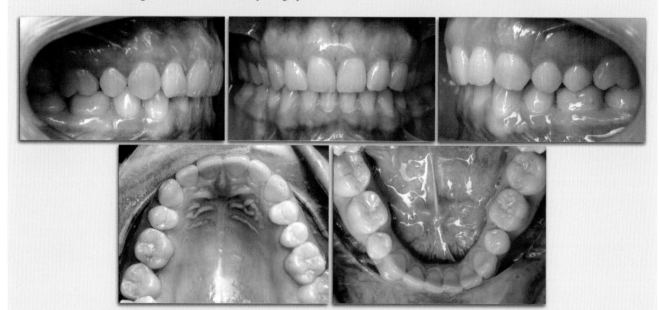

Fig. MSI 17–7. Posttreatment photographs.

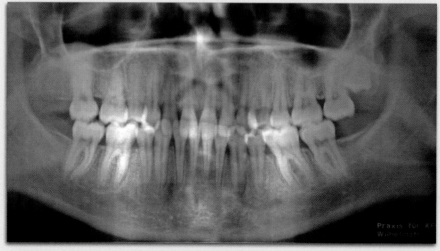

Fig. MSI 17–8. Posttreatment panoramic radiograph.

Table MSI 17-3.	Cephalometric Summary	
	Pretreatment	Posttreatment
SKELETAL		
SNA (degrees)	84.2	83.8
SNB (degrees)	80.7	81.1
ANB (degrees)	3.5	1.7
SN-ANS/PNS (degrees)	4.1	4.2
SN-GoMe (degrees)	27.4	28.4
N-ANS (mm)	51.7	51.9
ANS-Me (mm)	66.1	67.0
DENTAL		
U1-SN (degrees)	89.1	90.0
L1-GoMe (degrees)	92.1	89.4
U1-APo (mm)	3.0	3.6
L1-APo (mm)	0.0	0.9
SOFT TISSUE		
LS-PnPo′ (mm)	5.2	5.2
LI-PnPo′ (mm)	4.3	3.7

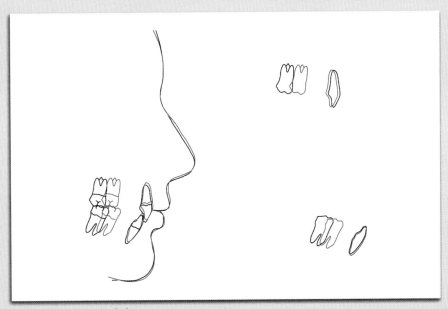

Fig. MSI 17–9. Cephalometric superimposition.

CR–MSI

Intrusion of a Supererupted Upper Molar and Uprighting of a Tipped Lower Molar for Placement and Restoration of a Lower Molar Implant

Jason B. Cope, Pedro F. Franco

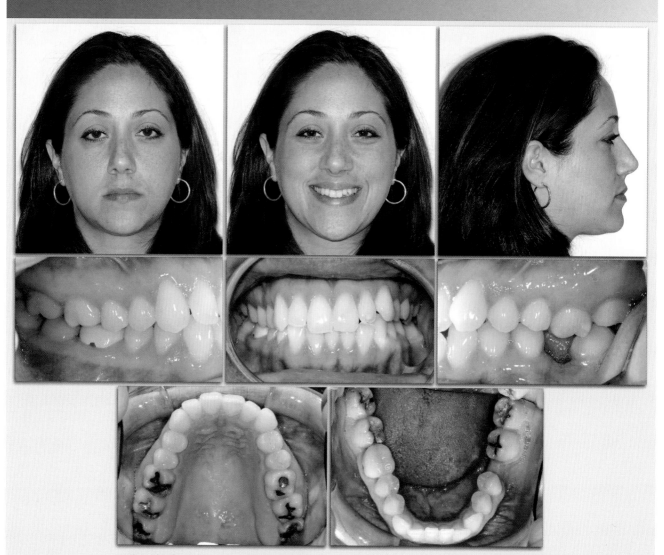

Fig. MSI 18–1. Pretreatment photographs.

The treatment plan was to extract the third molars (to allow for uprighting of the tipped lower left second molar) and the lower right central incisor (for protraction of the lower left buccal segment into a Class I relationship). At the time of the extractions, three Ortho Implants (IMTEC Corp., Ardmore, Oklahoma) were placed for differential anchorage. One was placed in the lower left retromolar region to distalize and slightly intrude the second molar.

The other two were placed on the facial and palatal, respectively, of the supererupted upper left first molar for intrusion. An 0.036-inch stainless steel wire was looped over the palatal miniscrew implant (MSI) and bonded to the upper left second premolar and second molar to prevent extrusion of these teeth upon initial arch wire placement. It became apparent that this fixed the distance between these teeth and would prevent intrusion of the first molar because of binding. Therefore, the distal component of the wire was sectioned and intrusion proceeded. After the lower molar was uprighted, the patient was to be reevaluated by her periodontist for a possible bone graft before implant dental placement and restoration.

The MSI placed in the lower left retromolar region was loose 14 days after placement. The MSI was replaced 3 weeks later with no further sequelae. The most probable reason for the failure was placement adjacent (lateral) to a recent extraction site. (See Chapter 5 for explanation.) To prevent this problem, the MSI should either be placed 2 to 3 weeks before extraction or 6 to 10 weeks after extraction.

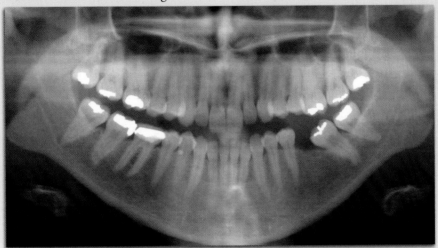

Fig. MSI 18-2. Pretreatment panoramic radiograph.

Table MSI 18-1.	Diagnosis and Treatment Goals	
	Diagnosis	Treatment Goals
SKELETAL		
Anteroposterior	Class I	Class I
Vertical	Normal	Normal
Transverse	Normal	Normal
DENTAL		
Right molar	Class I	Class I
Right canine	Class I	Class I
Left molar	End-on Class II	Class I
Left canine	Class II	Class I
Upper right	1 mm crowding	None
Upper left	1 mm crowding	None
Lower right	2 mm crowding	None
Lower left	3 mm crowding	None
Missing teeth	No. 36	No. 18, 28, 38, 41, 48
Restore teeth	N/A	No. 36
Overjet	3 mm	3 mm
Overbite	3 mm	3 mm
Upper ML	0 mm to facial ML	0 mm to facial ML
Lower ML	2.5 mm left of facial ML	No change
SOFT TISSUE		
Profile	Straight	Straight
Lips	Competent	Competent
PERIODONTIUM		
Inadequate KT/TT	None	None
Gingival recession	None	None
Bone loss	Mesioangular No. 36	Correct by uprighting

KT/TT, Keratinized tissue/thin tissue; *ML,* midline; *N/A,* not applicable.

Table MSI 18–2. Procedure	Temporary Anchorage Device Summary Data		
Appliances placed	10 Jun 2003		
TAD placed	10 Jun 2003	10 Jun 2003	17 Jul 2003*
Location of TAD	Distopalatal No. 26	Distofacial No. 26	Distal No. 37
Type of TAD	MSI	MSI	MSI
TAD loaded	26 Jun 2003	26 Jun 2003	23 Jul 2003
Healing duration	16 days	16 days	6 days
Force in grams	150-250	150-250	150-200
Mechanics used	Direct	Direct	Direct
TAD unloaded	24 Feb 2004	24 Feb 2004	5 Nov 2003
TAD loading duration	8 months	8 months	3½ months
TAD removed	24 Feb 2004	24 Feb 2004	5 Nov 2003
Appliances removed	24 Feb 2005		
Treatment duration	20½ months		

* Distal No. 37 miniscrew implant (MSI) was placed on 10 Jun 2003, but was loose on 26 Jun 2003, and was replaced on 17 Jul 2003. *TAD,* Temporary anchorage device.

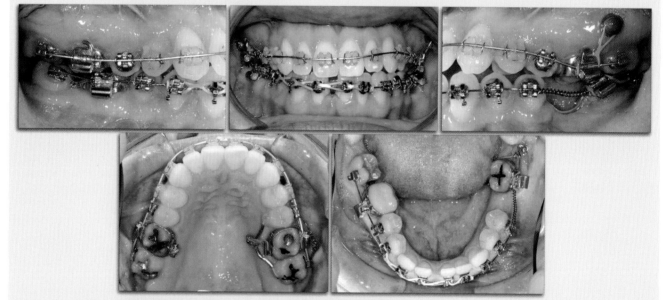

Fig. MSI 18-3. Initial temporary anchorage device (TAD) photographs.

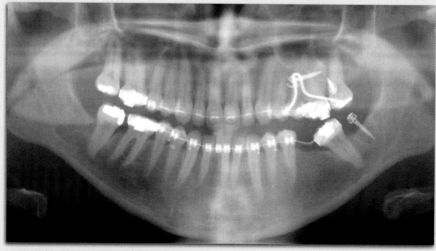

Fig. MSI 18-4. Initial TAD panoramic radiograph.

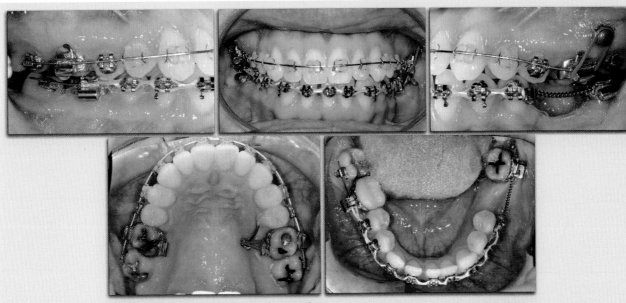

Fig. MSI 18-5. Progress TAD photographs.

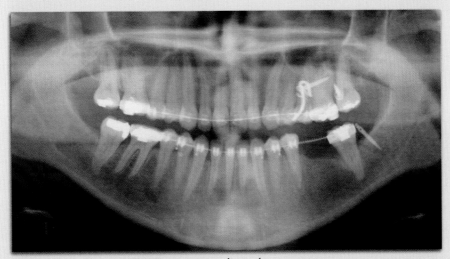

Fig. MSI 18-6. Progress TAD panoramic radiograph.

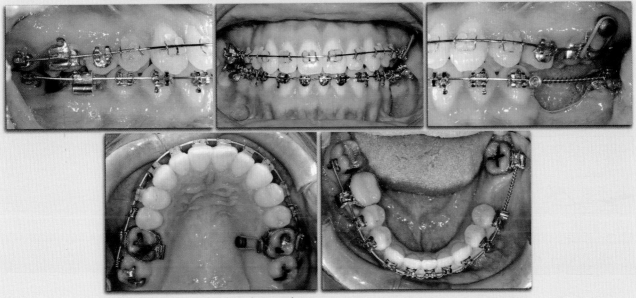

Fig. MSI 18-7. Final TAD photographs.

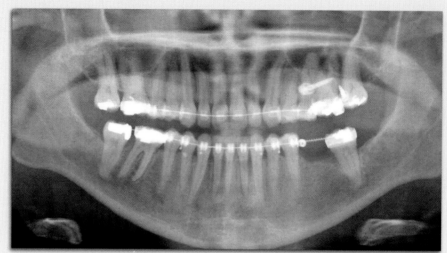

Fig. MSI 18-8. Final TAD panoramic radiograph.

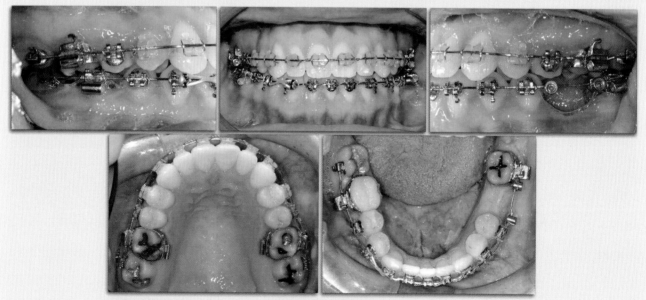

Fig. MSI 18-9. Progress treatment photographs.

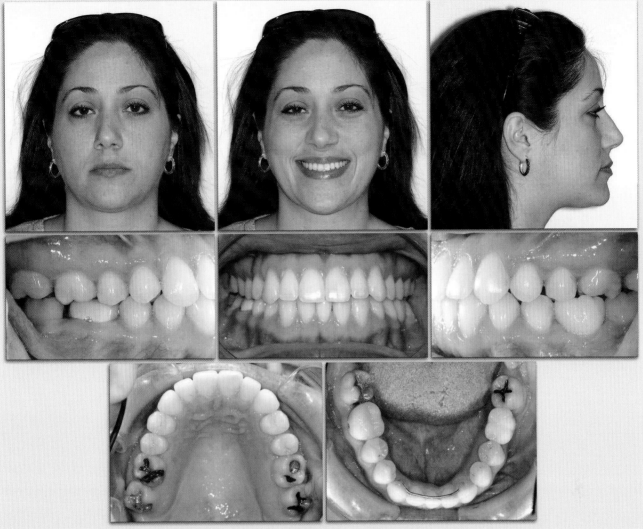

Fig. MSI 18-10. Posttreatment photographs.

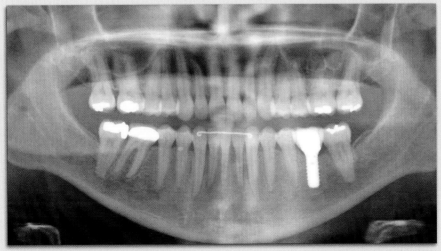

Fig. MSI 18-11. Posttreatment panoramic radiograph.

Table MSI 18-3.	Cephalometric Summary			
	Pretreatment	Pre-TAD	Post-TAD	Posttreatment
SKELETAL				
SNA (degrees)	79.4	78.0	80.8	78.0
SNB (degrees)	78.5	76.8	79.0	77.3
ANB (degrees)	1.0	1.2	1.7	0.7
SN-ANS/PNS (degrees)	14.7	14.5	13.0	14.7
SN-GoMe (degrees)	44.3	44.0	41.9	43.6
N-ANS (mm)	56.9	56.4	55.9	56.5
ANS-Me (mm)	68.3	67.9	67.4	67.6
DENTAL				
U1-SN (degrees)	109.0	108.5	108.3	111.4
L1-GoMe (degrees)	77.0	88.4	81.3	83.7
U1-APo (mm)	7.1	8.3	7.2	8.0
L1-APo (mm)	4.1	6.4	3.4	4.6
SOFT TISSUE				
LS-PnPo' (mm)	−7.5	−6.4	−7.6	−7.5
LI-PnPo' (mm)	−2.4	−2.0	−3.6	−3.5

TAD, Temporary anchorage device.

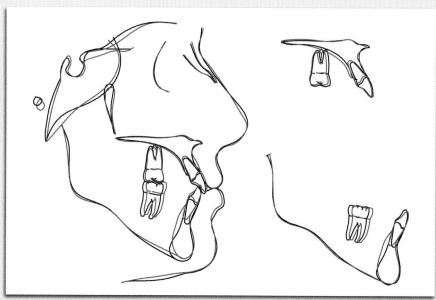

Fig. MSI 18-12. Cephalometric superimposition.

CR–MSI

Uprighting of Lower Second Molars for Placement and Restoration of Lower Implants

Jason B. Cope

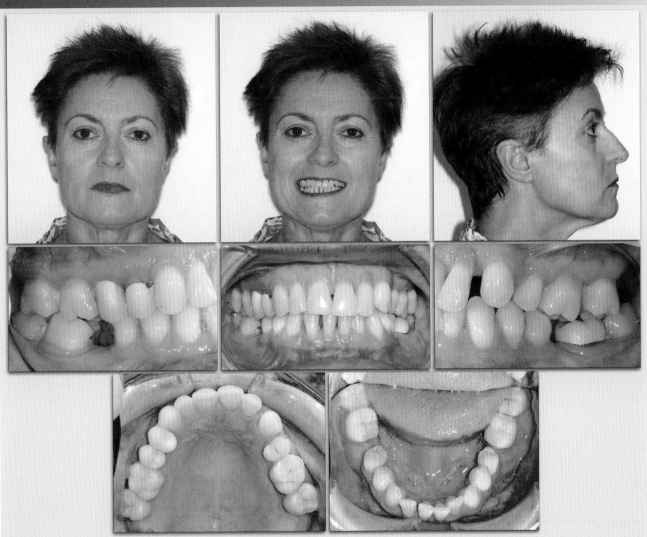

Fig. MSI 19-1. Pretreatment photographs.

The treatment plan was to extract the lower third molars to allow for uprighting of the tipped lower second molars. At the same time, Ortho Implants (IMTEC Corp., Ardmore, Oklahoma) placed in the lower retromolar areas would be used to distalize and slightly intrude the second molars, which would also correct the mesioangular bony defect on the lower left second molar. After the

lower molars were uprighted, the patient was to have dental implants placed by her periodontist, with restorations placed at the completion of orthodontic treatment.

The miniscrew implant (MSI) placed in the lower left retromolar region was loose 14 days after placement. The MSI was replaced the same day, but more posteriorly, with no further sequelae. The most probable reason for the failure was placement into the bony septum of the healing extraction site. At that point in time, the MSI had a rounded tip instead of a sharp tip and did not perforate the septum upon placement and therefore could not be placed any deeper. To prevent this problem, the MSI was redesigned with a sharp tip for drill-free placement. (See Chapter 9 for IMTEC Ortho Implant design.)

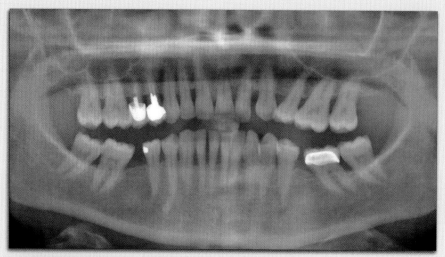

Fig. MSI 19-2. Pretreatment panoramic radiograph.

Table MSI 19-1.	Diagnosis and Treatment Goals	
	Diagnosis	Treatment Goals
SKELETAL		
Anteroposterior	Class I	Class I
Vertical	Normal	Normal
Transverse	Normal	Normal
DENTAL		
Right molar	Class I	Class I
Right canine	Class I	Class I
Left molar	Class II	Class II
Left canine	End-on Class III	Class I
Upper right	0 mm crowding	None
Upper left	2 mm spacing	None
Lower right	1 mm spacing	None
Lower left	0 mm crowding	None
Missing teeth	No. 18, 24, 28, 36, 46	No. 18, 24, 28, 38, 48
Restore teeth	N/A	No. 36, 46
Overjet	2 mm	2 mm
Overbite	3 mm	3 mm
Upper ML	2 mm right of facial ML	0 mm to facial ML
Lower ML	0 mm to facial ML	0 mm to facial ML
SOFT TISSUE		
Profile	Straight	Straight
Lips	Competent	Competent
PERIODONTIUM		
Inadequate KT/TT	None	None
Gingival recession	Generalized	Maintain
Bone loss	Generalized	Maintain

KT/TT, Keratinized tissue/thin tissue; *ML,* midline; *N/A,* not applicable.

| Table MSI 19-2. | Temporary Anchorage Device Summary | |
Procedure	Data	
Appliances placed	30 Sep 2002	
TAD placed	21 Jul 2003	4 Aug 2003*
Location of TAD	Distal No. 47	Distal No. 37
Type of TAD	MSI	MSI
TAD loaded	21 Jul 2003	4 Aug 2003
Healing duration	0 days	0 days
Force in grams	100-150	100-150
Mechanics used	Direct	Direct
TAD unloaded	2 Mar 2004	2 Mar 2004
TAD loading duration	7½ months	7 months
TAD removed	2 Mar 2004	2 Mar 2004
Appliances removed	6 Dec 2004	
Treatment duration	26 months	

*Distal No. 37 miniscrew implant (MSI) was placed on 21 Jul 2003, but was loose on 4 Aug 2003, and was replaced on 4 Aug 2003. *TAD,* Temporary anchorage device.

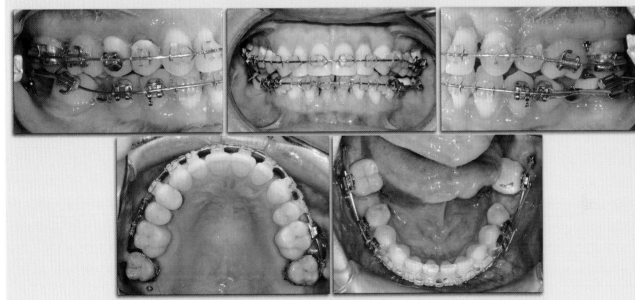

Fig. MSI 19-3. Initial temporary anchorage device (TAD) photographs.

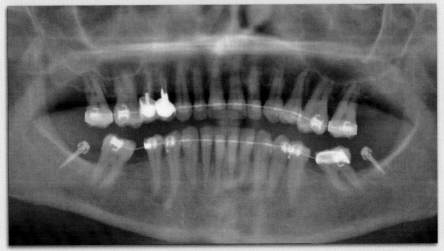

Fig. MSI 19-4. Initial TAD panoramic radiograph.

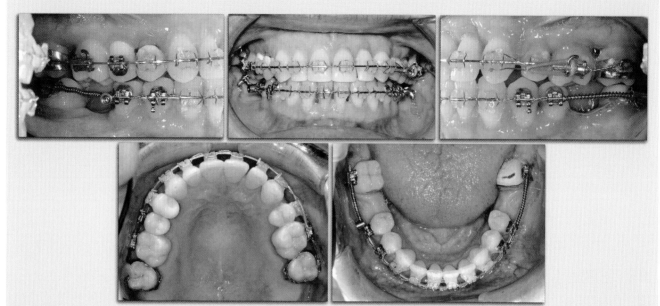

Fig. MSI 19-5. Final TAD photographs.

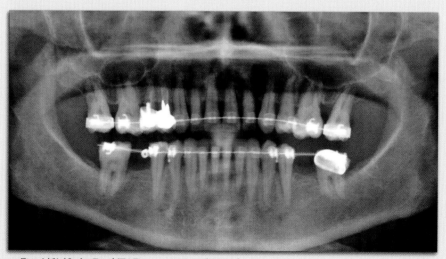

Fig. MSI 19-6. Final TAD panoramic radiograph.

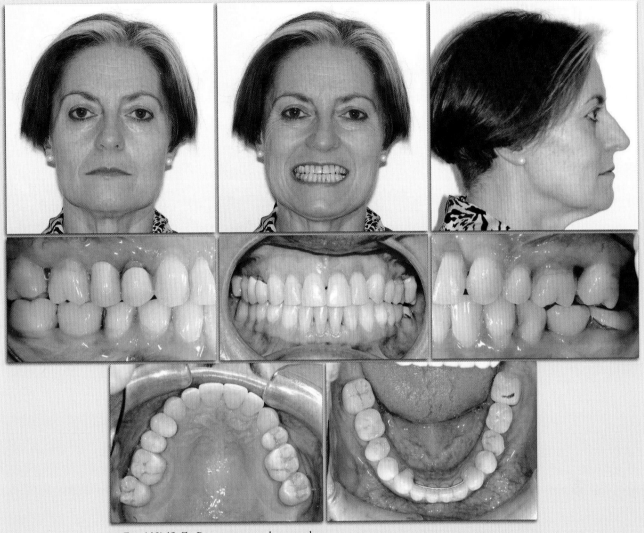

Fig. MSI 19-7. Posttreatment photographs.

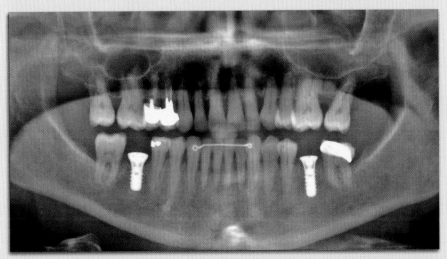

Fig. MSI 19-8. Posttreatment panoramic radiograph.

Table MSI 19-3.	Cephalometric Summary			
	Pretreatment	Pre-TAD	Post-TAD	Posttreatment
SKELETAL				
SNA (degrees)	86.7	85.8	85.6	85.5
SNB (degrees)	85.9	83.8	83.9	83.9
ANB (degrees)	0.9	2.0	1.7	1.6
SN-ANS/PNS (degrees)	4.7	6.5	6.7	6.6
SN-GoMe (degrees)	29.2	31.7	32.5	28.9
N-ANS (mm)	45.2	45.9	46.3	47.8
ANS-Me (mm)	61.2	63.1	63.9	62.7
DENTAL				
U1-SN (degrees)	112.7	109.6	110.8	112.4
L1-GoMe (degrees)	86.0	85.9	89.3	87.3
U1-APo (mm)	5.9	4.2	4.4	4.7
L1-APo (mm)	2.4	1.4	2.4	2.1
SOFT TISSUE				
LS-PnPo′ (mm)	–9.1	–8.2	–6.9	–7.4
LI-PnPo′ (mm)	–5.4	–4.9	–3.6	–3.8

TAD, Temporary anchorage device.

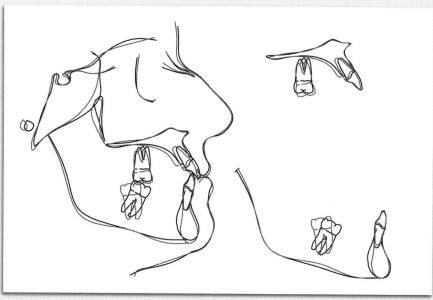

Fig. MSI 19-9. Cephalometric superimposition.

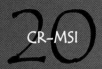

Intrusion of Upper Molars to Close a Skeletal Open Bite

Jason B. Cope

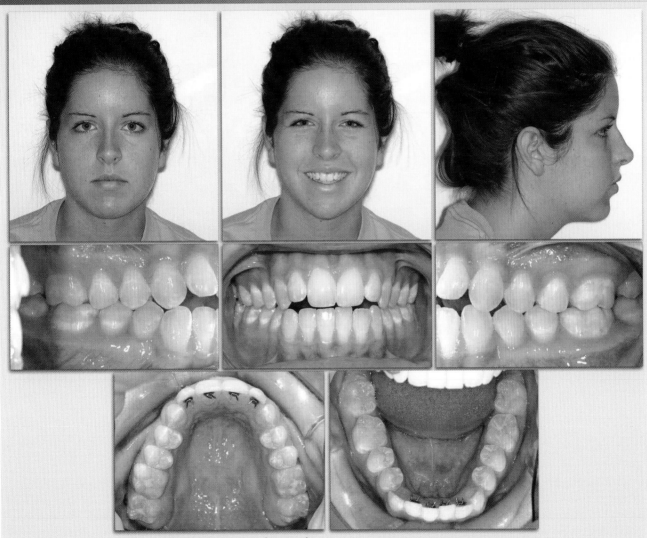

Fig. MSI 20-1. Pretreatment photographs.

The patient presented with an anterior open bite in the incisor region and a tongue thrust. She had previously undergone orthodontic treatment, which had subsequently relapsed anteriorly. Her original orthodontist gave her the retreatment option of orthognathic surgery. The family was uncomfortable with that option, however, and sought options from other orthodontists.

The treatment plan was to align the arches to remove any dental compensations and then to use two miniscrew implants (MSIs) in the palate to intrude the maxillary posterior teeth and allow the mandible to autorotate into an ideal Class I relationship and close the anterior open bite. The step in the occlusal plane between the maxillary lateral incisors and canines was maintained in the initial round and rectangular NiTi wires. The patient also began and completed myofunctional therapy during the first 6 months of orthodontic treatment to eliminate the tongue thrust. Once leveling and aligning had occurred, two Ortho Implants (IMTEC Corp., Ardmore, Oklahoma) were placed between the first and second molars and were attached to a transpalatal arch via power chain. The maxillary arch wire was sectioned at the step in the occlusal plane so that there were three maxillary sectional 0.017 × 0.025-inch NiTi arch wires—two posterior and one anterior. This was done so that the anterior teeth were not artificially extruded by continuous arch wire mechanics and that any bite closing would occur purely by posterior intrusion and mandibular autorotation. A lingual arch was placed on the mandibular dentition to prevent molar eruption into the intermaxillary growth space in an attempt to allow mandibular counterclockwise autorotation.

The reason that the palate was chosen as the location of the MSIs instead of the facial surface is anatomic. These cases usually have much higher palatal vaults and lingual cusps that hang lower than in normal cases. Moreover, there is no alveolar mucosa on the palate, so soft tissue concerns are not an issue. Therefore, the decision was made to place the MSIs at the depth of the palatal vault at a 45-degree angle to the occlusal plane. The forces then were connected directly to the transpalatal arch. This tended to seat the lingual cusps as the molars intruded and the bite closed while also maintaining the intermolar width.

Table MSI 20-1.	Diagnosis and Treatment Goals	
	Diagnosis	Treatment Goals
SKELETAL		
Anteroposterior	Class II	Class II
Vertical	Open bite	Normal
Transverse	Normal	Normal
DENTAL		
Right molar	End-on Class II	Class I
Right canine	End-on Class II	Class I
Left molar	End-on Class II	Class I
Left canine	End-on Class II	Class I
Upper right	0.5 mm crowding	None
Upper left	0 mm crowding	None
Lower right	1.5 mm crowding	None
Lower left	1.5 mm crowding	None
Missing teeth	No. 18, 28, 38, 48	No. 18, 28, 38, 48
Restore teeth	N/A	N/A
Overjet	4 mm	2 mm
Overbite	-2.0 mm	3 mm
Upper ML	0 mm to facial ML	0 mm to facial ML
Lower ML	0 mm to facial ML	0 mm to facial ML
SOFT TISSUE		
Profile	Convex	Convex
Lips	Competent	Competent
PERIODONTIUM		
Inadequate KT/TT	None	None
Gingival recession	None	None
Bone loss	None	None
OTHER	Tongue thrust	

KT/TT, Keratinized tissue/thin tissue; *ML*, midline; *N/A*, not applicable.

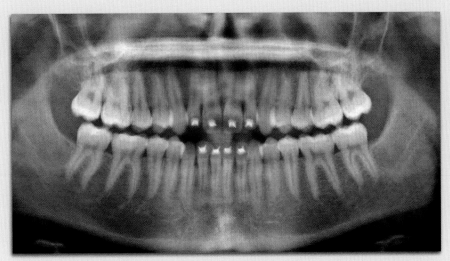

Fig. MSI 20-2. Pretreatment panoramic radiograph.

Table MSI 20-2.	Temporary Anchorage Device Summary	
Procedure	Data	
Appliances placed	27 Jul 2005	
TAD placed	17 Nov 2005	17 Nov 2005
Location of TAD	Distopalatal No. 16	Distopalatal No. 26
Type of TAD	MSI	MSI
TAD loaded	17 Nov 2005	17 Nov 2005
Healing duration	0 days	0 days
Force in grams	100-150	100-150
Mechanics used	Direct	Direct
TAD unloaded	22 Mar 2006	22 Mar 2006
TAD loading duration	4 months	4 months
TAD removed	21 Aug 2006	21 Aug 2006
Appliances removed	21 Aug 2006	
Treatment duration	13 months	

TAD, Temporary anchorage device; *MSI*, Miniscrew implant.

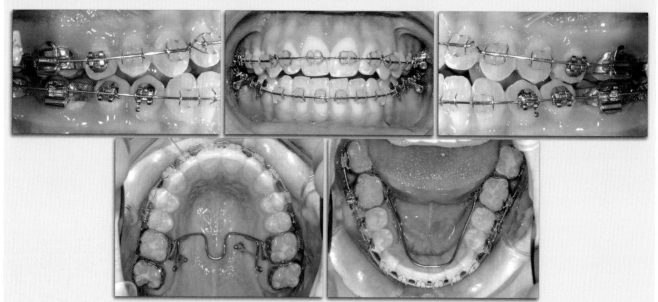

Fig. MSI 20-3. Initial temporary anchorage device (TAD) photographs.

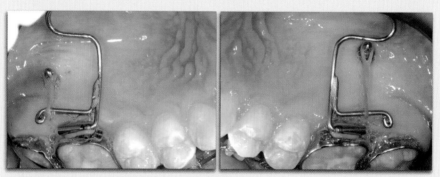

Fig. MSI 20-4. Initial TAD mechanics.

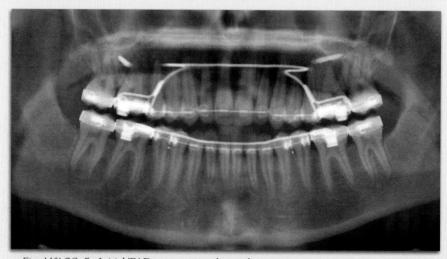

Fig. MSI 20-5. Initial TAD panoramic radiograph.

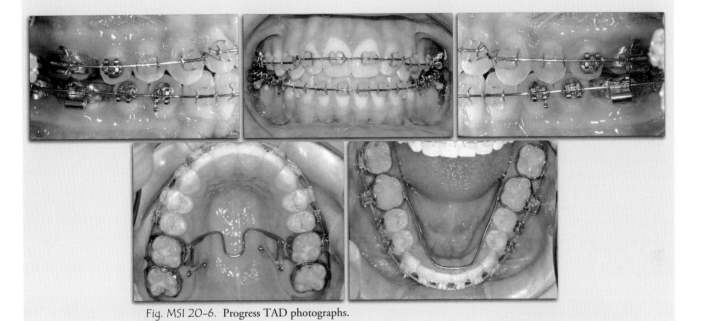

Fig. MSI 20-6. Progress TAD photographs.

Fig. MSI 20-7. Final TAD photographs.

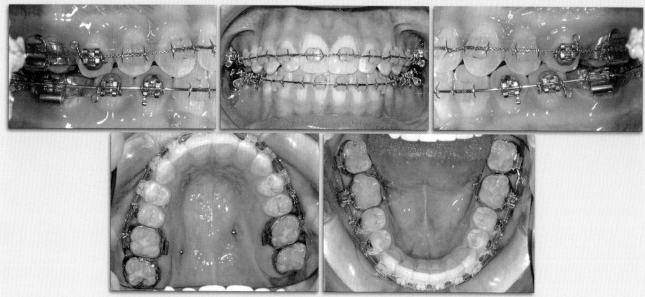

Fig. MSI 20–8. Progress photographs.

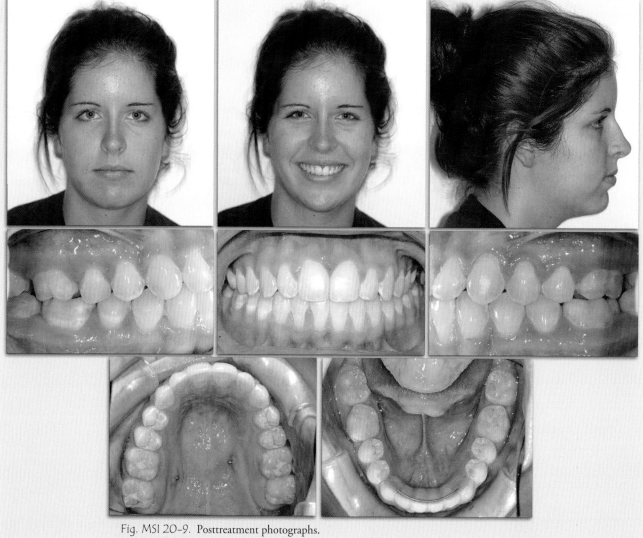

Fig. MSI 20–9. Posttreatment photographs.

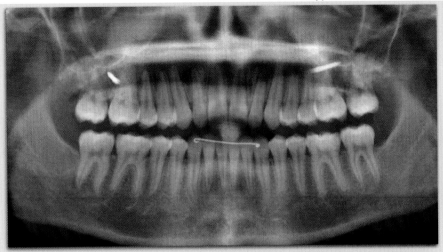

Fig. MSI 20-10. Posttreatment panoramic radiograph.

Table MSI 20-3.	Cephalometric Summary		
	Pretreatment	Pre-TAD	Posttreatment
SKELETAL			
SNA (degrees)	85.2	85.1	85.6
SNB (degrees)	79.5	78.1	79.8
ANB (degrees)	5.6	7.0	5.8
SN-ANS/PNS (degrees)	3.1	4.2	3.0
SN-GoMe (degrees)	30.8	35.1	31.6
N-ANS (mm)	48.2	49.2	48.4
ANS-Me (mm)	71.1	72.7	70.3
DENTAL			
U1-SN (degrees)	103.9	105.8	105.6
L1-GoMe (degrees)	99.5	99.3	101.4
U1-APo (mm)	5.2	5.9	5.0
L1-APo (mm)	1.1	3.0	3.0
SOFT TISSUE			
LS-PnPo' (mm)	–4.4	–4.2	–6.2
LI-PnPo' (mm)	–1.0	–0.2	–1.8

TAD, Temporary anchorage device.

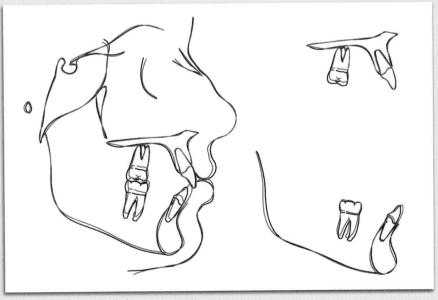

Fig. MSI 20-11. Cephalometric superimposition.

SECTION 6

PALATAL IMPLANT SYSTEM

CHAPTER 18

The OrthoSystem

Tomas Gedrange

Obtaining adequate orthodontic anchorage has been problematic since the infancy of the orthodontic specialty. Anchorage is even more difficult in patients with multiple missing teeth. In these cases, implant treatment has frequently been combined with orthodontic treatment in order to obtain an ideal functional and esthetic result. The implants in these cases often function as anchorage points for orthodontic purposes and are subsequently used for prosthetic reconstruction afterward.[1]

Although dental implants provide an alternative anchorage solution, they are only applicable in patients with missing teeth because they are too large to place in extraalveolar areas. Considering this, Straumann developed a miniaturized site-specific dental implant placed in the hard palate that functions as a complete system (Orthosystem®, Waldenburg, Switzerland). The palate was preferred in orthodontics as an anchorage site both because of its anatomy and its being a common location of other orthodontic appliances (Fig. 18-1). Insertion in the hard palate permits orthodontic tooth movement in the entire maxillary arch because the force is distributed to the entire maxilla.[2] More specifically, Triaca and colleagues[3] pointed out that the bone in the anterior palate is highly compact and provides good access for surgery and hygiene.

THE STRAUMANN ORTHOSYSTEM

The Orthosystem Palatal Implant is a one-piece titanium implant (Fig. 18-2).[4,5] The implant has two

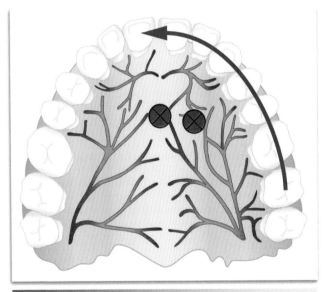

Fig. 18-1

Diagram of maxillary palatal bone and alveolar arch. Note that blue circles indicate possible palatal implant sites, and blue arrow indicates dental arch that prevents implant placement.

components; the upper is exposed to the oral cavity and the lower is submerged into the underlying bone. The upper component consists of a hexagonal abutment and a transmucosal collar. The hexagonal abutment permits the attachment of a stainless steel cap, which is retained by placing a screw through the cap and into an internally threaded hole in the implant. The hexagonal shape prevents rotation of the cap, which serves as the connection between the implant and the orthodontic appliances. The transmucosal collar protrudes through

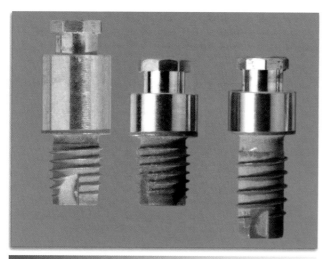

Fig. 18-2

The Orthosystem is a titanium screw-type implant with a threaded diameter of 3.3 mm, transmucosal collar lengths of 2.5 mm or 4.5 mm, and threaded lengths of 4.0 mm or 6.0 mm.

the mucous membrane and is available in two different lengths (2.5 or 4.5 mm) for different soft tissue depths. The upper component is polished to a high gloss to prevent bacterial colonization.

The lower component or threaded body lies completely within bone and is responsible for primary stability and osseointegration.[6] The threaded body is cylindrical with self-tapping threads. The demarcation between the upper and lower component is a supraperiosteal step, which creates a butt joint interface between the bone and the implant, thereby preventing overinsertion of the implant. The implant diameter is 3.3 mm with two lengths available (4.0 and 6.0 mm) for variations in bone depth. If the pilot hole is accidentally overenlarged or if the implant ever becomes mobile, an "emergency" palatal implant with a diameter of 4.0 mm is available for replacement.

Finite element studies[7] and animal experiments[8] suggest that the implant design of the Straumann palatal implant is significantly better in loading capacity compared with other implant designs with or without a supraperiosteal step. In spite of its relatively small size, the palatal implant handles force levels up to 100 N, which approximates masticatory force levels. Clinically, however, palatal implants are not required to handle forces nearly as high as this.

The long-term success of the palatal implant depends on its anatomic design and surface preparation.[9] The threaded body and supraperiosteal step provide initial stability to minimize micromotion, thereby increasing the potential for osseointegration.[5] Osseointegration is also enhanced by implant surface preparation (Fig. 18-3).[10] First, the implant surface is sandblasted with aluminum oxide particles and then is acid etched to reduce surface contamination. This process creates two distinct levels of surface roughness. Sandblasting creates a course roughness of 20 μm deep, and acid etching creates a finer roughness of 2 μm deep. This surface treatment leads to a considerable increase in surface area that is finally covered by a 5-μm thick oxide layer. Research indicates this to be an optimal condition for osseointegration.[10-12] This surface roughness also serves as an attachment latticework for human proteins and cells, which grow in and around the implant, thereby incorporating it into the body.

TREATMENT PLANNING

The first step in any type of treatment is patient evaluation. Patients must be evaluated to determine whether they are suitable candidates for treatment based on known indications and contraindications (see Chapter 5). Of particular concern with palatal implants is patient age. Because of incomplete fusion of the midpalatal suture, palatal implant placement is not indicated in the midpalatal suture in growing children. It may be possible to place palatal implants in

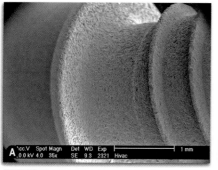
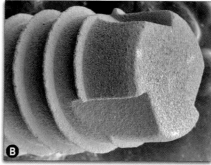
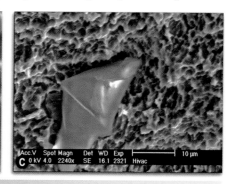

Fig. 18-3

Scanning electron micrographs of the Orthosystem. **A,** Polished transmucosal collar *(left)* and roughened SLA-treated (*s*andblasted, *l*arge grit, and *a*cid etched) threaded body *(right)*. **B,** The SLA-treated threaded apex. **C,** Higher magnification of roughened SLA-treated surface.

these patients lateral to the incompletely fused suture.

Treatment planning with palatal implants should be approached from an orthodontic and a surgical point of view. For orthodontics, the expected tooth movements and anchorage site should be clearly defined.[13,14] This also requires the clinician to determine the position and attachment locations of the orthodontic appliances. For surgery, placement location should consider the local anatomic constraints, such as tooth roots and incisive vessels anteriorly.

The use of diagnostic models helps determine ideal appliance design, insertion site, and transmucosal collar length for optimal access and attachment in the palatal vault. A longer transmucosal collar is often required in a high palatal vault for ease of access, whereas a shorter transmucosal collar can be used in a lower palatal vault. Because palatal vault anatomy and bone thickness varies from patient to patient and at different points within the hard palate, radiographic analysis should also be included in implant planning.[15-18] The site with the most available bone is the anterior palatal area (Fig. 18-4).

A lateral cephalometric radiograph is often sufficient to assess bone depth, anatomy, and any potential pathological condition (Fig. 18-5).[19] To avoid damaging the anterior tooth roots, the position of the incisors and the paranasal sinuses are traced on the cephalometric tracing. Frequently, a radiographic stent is used to assess the anticipated position and size of the palatal implant. If used, the acrylic stent is fabricated on the dental model. The stent has metal tubes equal to the diameter and length of the planned implant fixed in the planned implant position. These radiopaque markers appear on the radiograph and allow the clinician to confirm the planned implant position or move it to a better location. In some cases, computed tomography may be required to evaluate local bone

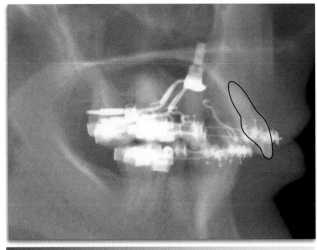

Fig. 18-5

Lateral cephalometric radiograph is used to determine the optimal insertion site and implant length. Note that bone depth, incisor position, and sinus anatomy are readily visible.

volume. Dental computed tomography of the alveolar process is well established for evaluating the alveolar bone volume before implant placement.[20] Dental computed tomography can also be used to assess the hard palate and is currently the most accurate tool for assessing the vertical bone volume at this site.

PRESURGICAL ORTHODONTICS

As a rule, orthodontic treatment before the placement of palatal implants is not necessary. However, because the implants require 8 to 12 weeks to osseointegrate, they should be placed during the leveling phase so that they can be loaded when leveling is completed.

SURGICAL PROCEDURE

After determining the exact location of the palatal implant, the surgical procedure is carried out under sterile conditions with a standardized instrument kit (Fig. 18-6).[4,21] Systemic antibiotic therapy before surgery is not indicated. The implants are delivered separately in sterile ampules. The procedure is relatively simple and straightforward and is routinely carried out under local anesthesia. The implant site in the hard palate is innervated from the greater palatine nerves bilaterally and nasopalatine nerve anteriorly. Therefore, all three nerves are anesthetized. For the nasopalatine nerve, about 0.1 mL of articain with 1:100,000 epinephrine is injected at the incisive foramen. For the greater palatine nerves, about 0.1 to 0.3 mL of articain with 1:100,000 epinephrine is injected at the greater palatine foramen. In both cases, penetration of the canal with the needle should be avoided. This limited anesthesia is sufficient for most patients.

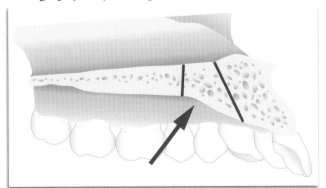

Fig. 18-4

Diagram of human palate in cross section. Note that the best available site is demarcated by blue lines and blue arrow.

In some patients, however, additional anesthesia is necessary. Depending on patient sensitivity, three different options are possible. First, if sensitivity is limited to the mucous membrane, additional infiltration can be injected into the palatal mucous membrane. Second, if the bone remains sensitive, intraosseous injection may be required. Finally, for overly sensitive patients, it may be necessary to anesthetize the floor of the nose. This entails placing cotton rolls soaked in epinephrine-free lidocaine into the nostrils to anesthetize the mucous membranes of the floor of the nose. After approximately 3 minutes, the cotton rolls

are removed and 0.1 to 0.3 mL articain with 1:100,000 epinephrine is injected into the floor of the nose.

The implant pilot hole can be prepared using two different techniques. The first technique involves free-handing the pilot hole based on local anatomy, such as papillary and tooth position. This, of course, requires some operator experience in order to achieve ideal results. The second method is based on using a surgical template. This technique uses a stent that is first made in the laboratory using the patient's diagnostic records. Regardless of the technique, after determining the entry point, the first step is to use the mucosal trephine (Fig. 18-7) in a slow-speed handpiece to incise the palatal mucosa (Fig. 18-8, *A*). The resulting circular plug (Fig. 18-8, *B*) of palatal mucosa is removed with a periosteal elevator (Fig. 18-8, *C*). Next, a 2.3-mm diameter round bur is used in a slow-speed handpiece to create a small indentation in the cortical bone (Fig. 18-9). The diameter of the resulting indentation is the same size as the subsequent pilot drill (Fig. 18-10). Finally, the pilot hole is created with a sharp pilot drill using a steady downward pressure with constant saline

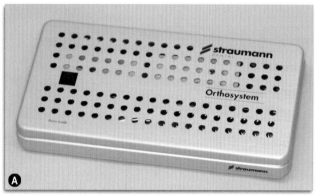

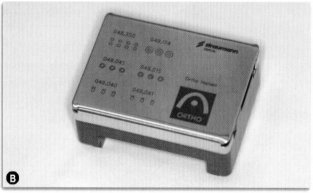

Fig. 18-6

The Orthosystem. **A,** Orthosystem aluminium anodized case. **B,** Orthosystem aluminium anodized screw container.

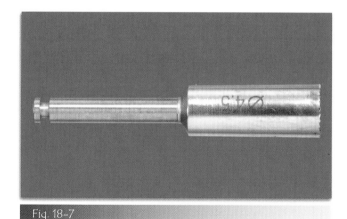

Fig. 18-7

Stainless steel Ortho mucosal trephine.

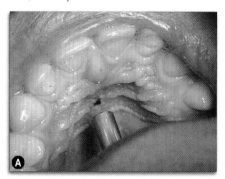
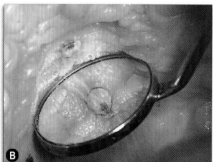
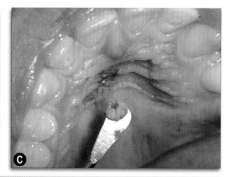

Fig. 18-8

Soft tissue removal procedure. **A,** Ortho mucosal trephine in slow-speed handpiece to perforate mucosa down to bone. **B,** Circular incision of palatal soft tissue. **C,** Removal of soft tissue with periosteal elevator.

irrigation cooled to 5° C at no more than 700 rpm. This continues until a complete osteotomy is created, preparing the supraperiosteal stop for the implant. It is important to not overenlarge the pilot hole because this will negatively affect primary stability. If the pilot hole is overenlarged or a 3.3-mm diameter palatal implant becomes mobile, an "emergency" implant with a 4.0-mm diameter is available. After the pilot hole has been prepared, the depth should be checked with a periodontal probe. The site should also be examined to ensure that the floor of the nose has not been perforated.[22]

The implant placement procedure begins by opening the outer ampule (Fig. 18-11, *A*) to expose the inner ampule (Fig. 18-11, *B*), which is removed and placed on a sterile towel. The palatal implant is maintained in the inner ampule by a spring. The ampule must be held vertically after the lid is removed, because the implant is no longer secure. The Ortho screwdriver is pressed onto the implant until it clicks audibly. To prevent screwdriver

aspiration, floss is tied around the screwdriver. Using the Ortho screwdriver (Fig. 18-11, *C* and *D*), the implant is transferred from the ampule (Fig. 18-11, *E*) to the mouth and then is screwed into the bone. The self-tapping palatal implant is inserted into the pilot hole and is screwed in as far as possible by hand. Next, the implant is slowly ratcheted to its final position (Fig. 18-12) with the torque-control device (Fig. 18-13).

Once the implant is placed, the Ortho healing cap (Fig. 18-14) or the SCS screw (Figs. 18-15 and 18-16, *A* and *B*) is placed to prevent collection of debris in the internal threads. To attach the healing cap, the special screwdriver with a retaining sleeve should be used (Fig. 18-16, *C*). The SCS occlusal screw is first picked up in the Ortho screwdriver, and then the retaining sleeve is pushed back and the healing cap is picked up and screwed into the implant at a torque of 15 N-cm. The screwdriver without a retaining sleeve (Fig. 18-16, *D* and *E*) is used for attachment of the SCS occlusal screw.

After placement, the implant should be allowed to heal without loading for 8 to 12 weeks in order to osseointegrate (Fig. 18-17). Soft tissue healing occurs within 8 days. We observe the healing process at four postoperative appointments at 24 hours, 1 week, 1 month, and 2 months. If no mobility or inflammation is seen, normal healing is assumed.

Unfortunately, radiographs are not conclusive in establishing a prognosis. Although no radiolucency may be evident around the implant, the traditional radiograph shows only a two-dimensional image; medial and lateral bone is not evident. The contribution of the lateral bone to implant stability cannot be determined. Because of this, we have used the Osstell™ gauge (Integration Diagnosis Company, Gothenburg, Sweden) to quantify implant stability.[23,24] The instrument uses resonance frequency analysis and provides better results than the implant percussion (Fig. 18-18). Resonance frequency

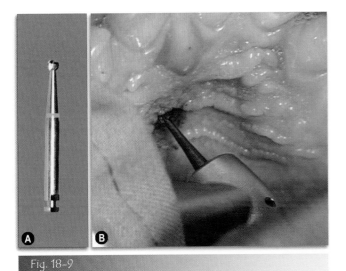

Fig. 18-9

Indenting the cortical bone. **A,** The 2.3-mm diameter stainless steel round bur. **B,** Bur is used in a slow-speed handpiece to create an indentation in the bone in preparation of pilot hole drilling.

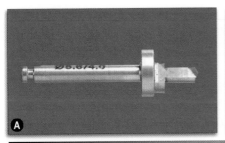
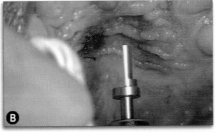
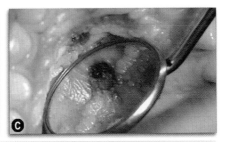

Fig. 18-10

Pilot hole preparation. **A,** Short Ortho profile drill for implants with 4.0 mm insertion depth. **B,** Ortho profile drill used to drill pilot hole. **C,** Pilot hole after preparation.

analysis was established as an additional method for implant stability evaluation.[25,26] The measurement is carried out with a transducer screwed onto the implant.

Once attached, the piezoelectric elements of the transducer begin to oscillate. The gauge records the resonance frequency at the bone-to-implant interface

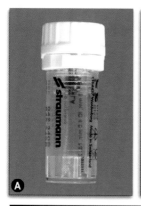 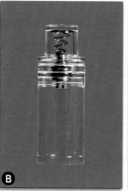 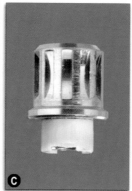 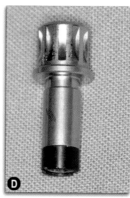 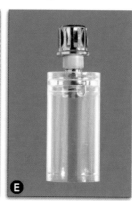

Fig. 18-11

Palatal implant delivery system. **A,** Nonsterile outer ampule with inner ampule and implant. **B,** Sterile inner ampule. Note that implant is held in inner ampule by spring. **C,** Short implant insertion device. **D,** Long implant insertion device. **E,** The short insertion device is pressed onto the implant until it engages and clicks audibly.

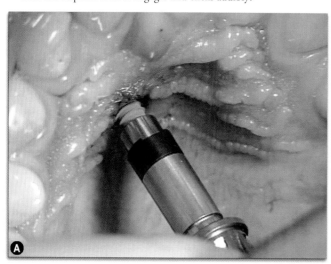 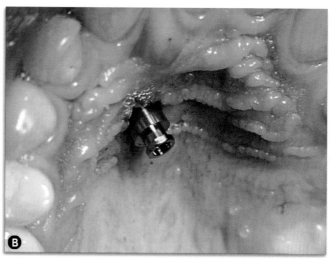

Fig. 18-12

Palatal implant placement. **A,** Insertion of the implant in the pilot hole. **B,** Final implant position.

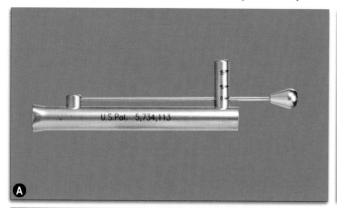 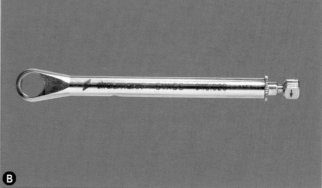

Fig. 18-13

Torque-control device for implant placement. **A,** Torque-control component with calibrated spring arm. **B,** Ratchet component that fits screwdriver.

(amplitude change over frequency band), and a graph is displayed.[24] The vibration response of the implant-transducer element documents the implant stability quotient, which is a measure of implant stability. Measurement comparisons from different healing stages provide information about implant stability.

In the immediate postoperative period, oral hygiene is critical, and the patient should be adequately educated. Also important is that the patient not touch the implant with the tongue during the first several weeks after placement operation. The implant should be cleaned with chlorhexidine rinses 3 times daily for the first 7 postoperative days. On day 8, the implant may be cleaned with a toothbrush. After the fourteenth day, the implant is cleaned with a toothbrush and an interdental brush 2 to 3 times daily. After that point, rinsing with chlorhexidine is no longer necessary. Analgesics are rarely required.

APPLIANCE FABRICATION

The palatal implant is generally allowed to heal for about 12 weeks before orthodontic loading. This is the time required to allow osseointegration. However, it is not necessary to wait 12 weeks to begin fabricating the orthodontic appliance that will be attached to the implant. Therefore, we usually see the patient after 9 weeks to take the impression for appliance construction. The procedure occurs as follows. First, the Ortho healing screw is removed from the implant. Next, an Ortho impression cap is screwed onto the top of the implant with an SCS occlusal screw (Fig. 18-19). Finally, an impression is taken of the maxillary arch.

Importantly, alginate material is often unsuitable material when orthodontic appliances are in place, because alginate usually causes tearing and distortion of the impression. Instead, a silicone-based material is often preferred because of its precision and stability. The most accurate technique involves a medium-body material as the base impression material with a light-body material injected directly around the implant. This provides the rigidity of the impression in general, with increased anatomic accuracy immediately adjacent to the implant.

After removal of the impression tray from the mouth,

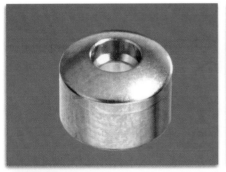

Fig. 18-14

Ortho healing cap with 6.0-mm diameter and 4.0-mm height.

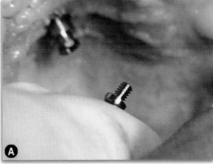
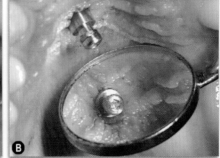

Fig. 18-15

Placement of SCS occlusal screw. **A,** Screw carried into mouth on screwdriver. **B,** Final position of screw.

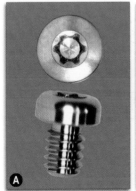
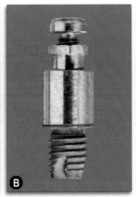
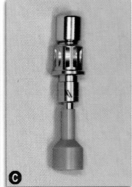
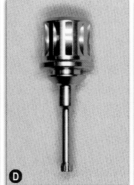
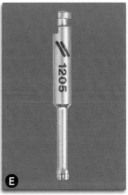

Fig. 18-16

SCS occlusal screw placement components. **A,** Superior and lateral aspects of screw. **B,** Screw in place to prevent debris accumulation in internal threads of implant. **C,** Ortho screwdriver with retaining sleeve for holding Ortho healing cap. **D,** Short manual screwdriver. **E,** Short handpiece screwdriver.

the Ortho impression cap is removed from the implant and screwed directly onto the Ortho Implant analog with the SCS occlusal screw (Fig. 18-20). At this point, the healing cap is replaced on the implant until loading commences 3 weeks later. The analog and impression cap are inserted into the impression and are poured in dental stone to create the working laboratory model. Once the stone is set, the Ortho impression cap is removed (Fig. 18-21) and replaced with the Ortho bonding base. The Ortho Implant analog in the working model is an exact duplicate of the intraoral implant.

At this point, it should be decided whether direct or indirect anchorage will be used. For indirect anchorage, the reactive segment is attached to and stabilized by the implant, and the reactive segment is used to move the active segment. For direct anchorage, the active segment is attached directly to the implant for tooth movement (see Chapter 1). In many patients, bands are used for the point of attachment from the implant to the teeth. In

these cases, bands are fit and impressed at the same time as the implant impression. The bands are not cemented at this time but are left in the impression for fabrication with the implant-based appliance (Fig. 18-22). This procedure has been described by in detail by Wehrbein and colleagues.[4]

Fabrication of the appliance begins with the laboratory technician marking the appliance design on the working model based on the prescription of the orthodontist. After confirming the construction and the mechanics for tooth movement, the appliance is fabricated. Depending on the planned use, the transpalatal arch (TPA) is made of standard stainless steel orthodontic wire (0.8 or 1.2 mm^2 or 0.036-inch) and is soldered to the Ortho bonding base (Fig. 18-23).

Two different methods of attaching the appliance to the teeth are bonded or banded. For the bonded technique, a wire mesh base is adapted to the teeth to be attached. The end of the TPA then is soldered to the wire mesh (Fig. 18-24, *A*). For the banded technique, the TPA is soldered directly to the bands on the working model (Fig. 18-24, *B*). Although bands provide a rigid connection, the disadvantage is that they are limited in postfabrication adjustments. The advantage of bands is that distalization appliances are easily fabricated, thereby taking advantage of the anchorage provided by the palatal implant in delivering a force through the center of resistance of the posterior teeth. The Distal Jet appliance (American Orthodontics, Sheboygan, Wisconsin) is one such example (Fig. 18-24, *C*).[27]

APPLIANCE DELIVERY

When the patient returns after the 12-week healing period, the Ortho healing screw is removed and the implant-based appliance is fit onto the implant. After verifying the fit, the cap is screwed to place with the

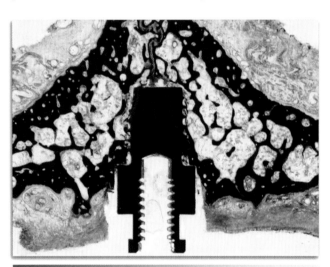

Fig. 18-17

Undecalcified cross section of implant in medial palatal suture (van Gieson's stain).

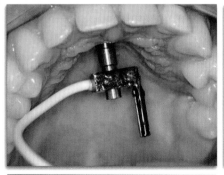

Fig. 18-18

Clinical photograph of transducer in situ. Note data transferred to PC for archiving.

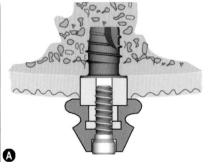

Fig. 18-19

Ortho impression cap. **A,** Diagram of Ortho impression cap and SCS occlusal screw in cross section. **B,** Ortho impression cap in place intraorally.

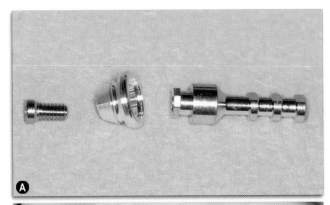

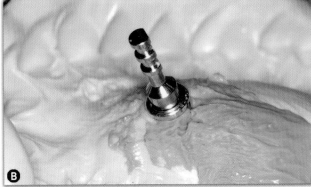

Fig. 18-20

Transfer technique. **A,** SCS occlusal screw, Ortho impression cap, and Ortho Implant analog. **B,** The impression cap and analog are transferred to impression before pouring in dental stone.

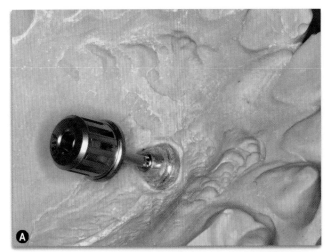

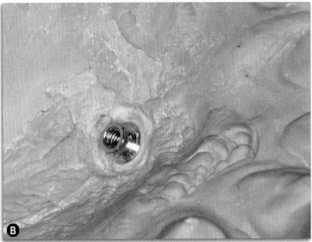

Fig. 18-21

Working dental model. **A,** The Ortho impression cap is removed. **B,** Final position of Ortho Implant analog.

SCS occlusal screw to a torque of 15 N-cm. If the appliance is bonded, the standard acid-etch technique is used. If the appliance is banded, then the appliance is seated as one unit with the bands loaded with cement. The bands are adapted to the teeth and are cleaned; then immediately thereafter the SCS occlusal screw is placed and tightened.

ORTHODONTIC MECHANICS

Depending on the clinical situation and the orthodontic treatment plan, palatal implants are loaded either directly or indirectly (Fig. 18-25). Using indirect anchorage, the teeth of the reactive segment are indirectly stabilized by the palatal implant, and the reactive segment is used to move the active segment. For example, the wires soldered on the implant can be bonded to stabilize the canines, which can then be used to distalize the buccal segments (Fig. 18-25. *A* to *C*). Using direct anchorage, the forces needed for the desired tooth movement of the active segment are directly applied from the implant. For example, the implant can be used to directly apply

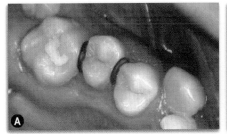

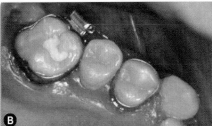

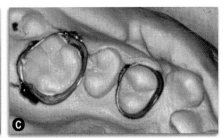

Fig. 18-22

Preparation for band placement. **A,** Placement of elastic separators. **B,** Placement of orthodontic bands. **C,** Placement of orthodontic bands in impression.

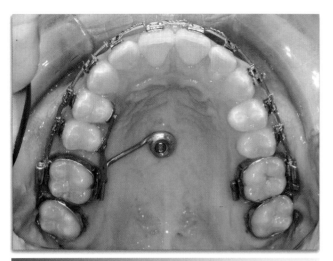

Fig. 18-23

Maxillary occlusal photograph of 0.036-inch stainless steel wire soldered to Ortho bonding base. Note sectional TPA is used to stabilize first molar indirectly as premolars are retracted. (Photograph courtesy Dr. Jason B. Cope.)

distalizing forces to the buccal segments (Fig. 18-25, *D* to *G*). Direct anchorage can also be used to protract posterior teeth (Fig. 18-25, *H* and *I*). Finally, indirect (Fig. 18-25, *J* and *K*) and direct (Fig. 18-25, *L*) forces can be applied from the same implant. In this case, indirect anchorage is applied on the facial surface, and direct anchorage is applied on the palatal surface.

REMOVAL PROCEDURE

After the palatal implant has been used for its intended purpose in orthodontic tooth movement, it can be removed. First, the TPA is removed and the implant is cleaned with chlorhexidine. Next, the region is anesthetized in the same way as for implant placement. Two additional components are available for implant removal: the Ortho explantation drill (Fig. 18-26, *A*) and the Ortho guiding cylinder (Fig. 18-26, *B*). The Ortho guiding cylinder is screwed onto the top of the implant and guides the Ortho explantation drill around the implant to the cortical bone surface (Fig. 18-26, *C*).

The process is carried out precisely at approximately 400 rpm and is cooled with sterile saline solution. It is important to drill perpendicular to the bone surface and parallel to the long axis of the implant because the Ortho explantation drill may break if angled to any degree (Fig. 18-26, *D*). Initially, the bone adjacent to about two thirds of the implant length is trephined to separate the compact bone from the implant. A pair of extraction forceps with gentle rotary motion is usually sufficient to extract the implant. If this is not possible, then trephining continues to the full depth of the implant, followed by implant removal. The Ortho explantation drill and the Ortho guiding cylinder should be discarded after one use.

After explantation, the wound heals as does a routine dental extraction. No sutures are necessary. Cotton gauze is used to compress the palatal tissue for the next 1 to 2 hours until the blood clot has formed. The patient is seen for routine follow-up care 1, 7, 30, and 60 days after explantation. Postoperative problems seldom occur and analgesics are rarely required.

POTENTIAL COMPLICATIONS

Few patients experience postoperative complications associated with the palatal implant. Although some failures have occurred, most of these involve implant loss during the healing phase shortly after implantation. If the implant does become loose, it should be removed immediately and replaced by an implant with a greater diameter. Implant loss rarely occurs during treatment. Similar to prosthetically restored dental implants, palatal implants are considered successful if they remain firmly fixed in the bone, are painless and without gingival irritation, and can be continually loaded until tooth movement is complete. The most common problem associated with any implantable device is soft tissue inflammation (Fig. 18-27). Inflammation is rarely a serious complication but should be addressed quickly with chlorhexidine rinses to prevent further problems.

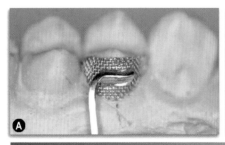
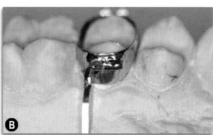
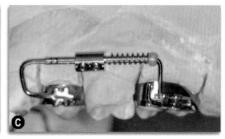

Fig. 18-24

Laboratory techniques. **A,** Wire mesh bases adapted to teeth followed by adaptation of TPA wires. **B,** TPA wires adapted to bands on working model. **C,** Distal Jet placed on facial surface of teeth and anchored to palatal implant on palatal surface (not shown) to move teeth distally.

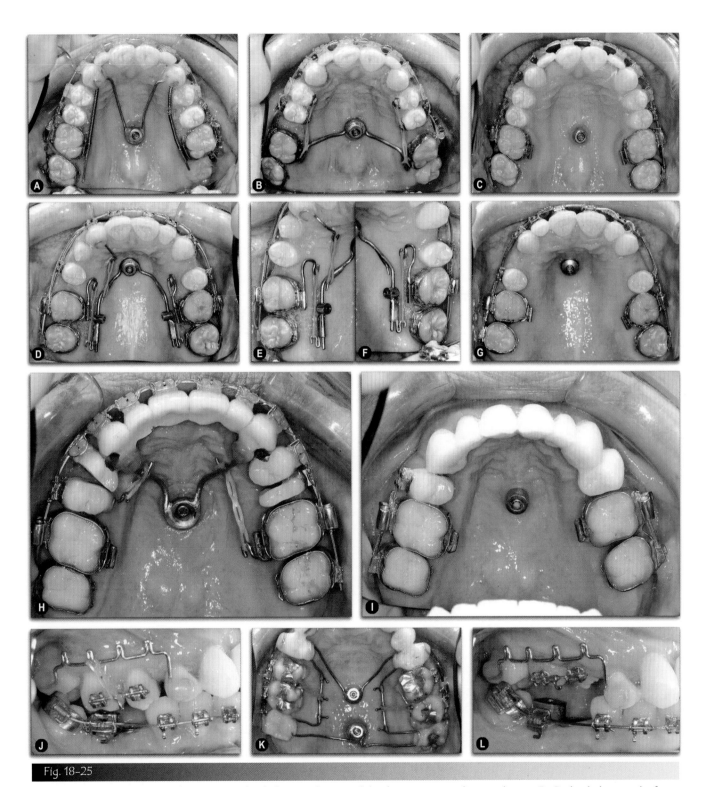

Fig. 18-25

Palatal implant treatment mechanics. **A,** Occlusal photograph at initial distalization using indirect anchorage. **B,** Occlusal photograph after distalization and start of retraction. **C,** Occlusal photograph after retraction. **D,** Occlusal photograph at initial distalization using direct anchorage. **E,** Right palatal mechanics. **F,** Left palatal mechanics. **G,** Occlusal photograph after distalization. **H,** Occlusal photograph at initial protraction using direct anchorage. **I,** Occlusal photograph after protraction. **J,** Buccal photograph at initial intrusion using indirect anchorage. **K,** Buccal photograph after overintrusion. **L,** Occlusal photograph at initial intrusion using direct anchorage. (Photographs courtesy Dr. Jason B. Cope.)

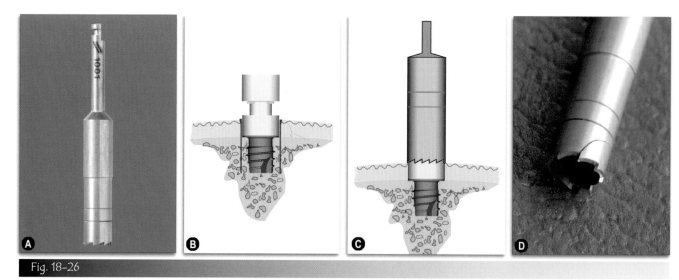

Fig. 18-26

Explantation procedure. **A,** Ortho explantation drill. **B,** Diagram of Ortho guiding cylinder on implant. **C,** Diagram of explantation drill placement around guiding cylinder to trephine bone. **D,** Fractured Ortho explantation drill.

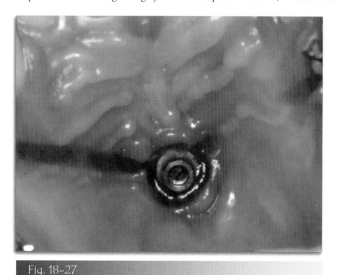

Fig. 18-27

Inflammation of palatal soft tissue.

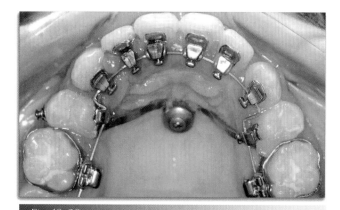

Fig. 18-28

Occlusal photograph of maxillary arch. Note final tooth position after extraction space closure with palatal implant and lingual orthodontic appliances.

Continuous bone pain after implantation may be a sign of an infection in the surrounding bone. In some cases, the bone may reject the implant slowly, like a foreign body. The reason is most likely inadequate cooling during bone preparation. The implant should be removed and replaced in this scenario also. However, because the local bone damage may have increased the diameter of the bony implant hole, replacement should be delayed for 3 to 4 months to allow bone deposition to decrease the size of the bony defect.

Although unlikely, it is possible to perforate the paranasal sinuses if the pilot hole drill deviates from its intended insertion point or if the pilot drill is too long. This situation may be noticed only if bone healing fails to occur. This is explained by the fact that implants placed into maxillary or nasal sinus mucosa are exposed to a higher risk of inflammation that may in turn lead to maxillary sinusitis. Radiographs can be used to determine whether the implant is too long. If so, the implant should be removed immediately.

SUMMARY

Because esthetics are increasingly important to patients,[7,28] the use of lingual intraoral anchorage is much better tolerated (Fig. 18-28).[29] Despite the rising increase in use of miniscrew implants for orthodontic anchorage, palatal implants are still widely used. Although the palatal implant is limited to use in the hard palate, it is broadly applicable to most any tooth movement in the maxilla. The Orthosystem is a well-designed yet simple system that is easy to use for maxillary tooth movement. Because of the low failure rate and the increased loading capacity, palatal implants remain a suitable choice for maxillary anchorage.

REFERENCES

1. Wehrbein H, Feifel H, Diedrich P. Palatal implant anchorage reinforcement of posterior teeth: a prospective study. *Am J Orthod Dentofacial Orthop.* 116(6):678-686, 1999.

2. Bernhart T, Vollgruber A, Gahleitner A, et al. Alternative to the median region of the palate for placement of an orthodontic implant. *Clin Oral Implants Res.* 11(6):595-601, 2000.

3. Triaca A, Antonini M, Wintermantel E. Ein neues Titan-Flachschrauben-Implantat zur orthodontischen Verankerung am anterioren Gaumen. *Inf Orthod Kieferorthop.* 24:251-257, 1992.

4. Wehrbein H, Glatzmaier J, Mundwiller U, Diedrich P. The Orthosystem—a new implant system for orthodontic anchorage in the palate. *J Orofac Orthop.* 57(3):142-153, 1996.

5. Wehrbein H, Merz BR, Diedrich P, Glatzmaier J. The use of palatal implants for orthodontic anchorage: design and clinical application of the orthosystem. *Clin Oral Implants Res.* 7(4):410-416, 1996.

6. Tada S, Stegaroiu R, Kitamura E, et al. Influence of implant design and bone quality on stress/strain distribution in bone around implants: a 3-dimensional finite element analysis. *Int J Oral Maxillofac Implants.* 18(3):357-368, 2003.

7. Gedrange T, Bourauel C, Kobel C, Harzer W. Three-dimensional analysis of endosseous palatal implants and bones after vertical, horizontal, and diagonal force application. *Eur J Orthod.* 25(2):109-115, 2003.

8. Gedrange T, Kobel C, Harzer W. Hard palate deformation in an animal model following quasi-static loading to stimulate that of orthodontic anchorage implants. *Eur J Orthod.* 23(4):349-354, 2001.

9. Wintermantel E, Ha S-W. *Biokompatible Werkstoffe und Bauweisen, Implantate für Medizin und Umwelt.* 2nd ed. Berlin, Heidelberg, New York: Springer, 1998.

10. Buser D, Schenk RK, Steinemann S, et al. Influence of surface characteristics on bone integration of titanium implants: a histomorphometric study in miniature pigs. *J Biomed Mater Res.* 25(7):889-902, 1991.

11. Wilke A, Orth J, Kraft M, Griss P. [Standardized infection model for the study of bony ingrowth dynamics of hydroxyapatite-coated and uncoated pure titanium mesh in swine femur]. *Z Orthop Ihre Grenzgeb.* 131(4):370-376, 1993.

12. Wilke A, Schroder G, Orth J, et al. [Evaluation of the biocompatibility of implant materials with human bone marrow cell cultures]. *Biomed Tech (Berl).* 38(6):126-129, 1993.

13. Bernhart T, Freudenthaler J, Dortbudak O, et al. Short epithetic implants for orthodontic anchorage in the paramedian region of the palate: a clinical study. *Clin Oral Implants Res.* 12(6):624-631, 2001.

14. Freudenthaler JW, Haas R, Bantleon HP. Bicortical titanium screws for critical orthodontic anchorage in the mandible: a preliminary report on clinical applications. *Clin Oral Implants Res.* 12(4):358-363, 2001.

15. Ferrario VF, Sforza C, Colombo A, et al. Three-dimensional hard tissue palatal size and shape in human adolescents and adults. *Clin Orthod Res.* 4(3):141-147, 2001.

16. Ferrario VF, Sforza C, Dellavia C, et al. Three-dimensional hard tissue palatal size and shape: a 10-year longitudinal evaluation in healthy adults. *Int J Adult Orthodon Orthognath Surg.* 17(1):51-58, 2002.

17. Ferrario VF, Sforza C, Schmitz JH, Colombo A. Quantitative description of the morphology of the human palate by a mathematical equation. *Cleft Palate Craniofac J.* 35(5):396-401, 1998.

18. Garg AK, Vicari A. Radiographic modalities for diagnosis and treatment planning in implant dentistry. *Implant Soc.* 5:7-11, 1995.

19. Wehrbein H, Merz BR, Diedrich P. Palatal bone support for orthodontic implant anchorage—a clinical and radiological study. *Eur J Orthod.* 21(1):65-70, 1999.

20. Lindh C, Petersson A, Klinge B. Measurements of distances related to the mandibular canal in radiographs. *Clin Oral Implants Res.* 6:96-103, 1995.

21. Tinsley D, O'Dwyer JJ, Benson PE, et al. Orthodontic palatal implants: clinical technique. *J Orthod.* 31(1):3-8, 2004.

22. Wetzel AC, Stich H, Caffesse RG. Bone apposition onto oral implants in the sinus area filled with different grafting materials: a histological study in beagle dogs. *Clin Oral Implants Res.* 6(3):155-163, 1995.

23. Balleri P, Cozzolino A, Ghelli L, et al. Stability measurements of osseointegrated implants using Osstell in partially edentulous jaws after 1 year of loading: a pilot study. *Clin Implant Dent Relat Res.* 4(3):128-132, 2002.

24. Gedrange T, Hietschold V, Mai R, et al. An evaluation of resonance frequency analysis for determination of the primary stability of orthodontic palatal implants: a study in human cadavers. *Clin Oral Implants Res.* 16(4):425-431, 2005.

25. Meredith N, Alleyne D, Cawley P. Quantitative determination of the stability of the implant-tissue interface using resonance frequency analysis. *Clin Oral Implants Res.* 7(3):261-267, 1996.

26. Sennerby L, Meredith N. Resonance frequency analysis: measuring implant stability and osseointegration. *Compend Contin Educ Dent.* 19(5):493-498, 1998.

27. Carano A, Testa M. The Distal Jet for upper molar distalization. *J Clin Orthod.* 30:374-380, 1996.

28. Gahleitner A, Podesser B, Schick S, et al. Dental CT and orthodontic implants: imaging technique and assessment of available bone volume in the hard palate. *Eur J Radiol.* 51(3):257-262, 2004.

29. Block MS, Hoffman DR. A new device for absolute anchorage for orthodontics. *Am J Orthod Dentofacial Orthop.* 107(3):251-258, 1995.

SECTION 7

PALATAL IMPLANT CASE REPORTS

CR-PI

Bilateral Distalization of Upper Buccal Segments to Place and Restore Lateral Incisor Implants

Jason B. Cope, Richard P. Harper

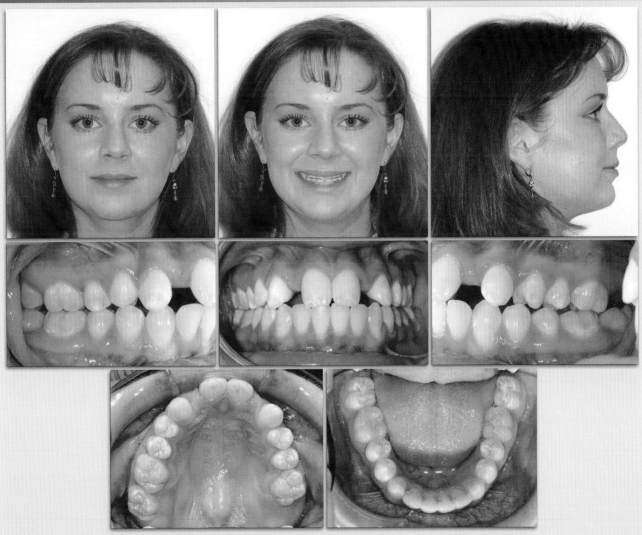

Fig. PI 1-1. Pretreatment photographs.

The patient was referred by an oral surgeon for creation of space for upper lateral incisor implants. The patient had been previously treated orthodontically with the treatment plan of dental implants for which there was inadequate room. Therefore, the treatment plan was to distalize the upper buccal segments from an end-on Class II malocclusion to a Class I occlusion with 6.5 to 7 mm of space for lateral incisor implants and restorations. The lower anterior teeth would be reduced in width by interproximal enamel reduction and retraction. At the time of palatal implant (Straumann Corp., Waldenburg, Switzerland) placement, the upper left second molar would be uncovered and extruded into its correct position in the upper arch.

Table PI 1-1.	Diagnosis and Treatment Goals	
	Diagnosis	Treatment Goals
SKELETAL		
Anteroposterior	Class I	Class I
Vertical	Normal	Normal
Transverse	Normal	Normal
DENTAL		
Right molar	End-on Class II	Class I
Right canine	End-on Class II	Class I
Left molar	End-on Class II	Class I
Left canine	End-on Class II	Class I
Upper right	2 mm crowding	None
Upper left	2 mm crowding	None
Lower right	0 mm crowding	None
Lower left	0 mm crowding	None
Missing teeth	No. 12, 22, 28, 38, 48	No. 18, 28, 38, 48
Restore teeth	N/A	No. 12, 22
Overjet	4 mm	2 mm
Overbite	1 mm	3 mm
Upper ML	0 mm to facial ML	0 mm to facial ML
Lower ML	0 mm to facial ML	0 mm to facial ML
SOFT TISSUE		
Profile	Straight	Straight
Lips	Competent	Competent
PERIODONTIUM		
Inadequate KT/TT	No. 13, 33, 34, 41, 43	Graft No. 13 with implants
Gingival recession	No. 33, 34, 41, 43	Maintain
Bone loss	None	None
OTHER	Prior orthodontics did not address No. 27	

KT/TT, Keratinized tissue/thin tissue; *ML,* midline; *N/A,* not applicable.

Table PI 1-2.	Temporary Anchorage Device Summary
Procedure	Data
Appliances placed	2 Apr 2002
TAD placed	9 Apr 2002
Location of TAD	Midpalatal No. 16-26
Type of TAD	PI
TAD loaded	9 Jul 2002
Healing duration	90 days
Force in grams	150-250
Mechanics used	Indirect
TAD unloaded	19 Nov 2003
TAD loading duration	16 months
TAD removed	3 Mar 2004
Appliances removed	2 Jun 2004
Treatment duration	26 months

TAD, Temporary anchorage device; *PI,* palatal implant.

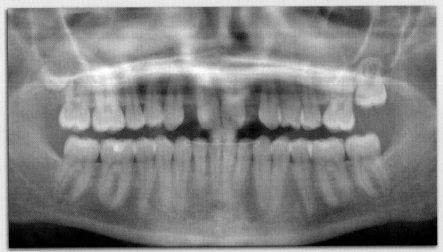

Fig. Pl 1-2. Pretreatment panoramic radiograph.

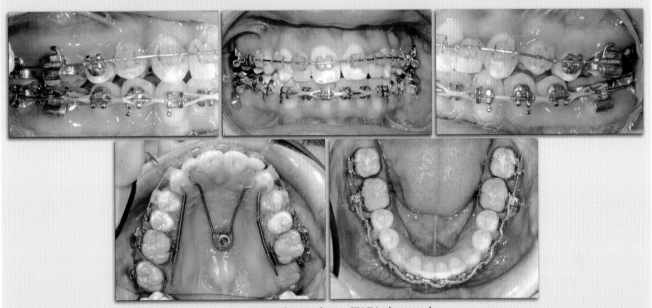

Fig. Pl 1-3.   Initial temporary anchorage device (TAD) photographs.

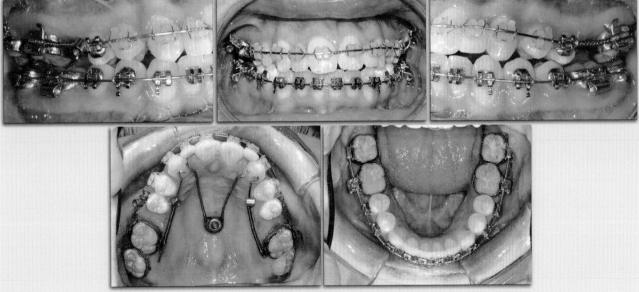

Fig. Pl 1-4.   First progress TAD photographs.

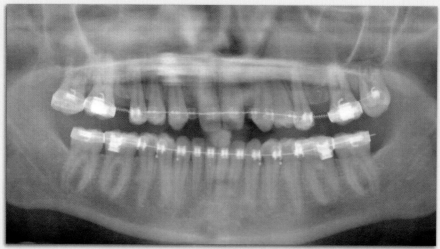

Fig. PI 1-5. First progress TAD panoramic radiograph.

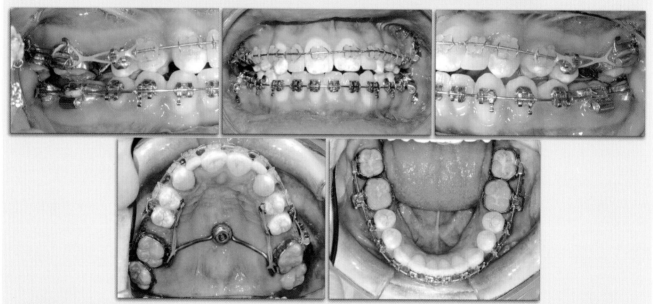

Fig. PI 1-6. Second progress TAD photographs.

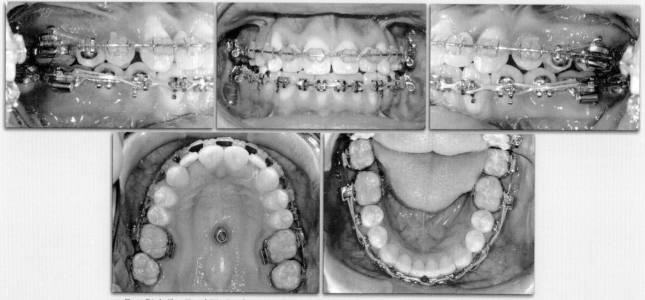

Fig. PI 1-7. Final TAD photographs.

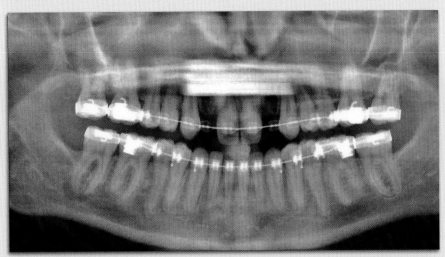

Fig. Pl 1-8. Final TAD panoramic radiograph.

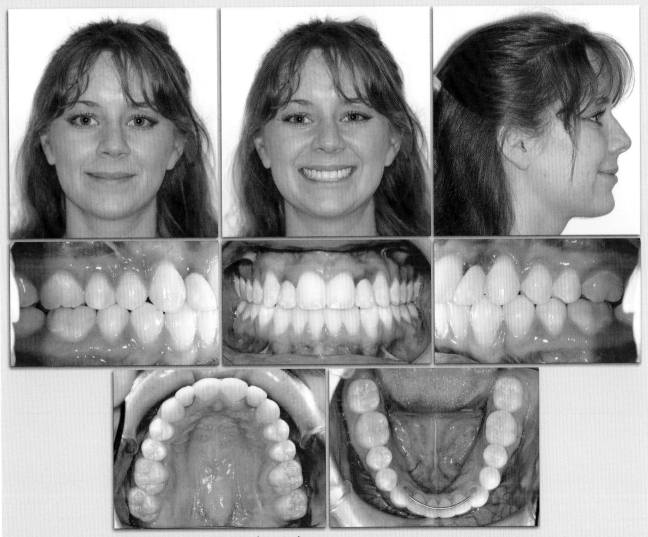

Fig. Pl 1-9. Posttreatment photographs.

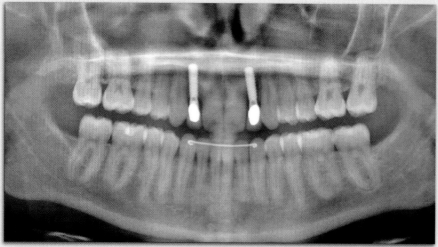

Fig. Pl 1-10. Posttreatment panoramic radiograph.

Table Pl 1-3.	Cephalometric Summary		
	Pretreatment	Post-TAD	Posttreatment
SKELETAL			
SNA (degrees)	75.7	77.0	76.3
SNB (degrees)	72.9	74.2	73.7
ANB (degrees)	2.7	2.8	2.6
SN-ANS/PNS (degrees)	10.9	9.3	9.6
SN-GoMe (degrees)	36.4	34.8	35.1
N-ANS (mm)	51.3	51.2	49.6
ANS-Me (mm)	57.6	57.6	56.1
DENTAL			
U1-SN (degrees)	102.6	99.4	100.0
L1-GoMe (degrees)	106.7	106.3	101.1
U1-APo (mm)	6.6	6.3	5.8
L1-APo (mm)	4.7	4.5	2.9
SOFT TISSUE			
LS-PnPo′ (mm)	−2.5	−3.5	−2.7
LI-PnPo′ (mm)	0.4	0.6	−1.9

TAD, Temporary anchorage device.

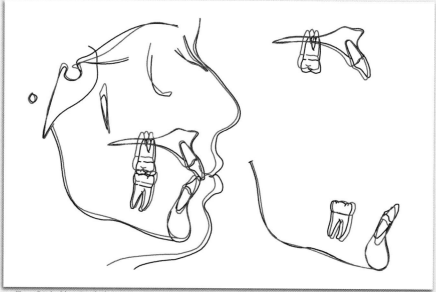

Fig. Pl 1-11. Cephalometric superimposition.

Bilateral Distalization of the Upper Arch to Eliminate Crowding and Obtain a Class I Occlusion

B. Giuliano Maino, Paola Mura

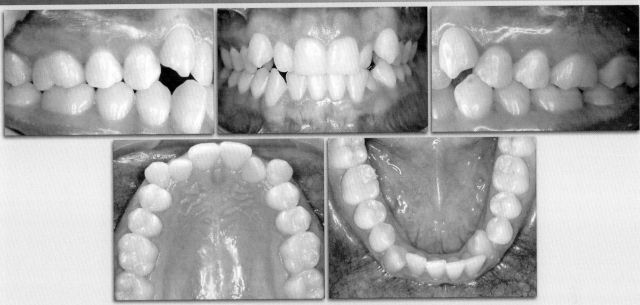

Fig. PI 2-1. Pretreatment photographs.

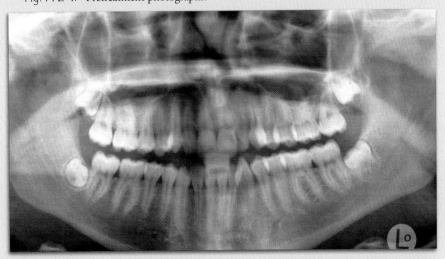

Fig. PI 2-2. Pretreatment panoramic radiograph.

The plan was to use a Midplant (HDC, Sarcedo [Vi], Italy) anchored Pendulum appliance to distalize the upper arch from an end-on Class II malocclusion with upper and lower crowding to a Class I occlusion without extractions. The lower anterior teeth would be reduced in width by interproximal enamel reduction. The upper molars would be distalized by the Pendulum appliance followed by retraction of the anterior teeth and premolars. Two Midplants were placed in case of failure of either. However, only one was used for the entire treatment period. Upon completion of treatment, the endosseous component of the Midplants was left in place with no apparent complication over a 2-year observation period.

Table PI 2-1.	Diagnosis and Treatment Goals	
	Diagnosis	Treatment Goals
SKELETAL		
Anteroposterior	Class I	Class I
Vertical	Normal	Normal
Transverse	Normal	Normal
DENTAL		
Right molar	End-on Class II	Class I
Right canine	End-on Class II	Class I
Left molar	End-on Class II	Class I
Left canine	End-on Class II	Class I
Upper right	4 mm crowding	None
Upper left	4 mm crowding	None
Lower right	2 mm crowding	None
Lower left	2 mm crowding	None
Missing teeth	None	None
Restore teeth	N/A	N/A
Overjet	2 mm	2 mm
Overbite	2 mm	2 mm
Upper ML	0 mm to facial ML	0 mm to facial ML
Lower ML	0 mm to facial ML	0 mm to facial ML
SOFT TISSUE		
Profile	Straight	Straight
Lips	Competent	Competent
PERIODONTIUM		
Inadequate KT/TT	None	None
Gingival recession	None	None
Bone loss	None	None

KT/TT, Keratinized tissue/thin tissue; *ML,* midline; *N/A,* not applicable.

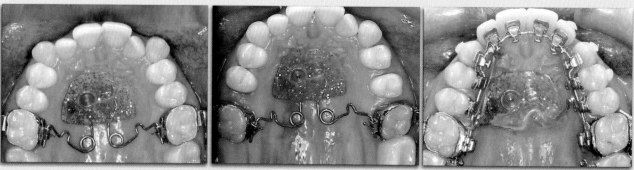

Fig. PI 2-3. Initial *(left)*, progress *(center)*, and final *(right)* temporary anchorage device (TAD) occlusal photographs.

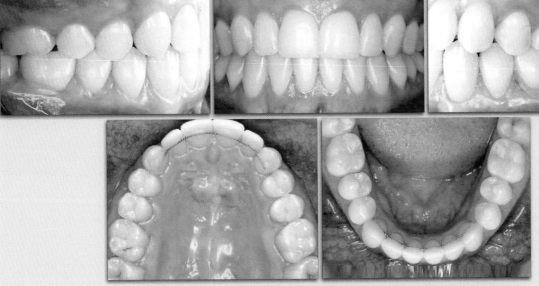

Fig. PI 2–4. Posttreatment photographs.

Table PI 2–2.	Temporary Anchorage Device Summary	
Procedure	Data	
Appliances placed	20 Mar 2001	
TAD placed	13 Dec 2000	13 Dec 2000
Location of TAD	Left parasagittal palatal No. 15-25*	Right parasagittal palatal No. 15-25
Type of TAD	PI	PI
TAD loaded	N/A	23 Apr 2001
Healing duration	N/A	112 days
Force in grams	N/A	450
Mechanics used	N/A	Indirect
TAD unloaded	N/A	3 Sep 2002
TAD loading duration	N/A	17 months
TAD removed	N/A	15 Oct 2002†
Appliances removed	21 Jan 2003	
Treatment duration	22 months	

* Two palatal implants (PI) were placed in case one failed, but only the right was used.
† Only the supramucosal components were removed; the endosseous components were
  left in place. *TAD,* Temporary anchorage device; *N/A,* not applicable.

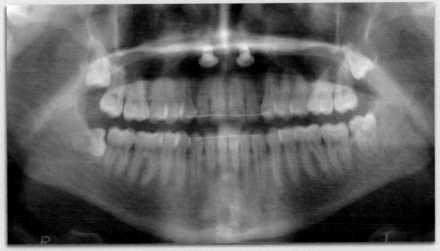

Fig. PI 2–5. Posttreatment panoramic radiograph.

Table PI 2–3.	Cephalometric Summary	
	Pretreatment	Posttreatment
SKELETAL		
SNA (degrees)	82.0	83.0
SNB (degrees)	80.0	81.0
ANB (degrees)	2.0	2.0
SN-ANS/PNS (degrees)	5.0	5.0
SN-GoMe (degrees)	32.0	32.0
N-ANS (mm)	52.0	54.0
ANS-Me (mm)	67.0	70.0
DENTAL		
U1-SN (degrees)	98.0	109.0
L1-GoMe (degrees)	80.0	87.0
U1-APo (mm)	2.0	4.0
L1-APo (mm)	–1.5	2.0
SOFT TISSUE		
LS-PnPo′ (mm)	–5.5	–5.5
LI-PnPo′ (mm)	–5.0	–5.0

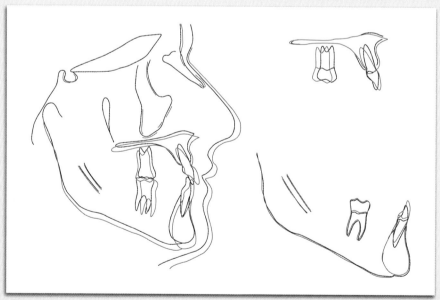

Fig. PI 2–6. Cephalometric superimposition.

Unilateral Distalization of an Upper Class II Buccal Segment

Jason B. Cope, Pedro F. Franco

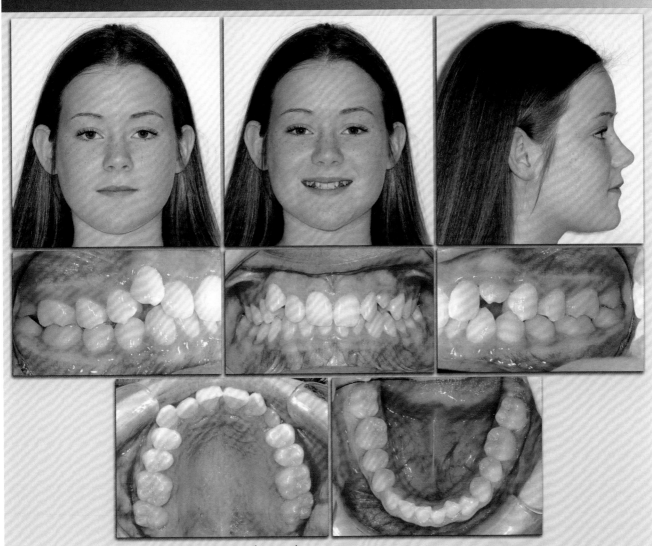

Fig. PI 3-1. Pretreatment photographs.

The patient had an end-on Class II buccal segment relationship on her right side. Upon consultation with the patient and parents, it was determined that cooperation would be inadequate to obtain an ideal Class I relationship.

Therefore, a palatal implant (Straumann Corp., Waldenburg, Switzerland) was to be placed for unilateral distalization of the right buccal segment. The lower third molars were to be extracted during palatal implant removal.

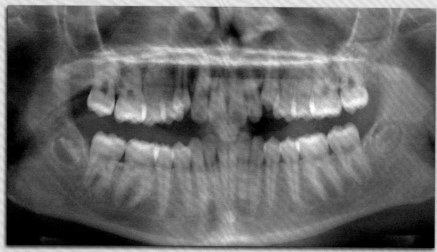

Fig. PI 3-2. Pretreatment panoramic radiograph.

Table PI 3-1.	Diagnosis and Treatment Goals	
	Diagnosis	Treatment Goals
SKELETAL		
Anteroposterior	Class I	Class I
Vertical	Normal	Normal
Transverse	Normal	Normal
DENTAL		
Right molar	End-on Class II	Class I
Right canine	Class II	Class I
Left molar	Class I	Class I
Left canine	End-on Class II	Class I
Upper right	2 mm crowding	None
Upper left	3 mm crowding	None
Lower right	1 mm crowding	None
Lower left	2 mm crowding	None
Missing teeth	No. 18, 28	No. 18, 28, 38, 48
Restore teeth	N/A	N/A
Overjet	2 mm	2 mm
Overbite	6 mm	3 mm
Upper ML	0 mm to facial ML	0 mm to facial ML
Lower ML	0 mm to facial ML	0 mm to facial ML
SOFT TISSUE		
Profile	Straight	Straight
Lips	Competent	Competent
PERIODONTIUM		
Inadequate KT/TT	None	None
Gingival recession	None	None
Bone loss	None	None

KT/TT, Keratinized tissue/thin tissue; *ML,* midline; *N/A,* not applicable.

Table PI 3-2.	Temporary Anchorage Device Summary
Procedure	Data
Appliances placed	7 May 2001
TAD placed	15 Aug 2001
Location of TAD	Midpalatal No. 15-25
Type of TAD	PI
TAD loaded	15 Nov 2001
Healing duration	90 days
Force in grams	150-250
Mechanics used	Indirect
TAD unloaded	11 Nov 2002
TAD loading duration	12 months
TAD removed	26 Nov 2002
Appliances removed	3 Mar 2003
Treatment duration	22 months

TAD, Temporary anchorage device; *PI*, palatal implant.

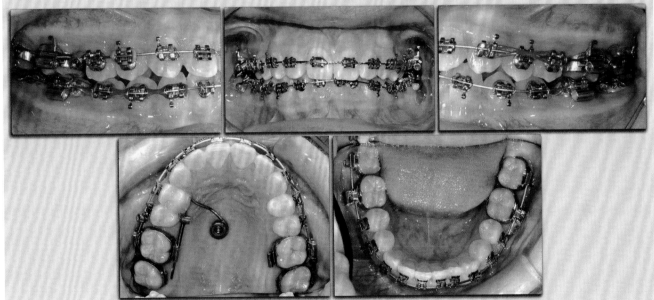

Fig. PI 3-3. Initial temporary anchorage device (TAD) photographs.

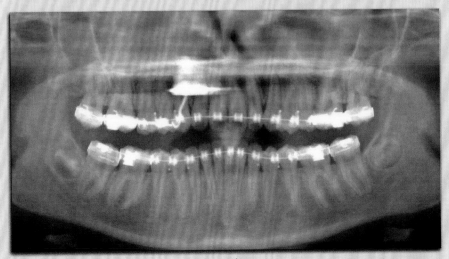

Fig. PI 3-4. Initial TAD panoramic radiograph.

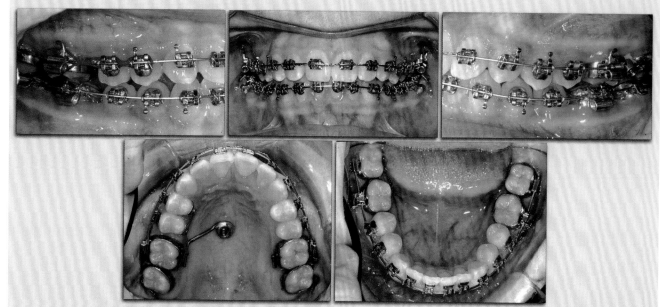

Fig. PI 3-5.   Progress TAD photographs.

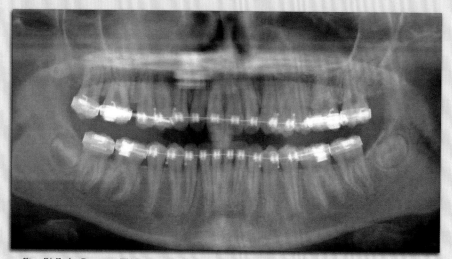

Fig. PI 3-6.   Progress TAD panoramic radiograph.

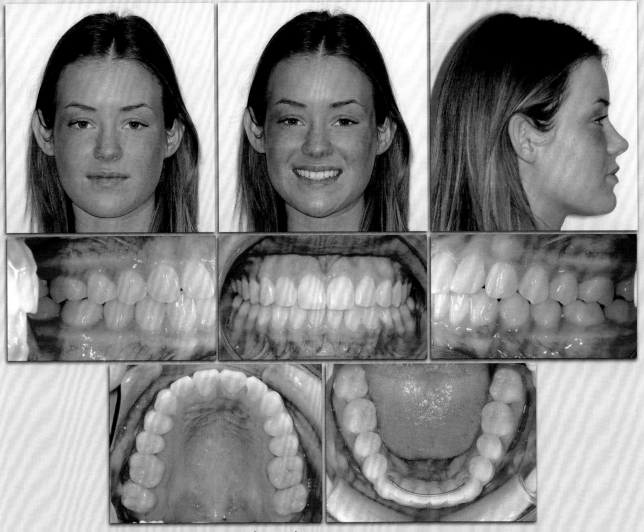

Fig. PI 3-7. Posttreatment photographs.

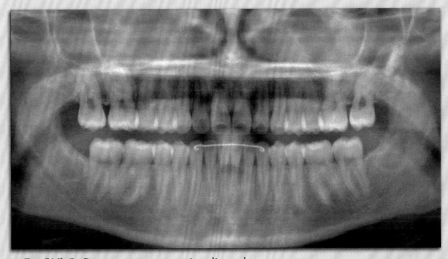

Fig. PI 3-8. Posttreatment panoramic radiograph.

Table PI 3-3.	Cephalometric Summary	
	Pretreatment	Posttreatment
SKELETAL		
SNA (degrees)	80.6	80.4
SNB (degrees)	79.0	79.7
ANB (degrees)	1.6	0.7
SN-ANS/PNS (degrees)	10.5	10.3
SN-GoMe (degrees)	35.0	31.6
N-ANS (mm)	50.3	50.5
ANS-Me (mm)	56.7	57.0
DENTAL		
U1-SN (degrees)	89.6	108.3
L1-GoMe (degrees)	80.3	96.7
U1-APo (mm)	1.8	5.8
L1-APo (mm)	–0.9	2.2
SOFT TISSUE		
LS-PnPo' (mm)	–6.0	–3.6
LI-PnPo' (mm)	–3.8	–2.3

TAD, Temporary anchorage device.

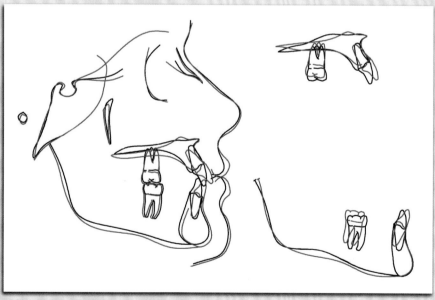

Fig. PI 3-9. Cephalometric superimposition.

Maximum Upper Anterior and Premolar Retraction to Correct a Class II Division II Malocclusion

Peter Goellner

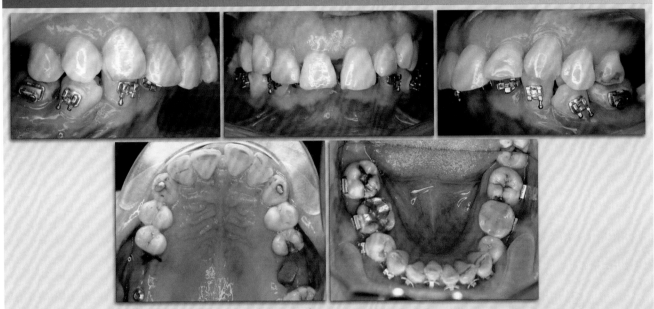

Fig. MPI 4–1. Pretreatment photographs.

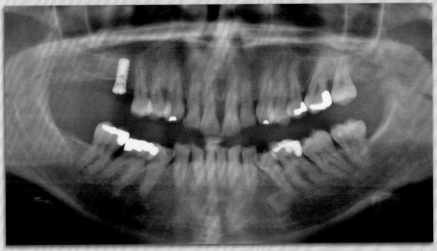

Fig. MSI 4–2. Pretreatment panoramic radiograph.

The treatment plan was to use a palatal implant (Straumann Corp., Waldenburg, Switzerland) and a dental implant in site No. 17 to retract the upper anterior segment and premolars maximally to eliminate the overjet.

The dental implant in the No. 16 site was placed too far mesially before orthodontic treatment and had to be removed and re-placed in the No. 17 site. Attempting such a difficult case with lingual appliances proved to be time consuming. Labial appliances may have taken less total treatment time.

Table PI 4-1.	Diagnosis	Treatment Goals
SKELETAL		
Anteroposterior	Class II	Class II
Vertical	Normal	Normal
Transverse	Normal	Normal
DENTAL		
Right molar	Class II	Class I
Right canine	Class II	Class I
Left molar	Class II	Class I
Left canine	Class II	Class I
Upper right	1 mm crowding	None
Upper left	1 mm crowding	None
Lower right	2 mm crowding	None
Lower left	3 mm crowding	None
Missing teeth	No. 16, 17, 18, 28, 34, 44, 48	No. 18, 28, 34, 44, 48
Restore teeth	N/A	No. 11, 12, 16, 17, 21, 22, 27, 31, 32, 41, 42
Overjet	9 mm	2 mm
Overbite	6 mm	2 mm
Upper ML	0 mm to facial ML	0 mm to facial ML
Lower ML	0 mm to facial ML	0 mm to facial ML
SOFT TISSUE		
Profile	Convex	Straight
Lips	Incompetent	Competent
PERIODONTIUM		
Inadequate KT/TT	None	None
Gingival recession	None	None
Bone loss	Around all teeth, No. 27 severe	Maintain
OTHER	Incorrect placement of No. 16 implant before orthodontics necessitated removal and re-placement more distally	

KT/TT, Keratinized tissue/thin tissue; *ML,* midline; *N/A,* not applicable.

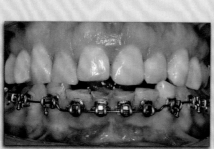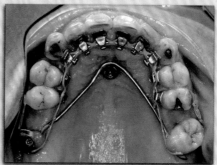

Fig. PI 4-3. Initial temporary anchorage device (TAD) photographs.

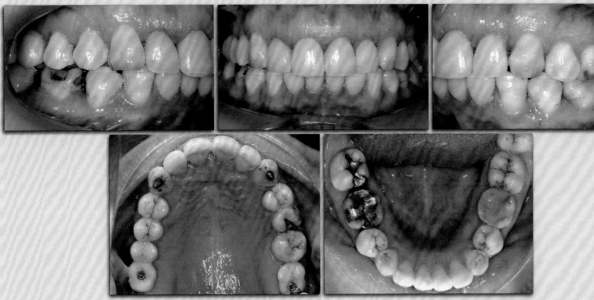

Fig. PI 4-4. Posttreatment photographs.

Table PI 4-2.	Temporary Anchorage Device Summary
Procedure	Data
Appliances placed	28 Oct 2000
TAD placed	5 Sep 2000
Location of TAD	Midpalatal No. 14-24
Type of TAD	PI
TAD loaded	26 Jan 2001
Healing duration	84 days
Force in grams	300
Mechanics used	Indirect
TAD unloaded	17 Apr 2003
TAD loading duration	27 months
TAD removed	10 Aug 2003
Appliances removed	10 Aug 2003
Treatment duration	34 months

TAD, Temporary anchorage device; *PI*, palatal implant.

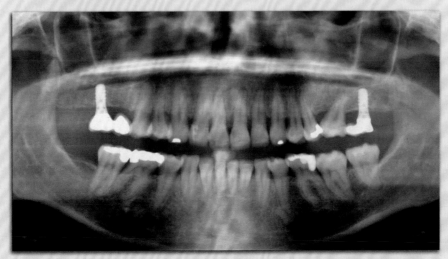

Fig. PI 4-5. Posttreatment panoramic radiograph.

Table PI 4–3.	Cephalometric Summary	
	Pretreatment	Posttreatment
SKELETAL		
SNA (degrees)	85.9	84.5
SNB (degrees)	80.3	77.8
ANB (degrees)	5.6	6.7
SN-ANS/PNS (degrees)	5.4	9.5
SN-GoMe (degrees)	33.6	35.7
N-ANS (mm)	61.3	60.1
ANS-Me (mm)	54.2	56.0
DENTAL		
U1-SN (degrees)	105.8	90.2
L1-GoMe (degrees)	101.6	112.4
U1-APo (mm)	14.0	8.3
L1-APo (mm)	4.7	5.7
SOFT TISSUE		
LS-PnPo′ (mm)	–1.0	–2.0
LI-PnPo′ (mm)	3.0	0.0

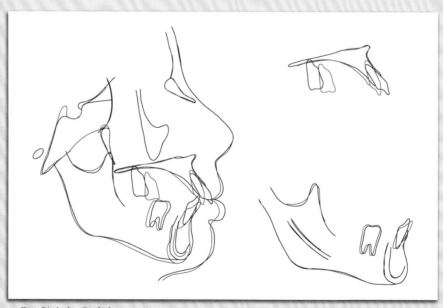

Fig. PI 4–6. Cephalometric superimposition.

Maximum Anterior Retraction and Third Molar Protraction after Premolar Extraction in a Bialveolar Protrusion Case

Aldo Giancotti, Claudio Arcuri

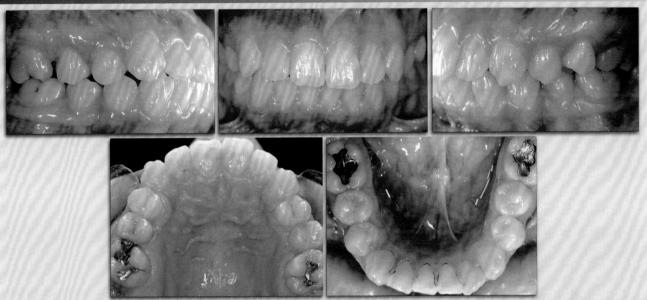

Fig. PI 5-1. Pretreatment photographs.

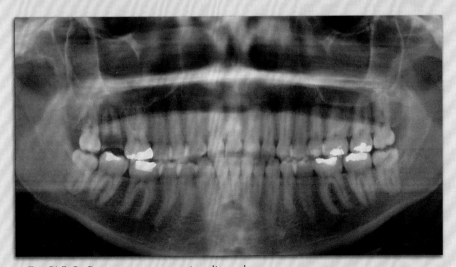

Fig. PI 5-2. Pretreatment panoramic radiograph.

The treatment plan was to eliminate bialveolar protrusion and lip protrusion by extracting upper and lower first premolars and the severely decayed upper right second molar. A palatal implant (Straumann Corp., Waldenburg, Switzerland) was to be used for maximum anterior retraction and protraction of the maxillary right third molar into the second molar position.

Table PI 5-1.	Diagnosis and Treatment Goals	
	Diagnosis	Treatment Goals
SKELETAL		
Anteroposterior	Class I	Class I
Vertical	Normal	Normal
Transverse	Normal	Normal
DENTAL		
Right molar	Class I	Class I
Right canine	Class I	Class I
Left molar	Class I	Class I
Left canine	Class I	Class I
Upper right	1 mm crowding	None
Upper left	1 mm crowding	None
Lower right	2 mm crowding	None
Lower left	2 mm crowding	None
Missing teeth	None	No. 14, 17, 24, 38, 34, 44
Restore teeth	N/A	N/A
Overjet	1.5 mm	1.5 mm
Overbite	2 mm	1.5 mm
Upper ML	1.5 mm left of facial ML	0 mm to facial ML
Lower ML	0 mm to facial ML	0 mm to facial ML
SOFT TISSUE		
Profile	Full	Straight
Lips	Incompetent	Competent
PERIODONTIUM		
Inadequate KT/TT	None	None
Gingival recession	None	None
Bone loss	None	None

KT/TT, Keratinized tissue/thin tissue; *ML*, midline; *N/A*, not applicable.

Table PI 5-2.	Temporary Anchorage Device Summary
Procedure	Data
Appliances placed	5 Oct 2002
TAD placed	25 Oct 2002
Location of TAD	Midpalatal No. 15-25
Type of TAD	PI
TAD loaded	10 Jan 2003
Healing duration	70 days
Force in grams	150-200
Mechanics used	Indirect
TAD unloaded	16 Dec 2003
TAD loading duration	11 months
TAD removed	20 Feb 2004
Appliances removed	30 Jul 2004
Treatment duration	22 months

TAD, Temporary anchorage device; *PI*, palatal implant.

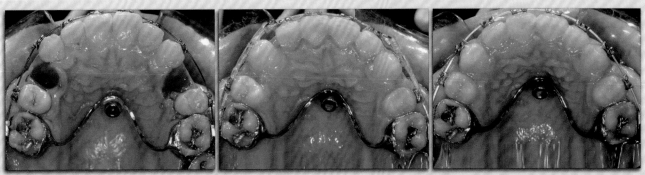

Fig. PI 5-3. Initial *(left)*, progress *(center)*, and final *(right)* temporary anchorage device (TAD) occlusal photographs.

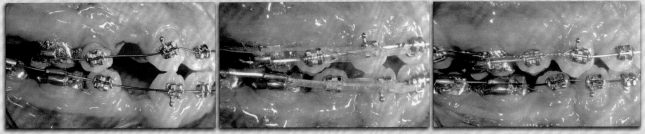

Fig. PI 5-4. Initial *(left)*, progress *(center)*, and final *(right)* TAD right buccal photographs.

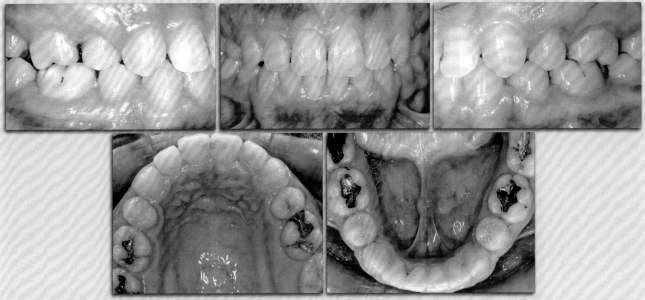

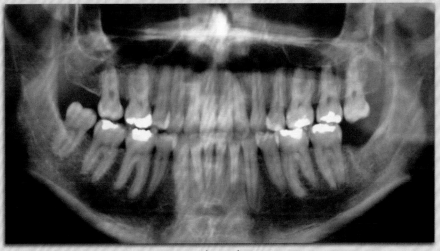

Fig. PI 5-5. Posttreatment photographs.

Fig. PI 5-6. Posttreatment panoramic radiograph.

Table PI 5-3.	Cephalometric Summary	
	Pretreatment	Posttreatment
SKELETAL		
SNA (degrees)	82.0	82.0
SNB (degrees)	79.0	77.0
ANB (degrees)	3.0	4.0
SN-ANS/PNS (degrees)	12.0	12.0
SN-GoMe (degrees)	42.0	43.0
N-ANS (mm)	60.0	60.0
ANS-Me (mm)	77.0	79.0
DENTAL		
U1-SN (degrees)	113.0	100.0
L1-GoMe (degrees)	95.0	87.0
U1-APo (mm)	14.0	8.0
L1-APo (mm)	11.0	6.0
SOFT TISSUE		
LS-PnPo′ (mm)	–2.0	–3.0
LI-PnPo′ (mm)	3.5	0.0

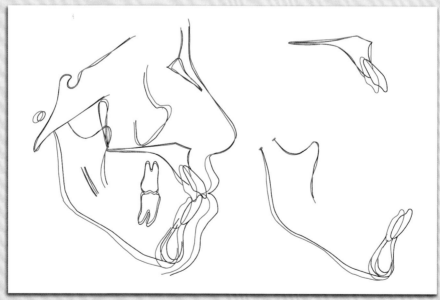

Fig. PI 5-7. Cephalometric superimposition.

Upper Left Retraction and Upper Right Protraction after Premolar Extraction for Midline Correction

Peter Goellner

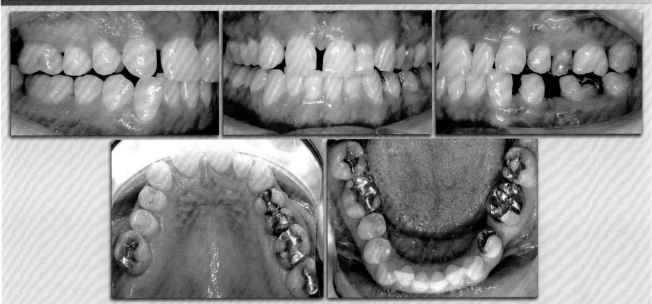

Fig. Pl 6-1. Pretreatment photographs.

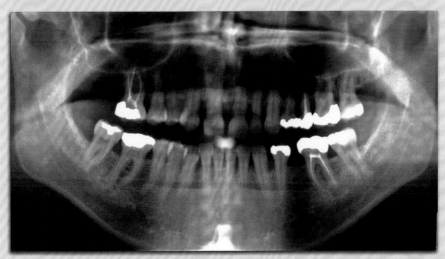

Fig. Pl 6-2. Pretreatment panoramic radiograph.

The plan was to extract the upper left second premolar and move the entire arch from the right to the left using a palatal implant (Straumann Corp., Waldenburg, Switzerland) for anchorage without retracting the upper incisors. Because of lack of patient compliance in wearing elastics, the left side remains in a slight end-on Class II relationship with the dental midlines slightly off.

Table PI 6-1.	Diagnosis and Treatment Goals	
	Diagnosis	Treatment Goals
SKELETAL		
Anteroposterior	Class I	Class I
Vertical	Normal	Normal
Transverse	Normal	Normal
DENTAL		
Right molar	End-on Class II	Class II
Right canine	End-on Class II	Class II
Left molar	Class I	Class I
Left canine	Class I	Class I
Upper right	6 mm crowding	None
Upper left	1 mm crowding	None
Lower right	2.5 mm crowding	None
Lower left	4 mm crowding	None
Missing teeth	No. 12, 17, 18, 28, 38, 35, 48	No. 12, 17, 18, 25, 28, 38, 35, 48
Restore teeth	N/A	N/A
Overjet	3 mm	2 mm
Overbite	3 mm	2 mm
Upper ML	4 mm right of facial ML	0 mm to facial ML
Lower ML	1 mm right of facial ML	0 mm to facial ML
SOFT TISSUE		
Profile	Straight	Straight
Lips	Competent	Competent
PERIODONTIUM		
Inadequate KT/TT	None	None
Gingival recession	None	None
Bone loss	No. 11, 12, 13, 16, 21, 22, 23, 26	Maintain

KT/TT, Keratinized tissue/thin tissue; *ML,* midline; *N/A,* not applicable.

Table PI 6-2.	Temporary Anchorage Device Summary
Procedure	Data
Appliances placed	10 Jan 2002
TAD placed	10 Jan 2002
Location of TAD	Midpalatal No. 15-25
Type of TAD	PI
TAD loaded	10 Jan 2002
Healing duration	0 days
Force in grams	150
Mechanics used	Indirect
TAD unloaded	13 Dec 2003
TAD loading duration	23 months
TAD removed	14 Mar 2004
Appliances removed	13 Feb 2004
Treatment duration	25 months

TAD, Temporary anchorage device; *PI,* palatal implant.

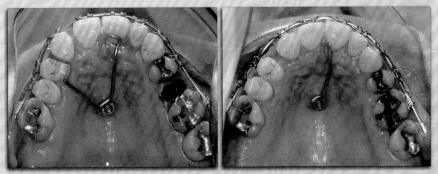

Fig. PI 6-3.   Initial *(left)* and final *(right)* temporary anchorage device (TAD) occlusal photographs.

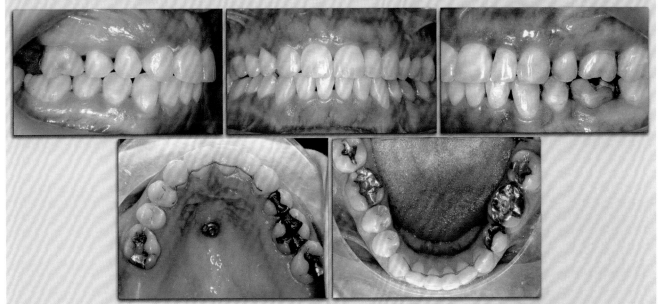

Fig. PI 6-4.   Posttreatment photographs.

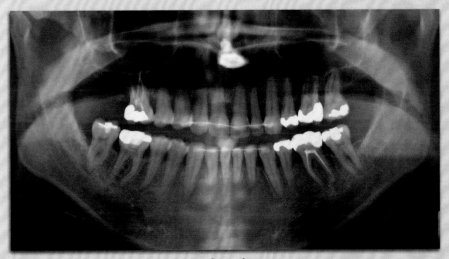

Fig. PI 6-5.   Posttreatment panoramic radiograph.

Table PI 6-3.	Cephalometric Summary	
	Pretreatment	Posttreatment
SKELETAL		
SNA (degrees)	81.5	80.0
SNB (degrees)	79.3	78.6
ANB (degrees)	2.2	1.3
SN-ANS/PNS (degrees)	5.4	4.6
SN-GoMe (degrees)	37.6	39.2
N-ANS (mm)	63.2	65.7
ANS-Me (mm)	55.3	53.3
DENTAL		
U1-SN (degrees)	100.9	103.0
L1-GoMe (degrees)	84.0	92.6
U1-APo (mm)	7.4	7.0
L1-APo (mm)	2.8	4.7
SOFT TISSUE		
LS-PnPo′ (mm)	–4.6	–5.2
LI-PnPo′ (mm)	–3.3	–3.9

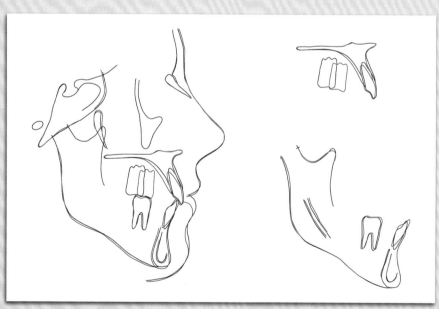

Fig. PI 6-6. Cephalometric superimposition.

Bilateral Protraction of the Entire Upper Arch to Substitute Central Incisors with Lateral Incisors

Peter Goellner

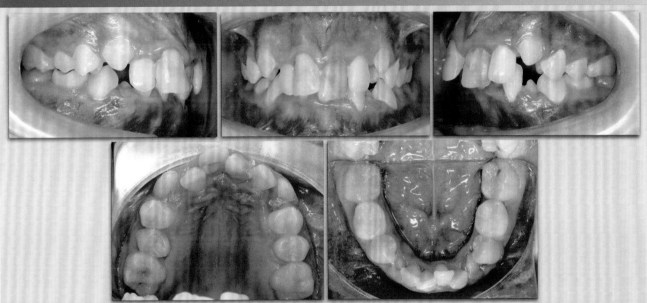

Fig. PI 7–1. Pretreatment photographs.

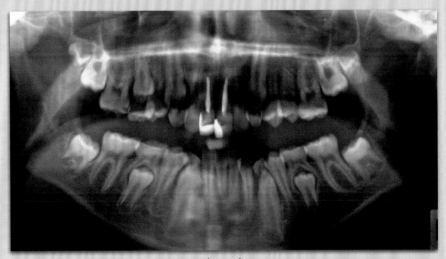

Fig. PI 7–2. Pretreatment panoramic radiograph.

The treatment plan was to initially align the upper arch to create space for placement of temporary central incisors after extraction of the failed endodontic treatment on the permanent central incisors. After a 6-month respite, a palatal implant (Straumann Corp., Waldenburg, Switzerland) would be placed with temporary central incisor crowns attached. Using the crowns as anchorage, the entire maxillary arch would be protracted to eliminate the space of the two missing incisors, eventually replacing them with the lateral incisors, which would be restored with laminate veneers.

Table PI 7-1.	Diagnosis and Treatment Goals	
	Diagnosis	Treatment Goals
SKELETAL		
Anteroposterior	Class II	Class II
Vertical	Deepbite	Normal
Transverse	Normal	Normal
DENTAL		
Right molar	Class II	Class II
Right canine	Class II	Class I
Left molar	Class II	Class II
Left canine	Class II	Class I
Upper right	1.5 mm crowding	None
Upper left	1.5 mm crowding	None
Lower right	3.5 mm crowding	None
Lower left	3 mm crowding	None
Missing teeth	No. 38, 48	No. 11, 21, 38, 48
Restore teeth	N/A	No. 12, 22
Overjet	9.5 mm	2 mm
Overbite	7.5 mm	2 mm
Upper ML	3 mm right of facial ML	0 mm to facial ML
Lower ML	0 mm to facial ML	0 mm to facial ML
SOFT TISSUE		
Profile	Convex	Convex
Lips	Competent	Competent
PERIODONTIUM		
Inadequate KT/TT	None	None
Gingival recession	None	None
Bone loss	None	None
OTHER	Because of previous trauma and failed endodontic treatment, No. 11 and 21 had to be extracted	

KT/TT, Keratinized tissue/thin tissue; *ML,* midline; *N/A,* not available.

Table PI 7-2.	Temporary Anchorage Device Summary
Procedure	Data
Appliances placed	18 Aug 2002
TAD placed	12 Dec 2001
Location of TAD	Midpalatal No. 15-25
Type of TAD	PI
TAD loaded	10 Feb 2002 (crowns); 15 Aug 2002 (ortho)
Healing duration	56 days
Force in grams	100
Mechanics used	Indirect
TAD unloaded	20 Aug 2004 (ortho)
TAD loading duration	24 months
TAD removed	20 Aug 2004
Appliances removed	20 Aug 2004
Treatment duration	24 months

TAD, Temporary anchorage device; *PI,* palatal implant.

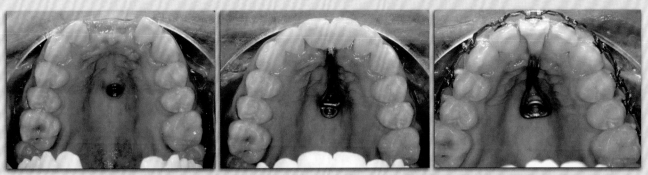

Fig. PI 7-3. Initial *(left)*, progress *(center)*, and final *(right)* temporary anchorage device (TAD) occlusal photographs.

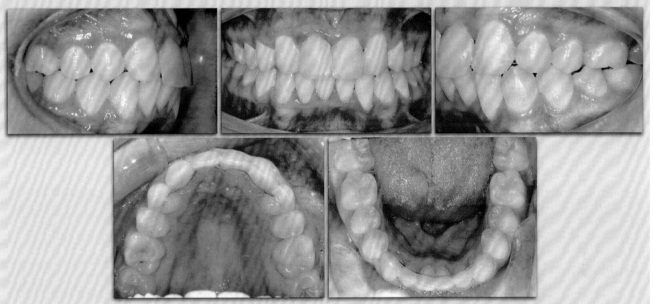

Fig. PI 7-4. Posttreatment photographs.

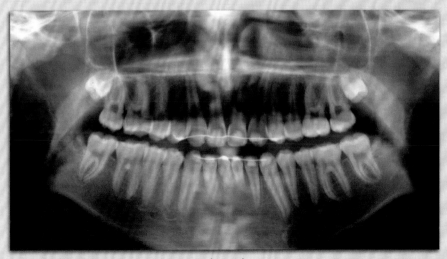

Fig. PI 7-5. Posttreatment panoramic radiograph.

Table PI 7–3.	Cephalometric Summary	
	Pretreatment	Posttreatment
SKELETAL		
SNA (degrees)	75.2	70.5
SNB (degrees)	70.3	70.3
ANB (degrees)	4.8	0.3
SN-ANS/PNS (degrees)	6.1	7.3
SN-GoMe (degrees)	39.1	40.8
N-ANS (mm)	59.0	58.9
ANS-Me (mm)	49.5	49.6
DENTAL		
U1-SN (degrees)	94.9	101.8
L1-GoMe (degrees)	87.4	97.5
U1-APo (mm)	9.9	9.7
L1-APo (mm)	0.4	7.3
SOFT TISSUE		
LS-PnPo′ (mm)	1.0	–5.0
LI-PnPo′ (mm)	2.0	–4.0

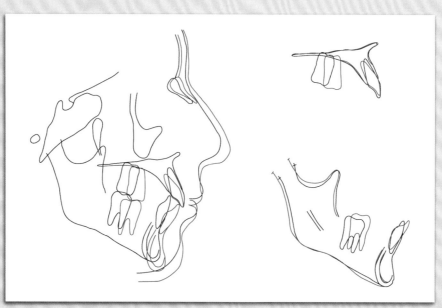

Fig. PI 7-6. Cephalometric superimposition.

Protraction of an Upper Second and Third Molar to Replace a Missing First Molar

Peter Goellner

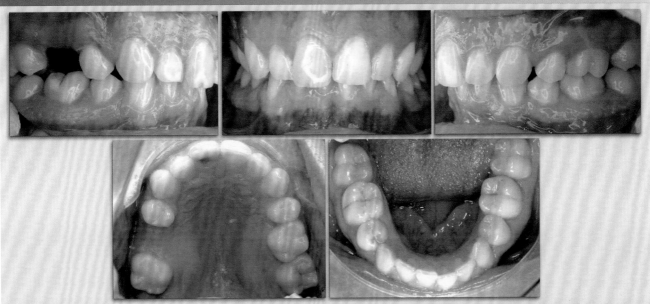

Fig. PI 8-1. Pretreatment photographs.

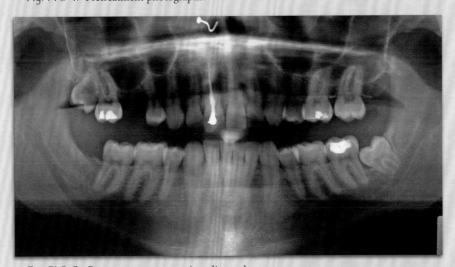

Fig. PI 8-2. Pretreatment panoramic radiograph.

The plan was to use a palatal implant (Straumann Corp., Waldenburg, Switzerland) to protract the upper right second and third molars to replace the missing first molar. The patient also had an end-on Class II buccal segment relationship from previous orthodontic treatment that was to be corrected. To move the upper right second molar through the sinus took longer than anticipated. The force had to be maintained at 100 g to prevent the crown of the tooth from tipping forward.

Table PI 8-1.	Diagnosis and Treatment Goals	
	Diagnosis	Treatment Goals
SKELETAL		
Anteroposterior	Class I	Class I
Vertical	Normal	Normal
Transverse	Normal	Normal
DENTAL		
Right molar	End-on Class II	Class I
Right canine	End-on Class II	Class I
Left molar	End-on Class I	Class I
Left canine	End-on Class I	Class I
Upper right	0 mm crowding	None
Upper left	0 mm crowding	None
Lower right	1 mm crowding	None
Lower left	1 mm crowding	None
Missing teeth	No. 15, 16, 25, 28, 35, 45	No. 15, 16, 25, 28, 38, 35, 45
Restore teeth	N/A	N/A
Overjet	4 mm	2 mm
Overbite	4.5 mm	2 mm
Upper ML	0 mm to facial ML	0 mm to facial ML
Lower ML	0 mm to facial ML	0 mm to facial ML
SOFT TISSUE		
Profile	Straight	Straight
Lips	Competent	Competent
PERIODONTIUM		
Inadequate KT/TT	None	None
Gingival recession	None	None
Bone loss	None	None

KT/TT, Keratinized tissue/thin tissue; *ML,* midline; *N/A,* not applicable.

Table PI 8-2.	Temporary Anchorage Device Summary
Procedure	Data
Appliances placed	10 Aug 2000
TAD placed	15 Jun 2000
Location of TAD	Midpalatal No. 14-24
Type of TAD	PI
TAD loaded	10 Aug 2000
Healing duration	56 days
Force in grams	100
Mechanics used	Indirect
TAD unloaded	14 Dec 2003
TAD loading duration	40 months
TAD removed	18 Jun 2004
Appliances removed	15 Jun 2004
Treatment duration	46 months

TAD, Temporary anchorage device; *PI,* palatal implant.

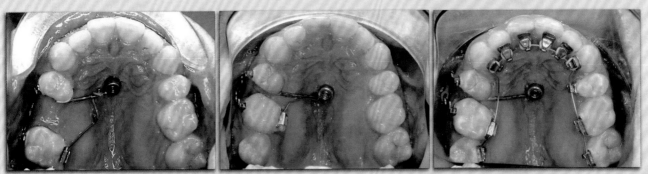

Fig. PI 8-3. Initial *(left)*, progress *(center)*, and final *(right)* temporary anchorage device (TAD) occlusal photographs.

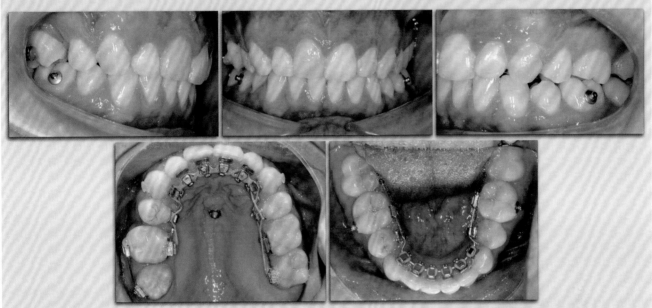

Fig. PI 8-4.   Final TAD photographs.

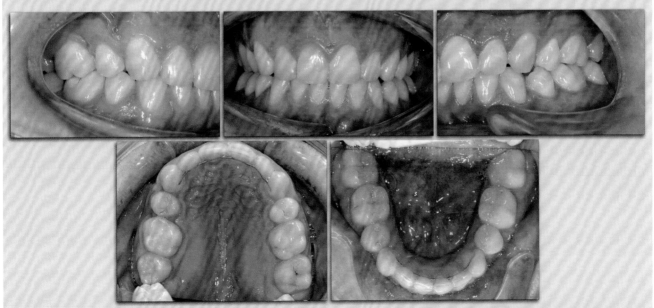

Fig. PI 8-5.   Posttreatment photographs.

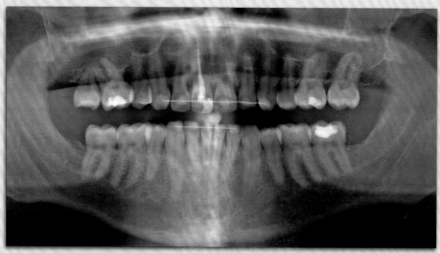

Fig. PI 8–6. Posttreatment panoramic radiograph.

Table PI 8–3.	Cephalometric Summary	
	Pretreatment	Posttreatment
SKELETAL		
SNA (degrees)	81.0	81.6
SNB (degrees)	77.2	76.9
ANB (degrees)	3.8	4.8
SN-ANS/PNS (degrees)	8.2	10.8
SN-GoMe (degrees)	29.0	30.1
N-ANS (mm)	63.3	63.5
ANS-Me (mm)	57.9	59.9
DENTAL		
U1-SN (degrees)	94.0	92.1
L1-GoMe (degrees)	87.9	93.2
U1-APo (mm)	4.7	2.9
L1-APo (mm)	–1.2	–0.4
SOFT TISSUE		
LS-PnPo′ (mm)	–6.8	–5.1
LI-PnPo′ (mm)	–4.3	–3.4

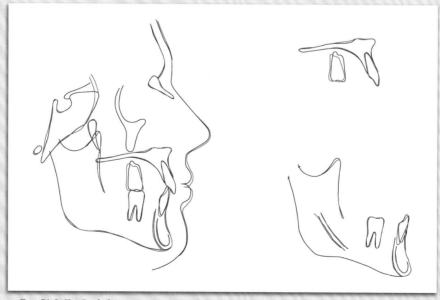

Fig. PI 8–7. Cephalometric superimposition.

Intrusion of Supererupted Upper Molars and Lower Molar Uprighting for Placement and Restoration of Lower Implants

Jason B. Cope, Thomas G. Wilson, Jr.

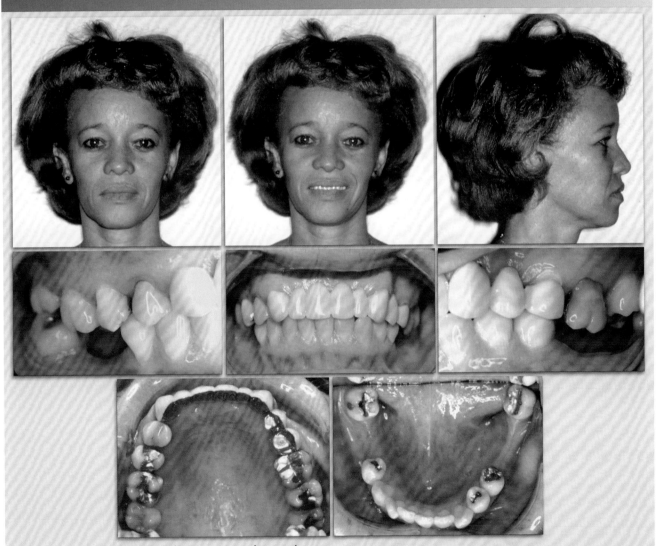

Fig. PI 9-1. Pretreatment photographs.

The treatment plan was to procline the lower incisors for crowding resolution and create an edge-to-edge overjet. The upper anterior bridge would then be remade as a provisional restoration with a normal overjet, thereby creating a more U-shaped upper anterior arch. Palatal implants (Straumann Corp., Waldenburg, Switzerland) were to be placed in the palate to facilitate intrusion of the upper supererupted teeth. Dental implants (Straumann

Corp., Waldenburg, Switzerland) were to be placed in the missing lower molar positions to upright and root correct the mesially tipped lower molars.

After 8 months of intrusion using the framework constructed on the palatal implants, the teeth had been overintruded. The four teeth were intruded an average of 5 to 6 mm each. The teeth also were rolled slightly to the palatal. This problem occurred because the forces were identical on the facial and palatal surfaces. However, it should be recalled that there is more resistance to intrusion on the facial surface because there are two facial roots and only one palatal root. It follows that palatal forces should be less than on the facial surface if pure intrusion without tipping is desired. Segmental mechanics were then used to extrude the teeth to ideal positions followed by prosthetic reconstruction.

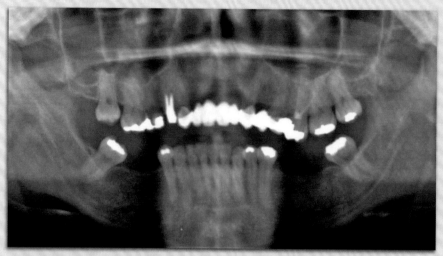

Fig. PI 9-2. Pretreatment panoramic radiograph.

Table PI 9-1.	Diagnosis and Treatment Goals	
	Diagnosis	Treatment Goals
SKELETAL		
Anteroposterior	Class I	Class I
Vertical	Normal	Normal
Transverse	Normal	Normal
DENTAL		
Right molar	Class II	Class II
Right canine	Class II	Class II
Left molar	Class I	Class I
Left canine	Class I	Class I
Upper right	4 mm crowding	None
Upper left	4 mm crowding	None
Lower right	2 mm crowding	None
Lower left	2 mm crowding	None
Missing teeth	No. 11, 12, 18, 21, 22, 24, 36, 37, 45, 46, 48	No. 18, 48
Restore teeth	N/A	No. 16-28, 35-37, 45-46
Overjet	3 mm	3 mm
Overbite	3 mm	3 mm
Upper ML	0 mm to facial ML	1 mm right of facial ML
Lower ML	5 mm right of facial ML	3 mm right of facial ML
SOFT TISSUE		
Profile	Full	Full
Lips	Competent	Competent
PERIODONTIUM		
Inadequate KT/TT	None	None
Gingival recession	No. 13, 16, 17, 23, 25, 26, 34, 45	Maintain
Bone loss	No. 12-22	Graft for implants

KT/TT, Keratinized tissue/thin tissue; *ML,* midline; *N/A,* not applicable.

Table PI 9-2.	Temporary Anchorage Device Summary	
Procedure	Data	
Appliances placed	16 Mar 2000	
TAD placed	1 Sep 2000	1 Sep 2000
Location of TAD	Midpalatal No. 16-26	Midpalatal No. 17-28
Type of TAD	PI	PI
TAD loaded	8 Dec 2000	8 Dec 2000
Healing duration	90 days	90 days
Force in grams	150-200	150-200
Mechanics used	Indirect	Indirect
TAD unloaded	19 Apr 2002	19 Apr 2002
TAD loading duration	16 months	16 months
TAD removed	21 Sep 2002	21 Sep 2002
Appliances removed	11 Oct 2002	
Treatment duration	31 months	

TAD, temporary anchorage device; *PI*, palatal implant.

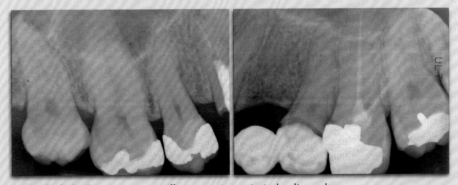

Fig. PI 9-3.   Pretreatment maxillary posterior periapical radiographs.

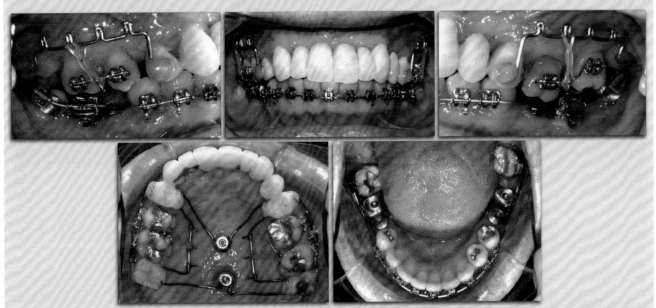

Fig. PI 9-4.   Initial temporary anchorage device (TAD) photographs.

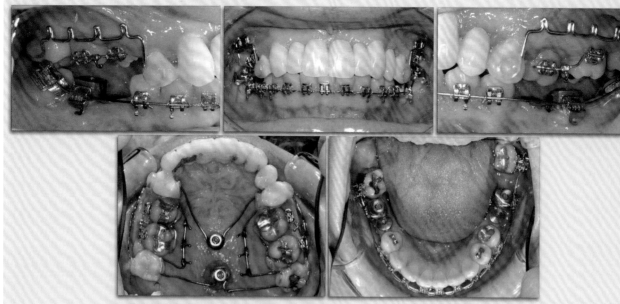

Fig. PI 9-5.   Progress TAD photographs.

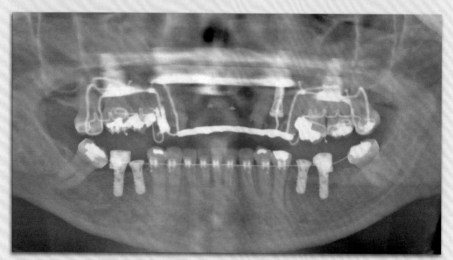

Fig. PI 9-6. Progress TAD panoramic radiograph.

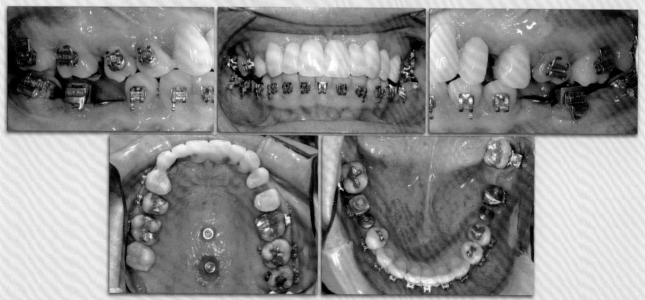

Fig. PI 9-7. Final TAD photographs.

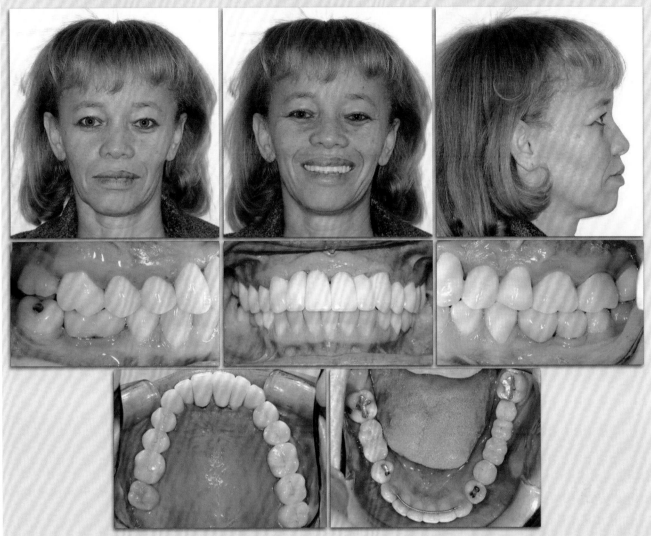

Fig. Pl 9-8. Posttreatment photographs.

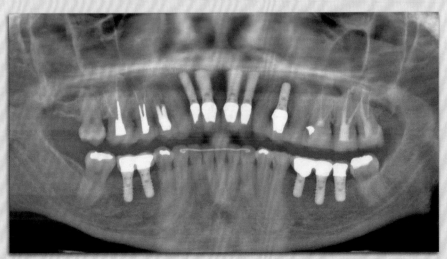

Fig. Pl 9-9. Posttreatment panoramic radiograph.

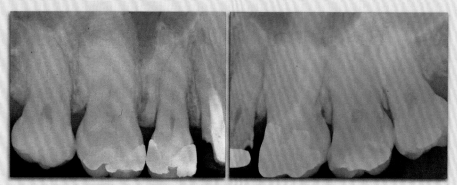

Fig. PI 9–10.   Posttreatment maxillary posterior periapical radiographs.

Table PI 9–3.	Cephalometric Summary	
	Pretreatment	Posttreatment
SKELETAL		
SNA (degrees)	81.6	81.9
SNB (degrees)	78.6	78.1
ANB (degrees)	3.0	3.7
SN-ANS/PNS (degrees)	7.7	7.5
SN-GoMe (degrees)	40.2	37.6
N-ANS (mm)	50.5	49.2
ANS-Me (mm)	70.3	66.9
DENTAL		
U1-SN (degrees)	101.0	117.0
L1-GoMe (degrees)	89.1	95.7
U1-APo (mm)	5.7	10.5
L1-APo (mm)	3.8	7.0
SOFT TISSUE		
LS-PnPo' (mm)	–2.5	0.3
LI-PnPo' (mm)	2.1	3.4

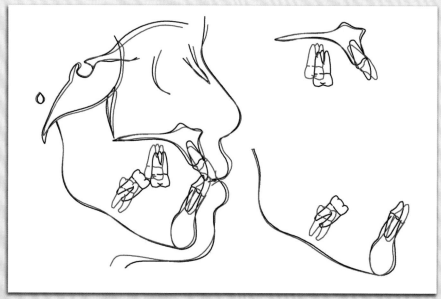

Fig. PI 9–11. Cephalometric superimposition.

SECTION 8

MiniPlate Implant Systems

CHAPTER

19

The C-Palatal Plate

Kyu-Rhim Chung, Seong-Hun Kim, Yoon-Ah Kook

To achieve direct translation of teeth requires a single force applied through the center of resistance.[1] Based on anatomy, lingual force application can be more efficiently directed through the center of resistance and may also more accurately control tooth movement than labial force application during en masse retraction of upper anterior teeth.[2-3] Our group has used the C-lingual retractor, an alternative method of segmental orthodontic mechanics, to effectively close extraction sites and control three-dimensional tooth movement.[4-6] In maximum anchorage cases, it is often necessary to incorporate complex dental mechanics, headgears, or transpalatal arches (TPA) to reinforce the posterior anchorage unit during en masse retraction of upper anterior teeth.[7] The limitation of these anchorage methods is that all provide unpredictable results because they are incapable of providing absolute anchorage. An alternative is to use implant anchorage on the palate, which enables clinicians to effectively retract the anterior teeth using a C-lingual retractor without the need for using posterior teeth for anchorage.

Placement of various types of orthodontic temporary anchorage devices in non–tooth-bearing areas, such as the palate and retromolar regions, is advantageous because it does not interfere with tooth movement. Because of the morphology and ease of access, palatal bone is a suitable anchorage area for placing implants.[8-9] To take advantage of the palatal anatomy, a new type of miniplate implant (MPI) has been developed. The C-palatal plate (C-plate®; KLS Martin LP, Jacksonville, Florida) eliminates the need for multiple individual miniscrew implants (MSI) for attachment mechanics by using a single plate designed specifically for use in the palate.[10]

THE C-PLATE
The C-plate consists of a T-shaped titanium miniplate (Fig. 19-1). The vertical plate has three holes to accommodate 1.5-mm diameter by 5-mm long miniscrews for fixation to the palatal bone. The most lateral extents of the horizontal plate are elevated from the vertical plate in order to be exposed into the oral cavity. The horizontal side arms can be used for retraction of anterior teeth (Fig. 19-2, *A*) and/or protraction of posterior teeth, for applying an intrusive force to individual or multiple teeth (Fig. 19-2, *B*), or for achieving rapid bodily movement of the anterior segment (Fig. 19-2, *C*) along with C-tube® (KLS Martin LP; see Chapter 20) or C-implant® (Cimplant Co., Seoul, Korea; see Chapter 17) mechanics.[11-13] The holes in the horizontal arms are for attaching springs or elastics to facilitate tooth movement. The C-plate is fixed to the midpalatal suture with two or three miniscrews in nongrowing patients whose midpalatal sutural growth is complete. The small size of the miniscrews avoids penetration of the nasal cavity and enables immediate application of orthodontic forces (Fig. 19-3).

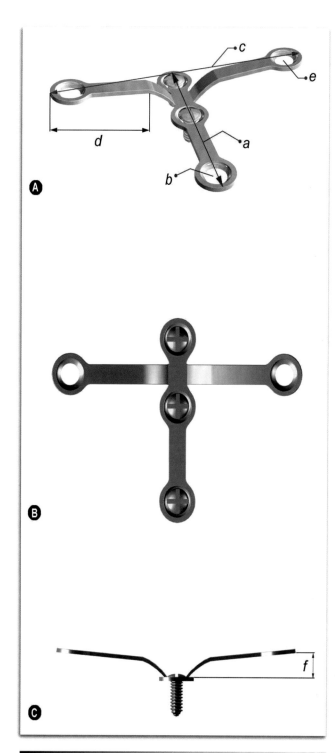

Fig. 19-1

Schematic illustration of titanium C-plate. **A,** Exploded view. The vertical arm *(a)* is 14 mm long and has three holes *(b)* for miniscrews. The horizontal arm *(c)* has two wings *(d)* with holes *(e)* that can be used for orthodontic or orthopedic traction. Two versions are available: short (13-mm wings) or long (20-mm wings). **B,** Superior view. C-plate is placed with two or three drill-free miniscrews. **C,** Anteroposterior view. The two wings of the horizontal arm are elevated 3 mm from the central joint *(f).*

The following are advantages of the C-plate:

1. The surgical procedure is relatively simple and quick because of direct vision and ease of access to the surgical field. The procedure is relatively risk-free because of the anatomy of the midpalate.
2. Immediate application of force is posssible.
3. Orthopedic force (up to 700 g) can be simultaneously applied in multiple directions.[14]
4. Potential complications such as loosening of the plate, pain, and inflammation are minimized.
5. More bodily retraction of the anterior segment is possible than with conventional mechanics.
6. Removal of the C-plate is as easy as placement.

TREATMENT PLANNING

The C-plate is usually used along with a C-lingual retractor in cases of upper anterior or bidentoalveolar protrusion. These cases are often treated with "Speedy Orthodontic Treatment" (a technique using a corticotomy to speed retraction), which requires an orthopedic force of 500 to 600 g. The design of the C-plate allows the clinician to modify its shape depending on the amount of force required for the particular case.

Presurgical radiographs and diagnostic models are necessary to determine the accurate moment:force ratio required. The lateral cephalometric radiograph is used to determine the center of resistance of the anterior segment and the point of force application. The occlusal radiograph is used to determine anteroposterior and mediolateral location of the C-plate. Model surgery (Fig. 19-4) is performed to predict the estimated movement and allows measurement of arch width discrepancies and the amount of retraction desired. C-plate placement location differs between growing and nongrowing patients. Placement of fixation screws in an incompletely fused midpalatal suture may lead to failure of the C-plate. To avoid this, the C-plate can be placed off-center to the midpalatal suture (Fig. 19-5).

PRESURGICAL ORTHODONTICS

The most important factor in presurgical orthodontics is to ensure that tooth movement with the C-plate will proceed uneventfully. This simply means ensuring that no interferences will occur during tooth movement. For example, during en masse retraction of upper anterior teeth, the first step is to align and derotate the anterior teeth based on the model surgery. This prevents upper and lower anterior dental premature contact during incisor retraction. For patients with treatment plans for en masse retraction, but who have narrow anterior

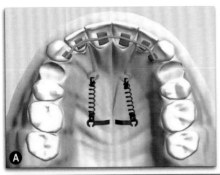 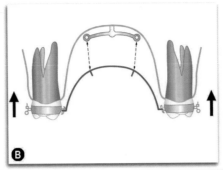 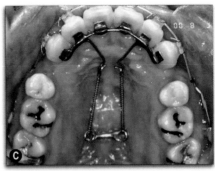

Fig. 19-2

Diagram of C-plate mechanics. **A,** Combined retraction using the C-plate and C-lingual retractor. **B,** Intrusion of molars. Note that molar intrusion requires a TPA between the molars to control torque during intrusion. **C,** Combined facial C-tube and palatal C-plate anterior retraction.

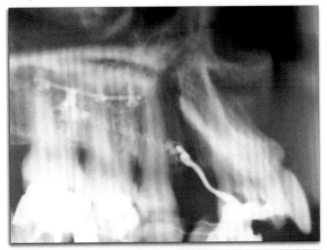

Fig. 19-3

Radiograph of C-plate inserted in the palatal vault with en masse retraction via a NiTi closed coil spring connected to the C-lingual retractor. Note that the small miniscrews do not penetrate the nasal floor.

maxillary arches or deep anterior overbites, treatment must be initiated by expanding the upper anterior dentition and/or intruding the lower anterior teeth before retraction.

SURGICAL PROCEDURE

The C-plate surgical kit (Fig. 19-6) is the same as for C-tube placement (see Chapter 20). Before the surgical procedure, the patient should rinse for 3 minutes with 0.2% chlorhexidine. Afterward, bend the C-plate to follow the palatal contour.

The surgical procedure for placement of the C-plate is as follows (Fig. 19-7):

1. Administer infiltration anesthesia (2% lidocaine with 1:100,000 epinephrine) to the palatal area.
2. Use a No. 15 blade to make an incision from the mesial of the upper first premolar to the distal of the upper first molar. The incision should be 3 mm to the right or left of the midpalatal suture to prevent the soft tissue line of

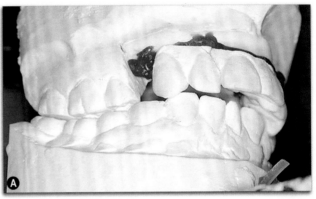

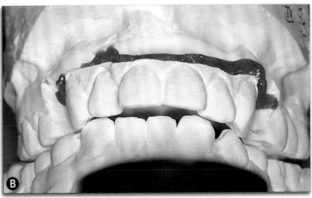

Fig. 19-4

Model surgery treatment planning for C-plate retraction. **A,** Lateral view indicates that a premature contact will occur between the upper and lower canines. **B,** Anterior view indicates that the upper intercanine width is too narrow, necessitating that the upper canines be widened before upper anterior retraction.

closure from falling directly over the vertical arm, which could cause delayed healing because of excessive pressure on the soft tissue.

3. Use a periosteal elevator to reflect a flap. Make a tunnel subperiosteally to the posterior aspect of the midpalatal suture.
4. Contour the vertical plate and position it on the bone surface using mosquito hemostats.
5. Place two or three miniscrews through the holes of the vertical plate. Because the screws are drill-free, a pilot hole

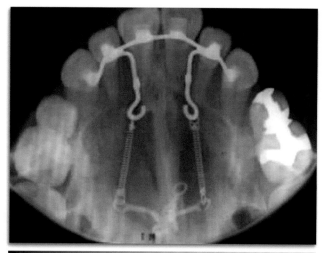

Fig. 19-5

Occlusal radiograph showing C-plate fixation with two miniscrews. Note that the C-plate is placed off center to the midpalatal suture in nongrowing patients to avoid screw failure caused by incomplete fusion of the midpalatal suture.

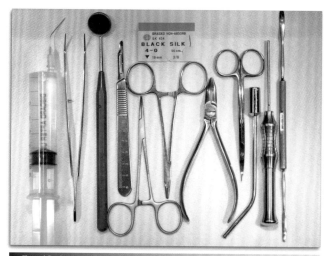

Fig. 19-6

C-plate surgical kit: irrigation syringe, cotton forceps, mouth mirror, No. 15 scalpel blade, 4-0 black silk suture, mosquito hemostats, Weingart pliers, Dean scissors, suction tip, screwdriver, needle holder, and periosteal elevator.

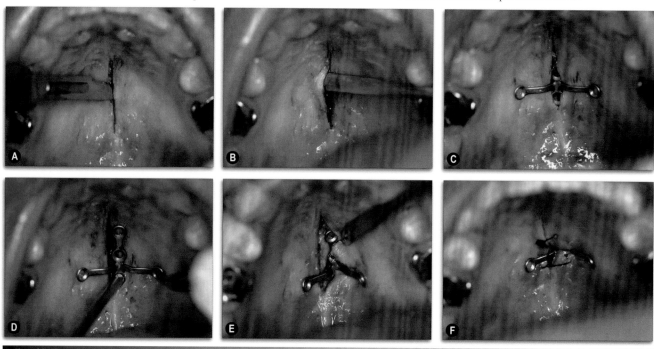

Fig. 19-7

Surgical procedure for C-plate placement without a pilot hole. **A,** Longitudinal incision along the midpalatal surface. **B,** Reflection of the soft tissue. **C,** Placement of the C-plate to check its position. **D,** Fixation of the C-plate with two drill-free miniscrews. **E,** Repositioning of the mucosa. **F,** Single-layer closure with sutures.

usually is not required, except in cases where the midpalatal bone is too dense (Fig. 19-8). Drill-free miniscrews with a Phillips head are preferred for placement because of their retention in the screwdriver tip during placement. Insert the screws using a Martin minidriver (Gebrüder Martin GmbH & Co., Tuttlingen, Germany) modified by adding acrylic to customize the handle for better control of the instrument (Fig. 19-9). However, take care to avoid the

patient swallowing the minidriver during surgery. To prevent this, attach floss to the handle of the minidriver.

6. Reposition the flap and close the incision with a standard single-layer closure. Then apply a periodontal surgical pack. Prescribe antibiotics for 3 days, and give the patient analgesics as necessary. The day after surgery, irrigate the sutured area with saline solution. Remove the sutures after a week.

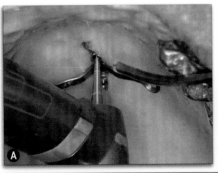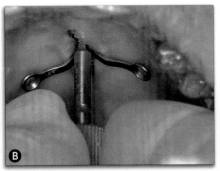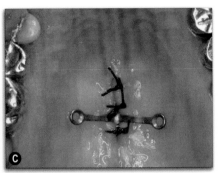

Fig. 19-8

Surgical procedure for C-plate placement with a pilot hole. **A,** After the flap is reflected, the wings are adjusted to the contour of mucosa and a low-speed No. 700 bur is used to drill the pilot hole through the screw hole. **B,** Fixation of the C-plate with three miniscrews. **C,** Single-layer closure with sutures.

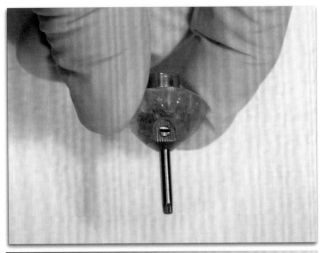

Fig. 19-9

Minidriver with a custom-made acrylic grip.

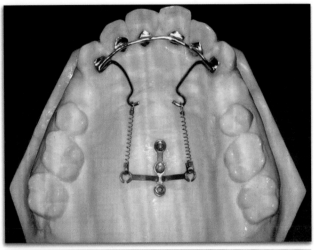

Fig. 19-10

Standard mechanics for combined C-plate and C-lingual retractor. Nickel-titanium closed coil springs are attached between the C-lingual retractor and C-plate to provide retraction force.

The C-plate is usually placed with the two screw holes positioned anteriorly. However, if heavy forces are anticipated or the bone demonstrates a decreased density anteriorly, the C-plate can be rotated 180 degrees and placed with the two screw holes in a posterior direction. Although there are three holes in the C-plate, in most cases only two miniscrews are required for retention.

In cases in which placement of the C-plate posterior to the first molar is desirable for mechanics, it is important to realize that access to the site may be difficult. Instead, it may be more practical to place the C-plate in a more anterior position but to bend the horizontal arms of the plate distally. This also allows the screws to be inserted perpendicularly to the palatal bone. A nonperpendicular screw angle is a major reason for screw failure.

ORTHODONTIC MECHANICS

To attach a closed coil spring to the C-plate, use a high-speed handpiece to cut a slit at the posterior aspect of each hole on the horizontal arm. The slit location depends on the position of the C-plate and the direction of retraction. A NiTi closed coil spring is usually applied to provide a retraction force of about 400 to 450 g per side (Fig. 19-10).

To treat anterior protrusion with crowding, bond lingual buttons on the lingual surface of the canines (Fig. 19-11). Use NiTi closed coil springs from the buttons to the C-plate to begin retraction and eliminate crowding. After elimination of crowding, take an impression for fabrication of the C-lingual retractor, which is connected to the C-plate with a NiTi closed coil spring to complete retraction. This procedure enables control of posterior teeth, leveling, and

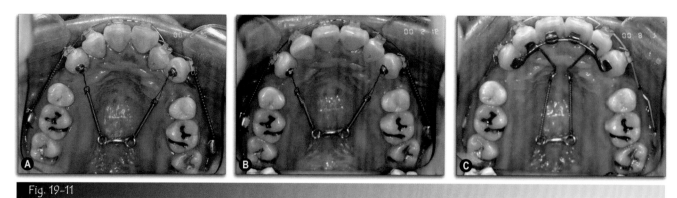

Fig. 19-11

Case with anterior protrusion and crowding. **A,** Lingual buttons on canines to eliminate crowding with NiTi closed coil springs. **B,** After initial resolution of crowding. **C,** C-lingual retractor attached to C-plate via NiTi closed coil springs.

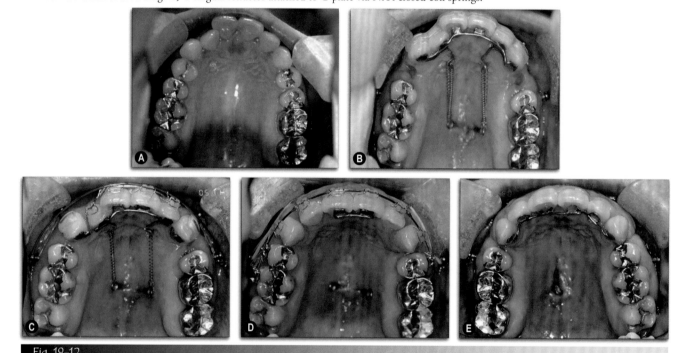

Fig. 19-12

Case combining C-lingual retractor, C-implant, and C-plate. **A,** Initial occlusal photograph **B,** En masse retraction is initiated with the C-lingual retractor and the C-plate. **C,** The C-lingual retractor is cut from the canines when retraction is almost complete, and 0.022 × 0.028-inch preadjusted brackets with an 0.016 × 0.022-inch stainless steel arch wire are used to initiate anterior alignment. **D,** After retraction of the upper incisors the C-retractor is removed and conventional orthodontic treatment is performed. **E,** After treatment a fixed retainer is bonded to the lingual side of the upper anterior teeth, and the C-plate is removed.

alignment. Once retraction is started, frequent adjustment of the C-plate is not necessary. This, in combination with constant force delivery by NiTi closed coil springs, significantly reduces chair time and the total number of appointments. In some cases (Fig. 19-12), when retraction is almost complete, remove the canine portion of the C-retractor and retract the upper central and lateral incisors further to finish closing the space.

During retraction of the upper anterior dentition using C-lingual retractor mechanics, the orthodontist should check for premature incisor contact about every 8 weeks. Once retraction is complete, remove the C-lingual retractor entirely and initiate routine orthodontic mechanics to complete treatment (Fig. 19-13). Although retraction is finished, the C-plate is left in place to control potential vertical movement of the posterior teeth if necessary.

REMOVAL PROCEDURE

Removal of the C-plate is as easy as placement despite the need for local anesthesia and an incision (Fig. 19-14). Make a linear incision over the vertical arm to expose the screw heads. Unscrew the screws and then remove the C-plate. Close the incision with sutures, which are removed a week later.

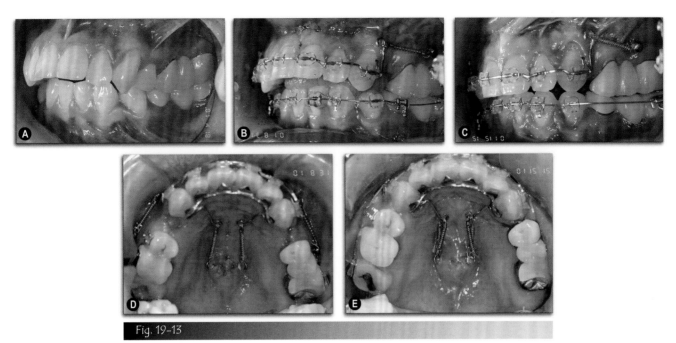

Fig. 19-13

A 37-year-old woman with upper anterior protrusion. **A,** Initial buccal photograph. **B,** Buccal photograph after 4 months. Note that an 0.018 × 0.025-inch stainless steel arch wire with an extension hook was used for labial retraction. **C,** Buccal photograph after 8 months. **D,** Occlusal photograph after 4 months. Note that a C-lingual retractor and a C-plate were used for lingual retraction. **E,** Occlusal photograph after 8 months. Note that the total treatment period was 10 months.

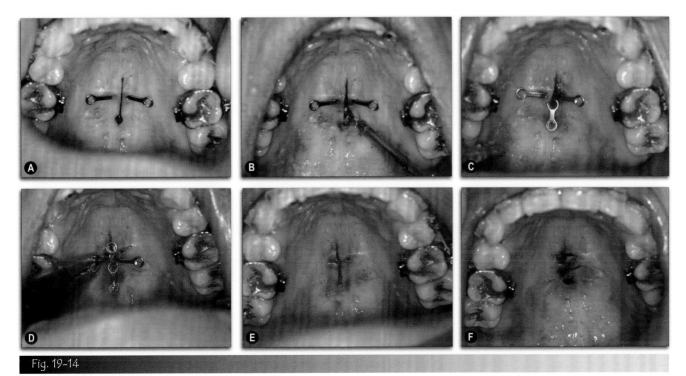

Fig. 19-14

C-plate removal. **A,** Make a vertical incision over the vertical arm. **B,** Slight periosteal elevation is required to expose and remove the miniscrews. **C,** Remove the remainder of the screws. **D,** Make an incision parallel to the horizontal arm and remove the C-plate using Howe pliers. **E,** Appearance after C-plate removal. **F,** Single-layer closure with sutures.

POTENTIAL COMPLICATIONS

Although complications are rare, the most common complication is soft tissue inflammation and/or overgrowth (Fig. 19-15). Another potential problem is failure or loosening of screws, which can usually be avoided by placing the screws perpendicular to the bone surface and in good-quality bone.

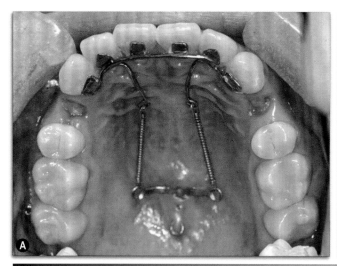 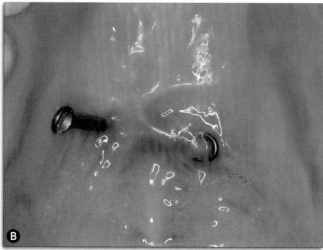

Fig. 19-15

Potential complications. **A,** The C-plate tends to cause inflammation in some cases, and the vertical plate and miniscrew heads might become exposed during traction. **B,** Eccentric force application to one side arm can cause the other side arm to be covered with soft tissue.

SUMMARY

The anatomy of the palate provides the most suitable site in non–tooth-bearing maxillary areas. The C-plate combined with the C-lingual retractor allows bodily en masse retraction of the upper six anterior teeth by directing the force through the center of resistance. This miniplate is recommended especially for speedy orthodontics or immediate loading of orthopedic force after a corticotomy. The C-plate is an excellent skeletal anchorage system because of its simplicity, ability to immediately apply force, and rigidity to withstand orthopedic forces.

ACKNOWLEDGMENTS

Supported in part by the Korean Society of Speedy Orthodontics.

REFERENCES

1. Burstone CJ. The segmented arch approach to space closure. *Am J Orthod.* 82:361-378, 1982.
2. Melsen B, Fotis V, Burstone CJ. Vertical force considerations in differential space closure. *J Clin Orthod.* 24:678-683, 1990.
3. Vanden Bulcke MM, Dermaut LR, Sachdeva RCL, et al. The center of resistance of anterior teeth during intrusion using the laser reflection technique and holographic interferometry. *Am J Orthod.* 90:211-220, 1986.
4. Lee HG, Chung KR. The vertical location of the center of resistance for maxillary six anterior teeth during retraction using three dimensional finite element analysis. *Korean J Orthod.* 31:425-438, 2001.
5. Kim SH, Park YG, Chung KR. Severe anterior open bite malocclusion with multiple odontoma treated by C-lingual retractor and horseshoe mechanics. *Angle Orthod.* 73:206-212, 2003.
6. Kim SH, Park YG, Chung KR. Severe anterior deep bite malocclusion treated by C-lingual retractor mechanics. *Angle Orthod.* 74:185-190, 2004.
7. Klontz H. Tweed-Merrifield sequential directional force treatment. *Semin Orthod.* 2:254-267, 1996.
8. Abels N, Schiel HJ, Hery-Langer G, et al. Bone condensing in the placement of endosteal palatal implants: a case report. *Int J Oral Maxillofac Implants.* 14:849-852, 1999.
9. Kyung SH, Hong SG, Park YC. Distalization of maxillary molars with a midpalatal miniscrew. *J Clin Orthod.* 37:22-26, 2003.
10. Chung KR. C-palatal plate. In: Chung KR, ed. *Textbook of Speedy Orthodontics.* Seoul, South Korea: Jeesung, 2001:99-113.
11. Chung KR, Kim YS, Linton JL, et al. The miniplate with tube for skeletal anchorage. *J Clin Orthod.* 36:407-412, 2002.
12. Chung KR, Kim SH, Kook YA: C-orthodontic microimplant. *J Clin Orthod.* 38:478-486, 2004.
13. Chung KR, Oh MY, Ko SJ. Corticotomy-assisted orthodontics. *J Clin Orthod.* 35:331-339, 2001.
14. Kim SJ, Lee YJ, Chung KR. An effect of immediate orthodontic force on palatal endosseous appliance (C-palatal plate) in beagle dog. *Korean J Orthod.* 33:91-102, 2003.

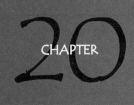

CHAPTER

The C-Tube

Kyu-Rhim Chung, Seong-Hun Kim, Yoon-Ah Kook

Despite the fact that a surgical flap is required, miniplate implants (MPIs) can withstand orthopedic force application immediately after placement. Moreover, they also show less adverse inflammation than conventional miniscrew implants (MSIs). Because of the small size of the miniscrews fixing the miniplate to the bone, the risk of sinus perforation or damage to the tooth roots or nerves is minimized.[1-3] Conventional MPIs have been only used for anchorage reinforcement by attaching force modules to the plate component exposed through the soft tissue into the oral cavity. These MPIs are limited in application primarily to simple mechanics. An MPI with a tube, however, could accommodate arch wires for sliding mechanics as would be necessary for anterior retraction. This would obviate the need for bonding or banding of posterior teeth, thereby maintaining an unaltered posterior occlusion and minimizing any periodontal breakdown or dental decalcification/decay caused by prolonged treatment times. To overcome the limitations of conventional MPIs and to achieve optimal immediate or early skeletal fixation, a new miniplate with a tube (C-tube®; KLS Martin LP, Jacksonville, Florida) was developed (Fig. 20-1).[4-7]

THE C-TUBE

The C-tube is basically an orthodontic tube attached to a commercially pure titanium miniplate and was designed to provide an alternative rigid anchorage system.[4] A round 0.036-inch diameter tube was

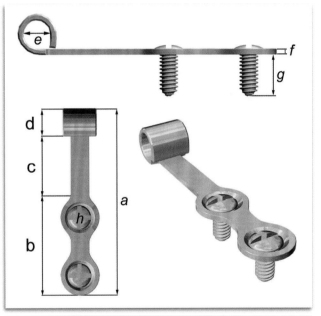

Fig. 20-1

Schematic illustration of titanium C-tube. The total plate length is 14 mm (*a*) broken down into a 7-mm plate with two screw holes (*b*), a 5-mm neck (*c*), and a 2-mm tube (*d*), which is 0.036 inch or 0.9 mm in diameter (*e*). The plate is 0.5 mm thick (*f*) with holes for four 5-mm long (*g*) by 1.5-mm diameter miniscrews (*h*).

created by rolling up one end of a miniplate to provide a housing for an orthodontic arch wire. The three shapes of C-tubes are the I-plate, L-plate, and T-plate (Fig 20-2). Whereas the Skeletal Anchorage System of Sugawara and others[8] (see Chapter 21) was originally designed to be fixed in the zygomatic buttress, the

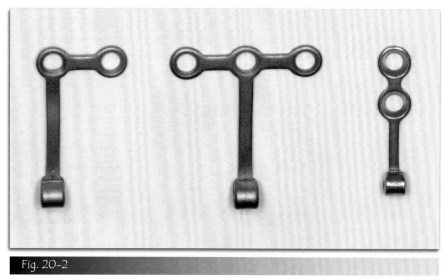

Fig. 20-2

C-tube variations. **A,** L-plate. **B,** T-plate. **C,** I-plate.

C-tube was designed to provide anchorage from a fixation point in cortical bone above the posterior dentition (Fig. 20-3). This placement site is also more accessible than the zygomatic buttress. The C-tube is fixed to bone by two drill-free miniscrews 1.5 mm in diameter and 5 mm long.

In a preliminary study, Chung and colleagues[7] evaluated the periimplant tissue responses to early orthodontic and orthopedic C-tube loading in a dog experiment. The results suggested that the C-tube can be used as a stable, firm osseous orthodontic and orthopedic anchorage unit loaded immediately after placement.

TREATMENT PLANNING

C-tubes are applied as independent treatment protocols without the need for banding or bonding of molars (Fig. 20-4). This biocreative therapy™ is appropriate for cases that require no loss of posterior anchorage, such as in patients who have an ideally intercuspated posterior occlusion in combination with anterior protrusion and crowding. C-tubes can also be used in cases with inadequate posterior anchorage caused by severe dental caries, advanced periodontal disease, or missing teeth. Finally, C-tubes can be used for simultaneous distalization of posterior teeth. C-tubes should not be used in cases of inadequate cortical bone thickness, poor oral hygiene, or in deciduous/mixed dentitions. Potential locations for C-tube placement include the buccal alveolar process, the anterior nasal spine region, the palate, the external oblique ridge, and the symphyseal region.

PRESURGICAL ORTHODONTICS

Because the C-tube is an orthodontic temporary anchorage device independent of other treatment appliances, presurgical orthodontic treatment, such as leveling the posterior dentition, is unnecessary. The ideal orientation of the C-tube is parallel to the occlusal plane and the buccal surface of the teeth. The C-tube

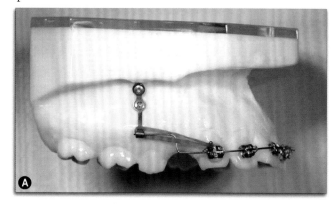

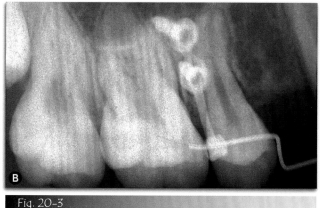

Fig. 20-3

The C-tube standard placement is in cortical bone above the posterior dentition.

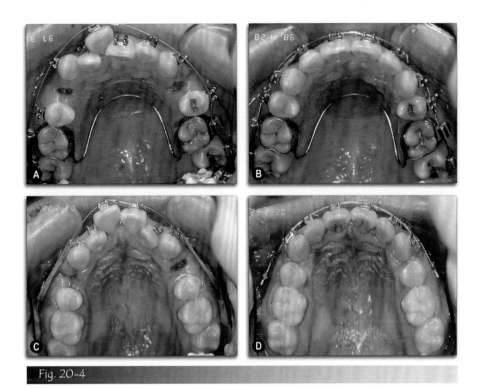

Fig. 20-4

Traditional anchorage vs. C-tube anchorage. **A,** Nance button before retraction. **B,** Nance button after en masse retraction. **C,** C-tube before retraction. **D,** C-tube after en masse retraction.

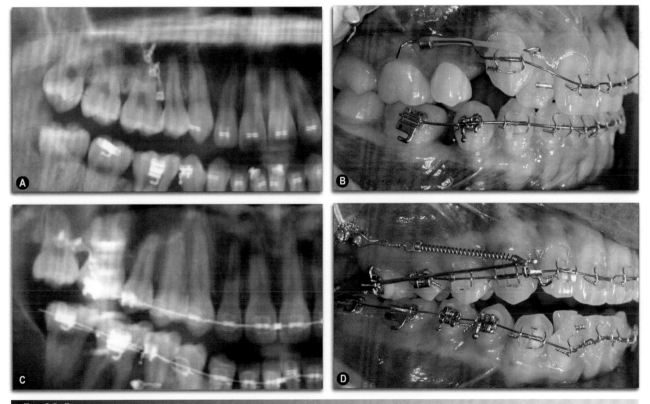

Fig. 20-5

C-tube placement location. **A,** Radiograph of tube placed parallel to occlusal plane for en masse retraction. **B,** Buccal photograph of tube placed parallel to occlusal plane for en masse retraction. **C,** Radiograph of tube placed posteriorly and diagonally to occlusal plane for simultaneous distalization of multiple posterior teeth. **D,** Buccal photograph of tube placed posteriorly and diagonally to occlusal plane for simultaneous distalization of multiple posterior teeth.

should be placed about 2 mm away from the gingiva and the cervical region to allow adequate hygiene and to prevent food impaction (Fig. 20-5, *A* and *B*). The miniscrew fixation site is determined by the orientation of the C-tube and local anatomy. For simultaneous distalization of multiple posterior teeth, place the C-tube posteriorly and diagonally to the occlusal plane (Fig. 20-5, *C* and *D*).

SURGICAL PROCEDURE

The preferred site for the C-tube is the alveolar or basal bone above the posterior dentition. The surgical procedure is simple, but the sites should be chosen carefully to prevent tooth damage and minimize soft tissue irritation. The surgical kit (Fig. 20-6) for C-tube placement includes a needle holder, 4-0 black silk suture, a screwdriver, a suction tip, a periosteal elevator, Weingart pliers, mosquito hemostats, a No. 15 scalpel blade, cotton forceps, a mouth mirror, a saline irrigation syringe, and Dean scissors. Before the surgical procedure, the patient should rinse for 3 minutes with 0.2% chlorhexidine. Afterward, bend the C-tube to prevent soft tissue irritation.

Perform the surgical implantation of the C-tube as follows (Fig. 20-7):

1. Administer infiltration anesthesia (2% lidocaine with 1:100,000 epinephrine) at the mucogingival junction and into the surgical area.

2. Determine the C-tube position based on evaluation of the periapical radiograph and intraoral anatomy.

3. Use a No. 15 blade to make a 1-cm semilunar incision at the fixation point.

4. Use a periosteal elevator to dissect and reflect the periosteum.

5. Contour the plate and position it on the bone surface using a mosquito hemostat.

6. Fix the C-tube with two drill-free miniscrews.

7. Reposition the soft tissue and close the incision with a standard single-layer closure. Prescribe antibiotics for 3 days, and give the patient analgesics as necessary. The day after surgery, irrigate the sutured area with saline solution. Remove the sutures after a week.

8. Immediate loading is possible; however, it is best to wait until the soft tissues have healed before loading.

ORTHODONTIC MECHANICS

Intrusion of anterior (Fig. 20-8) or posterior teeth (Figs. 20-9 and 20-10), molar uprighting (Fig 20-10) or protraction, and full dentition distalization (Fig. 20-9) are easily performed by directly applying elastics, power chain, NiTi closed coil spring, or elastic thread. In C-tube treatment mechanics, the controlled retraction of anterior teeth is important, not only for initial alignment and root angulation correction but also for continuing sliding mechanics effectively and efficiently (Fig. 20-11).[9-10] Canine and en masse retraction are usually initiated with 0.016-inch NiTi arch wires through the C-tubes with 3/16-inch, 3-oz elastics from the anterior segment to the C-tube (Fig. 20-12). Blue Elgiloy arch wire (0.016 × 0.022 inch; Elgiloy Specialty Metals, Elgin, Illinois) is used for en masse retraction during independent C-tube treatment mechanics. Torque control is possible by using soldered brass hooks on the arch wire with tip-back mechanics. Nickel-titanium closed coil springs are connected from the hooks to the C-tubes. Traditional fixed appliances, clear aligners, or tooth positioners can be used for final detailing.

REMOVAL PROCEDURE

After the completion of orthodontic treatment, initiate C-tube removal by performing a semilunar incision between the miniscrews in the plate (Figs. 20-13 and 20-14). Expose the plate around the

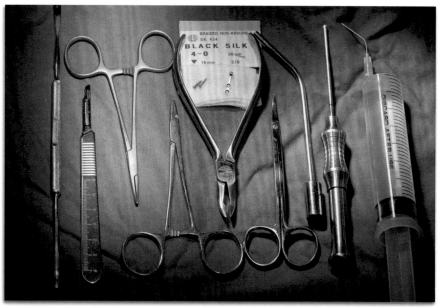

Fig. 20-6

C-tube surgical kit: periosteal elevator, No. 15 scalpel blade, mosquito hemostats, needle holder, 4-0 black silk suture, Weingart pliers, Dean scissors, suction tip, screwdriver, and irrigation syringe.

screws with a narrow periosteal elevator, and turn the screws counterclockwise for removal. Then remove the plate with mosquito hemostats followed by incision closure with a single-layer suture.

POTENTIAL COMPLICATIONS

Fixing C-tubes in the transitional area between the attached gingiva and the mucogingival tissue may cause soft tissue overgrowth. This complication can be avoided by bending the tube laterally away from the soft tissue. Loosening of the C-tube is also possible. This is usually only the case in thin cortical bone, which is sometimes seen overlying a pneumatized sinus. In this case, application of heavy forces may loosen the C-tube. If loosening occurs, the C-tube can be removed and re-placed in a different location. To enhance retention in these cases, select an L-plate or T-plate shaped C-tube.

Mechanical failure of C-tubes arises from excess forces on miniscrews inserted in thin cortical bone that cannot provide enough retention. Pathologic failure, however, is caused by bone resorption initiated by soft tissue infection around the miniscrew (Fig. 20-15). Any gap between the C-tube and miniscrews allows mobility, usually resulting in failure. To reduce the failure rate, bending of the C-tube for close adaptation to the bone surface is essential.

SUMMARY

The C-tube design facilitates placement and provides a simpler procedure than conventional MPIs. Because the C-tube is immediately loadable and applicable without banding or bonding of posterior teeth, treatment is often simplified considerably and treatment time is reduced.

ACKNOWLEDGMENTS

Supported in part by the Korean Society of Speedy Orthodontics.

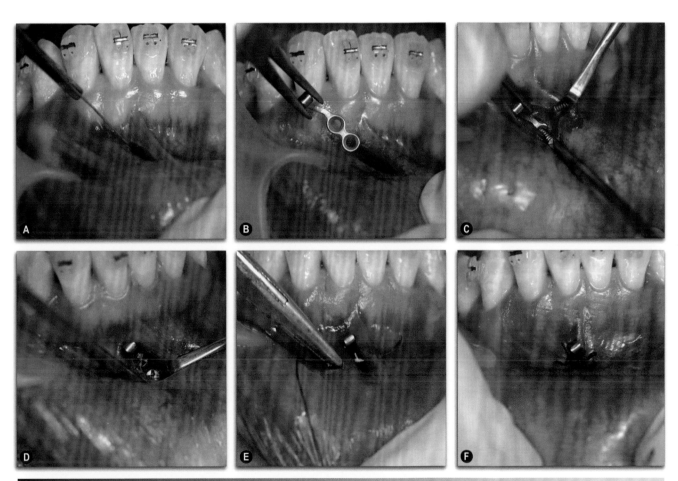

Fig. 20-7

Surgical procedure for C-tube placement for lower anterior intrusion. **A,** Vertical 1-cm incision using No. 15 blade. **B,** Placement of C-tube to check its position. **C,** Fixation of C-tube with two drill-free miniscrews. **D,** Repositioning of the mucosa. **E,** Initial suture placement. **F,** Single-layer closure with sutures.

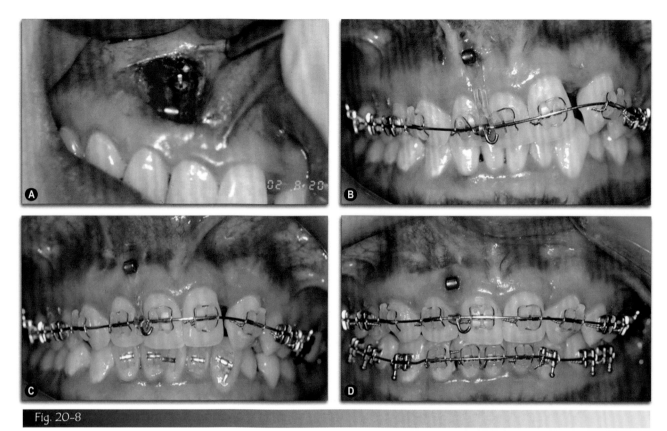

Fig. 20-8

Upper anterior intrusion. **A,** C-tube placed superior to the upper right lateral incisor. **B,** Power chain attached for intrusion. **C,** Intrusion partially complete. **D,** Intrusion complete.

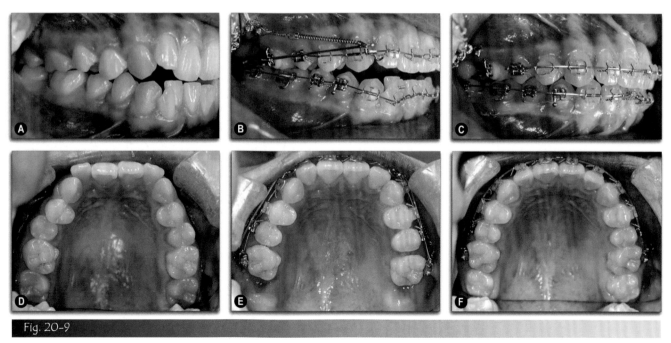

Fig. 20-9

Simultaneous distalization of posterior teeth. **A,** Initial buccal photograph. **B,** Progress buccal photograph. **C,** Final buccal photograph. **D,** Initial occlusal photograph. **E,** Progress occlusal photograph. **F,** Final occlusal photograph. Note that final photographs were taken at 8 months.

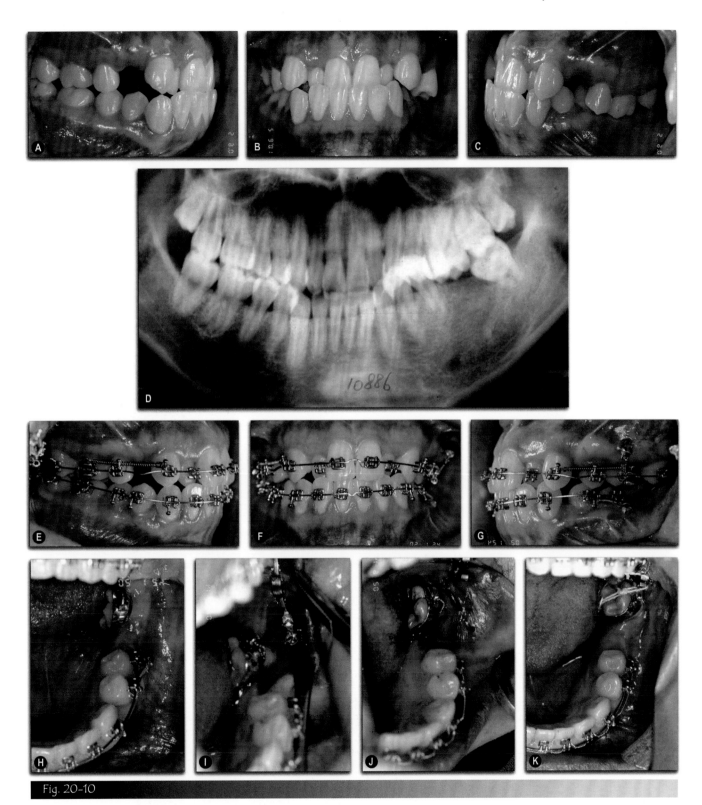

Fig. 20-10

Class III scissor bite with upper posterior supereruption and lower molar dumping. **A,** Initial right buccal photograph. **B,** Initial anterior photograph. **C,** Initial left buccal photograph. **D,** Initial panoramic radiograph. **E,** Postintrusion right buccal photograph. **F,** Postintrusion anterior photograph. **G,** Postintrusion left buccal photograph. Note that intrusion took 8 months. **H,** Preuprighting occlusal photograph. **I,** C-tube placement in retromolar region. **J,** Postoperative occlusal photograph. **K,** Postuprighting occlusal photograph. Note that uprighting took 2 months. *(continued)*

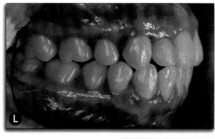
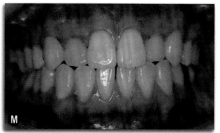
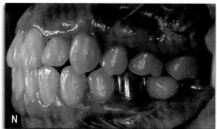

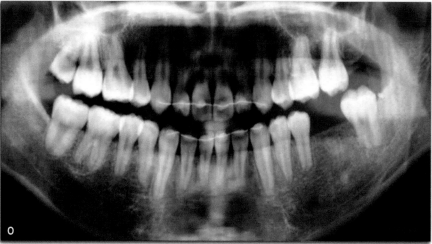

Fig. 20-10 (continued)

L, Final right buccal photograph. M, Final anterior photograph. N, Final left buccal photograph. O, Final panoramic radiograph. Note that total treatment time was 19 months.

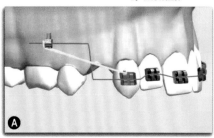
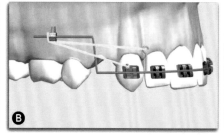
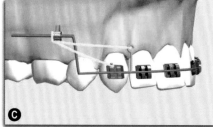

Fig. 20-11

Treatment mechanics using a C-tube as substitute for posterior anchorage teeth. **A,** Initial leveling and canine retraction using blue Elgiloy arch wire (0.016 × 0.022 inch) and ³/₁₆-inch, 3.5-oz elastics. **B,** Soldered extension hooks added to arch wire for en masse retraction (¼-inch, 3.5-oz elastics). **C,** Space closure complete.

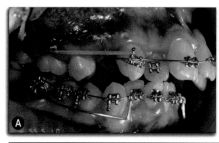
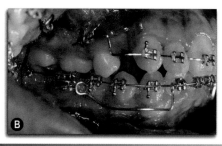
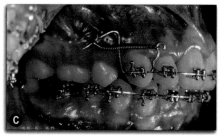

Fig. 20-12

C-tube independent en masse retraction. **A,** Upper: 0.016-inch NiTi with ³/₁₆-inch, 3-oz elastics. Lower: 0.014-inch NiTi with 0.019 × 0.025-inch uprighting sectional stainless steel arch wire for 5 months. **B,** Upper: 0.017 × 0.022-inch blue Elgiloy arch wire with NiTi closed coil spring. Lower: 0.017 × 0.025-inch NiTi with uprighting sectional stainless steel arch wire for 12 months. **C,** Upper: 0.017 × 0.022-inch blue Elgiloy arch wire with soldered hooks and NiTi closed coil spring.

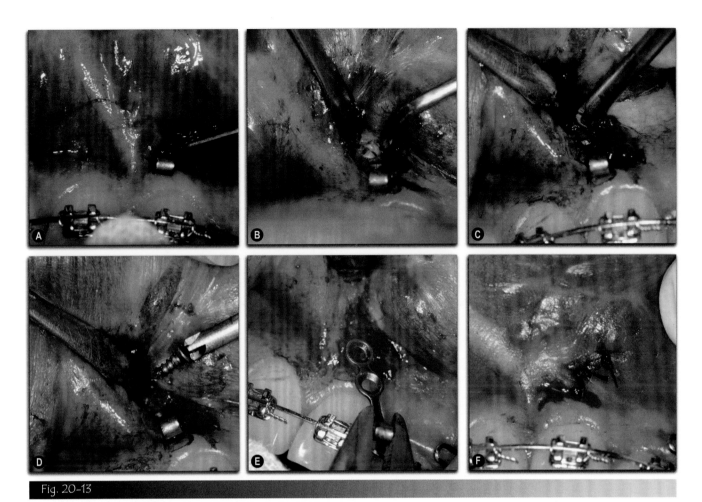

Fig. 20-13

C-tube removal in upper anterior region. **A,** A vertical incision is performed between the screws. **B,** A narrow periosteal elevator is used to expose the plate around the screws. **C,** The screws are rotated counterclockwise. **D,** The screws are removed. **E,** The C-tube is removed. **F,** Single-layer closure with sutures.

REFERENCES

1. Umemori M, Sugawara J, Mitani H, et al. Skeletal anchorage system for open-bite correction. *Am J Orthod Dentofacial Orthop.* 115:166-174, 1999.

2. Sherwood KH, Burch JG, Thompson WJ. Closing anterior open bites by intruding molars with titanium mini-plate anchorage. *Am J Orthod Dentofacial Orthop.* 122:593-600, 2002.

3. Sugawara J, Daimaruya T, Umemori M, et al. Distal movement of mandibular molars in adult patients with the skeletal anchorage system. *Am J Orthod Dentofacial Orthop.* 125:130-138, 2004.

4. Chung KR. Implant orthodontics in the future. In: Chung KR, ed. *Textbook of Speedy Orthodontics.* Seoul, South Korea: Jeesung, 2001:331-337.

5. Chung KR, Kim YS, Linton JL, et al. The mini-plate with tube for skeletal anchorage. *J Clin Orthod.* 36:407-412, 2002.

6. Chung KR, Kim SH, Mo SS, et al. Severe Class II division 1 malocclusion treated by orthodontic mini-plate with tube. *Prog Orthod.* 6:172-186, 2005.

7. Chung YG, Lee YJ, Chung KR. The experimental study of early loading on the mini-plate in the beagle dog. *Korean J Orthod.* 33:307-317, 2003.

8. Sugawara J, Baik UB, Umemori M, et al. Treatment and posttreatment dentoalveolar changes following intrusion of mandibular molars with application of a skeletal anchorage system (SAS) for open bite correction. *Int J Adult Orthodon Orthognath Surg.* 17:243-253, 2002.

9. Dermaut LR, De Pauw G. Biomechanical aspects of Class II mechanics with special emphasis in deep bite correction as part of the treatment goal. In: Nanda R, ed. *Biomechanics in Clinical Orthodontics.* Philadelphia, Pa: Saunders, 1997:86-98.

10. Burstone CJ. The segmented arch approach to space closure. *Am J Orthod.* 82:361-378, 1982.

(Figs. 20-14 to 20-15 continued on next page)

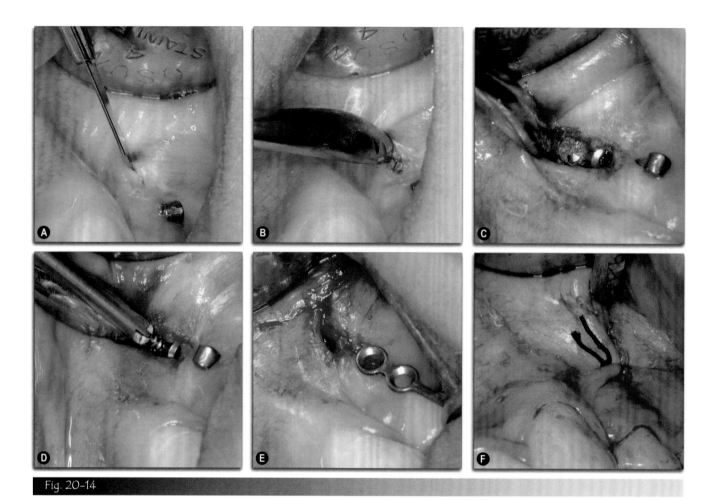

Fig. 20-14

C-tube removal in upper posterior region. **A,** A vertical incision is performed between the screws. **B,** A narrow periosteal elevator is used to expose the plate around the screws. **C,** The screws are rotated counterclockwise. **D,** The screws are removed. **E,** The C-tube is removed. **F,** Single-layer closure with sutures.

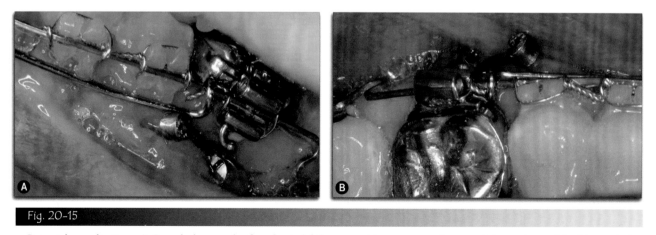

Fig. 20-15

Potential complications. **A,** Buccal photograph of mechanical failure caused by excess traction on miniscrew inserted in thin cortical bone. **B,** Occlusal photograph of same failure.

The Skeletal Anchorage System

Junji Sugawara, Mikako Umemori, Ichiro Takahashi,
Hiroshi Nagasaka, Hiroshi Kawamura

Skeletal anchorage was introduced to orthodontics through orthognathic surgery and originally was developed as an adjunct to *dental* anchorage for intermaxillary fixation after jaw surgery. The first clinical report using skeletal anchorage for orthodontic treatment appeared in 1983, when Creekmore and Eklund[1] demonstrated the successful treatment of a severe deep bite using a surgical Vitallium bone screw temporarily inserted just below the anterior nasal spine to intrude the anterior teeth. The second clinical report was published by Jenner and Fitzpatrick[2] in 1985. They fixed a bone plate to the ascending ramus to distalize a lower first molar into the missing second molar position to resolve premolar crowding. Although no complications were reported with either of these cases, little interest developed in using temporary anchorage devices for orthodontics. These and other reports stimulated our group to develop the skeletal anchorage system (SAS) about 12 years ago.[3-8]

THE SKELETAL ANCHORAGE SYSTEM

The SAS consists of modified miniplate implants (MPIs) and monocortical screws. The system was initially developed as an adjunctive treatment modality for difficult adult orthodontics. The plates are made of pure titanium and have three components: a head, an arm, and a body (Fig. 21-1). The head is exposed intraorally and is positioned away from the dentition so that it does not interfere with tooth movement. Each head component has three hooks

for application of orthodontic force. The hooks are oriented in only one direction; therefore, both a left- and a right-sided plate are required for universal use. The arm is located transmucosally and is available in three lengths—short (10.5 mm), medium (13.5 mm), and long (16.5 mm)—to allow for individual patient variation and different tooth movement situations. The body is located subperiosteally. The underlying surface of the MPI that is in contact with bone is sandblasted to increase its osseointegration potential. All other surfaces are machine polished and smooth. The three basic MPI designs are the T-type (Fig. 21-2, *A*), the Y-type (Fig. 21-2, *B*), and the I-type (Fig. 21-2, *C*). The T-type plate can be modified for use as an L-type plate by cutting off one of the screw holes. The variations in design broaden the application to many different anatomic sites in the oral cavity, such that the appropriate anchor plate can be chosen based on anatomic location, bony contour, and distance from the point of force application to the implant site.

The specific anatomic locations for the various plate designs are as follows. The Y-type plates are usually placed on the zygomatic buttress to intrude or distalize upper molars. Although the lateral wall of the maxilla might be closer to the point of force application in these types of cases, it is generally too thin for screw fixation. The I-type plates are usually placed on the anterior ridge of the piriform rim to intrude upper anterior teeth or protract upper molars. The T-type and

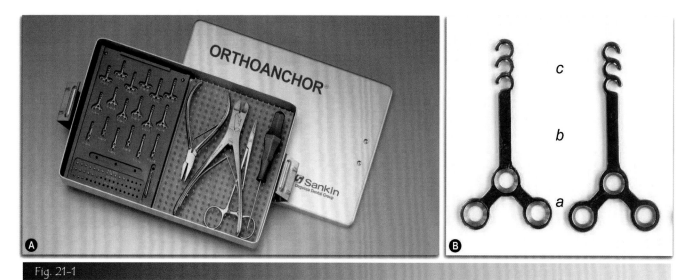

Fig. 21-1

The Super Mini Anchor Plate system (Dentsply-Sankin, Tokyo, Japan) referred to as the skeletal anchorage system (SAS). **A,** Kit of instruments, miniplates, and screws. **B,** Miniplate implant components. *(a)* Head; *(b)* body; *(c)* arm.

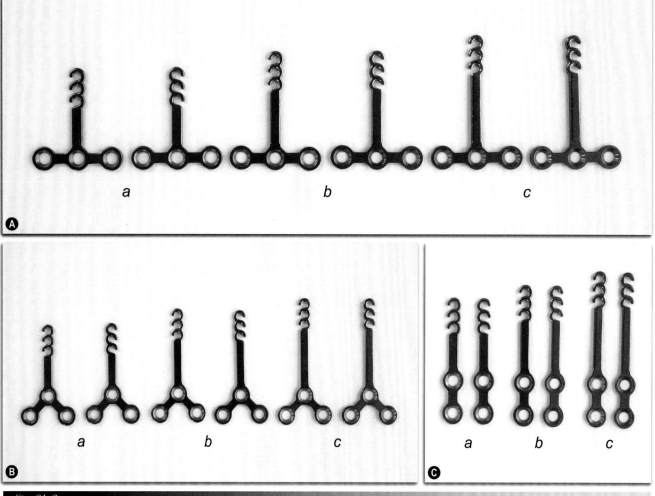

Fig. 21-2

Different designs of miniplates. **A,** T-type plates. **B,** Y-type plates. **C,** I-type plates. *(a)* Short; *(b)* medium; *(c)* long.

L-type plates are usually placed in the mandibular body to intrude, protract, or distalize lower molars or at the anterior border of the mandibular ramus to upright impacted molars. The thickness of the mandibular facial cortical bone is generally sufficient for screw fixation except around the mental foramen.

When determining the location for the MPI, the main criterion is that the implant site must have enough cortical bone thickness (at least 2 mm) to fix the miniplates using monocortical screws. The screws are also pure titanium and have a self-tapping thread. They are placed with a manual screwdriver that attaches to the screw head via a tapered recessed hole that is square shaped. The screw diameter is 2 mm, and the screw is available in lengths of 5 mm and 7 mm. In cases in which a screw becomes loose or bent, an emergency screw with a 2.2 mm diameter is available.

The surgical site around the MPIs is allowed to heal for about 3 weeks before force application. This is mainly for soft tissue swelling and inflammation and not to allow osseointegration. Upon completion of orthodontic treatment, the MPIs are removed immediately.

TREATMENT PLANNING
To introduce our treatment planning methodology for SAS mechanotherapy, a recently completed case will be presented.

Problem List
A 16-year-old Japanese boy (Fig. 21-3) had a chief complaint of anterior open bite and difficulty chewing food. Initial clinical examination revealed a long lower anterior facial height and a large interlabial gap. The

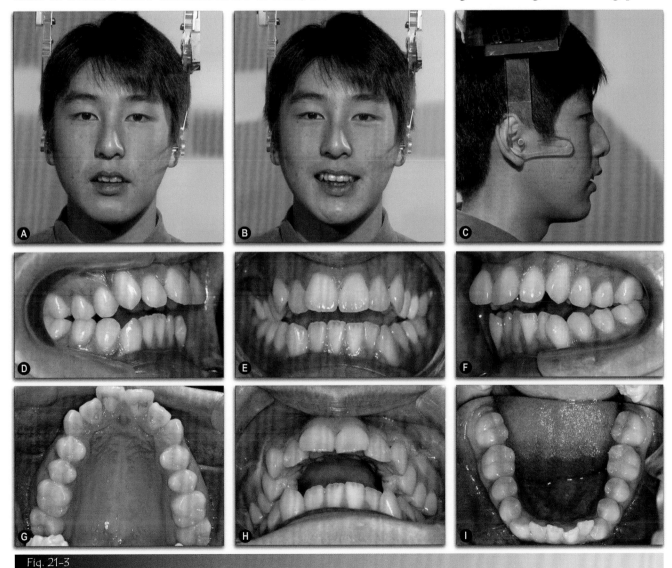

Fig. 21-3

Pretreatment photographs. **A,** Facial photograph. **B,** Facial smiling photograph. **C,** Lateral facial photograph. **D,** Right buccal photograph. **E,** Anterior photograph. **F,** Left buccal photograph. **G,** Upper occlusal photograph. **H,** Overjet photograph. **I,** Lower occlusal photograph.

posteroanterior cephalometric radiograph indicated a dental midline deviation but no facial asymmetry. The lateral cephalometric radiograph was taken with natural head posture, a relaxed lip posture, and in centric relation. The cephalometric analysis (referred to as the craniofacial drawing standards analysis),[9] indicated that the major problems were vertical maxillary excess, a steep mandibular plane, a short ramus, skeletal Class II tendency, and a large interlabial gap. The panoramic radiograph revealed four unerupted third molars (Fig. 21-4). The dental problems were anterior open bite, upper incisor proclination, lower incisor crowding, lower dental midline deviation, dental Class II relationship, and a narrow upper arch (Box 21-1).

Diagnosis
Based on the problem list, the diagnosis was skeletal Class I (Class II tendency): long facial type accompanied by a large interlabial gap, anterior open bite, dental Class II relationship, lower dental midline deviation, and lower arch length deficiency. Traditionally, the treatment plan would have most likely been surgical orthodontics. However, the incorporation of the SAS allows similar treatment results without the surgical risks associated with orthognathic surgery.

Treatment Goals
The skeletal goal was to intrude the upper posterior teeth 3.0 mm with the SAS (Fig. 21-5). Following posterior intrusion, a counterclockwise mandibular rotation would automatically occur, thereby allowing simultaneous correction of the excessive lower facial height, large interlabial gap, anterior open bite, and Class II profile.

The dental treatment goal was to correct upper incisor proclination, lower anterior crowding, and lower dental midline deviation. To correct the upper incisor proclination, the upper incisors needed to be moved palatally 5 mm. In addition, the lower incisors needed to move facially 1 mm to achieve a normal overjet and overbite. This would require distalization of the upper and lower molars by 3 mm and 4 mm, respectively (Box 21-2).

PRESURGICAL ORTHODONTICS
SAS mechanics have been used primarily (92%) for distalization, intrusion, and protraction of the posterior teeth in adult patients. Generally, these cases are leveled and aligned and in 0.018 × 0.025-inch stainless steel wires (0.022-inch preadjusted brackets) before MPI placement, because sliding mechanics are frequently used for distalization or protraction of the posterior teeth. In addition, the third molars should be extracted at least a month before MPI placement because the third molars prevent distalization and intrusion of molars.

SURGICAL PROCEDURE
The entire surgical procedure is carried out under intravenous sedation.[10] Before the procedure, a skin marker is used to draw the intended incision line (Figs. 21-6, *A,* and 21-7, *A*). A vertical incision is usually made in the maxilla, whereas a horizontal incision is made in the mandible. The incision is made at the vestibular extent of the implant site on the facial bone surface. A mucoperiosteal flap is elevated, followed by complete exposure of the cortical bone

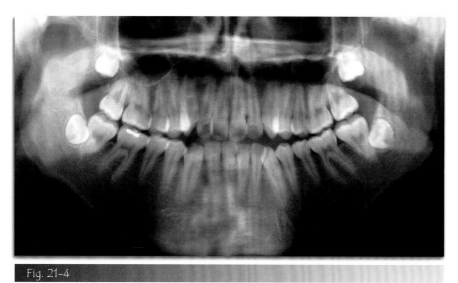

Fig. 21-4
Pretreatment panoramic radiograph.

(Figs. 21-6, *B,* and 21-7, *B*). Next, the appropriate plate design is selected based on the anatomic site, the bony contour, and the distance from the point of force application. The presurgical panoramic radiograph is helpful in this decision. The selected plate is then bent and contoured to fit the bone surface. The position of the initial pilot hole is then marked on the bone through a hole in the bone plate (Figs. 21-6, *C,* and 21-7, *C*). This is followed by drilling of the initial pilot hole (Figs. 21-6, *D,* and 21-7, *D*), and one self-tapping monocortical screw is inserted. After the initial screw is in place, the remaining pilot holes

are drilled and screws are inserted to firmly attach the MPI (Figs. 21-6, *E,* and 21-7, *E*). Finally, the incision is closed and sutured with resorbable sutures (Figs. 21-6, *F,* and 21-7, *F*). The surgical procedure takes about 10 to 15 minutes for each MPI.

ORTHODONTIC MECHANICS
Biomechanics
A significant advantage of the SAS is that it allows predictable three-dimensional posterior tooth movement. Tooth movement includes distalization, protraction, intrusion, extrusion, facial movement, and lingual movement. To date, we have treated more than 500 patients with the SAS in our clinic. In those cases, approximately 85% of all patients underwent distalization and intrusion of posterior teeth.

It is extremely difficult, if not impossible, to intrude upper and lower molars with traditional orthodontic mechanotherapies. Even with orthognathic surgery, segmentally impacting posterior teeth has risks associated with treatment in that neurovascular damage is possible. SAS mechanics, however, make possible the intrusion of posterior teeth, thereby enabling the correction of severe open bites without orthognathic surgery or iatrogenic side effects. Typically, upper posterior intrusion is accomplished by first leveling and aligning the upper posterior teeth (Fig. 21-8). The SAS is then placed to intrude the upper posterior teeth segmentally. After the teeth are intruded to the level of the anterior teeth, a continuous arch wire is placed to finish the case. During this phase, the upper posterior teeth are often ligated to the MPI for retention and to prevent extrusion. Similar mechanics are used to intrude lower posterior teeth (Fig. 21-9).

Distalization of the upper or lower posterior teeth is also difficult. Traditionally, this has been attempted with auxiliary appliances, such as headgears. However, with today's uncooperative patients, ideal results are rarely possible. Uncooperativeness is an even bigger

Box 21-1.	Problem List

1. Long lower anterior height
2. Large interlabial gap
3. Skeletal Class II tendency
4. High mandibular plane angle
5. Lower dental midline deviation
6. Upper incisor proclination
7. Dental Class II relationship
8. Lower anterior crowding
9. Narrow upper arch

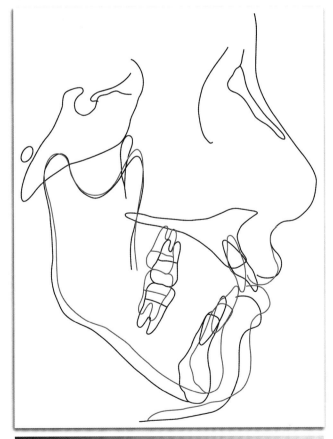

Fig. 21-5

Cephalometric prediction tracing of treatment goals. *Black line:* Pretreatment. *Red line:* Treatment goal.

Box 21-2.	Treatment Plan

1. Extraction (17, 27, 38, 48)
2. Banding (16, 26)
3. Transpalatal arch for distal rotation of 16 and 26
4. Implantation of miniplates (zygomatic buttress, mandibular body)
5. Intrusion and distalization of upper and lower posterior teeth
6. Coordination of upper and lower arches
7. Detailing and finishing
8. Debonding
9. Retention (upper wraparound retainer, lower lingual bonded retainer)

problem in adults, who usually refuse to wear headgears. By using SAS mechanics, it is now possible to achieve en masse distalization of the posterior teeth, which allows the correction of severe crowding, upper protrusion, anterior crossbite, and asymmetries without resorting to premolar extraction. Moreover, this

requires little cooperation on the part of the patient. Typically, upper distalization is accomplished by first extracting third molars if present and leveling and aligning the upper teeth (Fig. 21-10). The SAS is then placed to distalize the posterior segment from the first premolar back. After the posterior teeth are distalized,

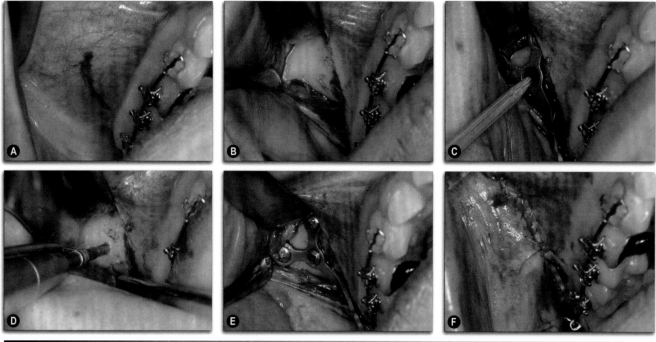

Fig. 21-6

Maxillary surgical procedure. **A,** Incision line drawn with skin marker. **B,** Mucoperiosteal flap. **C,** Marking of pilot hole. **D,** Drilling of pilot hole. **E,** Insertion of monocortical screws. **F,** Soft tissue closure with sutures.

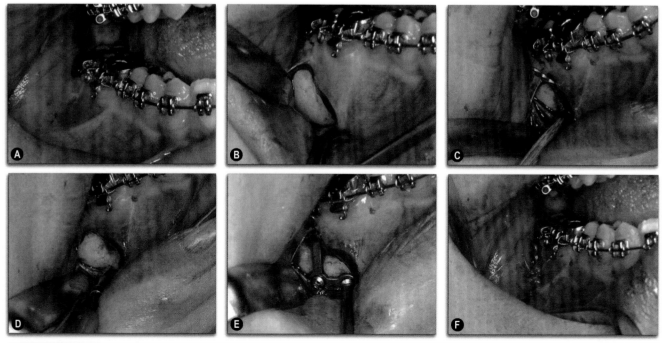

Fig. 21-7

Mandibular surgical procedure. **A,** Incision line drawn with skin marker. **B,** Mucoperiosteal flap. **C,** Marking of pilot hole. **D,** Drilling of pilot hole. **E,** Insertion of monocortical screws. **F,** Soft tissue closure with sutures.

the anterior teeth are retracted en masse into the newly created space by sliding mechanics. Afterward, the case is finished and detailed as usual. Similar mechanics are used to distalize the lower arch (Fig. 21-11).

Treatment Progress

To intrude the upper and lower molars, two MPIs were placed on the zygomatic buttress and another two were placed on mandibular body (Figs. 21-12 and 21-13). After placing a rigid rectangular arch wire, intrusive forces were generated to the upper molars via 400- to 500-g elastic modules from the Y-type plates. The lower molars were not actively intruded, but were merely held in place via stainless steel ligatures from the molars to the L-type plates. Orthodontic force

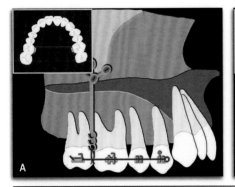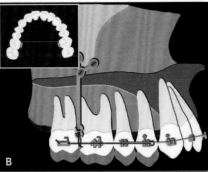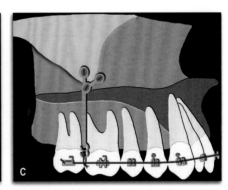

Fig. 21-8

Biomechanics of maxillary posterior intrusion. **A,** Leveling and aligning of upper posterior teeth followed by placement of Y-type plate implanted at the zygomatic buttress and active intrusion. Note the two occlusal planes and transpalatal arch used to prevent facial flaring of the posterior teeth. **B,** Mechanical retention of posterior intrusion by ligating from Y-type plate to molars. Note grey teeth represent pretreatment position. **C,** Leveling and aligning of the entire dentition after intrusion of the posterior teeth.

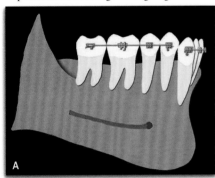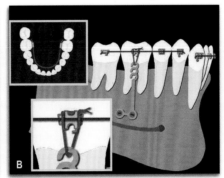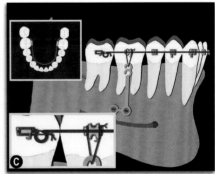

Fig. 21-9

Biomechanics of mandibular posterior intrusion. **A,** Leveling and aligning of lower posterior teeth. Note the two occlusal planes. **B,** Intrusion of posterior teeth with L-type plate implanted at the mandibular body. Note that lingual arch is used to prevent facial flaring of the posterior teeth. **C,** Mechanical retention is obtained by ligaturing arch wire to miniplate.

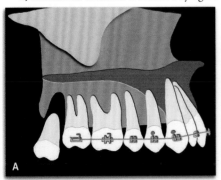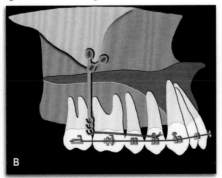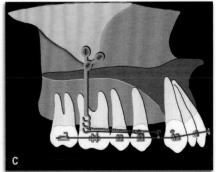

Fig. 21-10

Biomechanics of maxillary posterior distalization. **A,** Extraction of third molars before distalization of upper posterior teeth. **B,** En masse distalization of upper posterior teeth using Y-type anchor plate implanted at the zygomatic buttress. **C,** En masse retraction of the anterior teeth via sliding mechanics after posterior distalization.

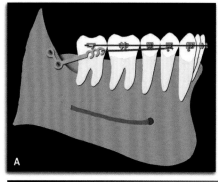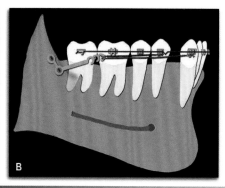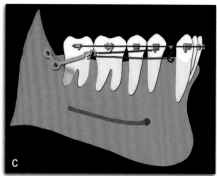

Fig. 21-11

Biomechanics of mandibular posterior distalization. **A,** Extraction of third molars before distalization of lower posterior teeth. **B,** En masse distalization of lower posterior teeth using L-type anchor plate implanted at the anterior border of the ramus followed by individual canine retraction. **C,** En masse retraction of the anterior teeth via sliding mechanics after posterior distalization.

application was initiated 3 weeks after implant surgery, waiting to allow for completion of postoperative swelling and ideal oral hygiene.

Because of the difficulty in accessing the upper third molars, the upper second molars were extracted instead before orthodontic treatment. A preadjusted 0.022-inch appliance was placed to begin leveling and aligning. The posterior teeth were aligned independently with segmental arch wires, whereas passive segmental rectangular wires were placed in the anterior brackets (Figs. 21-14, *A,* and 21-15, *A*). Upper expansion was initiated with the arch wires and a transpalatal arch. After 3 months of treatment, the SAS plates were implanted. After placing 0.018 × 0.025-inch stainless steel arch wires, molar intrusion and distalization was initiated by en masse mechanics with approximately 400 g of force per segment (Figs. 21-14, *B,* and 21-15, *B*). After the upper and lower posterior teeth were distalized, the anterior teeth were leveled and aligned as intrusion of the upper posterior teeth continued (Figs. 21-14, *C,* and 21-15, *C*). The anterior

open bite was almost corrected within 10 months of initiating SAS treatment (Figs. 21-14, *D,* and 21-15, *D*). Following posterior intrusion, occlusal interference occurred in the incisor region. Because of this, the upper incisors were intruded using an auxiliary arch of 0.017 × 0.025-inch titanium molybdenum alloy (TMA), which was inserted into buccal tubes bonded directly to the SAS plates (Figs. 21-14, *E,* and 21-15, *E*). The case was finished and detailed as usual (Figs. 21-14, *F,* and 21-15, *F*). The SAS plates were left in place and were used for mechanical retention during the finishing and detailing stage.

Treatment Results

The active treatment period was 20 months total. An upper wraparound retainer and a lower canine-to-canine bonded retainer were used for retention. As an additional step for stability, eight 3-mm long palatal spurs were bonded to the upper incisor cingula to minimize pressure from the tongue thrust.[11] The SAS plates were removed a month after appliance removal. An appealing facial result with good posterior support,

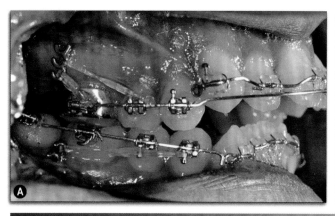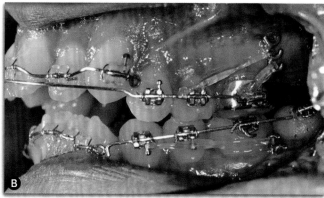

Fig. 21-12

Initial implantation and loading of SAS plates. **A,** Right buccal photograph. **B,** Left buccal photograph.

anterior guidance, and maximum intercuspation was achieved (Fig. 21-16).

Based on the occlusogram, the lower first molars were distalized 2 mm. The upper right and left first molars were distalized 5 mm and 6 mm, respectively. No root resorption was apparent on the posttreatment panoramic radiograph (Fig. 21-17).

The cephalometric super-imposition (Fig. 21-18) revealed that the anterior open bite was successfully corrected by intrusion of the upper posterior teeth. However, mandibular autorotation

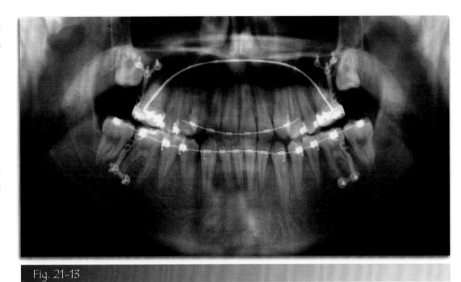

Fig. 21-13

Panoramic radiograph at initial SAS implantation.

was less than initially predicted would occur. This may be attributed to excessive retroclination of the upper incisors following en masse distalization of the upper posterior teeth.

REMOVAL PROCEDURE

The SAS plates are removed immediately after the completion of orthodontic treatment. First, an incision is made over the bone plate, and a mucoperiosteal flap is reflected (Figs. 21-19, *A,* and 21-20, *A*). Next, all soft tissue is removed to expose the plate. It is not uncommon for a thin layer newly formed

bone to cover parts of the plate (Figs. 21-19, *B,* and 21-20, *B*). After careful removal of the new bone, all of the monocortical screws are removed with the manual screwdriver by counterrotating the screws (Figs. 21-19, *C,* and 21-20, *C*). Because of the frequent integration of the plate undersurface, even though the screws are removed, the plate is often firmly attached to the bone surface. After removing the SAS plate, an indention of the plate is seen where bone had grown around the edges of the plate (Figs. 21-19, *D,* and 21-20, *D*). Finally, the wound is closed and sutured (Figs. 21-19, *E,* and 21-20, *E*).

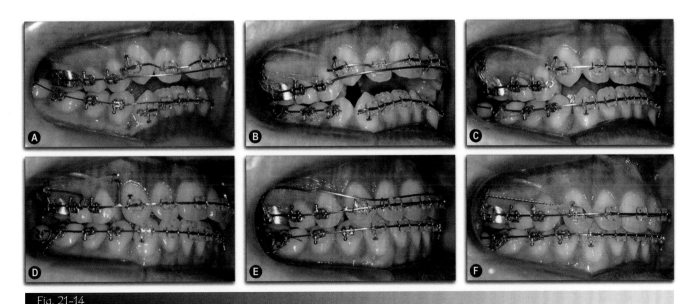

Fig. 21-14

Progress treatment right buccal photographs. **A,** Leveling of posterior teeth. **B,** Intrusion and distalization of posterior teeth with initial leveling of the anterior teeth. **C,** Continued posterior intrusion and distalization. **D,** Retraction of upper anterior teeth. **E,** Intrusion of the upper incisors. **F,** Detailing and finishing.

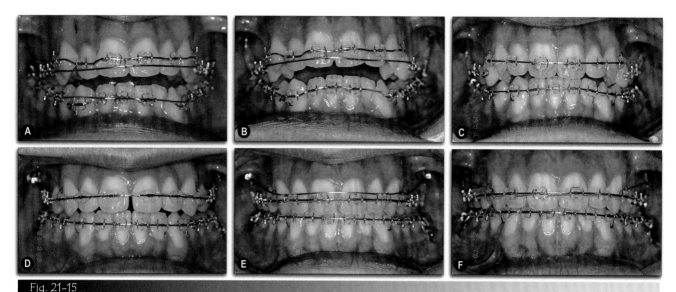

Fig. 21-15

Progress treatment anterior photographs. **A,** Leveling of posterior teeth. **B,** Intrusion and distalization of posterior teeth with initial leveling of the anterior teeth. **C,** Posterior intrusion and distalization. **D,** Retraction of upper anterior teeth. **E,** Intrusion of the upper incisors. **F,** Detailing and finishing.

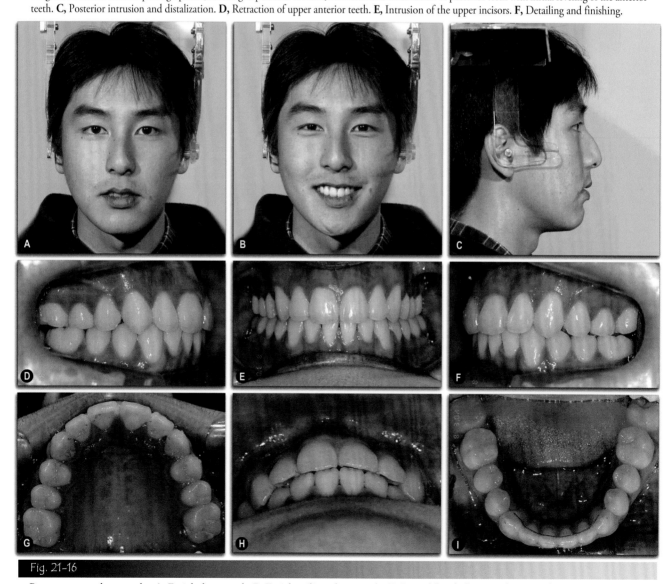

Fig. 21-16

Posttreatment photographs. **A,** Facial photograph. **B,** Facial smiling photograph. **C,** Lateral facial photograph. **D,** Right buccal photograph. **E,** Anterior photograph. **F,** Left buccal photograph. **G,** Upper occlusal photograph. **H,** Overjet photograph. **I,** Lower occlusal photograph.

POTENTIAL COMPLICATIONS

Most patients who undergo the SAS implant surgery show mild to moderate facial swelling for several days after the procedure. Although infrequent, infection occurs in less than 10% of patients, for which antibiotics are required. Mild inflammation is easily controlled with antiseptic mouth rinses and meticulous brushing. Clinicians must instruct patients in thorough oral hygiene procedures and professionally clean the plates at each routine orthodontic appointment. Initiating this regimen has greatly reduced postsurgical infection in our clinic. Other potential complications include loosening of plates and screws, fracture of plates, and mucosal overgrowth of the head component of the plates. The only one of these that we have experienced has been plates loosening, which has occurred in only 1% of our cases.

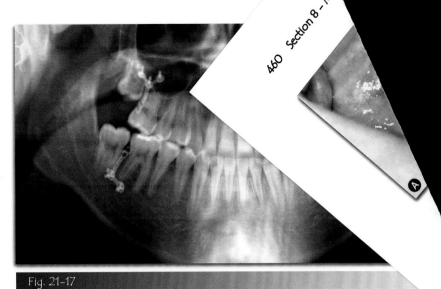

Fig. 21-17

Posttreatment panoramic radiograph.

SUMMARY

The SAS is a recently developed orthodontic anchorage system using titanium miniplates and monocortical screws that are temporarily implanted in the maxilla and/or mandible as temporary absolute orthodontic anchorage. The most distinguishing feature of the SAS is that it allows predictable intrusion and distalization of the upper and lower posterior teeth with ease. Therefore, the SAS expands the scope of orthodontics in overcoming the limitations associated with nonsurgical correction of skeletal malocclusion and allows the treatment of many malocclusions characterized by upper or lower protrusion and anterior crowding without dental extractions.

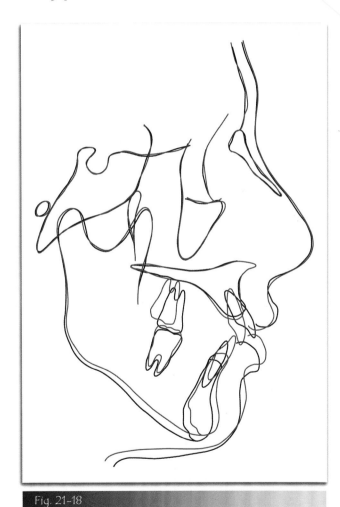

Fig. 21-18

Cephalometric superimposition. *Black line:* Pretreatment. *Red line:* Posttreatment.

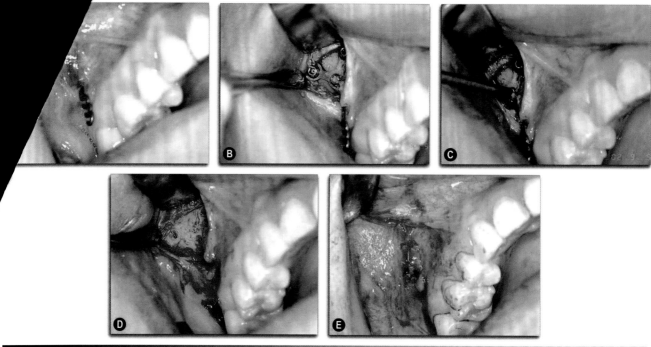

Fig. 21-19

Removal of Y-type plate in the maxilla. **A,** Incision line drawn with skin marker. **B,** Mucoperiosteal incision and subperiosteal reflection. **C,** Removal of monocortical screws. **D,** Removal of plate. Note bone growth around margins of bone plate. **E,** Soft tissue closure with sutures.

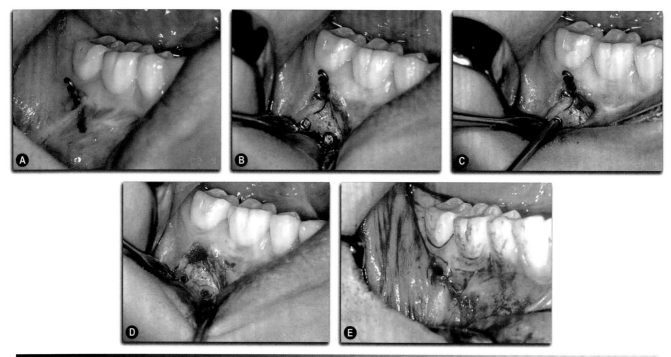

Fig. 21-20

Removal of L-type plate in the mandible. **A,** Incision line drawn with skin marker. **B,** Mucoperiosteal incision and subperiosteal reflection. **C,** Removal of monocortical screws. **D,** Removal of plate. Note bone growth around margins of bone plate. **E,** Soft tissue closure with sutures.

REFERENCES

1. Creekmore TD, Eklund MK. The possibility of skeletal anchorage. *J Clin Orthod.* 17:266-269, 1983.
2. Jenner JD, Fitzpatrick BN. Skeletal anchorage utilizing bone plates. *Aust Orthod J.* 9:231-233, 1985.
3. Sugawara J, Umemori M, Mitani H, et al. Orthodontic treatment system for Class III malocclusion using a titanium miniplate as an anchorage. *Orthodontic Waves.* 57:25-35, 1998.
4. Sugawara J. JCO interviews, Dr. Junji Sugawara on the skeletal anchorage system. *J Clin Orthod.* 33:689-696, 2000.
5. Umemori M, Sugawara J, Mitani H, et al. Skeletal anchorage system for open-bite correction. *Am J Orthod Dentofacial Orthop.* 115:166-174, 1999.
6. Sugawara J, Un Bong Baik, Umemori M, et al. Treatment and posttreatment dentoalveolar changes following intrusion of mandibular molars with application of a skeletal anchorage system (SAS) for open bite correction. *Int J Adult Orthodon Orthognath Surg.* 17:243-253, 2002.
7. Sugawara J, Daimaruya T, Umemori M, et al. Distal movement of mandibular molars in adult patients with the skeletal anchorage system. *Am J Orthod Dentofacial Orthop.* 125:130-138, 2004.
8. Sugawara J, Kanzaki R, Takahashi I, et al. Distal movement of the maxillary molars in nongrowing patients with the skeletal anchorage system. *Am J Orthod Dentofacial Orthop.* 129(6):723-733, 2006.
9. Sugawara J, Soya T, Kawamura H, Kanamori Y. Analysis of craniofacial morphology using craniofacial drawing standards (CDS): application for orthognathic surgery. *Nippon Kyosei Shika Gakkai Zasshi [Journal of the Japan Orthodontic Society]* 47:394-408, 1988.
10. Huang BGJ, Justus R, Kennedy D, Kokich VG. Stability of anterior openbite treated with crib therapy. *Angle Orthod.* 60:17-24, 1990.
11. Nagasaka H, Sugawara J, Kawamura H, et al. A clinical evaluation on the efficacy of titanium miniplates as orthodontic anchorage. *Orthodontic Waves.* 58:136-147, 1999.

SECTION 9

MiniPlate Implant Case Reports

CR–MPI 1

Distalization of Upper and Lower Molars to Eliminate Crowding and Correct an Asymmetric Midline

Renya Sato, Shuichi Saeki

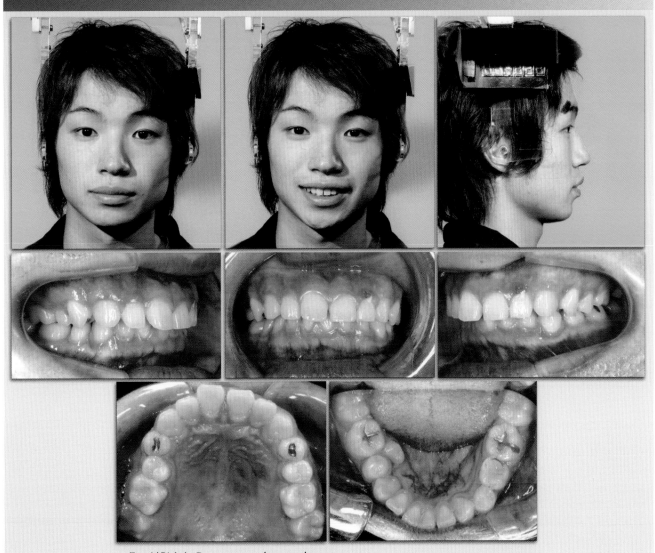

Fig. MPI 1-1. Pretreatment photographs.

The treatment plan was to extract all four third molars in order to create posterior space for distalization of the upper and lower arches. The Skeletal Anchorage System would then be used to distalize the upper and lower molars to create space for the blocked-out lower right second premolar and to correct the deviated dental midlines, which were to be corrected by asymmetric distalization of the lower posterior teeth.

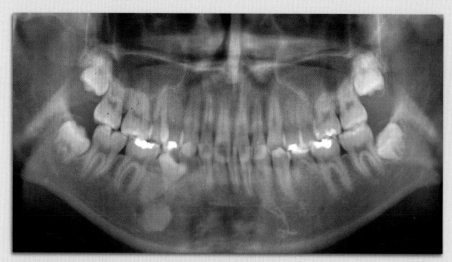

Fig. MPI 1–2. Pretreatment panoramic radiograph.

Table MPI 1-1.	Diagnosis and Treatment Goals	
	Diagnosis	Treatment Goals
SKELETAL		
Anteroposterior	Class I	Class I
Vertical	Normal	Normal
Transverse	Normal	Normal
DENTAL		
Right molar	Class I	Class I
Right canine	Class II	Class I
Left molar	Class I	Class I
Left canine	Class II	Class I
Upper right	1.5 mm crowding	None
Upper left	2 mm crowding	None
Lower right	5 mm crowding	None
Lower left	2 mm crowding	None
Missing teeth	No. 35	No. 18, 28, 35, 38, 48
Restore teeth	N/A	N/A
Overjet	6 mm	3.5 mm
Overbite	4 mm	2.5 mm
Upper ML	1 mm right of facial ML	0 mm to facial ML
Lower ML	5 mm right of facial ML	0 mm to facial ML
SOFT TISSUE		
Profile	Convex	Convex
Lips	Competent	Competent
PERIODONTIUM		
Inadequate KT/TT	None	None
Gingival recession	None	None
Bone loss	None	None

KT/TT, Keratinized tissue/thin tissue; *ML*, midline; *N/A*, not applicable.

Table MPI 1–2.	Temporary Anchorage Device Summary			
Procedure	Data			
Appliances placed	28 Jun 2001			
TAD placed	29 Oct 2001	29 Oct 2001	29 Oct 2001	29 Oct 2001
Location of TAD	Zygomatic buttress apical No. 16	Zygomatic buttress apical No. 26	External oblique ridge apical No. 36	External oblique ridge apical No. 46
Type of TAD	MPI	MPI	MPI	MPI
TAD loaded	29 Nov 2001	29 Nov 2001	29 Nov 2001	29 Nov 2001
Healing duration	28 days	28 days	28 days	28 days
Force in grams	400	400	400	400
Mechanics used	Direct	Direct	Direct	Direct
TAD unloaded	16 May 2003	16 May 2003	16 May 2003	16 May 2003
TAD loading duration	18 months	18 months	18 months	18 months
TAD removed	20 Feb 2004	20 Feb 2004	20 Feb 2004	20 Feb 2004
Appliances removed	26 Jan 2004			
Treatment duration	31 months			

TAD, Temporary anchorage device; *MPI*, miniplate implant.

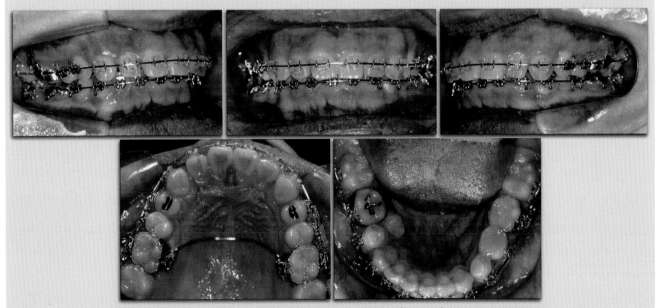

Fig. MPI 1–3. Initial temporary anchorage device (TAD) photographs.

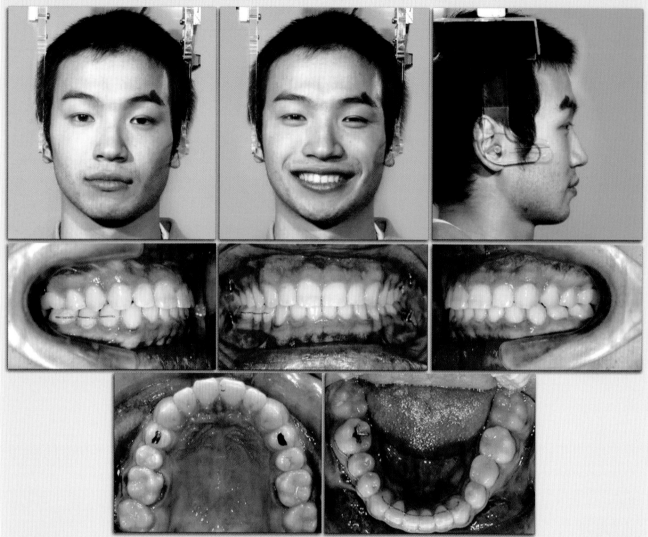

Fig. MPI 1–4. Posttreatment photographs.

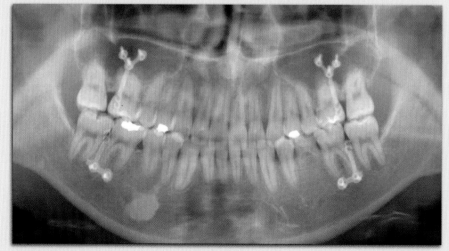

Fig. MPI 1–5. Posttreatment panoramic radiograph.

Table MPI 1-3.	Cephalometric Summary	
	Pretreatment	Posttreatment
SKELETAL		
SNA (degrees)	79.0	78.5
SNB (degrees)	76.0	76.0
ANB (degrees)	3.0	2.5
SN-ANS/PNS	10.0	10.0
SN-GoMe (degrees)	32.0	32.0
N-ANS (mm)	60.5	60.5
ANS-Me (mm)	72.0	72.0
DENTAL		
U1-SN (degrees)	114.0	110.0
L1-GoMe (degrees)	104.5	102.0
U1-APo (mm)	13.0	10.0
L1-APo (mm)	8.0	7.0
SOFT TISSUE		
LS-PnPo' (mm)	0.0	–1.0
LI-PnPo' (mm)	3.0	2.0

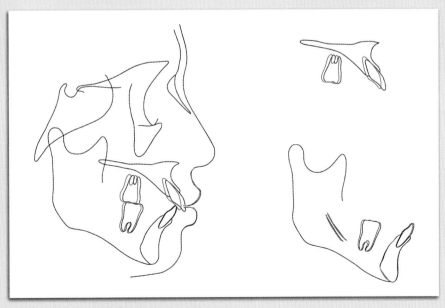

Fig. MPI 1–6. Cephalometric superimposition.

CR-MPI 2

Distalization of Upper Molars to Correct a Class II, Division 2 Malocclusion

Satoshi Yamada, Junji Sugawara

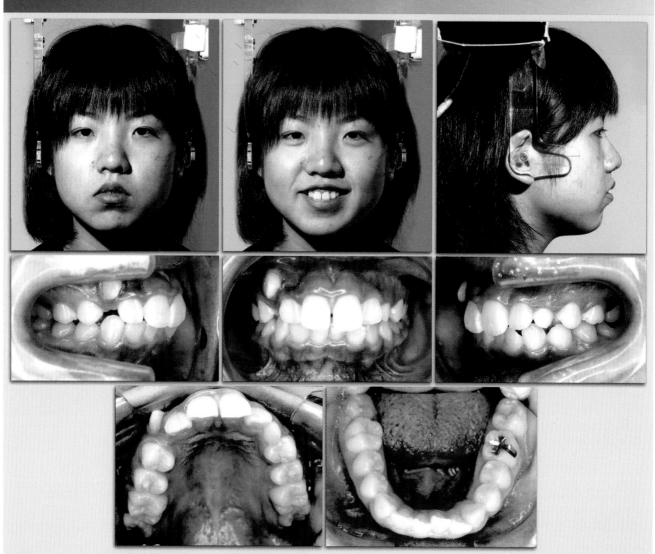

Fig. MPI 2-1.   Pretreatment photographs.

The plan was to use the Skeletal Anchorage System (SAS) to distalize the upper posterior teeth bilaterally to create space for the upper right blocked-out and upper left palatally impacted canines and to correct the Class II malocclusion. To create space for distalization of the upper dentition, the upper second molars would be extracted. The upper third molars demonstrated normal crown and root development, so it was planned that they eventually would erupt into the position of the second molars.

Initially, the upper arch was aligned, then the SAS was applied to distalize the upper first molars directly from a hook and open coil spring on the arch wire. After the molars were distalized, the premolars were retracted en masse to a Class I relationship, followed by uncovering and retracting the palatally impacted canine into position. The lower right buccal segment was also distalized simultaneously.

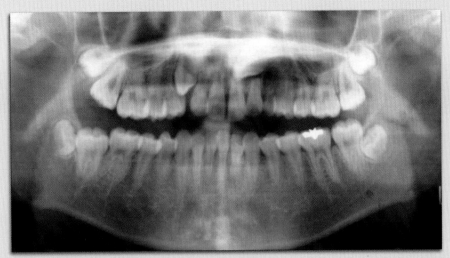

Fig. MPI 2–2. Pretreatment panoramic radiograph.

Table MPI 2-1.	Diagnosis and Treatment Goals	
	Diagnosis	Treatment Goals
SKELETAL		
Anteroposterior	Class II	Class II
Vertical	Normal	Normal
Transverse	Normal	Normal
DENTAL		
Right molar	End-on Class II	Class I
Right canine	End-on Class II	Class I
Left molar	End-on Class II	Class I
Left canine	End-on Class II	Class I
Upper right	4 mm crowding	None
Upper left	2.3 mm crowding	None
Lower right	0 mm crowding	None
Lower left	1.0 mm crowding	None
Missing teeth	None	No. 17, 27
Restore teeth	N/A	N/A
Overjet	3.0 mm	3.0 mm
Overbite	3.0 mm	3.0 mm
Upper ML	0.5 mm right of facial ML	0 mm to facial ML
Lower ML	1.0 mm left of facial ML	0 mm to facial ML
SOFT TISSUE		
Profile	Convex	Convex
Lips	Competent	Competent
PERIODONTIUM		
Inadequate KT/TT	None	None
Gingival recession	None	None
Bone loss	None	None
OTHER	No. 23 impacted	

KT/TT, Keratinized tissue/thin tissue; *ML,* midline; *N/A,* not applicable.

Table MPI 2-2. Procedure	Temporary Anchorage Device Summary Data		
Appliances placed	29 Feb 2000		
TAD placed	17 Apr 2000	17 Apr 2000	18 Mar 2002
Location of TAD	Zygomatic buttress apical No. 16	Zygomatic buttress apical No. 16	External oblique ridge apical No. 46
Type of TAD	MPI	MPI	MPI
TAD loaded	18 May 2000	18 May 2000	18 May 2000
Healing duration	28 days	28 days	28 days
Force in grams	300	300	300
Mechanics used	Direct	Direct	Direct
TAD unloaded	15 Jan 2001	15 Jan 2001	19 Aug 2002
TAD loading duration	8 months	8 months	3 months
TAD removed	13 May 2003	13 May 2003	13 May 2003
Appliances removed	6 May 2003		
Treatment duration	39 months		

TAD, Temporary anchorage device; *MPI*, miniplate implant.

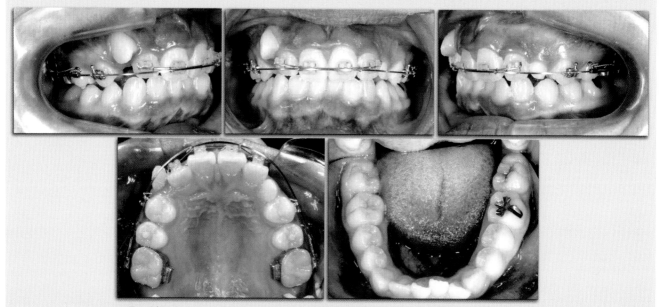

Fig. MPI 2-3. Initial temporary anchorage device (TAD) photographs.

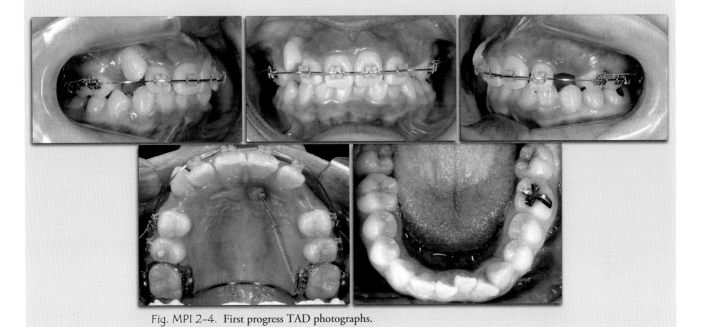

Fig. MPI 2-4. First progress TAD photographs.

Fig. MPI 2-5. Second progress TAD photographs.

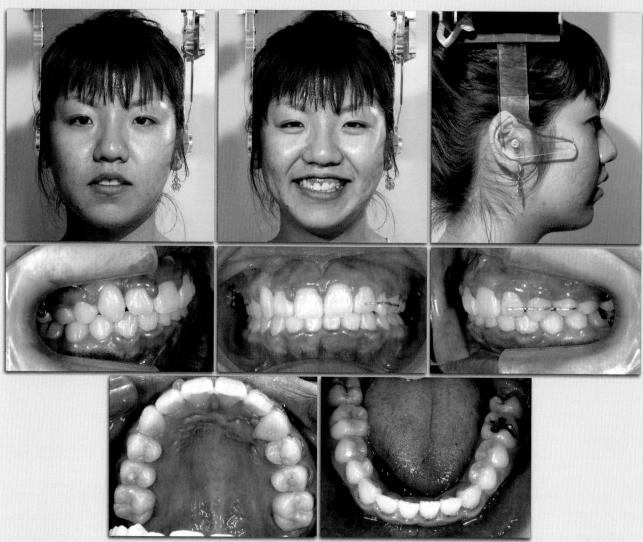

Fig. MPI 2-6. Posttreatment photographs.

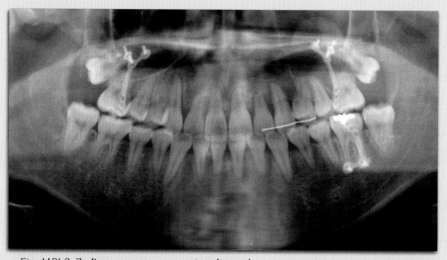

Fig. MPI 2-7. Posttreatment panoramic radiograph.

Table MPI 2-3.	Cephalometric Summary		
	Pretreatment	Posttreatment	1 Year Posttreatment
SKELETAL			
SNA (degrees)	79.7	80.0	79.6
SNB (degrees)	73.3	73.5	73.5
ANB (degrees)	6.5	6.5	6.1
SN-ANS/PNS (degrees)	8.3	8.2	8.0
SN-GoMe (degrees)	37.6	37.2	37.1
N-ANS (mm)	53.2	52.6	53.1
ANS-Me (mm)	74.0	77.6	75.6
DENTAL			
U1-SN (degrees)	95.8	90.2	93.8
L1-GoMe (degrees)	103.4	100.8	104.0
U1-APo (mm)	9.5	7.2	8.3
L1-APo (mm)	5.8	4.3	6.0
SOFT TISSUE			
LS-PnPo' (mm)	1.0	3.5	3.0
LI-PnPo' (mm)	4.5	4.0	4.0

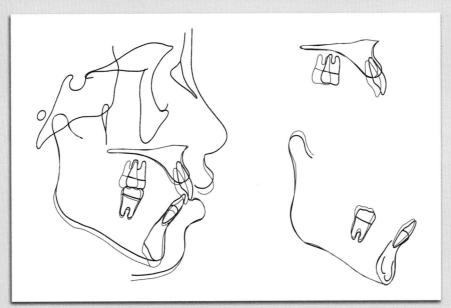

Fig. MPI 2-8. Cephalometric superimposition.

CR-MPI

Distalization of the Entire Lower Arch to Treat a Skeletal Class III Malocclusion Dentally

Junji Sugawara, Tadashi Yamada

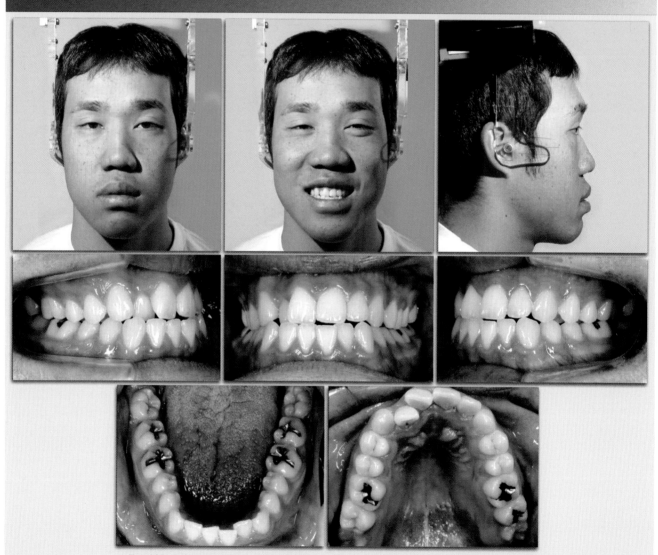

Fig. MPI 3-1. Pretreatment photographs.

The plan was to use the extraction space of the lower third molars to distalize the entire lower arch via en masse distalization for Class III denture correction with the application of the Skeletal Anchorage System (SAS). The entire lower arch was distalized from an edge-to-edge Class III relationship to a normal Class I occlusion. The treatment appears stable 1 year after the orthodontic appliances were removed.

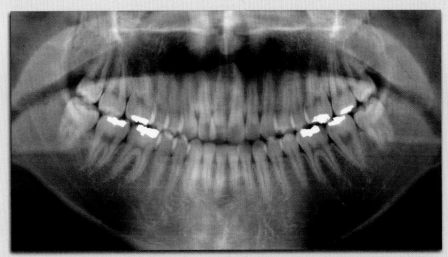

Fig. MPI 3-2. Pretreatment panoramic radiograph.

| Table MPI 3-1. | Diagnosis and Treatment Goals | |
	Diagnosis	Treatment Goals
SKELETAL		
Anteroposterior	Class III	Class III
Vertical	Open bite tendency	Normal
Transverse	Normal	Normal
DENTAL		
Right molar	Class I	Class I
Right canine	Class I	Class I
Left molar	Class III	Class I
Left canine	Class III	Class I
Upper right	2.0 mm crowding	None
Upper left	0.5 mm crowding	None
Lower right	0 mm crowding	None
Lower left	1.5 mm crowding	None
Missing teeth	None	No. 18, 28, 38, 48
Restore teeth	N/A	N/A
Overjet	−1.0 mm	2.5 mm
Overbite	−0.5 mm	2.0 mm
Upper ML	0 mm to facial ML	0 mm to facial ML
Lower ML	0 mm to facial ML	0 mm to facial ML
SOFT TISSUE		
Profile	Concave	Concave
Lips	Competent	Competent
PERIODONTIUM		
Inadequate KT/TT	None	None
Gingival recession	None	None
Bone loss	None	None

KT/TT, Keratinized tissue/thin tissue; *ML,* midline; *N/A,* not applicable.

Table MPI 3-2.	Temporary Anchorage Device Summary	
Procedure	Data	
Appliances placed	26 Jul 2000	
TAD placed	8 May 2000	8 May 2000
Location of TAD	Anterior ascending ramus distal No. 37	Anterior ascending ramus distal No. 47
Type of TAD	MPI	MPI
TAD loaded	26 Jul 2000	26 Jul 2000
Healing duration	90 days	90 days
Force in grams	400	400
Mechanics used	Direct	Direct
TAD unloaded	10 Jan 2001	10 Jan 2001
TAD loading duration	6 months	6 months
TAD removed	6 Aug 2001	6 Aug 2001
Appliances removed	4 Jul 2001	
Treatment duration	12 months	

TAD, Temporary anchorage device; *MPI,* miniplate implant.

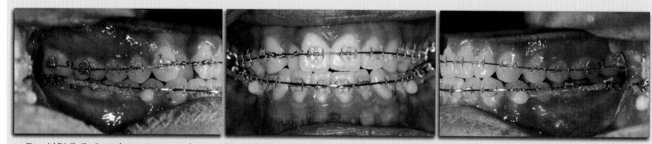

Fig. MPI 3-3. Initial temporary anchorage device (TAD) photographs.

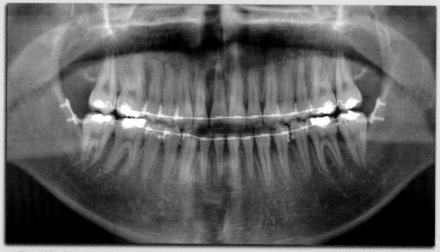

Fig. MPI 3-4. Initial TAD panoramic

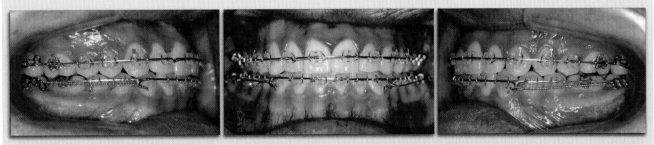

Fig. MPI 3-5. Progress TAD photographs.

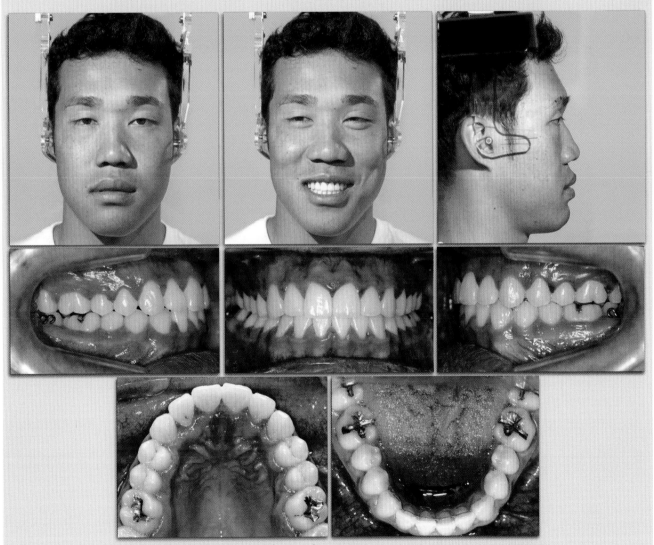

Fig. MPI 3-6. Posttreatment photographs.

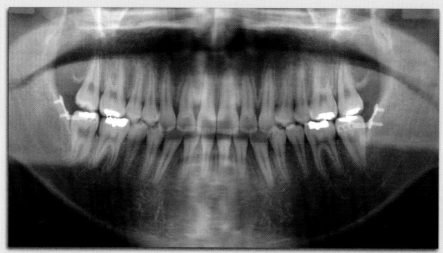

Fig. MPI 3-7. Posttreatment panoramic radiograph.

Table MPI 3-3.	Cephalometric Summary		
	Pretreatment	Posttreatment	1 Year Posttreatment
SKELETAL			
SNA (degrees)	81.5	81.5	81.5
SNB (degrees)	82.0	82.0	82.0
ANB (degrees)	–0.5	–0.5	–0.5
SN-ANS/PNS (degrees)	8.5	8.5	8.5
SN-GoMe (degrees)	37.0	37.0	37.5
N-ANS (mm)	63.5	63.5	63.5
ANS-Me (mm)	85.0	85.0	85.0
DENTAL			
U1-SN (degrees)	107.0	107.0	107.0
L1-GoMe (degrees)	92.0	81.0	85.5
U1-APo (mm)	8.0	9.0	8.5
L1-APo (mm)	8.5	6.0	6.5
SOFT TISSUE			
LS-PnPo′ (mm)	2.5	2.0	2.0
LI-PnPo′ (mm)	4.0	2.0	2.0

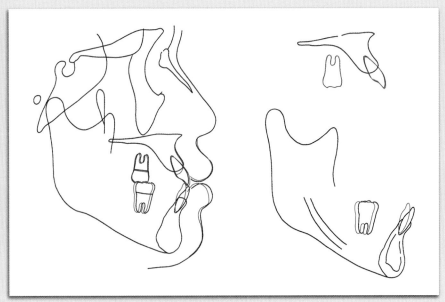

Fig. MPI 3-8. Cephalometric superimposition.

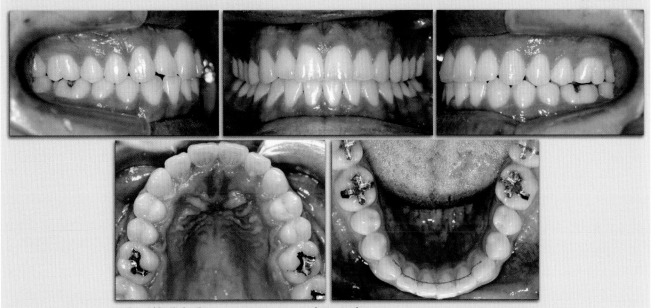

Fig. MPI 3-9. One-year posttreatment photographs.

Nonextraction Unilateral Molar Distalization Using a Bone Plate for Correction of an End-on Class II Molar Relationship

Ryoon-Ki Hong

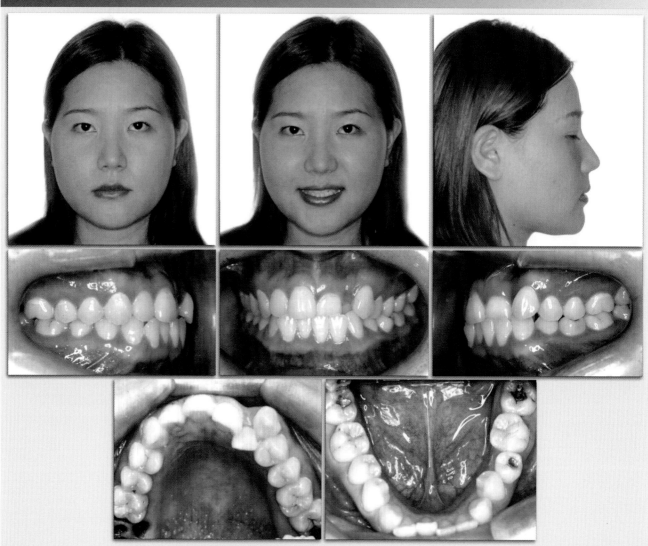

Fig. MPI 4-1. Pretreatment photographs.

The treatment plan was to use a bone plate in the upper left zygomatic region to distalize the buccal segment from an end-on Class II to Class I without the need for extraction. Treatment proceeded as planned.

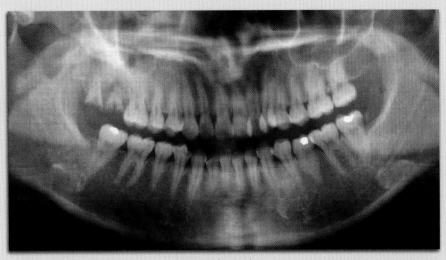

Fig. MPI 4-2. Pretreatment panoramic radiograph.

Table MPI 4-1.	Diagnosis and Treatment Goals	
	Diagnosis	Treatment Goals
SKELETAL		
Anteroposterior	Class I	Class I
Vertical	Normal	Normal
Transverse	Normal	Normal
DENTAL		
Right molar	Class I	Class I
Right canine	Class I	Class I
Left molar	End-on Class II	Class I
Left canine	End-on Class II	Class I
Upper right	0 mm crowding	None
Upper left	6.9 mm crowding	None
Lower right	2 mm crowding	None
Lower left	2 mm crowding	None
Missing teeth	No. 17, 18, 28, 38, 48	No. 17, 18, 28, 38, 48
Restore teeth	N/A	N/A
Overjet	2 mm	3 mm
Overbite	2 mm	2 mm
Upper ML	1 mm left of facial ML	0 mm to facial ML
Lower ML	0 mm to facial ML	0 mm to facial ML
SOFT TISSUE		
Profile	Straight	Straight
Lips	Competent	Competent
PERIODONTIUM		
Inadequate KT/TT	None	None
Gingival recession	None	None
Bone loss	None	None
OTHER	Root tips No. 17 and 18 to be removed; Crossbite No. 21 and 22	

KT/TT, Keratinized tissue/thin tissue; *ML,* midline; *N/A,* not applicable.

Table MPI 4–2.	Temporary Anchorage Device Summary
Procedure	Data
Appliances placed	16 Dec 2000
TAD placed	9 Apr 2001
Location of TAD	Zygomatic buttress apical No. 26
Type of TAD	MPI
TAD loaded	16 Apr 2001
Healing duration	7 days
Force in grams	200
Mechanics used	Indirect
TAD unloaded	23 Sep 2002
TAD loading duration	17 months
TAD removed	12 Jan 2004
Appliances removed	7 Jan 2004
Treatment duration	39 months

TAD, Temporary anchorage device; *MPI,* miniplate implant.

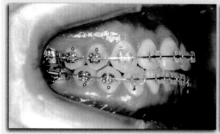 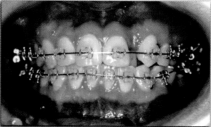 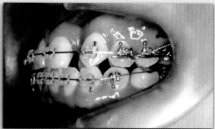

Fig. MPI 4-3. Initial temporary anchorage device (TAD) photographs.

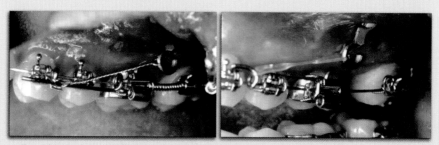

Fig. MPI 4-4. Initial *(left)* and progress *(right)* TAD buccal photographs.

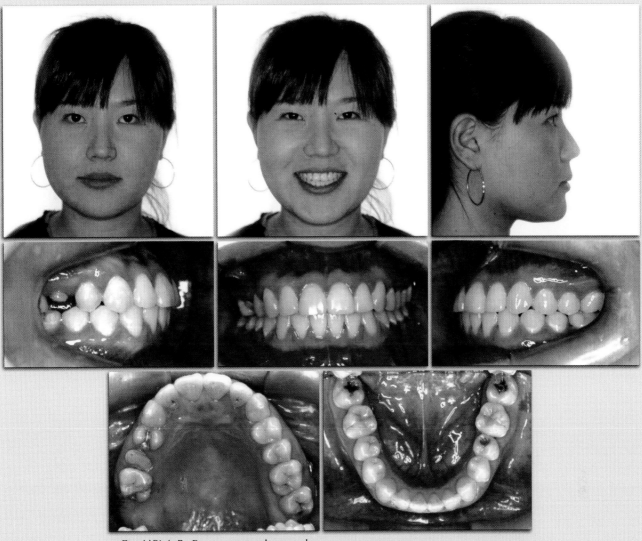

Fig. MPI 4-5. Posttreatment photographs.

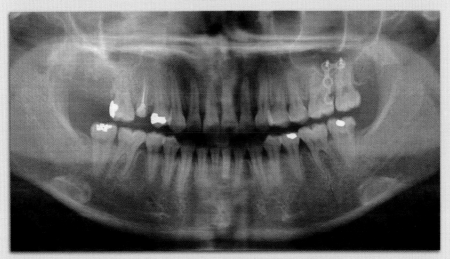

Fig. MPI 4-6. Posttreatment panoramic radiograph.

Table MPI 4-3.	Cephalometric Summary	
	Pretreatment	Posttreatment
SKELETAL		
SNA (degrees)	83.1	83.5
SNB (degrees)	81.0	81.2
ANB (degrees)	2.1	2.3
SN-ANS/PNS (degrees)	11.3	10.9
SN-GoMe (degrees)	32.9	32.6
N-ANS (mm)	58.2	58.1
ANS-Me (mm)	70.6	71.4
DENTAL		
U1-SN (degrees)	104.3	109.5
L1-GoMe (degrees)	93.0	103.0
U1-APo (mm)	7.0	9.7
L1-APo (mm)	4.5	6.8
SOFT TISSUE		
LS-PnPo' (mm)	–3.0	–3.0
LI-PnPo' (mm)	–3.0	–3.0

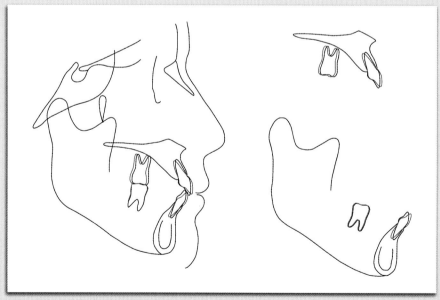

Fig. MPI 4-7. Cephalometric superimposition.

CR–MPI

En Masse Retraction of Upper Anterior Teeth Using the C-Lingual Retractor and C-Palatal Plate

Kyu-Rhim Chung, Seong-Hun Kim

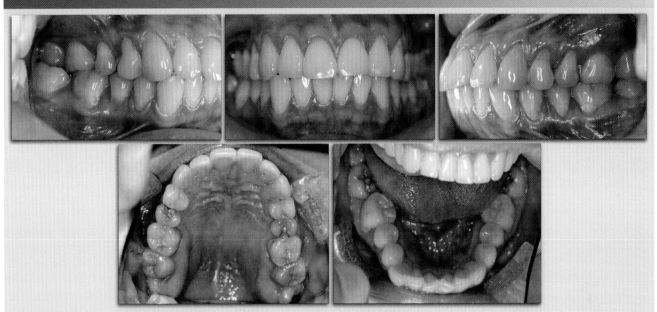

Fig. MPI 5–1. Pretreatment photographs.

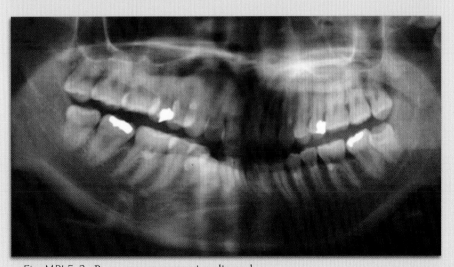

Fig. MPI 5–2. Pretreatment panoramic radiograph.

Because of the poor oral hygiene and gingival recession, the first step in treatment was to perform periodontal scaling and gingival grafts. After periodontal healing, the plan was to extract the upper first premolars in order to correct the anterior protrusion via anterior retraction using a C-lingual retractor and a C-plate (KLS Martin LP, Jacksonville, Florida). Conventional orthodontic treatment was to be performed in the lower left for correcting the molar relationship, and independent C-tube (KLS Martin LP) anterior retraction was to be performed on the lower right. A positioner was planned for final detailing.

After initial leveling and aligning and en masse retraction of the lower anterior teeth, 6 months of conventional orthodontic treatment was performed for molar relationship control. An 0.018 × 0.025-inch sectional arch wire was added between the C-tube and the lower right second molar for uprighting. After en masse retraction of the upper anterior teeth, a slight bite opening tendency was seen in the upper canine region because of the retraction force being applied slightly apical to the center of resistance. To correct this, clear buttons were bonded on the facial of the upper canines, and triangular elastics (3 oz, ³/₁₆ inch) were used to close the bite in the canine region.

Table MPI 5-1.	Diagnosis and Treatment Goals	
	Diagnosis	Treatment Goals
SKELETAL		
Anteroposterior	Class II	Class II
Vertical	Normal	Normal
Transverse	Normal	Normal
DENTAL		
Right molar	Class I	Class I
Right canine	Class I	Class I
Left molar	End-on Class II	Class I
Left canine	End-on Class II	Class I
Upper right	0 mm crowding	None
Upper left	0 mm crowding	None
Lower right	1 mm crowding	None
Lower left	1 mm crowding	None
Missing teeth	None	No. 14, 18, 24, 28, 34, 38, 44, 48
Restore teeth	N/A	N/A
Overjet	3.5 mm	2 mm
Overbite	1.5 mm	2 mm
Upper ML	0 mm to facial ML	0 mm to facial ML
Lower ML	1 mm right of facial ML	0 mm to facial ML
SOFT TISSUE		
Profile	Convex	Straight
Lips	Incompetent	Competent
PERIODONTIUM		
Inadequate KT/TT	None	None
Gingival recession	No. 13-15, 23-25, 34-36, 44-46	None because of gingival grafts
Bone loss	None	None
OTHER	Cervical abrasion, poor oral hygiene	

KT/TT, Keratinized tissue/thin tissue; *ML*, midline; *N/A*, not applicable.

| Table MPI 5-2. | Temporary Anchorage Device Summary | |
Procedure	Data	
Appliances placed	16 Nov 2002	1 Feb 2003
TAD placed	2 Nov 2002	25 Jan 2003
Location of TAD	Buccal No. 45-46	Midpalatal No. 16-26
Type of TAD	MPI (C-tube)	MPI (C-plate)
TAD loaded	16 Nov 2002	2 Feb 2003
Healing duration	14 days	7 days
Force in grams	150-300	300-600
Mechanics used	Direct	Direct
TAD unloaded	25 Nov 2003	20 May 2004
TAD loading duration	12 months	15 months
TAD removed	30 Nov 2003	30 Jun 2004
Appliances removed	10 Jun 2004	
Treatment duration	19 months	

TAD, Temporary anchorage device; *MPI*, miniplate implant.

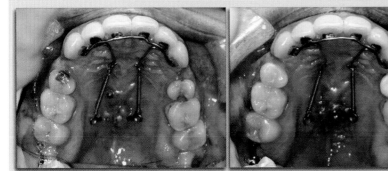
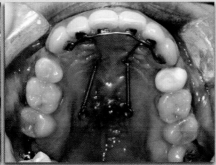
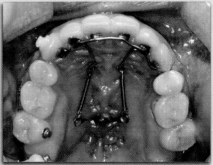

Fig. MPI 5-3. Initial *(left)*, progress *(center)*, and final *(right)* temporary anchorage device (TAD) occlusal photographs.

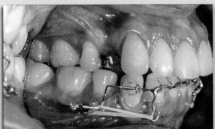
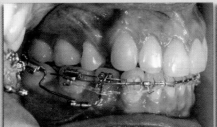
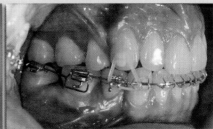

Fig. MPI 5-4. Initial *(left)*, progress *(center)*, and final *(right)* TAD buccal photographs.

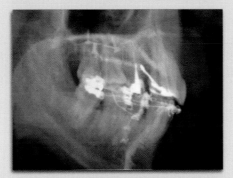

Fig. MPI 5-5. Progress TAD
cephalometric radiograph.

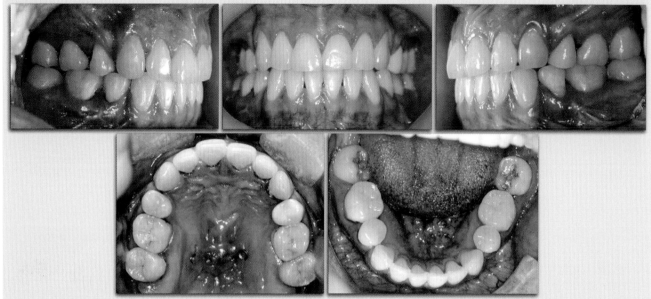

Fig. MPI 5-6. Posttreatment photographs.

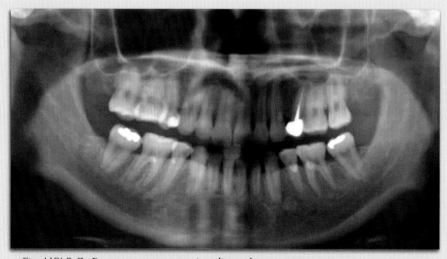

Fig. MPI 5-7. Posttreatment panoramic radiograph.

Table MPI 5-3.	Cephalometric Summary	
	Pretreatment	Posttreatment
SKELETAL		
SNA (degrees)	78.0	78.0
SNB (degrees)	73.0	73.0
ANB (degrees)	5.0	5.0
SN-ANS/PNS (degrees)	15.0	15.0
SN-GoMe (degrees)	42.0	42.0
N-ANS (mm)	65.0	65.0
ANS-Me (mm)	65.0	65.5
DENTAL		
U1-SN (degrees)	105.0	92.0
L1-GoMe (degrees)	107.0	89.5
U1-APo (mm)	15.0	9.0
L1-APo (mm)	10.5	5.0
SOFT TISSUE		
LS-PnPo' (mm)	4.0	1.0
LI-PnPo' (mm)	6.5	3.0

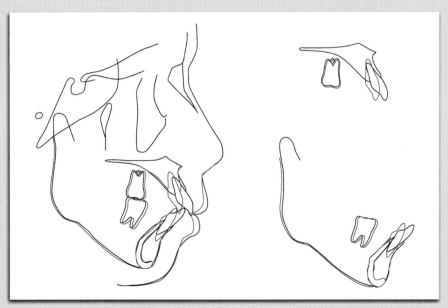

Fig. MPI 5-8. Cephalometric superimposition.

Maximum Anterior Retraction Using a C-Palatal Plate and C-Tubes for Bidentoalveolar Protrusion

Seong-Hun Kim, Kyu-Rhim Chung, Yoon-Ah Kook

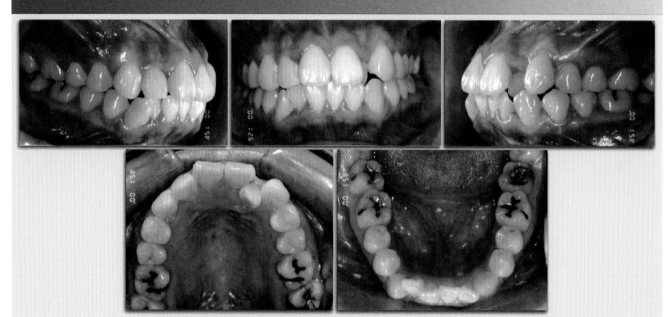

Fig. MPI 6-1. Pretreatment photographs.

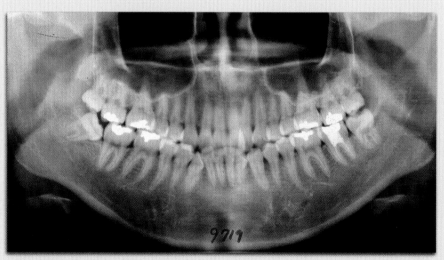

Fig. MPI 6-2. Pretreatment panoramic radiograph.

The treatment plan was to extract all first premolars, followed by maximum anterior retraction with an upper C-lingual retractor and a C-plate (KLS Martin LP, Jacksonville, Florida) in combination with upper and lower buccal C-tubes (KLS Martin LP) for decrowding and anterior retraction without the placement of posterior appliances.

After en masse retraction of the upper and lower anterior teeth, a slight bite opening tendency was seen in the canine region because of the retraction force being applied apical to the center of resistance. To correct this, clear buttons were bonded on the facial of the canines, and triangular elastics (3 oz, 3/16 inch) were used to close the bite in the canine region.

All photos herein reprinted from Chung K-R. Speedy Orthodontics, 2001, with permission from JeeSung Publishing Company.

Table MPI 6-1.	Diagnosis and Treatment Goals	
	Diagnosis	Treatment Goals
SKELETAL		
Anteroposterior	Class I	Class I
Vertical	Normal	Normal
Transverse	Normal	Normal
DENTAL		
Right molar	Class III	Class I
Right canine	Class III	Class I
Left molar	Class I	Class I
Left canine	Class II	Class I
Upper right	1 mm crowding	None
Upper left	3 mm crowding	None
Lower right	3 mm crowding	None
Lower left	3 mm crowding	None
Missing teeth	None	No. 14, 24, 34, 44
Restore teeth	N/A	No. 16, 17, 26, 27, 36-38, 46, 47
Overjet	2 mm	2 mm
Overbite	2 mm	2 mm
Upper ML	1 mm left of facial ML	0 mm to facial ML
Lower ML	1 mm right of facial ML	0 mm to facial ML
SOFT TISSUE		
Profile	Convex	Straight
Lips	Incompetent	Competent
PERIODONTIUM		
Inadequate KT/TT	None	None
Gingival recession	None	None
Bone loss	None	None
OTHER	No. 12 blocked out lingually; No. 37 inadequate restoration	

KT/TT, Keratinized tissue/thin tissue; *ML*, midline; *N/A*, not applicable.

Table MPI 6–2. Procedure	Temporary Anchorage Device Summary Data				
Appliances placed	21 Mar 2000				
TAD placed	7 Mar 2000	7 Mar 2000	7 Mar 2000	7 Mar 2000	14 Mar 2000
Location of TAD	Buccal No. 35-36	Buccal No. 45-46	Buccal No. 16-17	Buccal No. 26-27	Midpalatal No. 16-26
Type of TAD	MPI (C-tube)	MPI (C-tube)	MPI (C-tube)	MPI (C-tube)	MPI (C-plate)
TAD loaded	21 Mar 2000	21 Mar 2000	21 Mar 2000	21 Mar 2000	16 Apr 2000
Healing duration	14 days	14 days	14 days	14 days	28 days
Force in grams	250	250	250	250	450-800
Mechanics used	Direct	Direct	Direct	Direct	Direct
TAD unloaded	28 Sep 2001	28 Sep 2001	28 Sep 2001	28 Sep 2001	28 Sep 2001
TAD loading duration	18 months	18 months	18 months	18 months	17 months
TAD removed	27 Nov 2001	27 Nov 2001	27 Nov 2001	27 Nov 2001	27 Nov 2001
Appliances removed	23 Oct 2001				
Treatment duration	19 months				

TAD, Temporary anchorage device; *MPI*, miniplate implant.

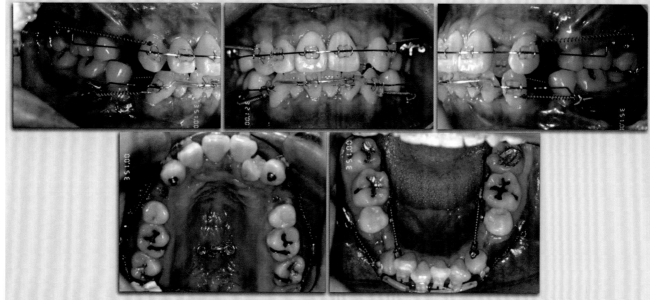

Fig. MPI 6-3. Initial temporary anchorage device (TAD) photographs.

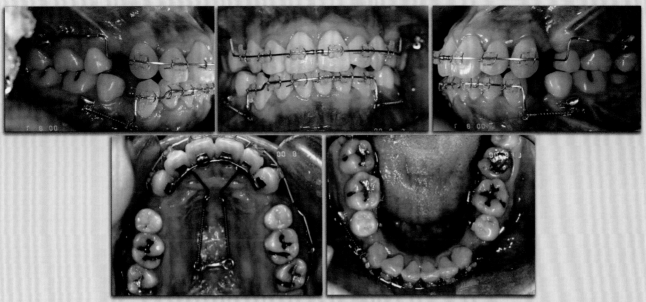

Fig. MPI 6-4. Progress TAD photographs.

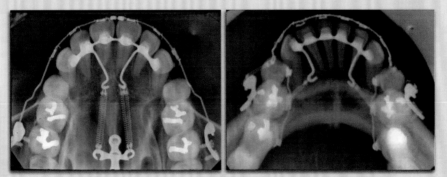

Fig. MPI 6-5. Progress TAD occlusal radiographs.

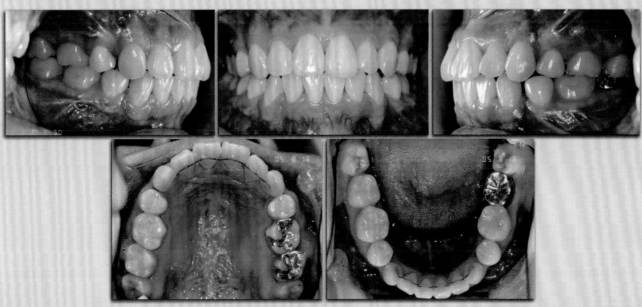

Fig. MPI 6-6. Posttreatment photographs.

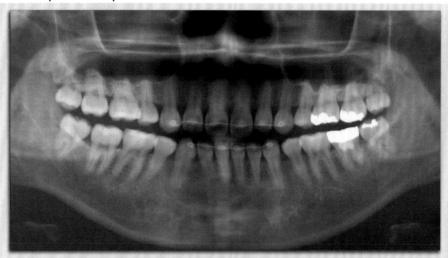

Fig. MPI 6-7. Posttreatment panoramic radiograph.

Table MPI 6-3.	Cephalometric Summary	
	Pretreatment	Posttreatment
SKELETAL		
SNA (degrees)	85.0	82.5
SNB (degrees)	79.0	79.0
ANB (degrees)	6.0	3.5
SN-ANS/PNS (degrees)	7.0	7.0
SN-GoMe (degrees)	38.0	38.0
N-ANS (mm)	60.0	60.0
ANS-Me (mm)	77.0	77.0
DENTAL		
U1-SN (degrees)	115.5	104.5
L1-GoMe (degrees)	103.0	97.5
U1-APo (mm)	14.0	9.0
L1-APo (mm)	9.0	6.0
SOFT TISSUE		
LS-PnPo' (mm)	1.0	–1.5
LI-PnPo' (mm)	5.5	2.0

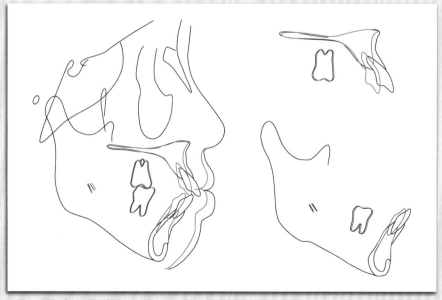

Fig. MPI 6-8. Cephalometric superimposition.

Blocked-out Upper Canines Treated via C-Tube Mechanics without Posterior Appliances

Kyu-Rhim Chung, Yoon-Ah Kook

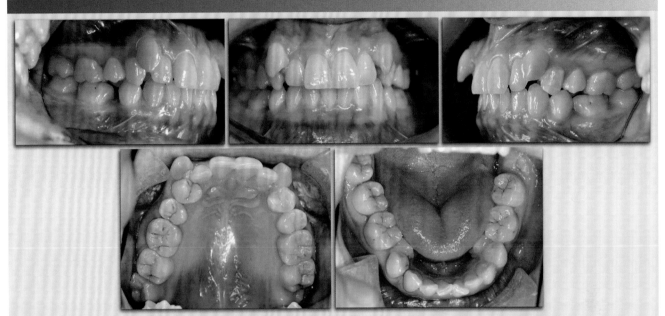

Fig. MPI 7-1. Pretreatment photographs.

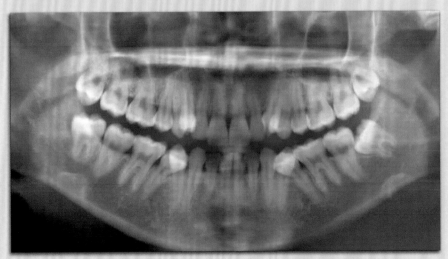

Fig. MPI 7-2. Pretreatment panoramic radiograph.

The treatment plan was to extract the upper first and lower second premolars. Because the posterior occlusion was an ideal Class I relationship and the lower premolars were completely blocked out of the arch to the lingual, the upper molars could not slip forward at all. Therefore, C-tubes (KLS Martin LP, Jacksonville, Florida) were to be placed in the upper arch for maximum retraction without upper posterior appliances. Conventional appliances were to be used on the lower arch.

Table MPI 7-1.	Diagnosis and Treatment Goals	
	Diagnosis	Treatment Goals
SKELETAL		
Anteroposterior	Class I	Class I
Vertical	Normal	Normal
Transverse	Normal	Normal
DENTAL		
Right molar	Class I	Class I
Right canine	End-on Class II	Class I
Left molar	Class I	Class I
Left canine	Class II	Class I
Upper right	8.5 mm crowding	None
Upper left	7 mm crowding	None
Lower right	7.5 mm crowding	None
Lower left	8.5 mm crowding	None
Missing teeth	None	No. 14, 24, 35, 45
Restore teeth	N/A	N/A
Overjet	3.5 mm	3 mm
Overbite	3 mm	2.5 mm
Upper ML	0 mm to facial ML	0 mm to facial ML
Lower ML	0 mm to facial ML	0 mm to facial ML
SOFT TISSUE		
Profile	Straight	Straight
Lips	Competent	Competent
PERIODONTIUM		
Inadequate KT/TT	None	None
Gingival recession	None	None
Bone loss	None	None
OTHER	Blocked out No. 13, 23, 35, 45	

KT/TT, Keratinized tissue/thin tissue; *ML,* midline; *N/A,* not applicable.

Table MPI 7-2.	Temporary Anchorage Device Summary	
Procedure	Data	
Appliances placed	8 Jan 2003	
TAD placed	7 Feb 2003	7 Feb 2003
Location of TAD	Buccal No. 15-16	Buccal No. 25-26
Type of TAD	MPI (C-tube)	MPI (C-tube)
TAD loaded	7 Feb 2003	7 Feb 2003
Healing duration	10 days	10 days
Force in grams	200-350	200-350
Mechanics used	Direct	Direct
TAD unloaded	26 Nov 2003	26 Nov 2003
TAD loading duration	10 months	10 months
TAD removed	5 Dec 2003	5 Dec 2003
Appliances removed	26 Nov 2003	
Treatment duration	10 months	

TAD, Temporary anchorage device; *MPI,* miniplate implant.

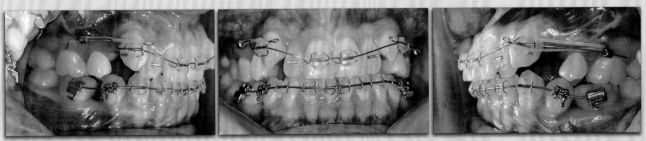

Fig. MPI 7–3. Initial temporary anchorage device (TAD) photographs.

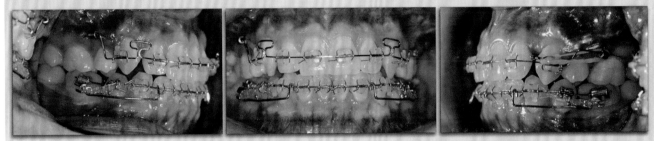

Fig. MPI 7–4. Progress TAD photographs.

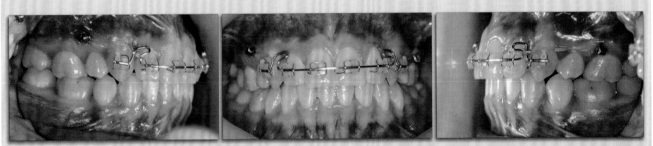

Fig. MPI 7–5. Final TAD photographs.

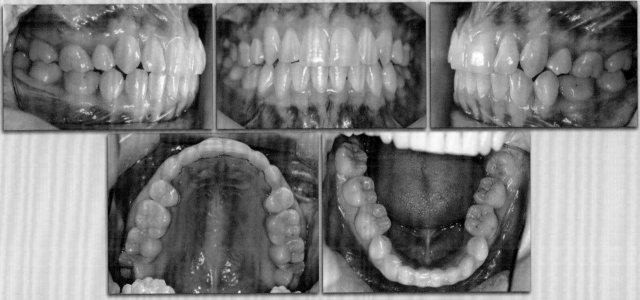

Fig. MPI 7–6. Posttreatment photographs.

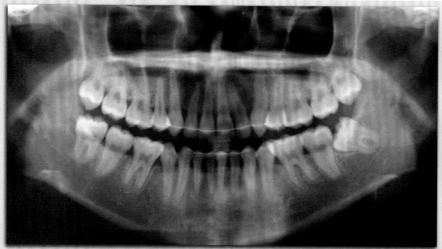

Fig. MPI 7–7. Posttreatment panoramic radiograph.

Table MPI 7-3.	Cephalometric Summary	
	Pretreatment	Posttreatment
SKELETAL		
SNA (degrees)	77.0	77.0
SNB (degrees)	71.0	70.5
ANB (degrees)	6.0	6.5
SN-ANS/PNS (degrees)	10.5	11.0
SN-GoMe (degrees)	43.0	44.0
N-ANS (mm)	60.0	61.0
ANS-Me (mm)	71.0	71.0
DENTAL		
U1-SN (degrees)	119	114.0
L1-GoMe (degrees)	91.0	91.0
U1-APo (mm)	7.0	7.0
L1-APo (mm)	4.0	4.0
SOFT TISSUE		
LS-PnPo' (mm)	–0.5	–1
LI-PnPo' (mm)	1.5	2

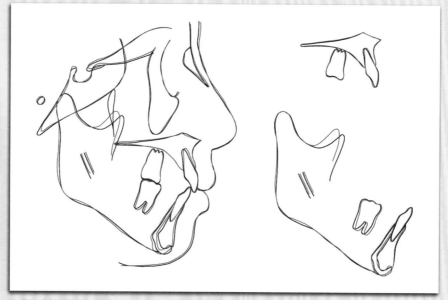

Fig. MPI 7–8. Cephalometric superimposition.

Protraction of Lower Posterior Teeth for Decompensation of Lower Incisors in a Retreatment Skeletal Class III Surgery Case

Junji Sugawara, Shiori Hashimoto

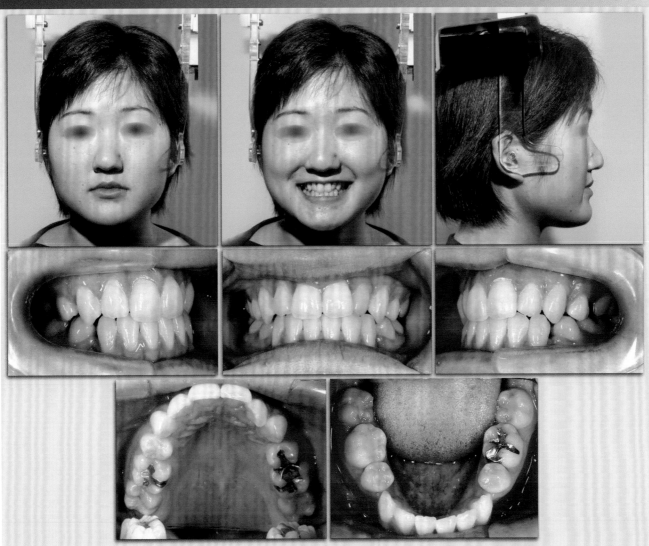

Fig. MPI 8-1. Pretreatment photographs.

The patient presented with an unstable jaw position, temporomandibular joint disorder, and a mandibular prognathic profile. She had previously undergone orthodontic treatment that included the extraction of four premolars. The treatment plan was to decompensate the lower incisors followed by en masse protraction of lower posterior teeth using the Skeletal Anchorage System (SAS).

After the lower arch was aligned, a negative overjet was anticipated, which would be subsequently corrected by a mandibular setback osteotomy.

The soft tissue surrounding the left anchor plate was infected on several occasions; however, the infections were controlled using routine antibiotics.

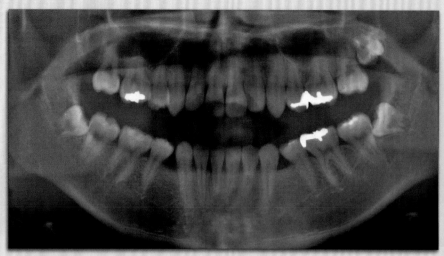

Fig. MPI 8–2. Pretreatment panoramic radiograph.

Table MPI 8-1.	Diagnosis and Treatment Goals	
	Diagnosis	Treatment Goals
SKELETAL		
Anteroposterior	Class III	Class I
Vertical	Normal	Normal
Transverse	Normal	Normal
DENTAL		
Right molar	Class III	Class I
Right canine	Class III	Class I
Left molar	Class III	Class I
Left canine	Class III	Class I
Upper right	0 mm crowding	None
Upper left	0 mm crowding	None
Lower right	1 mm spacing	None
Lower left	1 mm spacing	None
Missing teeth	No. 14, 24, 34, 44	No. 14, 24, 34, 44
Restore teeth	N/A	N/A
Overjet	1.5 mm	2.5 mm
Overbite	1.5 mm	2 mm
Upper ML	0.5 mm left of facial ML	0 mm to facial ML
Lower ML	0 mm to facial ML	0 mm to facial ML
SOFT TISSUE		
Profile	Concave	Straight
Lips	Competent	Competent
PERIODONTIUM		
Inadequate KT/TT	None	None
Gingival recession	None	None
Bone loss	None	None

KT/TT, Keratinized tissue/thin tissue; *ML,* midline; *N/A,* not applicable.

Table MPI 8-2.	Temporary Anchorage Device Summary	
Procedure	Data	
Appliances placed	21 Jan 2000	
TAD placed	19 Jun 2000	19 Jun 2000
Location of TAD	Buccal No. 35	Buccal No. 45
Type of TAD	MPI	MPI
TAD loaded	21 Jul 2000	21 Jul 2000
Healing duration	28 days	28 days
Force in grams	400	400
Mechanics used	Direct	Direct
TAD unloaded	3 Aug 2001	3 Aug 2001
TAD loading duration	12 months	12 months
TAD removed	18 Nov 2002	18 Nov 2002
Appliances removed	16 Apr 2003	
Treatment duration	39 months	

TAD, Temporary anchorage device; *MPI*, miniplate implant.

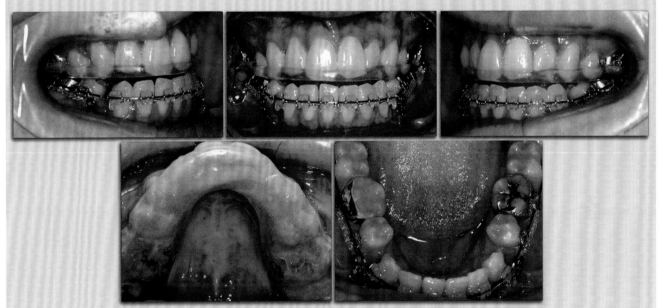

Fig. MPI 8-3. Initial temporary anchorage device (TAD) photographs.

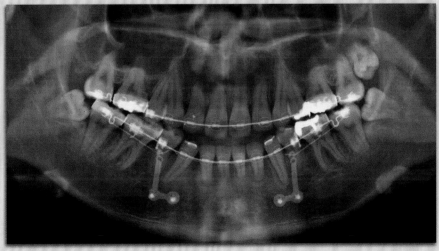

Fig. MPI 8-4. Initial TAD panoramic radiograph.

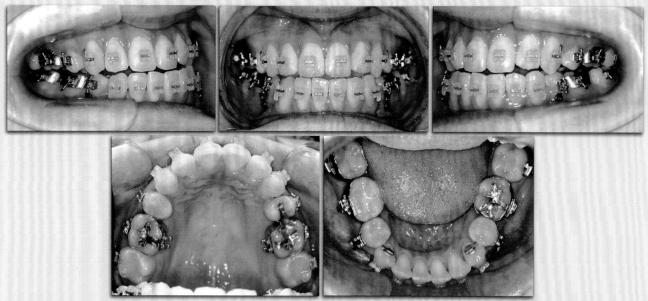

Fig. MPI 8-5. Progress TAD photographs.

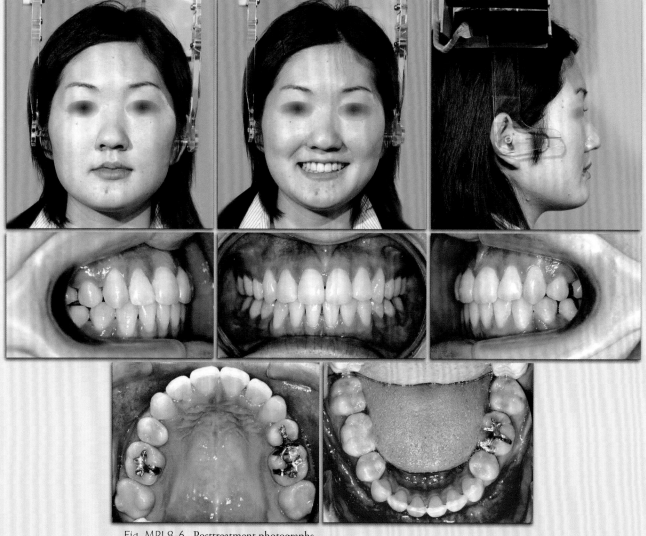

Fig. MPI 8-6. Posttreatment photographs.

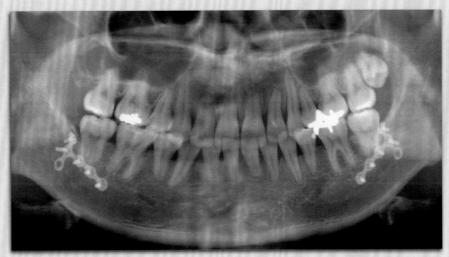

Fig. MPI 8-7. Posttreatment panoramic radiograph.

Table MPI 8-3.	Cephalometric Summary		
	Pretreatment	Posttreatment	1 Year Posttreatment
SKELETAL			
SNA (degrees)	83.0	83.0	83.0
SNB (degrees)	84.0	80.5	81.0
ANB (degrees)	–1.0	2.5	2.0
SN-ANS/PNS (degrees)	6.0	6.0	6.0
SN-GoMe (degrees)	25.5	26.5	26.0
N-ANS (mm)	55.5	55.5	55.5
ANS-Me (mm)	68.0	69.0	69.0
DENTAL			
U1-SN (degrees)	101.0	100.0	100.0
L1-GoMe (degrees)	81.5	94.0	93.0
U1-APo (mm)	1.0	2.0	2.0
L1-APo (mm)	–0.5	–1.0	–1.0
SOFT TISSUE			
LS-PnPo' (mm)	–6.0	–6.0	–6.0
LI-PnPo' (mm)	–4.0	–5.5	–5.5

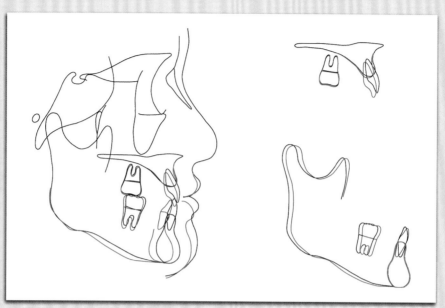

Fig. MPI 8-8. Cephalometric superimposition.

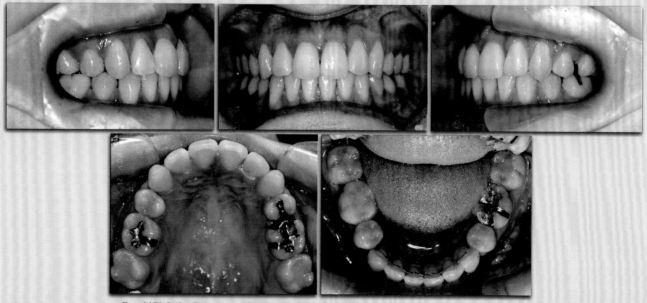

Fig. MPI 8-9. One-year posttreatment photographs.

CR-MPI

9

Protraction of Lower Molars to Avoid Dental Implants and Restorations

Ryoon-Ki Hong

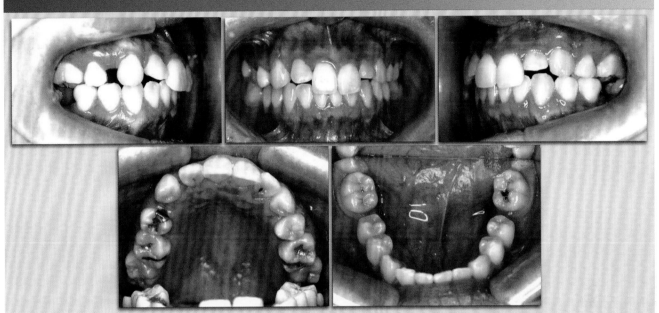

Fig. MPI 9-1. Pretreatment photographs.

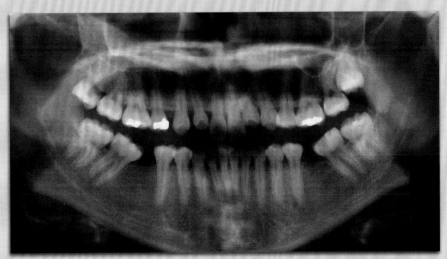

Fig. MPI 9-2. Pretreatment panoramic radiograph.

The patient had multiple missing teeth, considerable lip protrusion, and a midline discrepancy. To minimize restorative costs, the plan was to protract the lower second and third molars into the position of the first and second molars using miniplate implants (MPIs). Conventional mechanics were to be used on the upper arch.

During protraction of the lower right molars, the MPI became loose, and a miniscrew implant was placed on the facial surface between teeth No. 44 and 45 to complete protraction.

Table MPI 9-1.	Diagnosis and Treatment Goals	
	Diagnosis	Treatment Goals
SKELETAL		
Anteroposterior	Class I	Class I
Vertical	Normal	Normal
Transverse	Normal	Normal
DENTAL		
Right molar	Class II	Class I
Right canine	End-on Class III	Class I
Left molar	Class II	Class I
Left canine	End-on Class II	Class I
Upper right	4.2 mm spacing	None
Upper left	0 mm crowding	None
Lower right	5.7 mm spacing	None
Lower left	5.9 mm spacing	None
Missing teeth	No. 14, 24, 36, 46	No. 18, 28, 38, 48
Restore teeth	N/A	No. 17, 37, 47
Overjet	3.5 mm	3.5 mm
Overbite	3 mm	2.5 mm
Upper ML	2 mm left of facial ML	0 mm to facial ML
Lower ML	0 mm to facial ML	0 mm to facial ML
SOFT TISSUE		
Profile	Convex	Straight
Lips	Competent	Competent
PERIODONTIUM		
Inadequate KT/TT	None	None
Gingival recession	None	None
Bone loss	None	None

KT/TT, Keratinized tissue/thin tissue; *ML,* midline; *N/A,* not applicable.

Table MPI 9-2.	Temporary Anchorage Device Summary	
Procedure	Data	
Appliances placed	22 Mar 2000	
TAD placed	17 Mar 2001	17 Mar 2001
Location of TAD	Buccal No. 44-45	Buccal No. 34-35
Type of TAD	MPI	MPI
TAD loaded	7 Apr 2001	7 Apr 2001
Healing duration	21 days	21 days
Force in grams	200	200
Mechanics used	Direct	Direct
TAD unloaded	28 Apr 2003	28 Apr 2003
TAD loading duration	25 months	25 months
TAD removed	20 Aug 2003	20 Aug 2003
Appliances removed	10 Jul 2003	
Treatment duration	40 months	

TAD, Temporary anchorage device; *MPI,* miniplate implant.

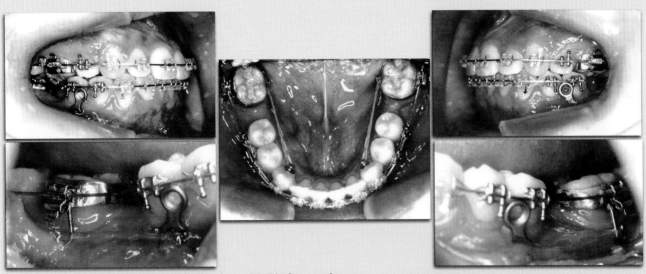

Fig. MPI 9-3. Initial temporary anchorage device (TAD) photographs.

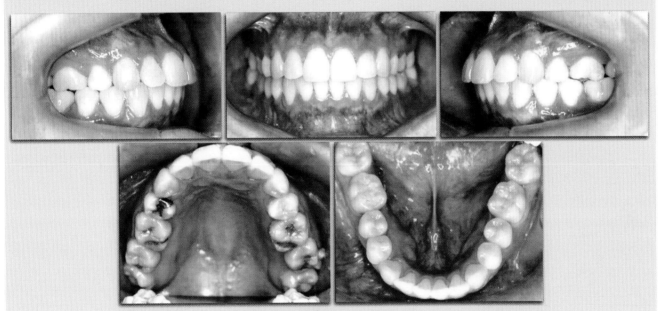

Fig. MPI 9-4. Posttreatment photographs.

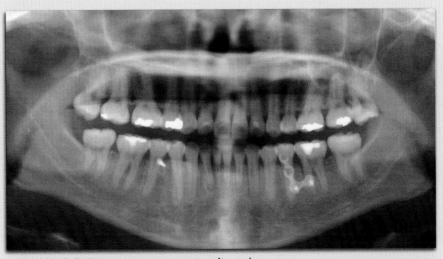

Fig. MPI 9-5. Posttreatment panoramic radiograph.

Table MPI 9-3.	Cephalometric Summary	
	Pretreatment	Posttreatment
SKELETAL		
SNA (degrees)	77.0	76.8
SNB (degrees)	75.2	74.1
ANB (degrees)	1.8	2.7
SN-ANS/PNS (degrees)	13.0	13.0
SN-GoMe (degrees)	43.5	43.5
N-ANS (mm)	58.0	58.0
ANS-Me (mm)	73.0	73.0
DENTAL		
U1-SN (degrees)	107.0	106.0
L1-GoMe (degrees)	80.5	94.0
U1-APo (mm)	10.5	9.5
L1-APo (mm)	5.0	6.0
SOFT TISSUE		
LS-PnPo' (mm)	3.0	2.5
LI-PnPo' (mm)	5.5	3.0

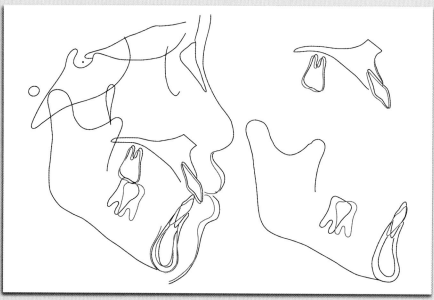

Fig. MPI 9–6. Cephalometric superimposition.

CR-MPI

Simultaneous Intrusion and Distalization of Upper and Lower Posterior Teeth for Correction of a Skeletal Open Bite

Junji Sugawara, Minayo Funatsu

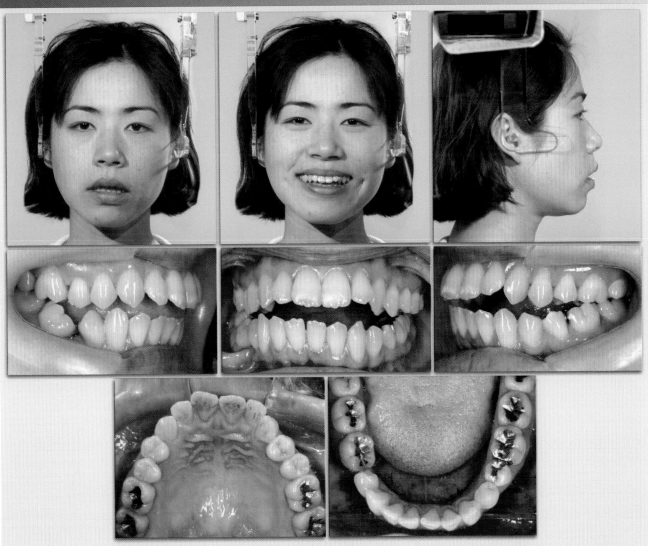

Fig. MPI 10-1. Pretreatment photographs.

The treatment plan was to use the Skeletal Anchorage System (SAS) to intrude the upper and lower posterior teeth and allow mandibular autorotation for open bite correction. The SAS would also be used for differential molar distalization to correct the deviated mandibular dental midline and to upright the lower right second and third molars to create space for the missing first molar.

Although minor, it appears that some relapse has occurred in the anterior overbite a year after the appliances were removed.

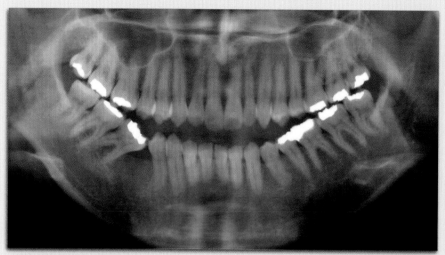

Fig. MPI 10-2. Pretreatment panoramic radiograph.

Table MPI 10-1.	Diagnosis and Treatment Goals	
	Diagnosis	Treatment Goals
SKELETAL		
Anteroposterior	Class II	Class I
Vertical	Open bite	Normal
Transverse	Normal	Normal
DENTAL		
Right molar	Class III	Class I
Right canine	Class II	Class I
Left molar	Class III	Class I
Left canine	Class I	Class I
Upper right	1 mm crowding	None
Upper left	1.5 mm crowding	None
Lower right	5 mm crowding	None
Lower left	4 mm crowding	None
Missing teeth	No. 45	No. 18, 28, 38, 45, 48
Restore teeth	N/A	No. 45
Overjet	4 mm	2.5 mm
Overbite	3-mm open bite	2 mm
Upper ML	0 mm to facial ML	0 mm to facial ML
Lower ML	4 mm right of facial ML	0 mm to facial ML
SOFT TISSUE		
Profile	Convex	Straight
Lips	Incompetent	Competent
PERIODONTIUM		
Inadequate KT/TT	None	None
Gingival recession	No. 16, 26, 44	Maintain
Bone loss	No. 46	Maintain
OTHER	Temporomandibular joint clicking	

KT/TT, Keratinized tissue/thin tissue; *ML,* midline; *N/A,* not applicable.

Table MPI 10-2. Procedure	Temporary Anchorage Device Summary Data			
Appliances placed	5 Jun 1996			
TAD placed	25 Nov 1996	25 Nov 1996	25 Nov 1996	25 Nov 1996
Location of TAD	Zygoma apical No. 16-17	Zygoma apical No. 26-27	Buccal apical No. 37	Buccal apical No. 47
Type of TAD	MPI	MPI	MPI	MPI
TAD loaded	7 mar 1997	7 mar 1997	7 mar 1997	7 mar 1997
Healing duration	90 days	90 days	90 days	90 days
Force in grams	500	500	500	500
Mechanics used	Direct	Direct	Direct	Direct
TAD unloaded	17 Jun 1998	17 Jun 1998	17 Jun 1998	17 Jun 1998
TAD loading duration	15 months	15 months	15 months	15 months
TAD removed	1 Sep 1998	1 Sep 1998	1 Sep 1998	1 Sep 1998
Appliances removed	14 Sep 1998			
Treatment duration	27 months			

TAD, Temporary anchorage device; *MPI*, miniplate implant.

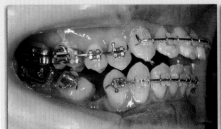 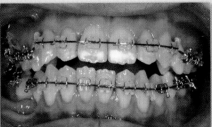 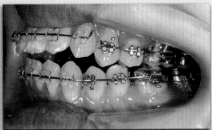

Fig. MPI 10-3. Initial temporary anchorage device (TAD) photographs.

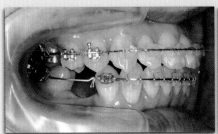 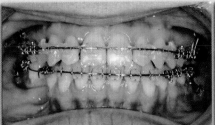 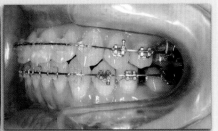

Fig. MPI 10-4. Progress TAD photographs.

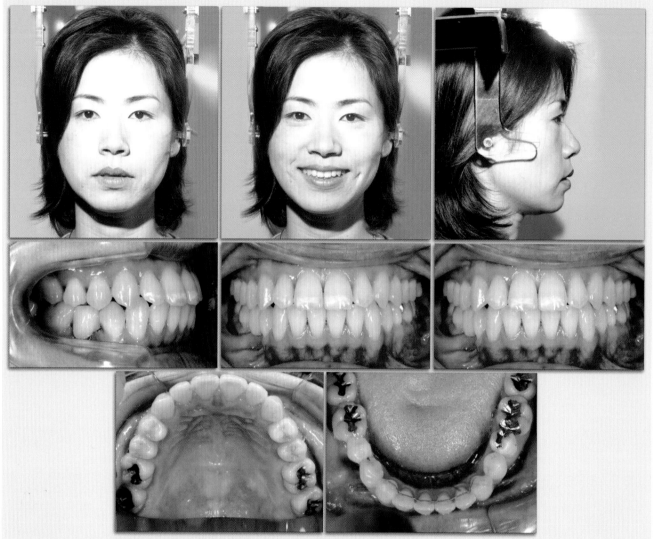

Fig. MPI 10–5. Posttreatment photographs.

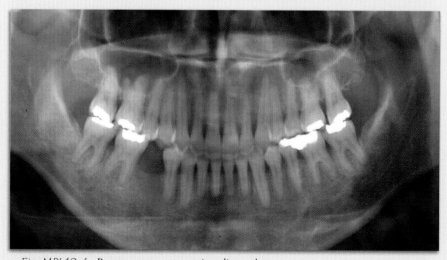

Fig. MPI 10–6. Posttreatment panoramic radiograph.

Table MPI 10-3.	Cephalometric Summary		
	Pretreatment	Posttreatment	1 Year Posttreatment
SKELETAL			
SNA (degrees)	84.0	84.0	84.0
SNB (degrees)	76.4	78.7	78.3
ANB (degrees)	7.6	5.3	5.7
SN-ANS/PNS (degrees)	13.5	13.5	13.5
SN-GoMe (degrees)	45.0	41.0	41.5
N-ANS (mm)	58.6	58.6	58.6
ANS-Me (mm)	76.8	71.8	72.0
DENTAL			
U1-SN (degrees)	108.5	109.5	108.5
L1-GoMe (degrees)	100.1	96.5	98.7
U1-APo (mm)	12.5	10.5	11.5
L1-APo (mm)	8.5	8.0	9.0
SOFT TISSUE			
LS-PnPo' (mm)	2.0	2.0	2.0
LI-PnPo' (mm)	6.5	6.0	6.0

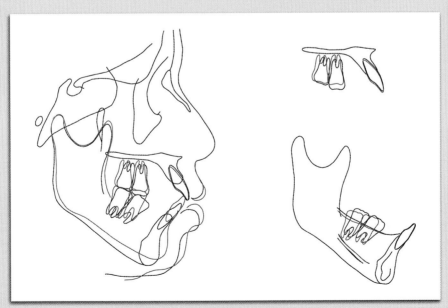

Fig. MPI 10-7. Cephalometric superimposition.

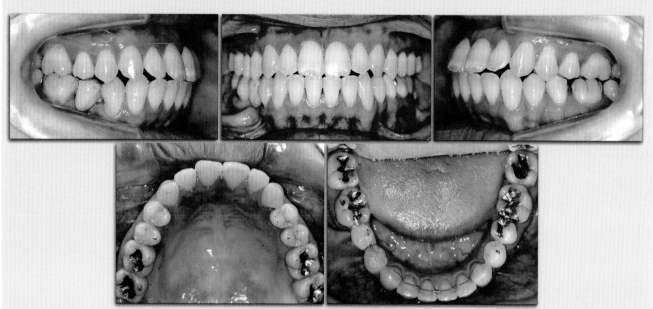

Fig. MPI 10-8. One-year posttreatment photographs.

CR–MPI

Upper and Lower Premolar Extraction Combined with Upper Posterior Intrusion to Correct a Skeletal Class III Malocclusion

Ryoon-Ki Hong

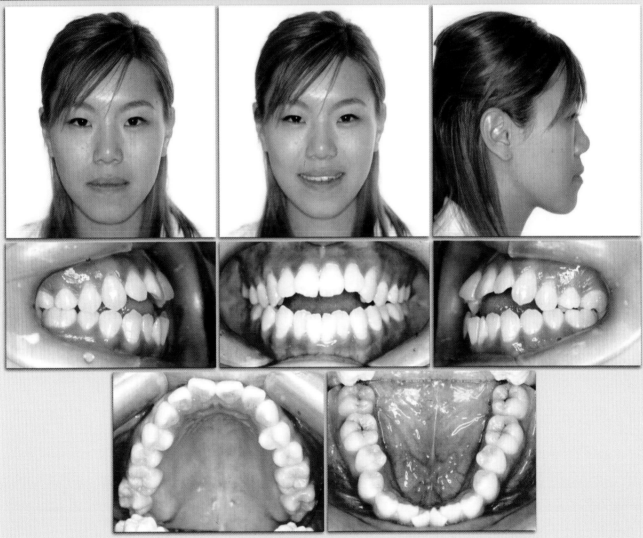

Fig. MPI 11-1. Pretreatment photographs.

The treatment plan was to use miniplate implants to intrude the upper posterior teeth and allow autorotation of the mandible. After upper posterior intrusion, the upper second and lower first premolars were to be extracted to finish correcting the buccal segment relationship.

Although the dental occlusion was improved, mandibular autorotation caused a decrease in ANB to a more Class III skeletal relationship. Frequent missed appointments by the patient made the total treatment time excessively prolonged.

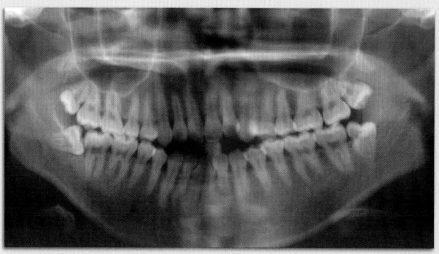

Fig. MPI 11-2. Pretreatment panoramic radiograph.

Table MPI 11-1.	Diagnosis and Treatment Goals	
	Diagnosis	Treatment Goals
SKELETAL		
Anteroposterior	Class III	Class III
Vertical	Open bite	Normal
Transverse	Normal	Normal
DENTAL		
Right molar	Class III	Class I
Right canine	Class III	Class I
Left molar	Class II	Class I
Left canine	Class III	Class I
Upper right	2.7 mm crowding	None
Upper left	2.3 mm crowding	None
Lower right	2.7 mm crowding	None
Lower left	2.4 mm crowding	None
Missing teeth	None	No. 15, 18, 25, 28, 34, 38, 44, 48
Restore teeth	N/A	No. 16, 17, 26, 27
Overjet	2 mm	3 mm
Overbite	3 mm open bite	2.5 mm
Upper ML	0 mm to facial ML	0 mm to facial ML
Lower ML	1 mm left of facial ML	0 mm to facial ML
SOFT TISSUE		
Profile	Concave	Concave
Lips	Incompetent	Competent
PERIODONTIUM		
Inadequate KT/TT	None	None
Gingival recession	None	None
Bone loss	None	None

KT/TT, Keratinized tissue/thin tissue; *ML,* midline; *N/A,* not applicable.

Table MPI 11-2.	Temporary Anchorage Device Summary	
Procedure	**Data**	
Appliances placed	30 Apr 2001	
TAD placed	10 Oct 2001	10 Oct 2001
Location of TAD	Buccal apical No. 15-17	Buccal apical No. 25-27
Type of TAD	MPI	MPI
TAD loaded	23 Oct 2001	23 Oct 2001
Healing duration	14 days	14 days
Force in grams	200	200
Mechanics used	Direct	Direct
TAD unloaded	22 Mar 2002	22 Mar 2002
TAD loading duration	5 months	5 months
TAD removed	7 Nov 2003	7 Nov 2003
Appliances removed	7 Nov 2003	
Treatment duration	31 months	

TAD, Temporary anchorage device; *MPI*, miniplate implant.

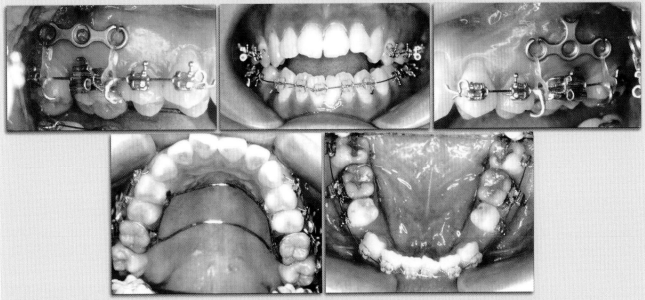

Fig. MPI 11-3. Initial temporary anchorage device (TAD) photographs.

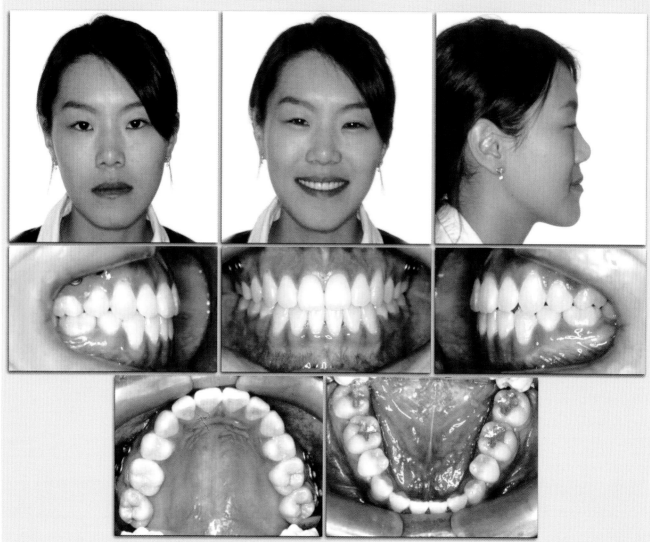

Fig. MPI 11-4. Posttreatment photographs.

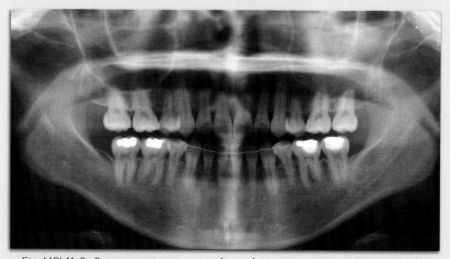

Fig. MPI 11-5. Posttreatment panoramic radiograph.

Table MPI 11–3.	Cephalometric Summary		
	Pretreatment	Posttreatment	1 Year Posttreatment
SKELETAL			
SNA (degrees)	78.2	78.1	78.1
SNB (degrees)	78.0	79.2	78.5
ANB (degrees)	0.2	–0.9	–0.4
SN-ANS/PNS (degrees)	7.0	7.0	7.0
SN-GoMe (degrees)	47.5	45.9	46.0
N-ANS (mm)	51.0	51.0	50.5
ANS-Me (mm)	81.6	79.4	79.6
DENTAL			
U1-SN (degrees)	111.8	111.7	94.8
L1-GoMe (degrees)	83.2	74.4	73.4
U1-APo (mm)	11.2	9.6	5.6
L1-APo (mm)	8.5	4.5	2.5
SOFT TISSUE			
LS-PnPo′ (mm)	0.0	0.0	–2.5
LI-PnPo′ (mm)	1.5	2.0	–0.5

TAD, Temporary anchorage device.

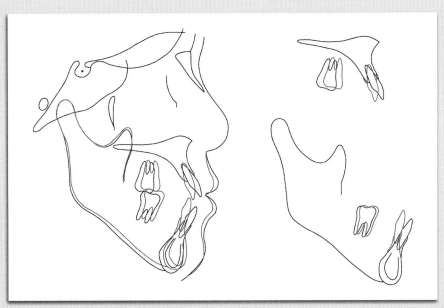

Fig. MPI 11–6. Cephalometric superimposition.

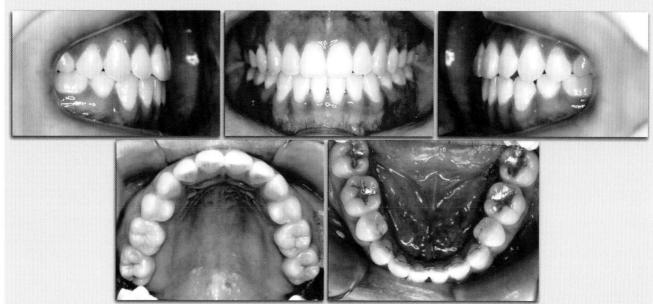

Fig. MPI 11-7. One-year posttreatment photographs.

CR–MPI

Intrusion of Overerupted Upper Anterior Teeth in a Skeletal Class II Deep Bite Case

Junji Sugawara, Makoto Nishimura

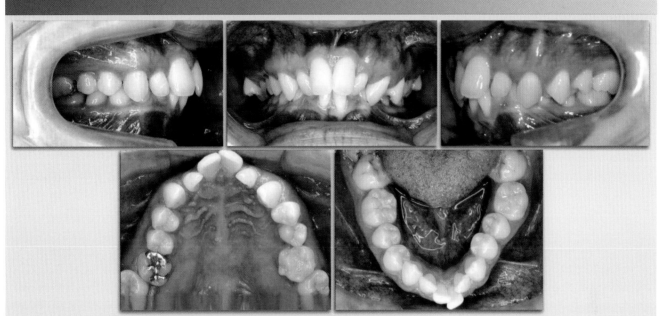

Fig. MPI 12-1. Pretreatment photographs.

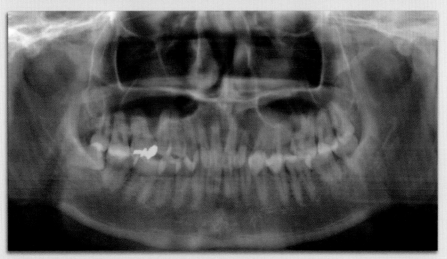

Fig. MPI 12-2. Pretreatment panoramic radiograph.

The plan was to use the Skeletal Anchorage System (SAS) to intrude and retract the overerupted upper anterior teeth. A traditional fixed bite plane was to be used to open the bite for correction of the bilateral buccal crossbite of the upper second molars. After the anterior teeth were intruded, the same miniplate implants would be used to retract the anterior teeth into a normal overjet relationship.

Table MPI 12-1.	Diagnosis and Treatment Goals	
	Diagnosis	Treatment Goals
SKELETAL		
Anteroposterior	Class II	Class I
Vertical	Deep bite	Normal
Transverse	Normal	Normal
DENTAL		
Right molar	End-on Class II	Class I
Right canine	Class II	Class I
Left molar	Class I	Class I
Left canine	Class II	Class I
Upper right	0.4 mm spacing	None
Upper left	0.9 mm crowding	None
Lower right	0.9 mm crowding	None
Lower left	1.2 mm crowding	None
Missing teeth	None	No. 18, 28, 38, 48
Restore teeth	N/A	N/A
Overjet	5 mm	3 mm
Overbite	6 mm	3.5 mm
Upper ML	0 mm to facial ML	0 mm to facial ML
Lower ML	0 mm to facial ML	0 mm to facial ML
SOFT TISSUE		
Profile	Convex	Convex
Lips	Competent	Competent
PERIODONTIUM		
Inadequate KT/TT	None	None
Gingival recession	None	None
Bone loss	None	None
OTHER	Bilateral buccal crossbite of No. 17 and 27	

KT/TT, Keratinized tissue/thin tissue; *ML,* midline; *N/A,* not applicable.

Table MPI 12-2.	Temporary Anchorage Device Summary	
Procedure	Data	
Appliances placed	13 May 2002	
TAD placed	20 May 2002	20 May 2002
Location of TAD	Piriform rim No. 13-14	Piriform rim No. 23-24
Type of TAD	MPI	MPI
TAD loaded	3 Jul 2002	3 Jul 2002
Healing duration	42 days	42 days
Force in grams	160	160
Mechanics used	Direct	Direct
TAD unloaded	13 Feb 2004	13 Feb 2004
TAD loading duration	18 months	18 months
TAD removed	4 Jun 2004	4 Jun 2004
Appliances removed	19 Mar 2004	
Treatment duration	22 months	

TAD, Temporary anchorage device; *MPI,* miniplate implant.

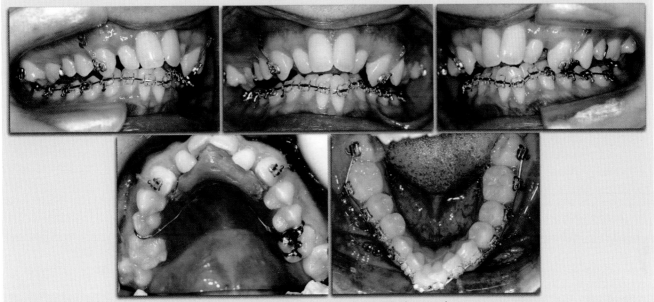

Fig. MPI 12-3. Initial temporary anchorage device (TAD) photographs.

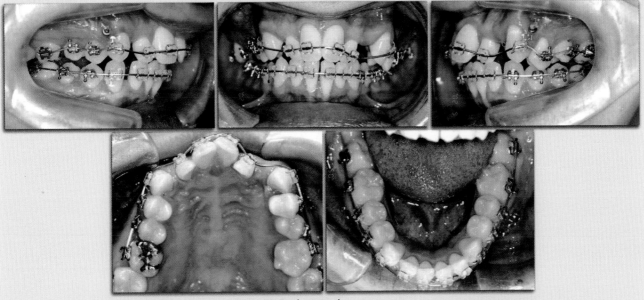

Fig. MPI 12-4. First progress TAD photographs.

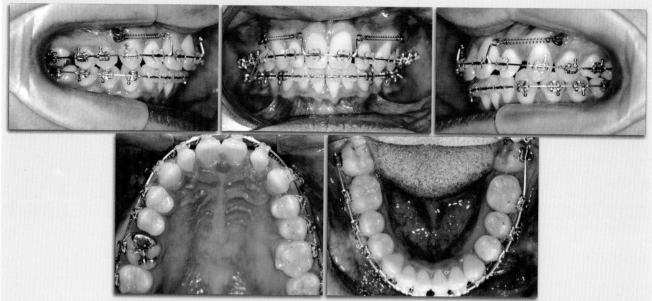

Fig. MPI 12-5. Second progress TAD photographs.

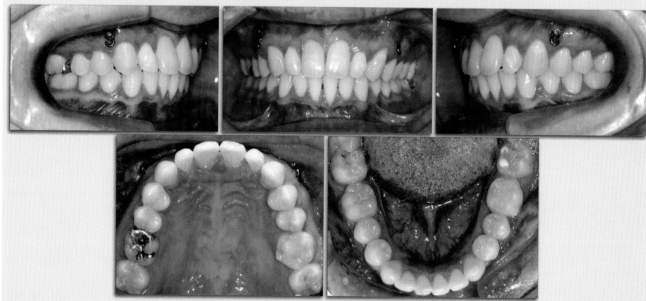

Fig. MPI 12-6. Posttreatment photographs.

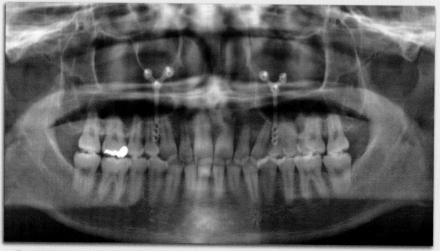

Fig. MPI 12-7. Posttreatment panoramic radiograph.

Table MPI 12-3.	Cephalometric Summary	
	Pretreatment	Posttreatment
SKELETAL		
SNA (degrees)	82.8	82.5
SNB (degrees)	78.9	78.4
ANB (degrees)	3.9	4.1
SN-ANS/PNS (degrees)	11.0	11.0
SN-GoMe (degrees)	20.0	20.9
N-ANS (mm)	59.9	60.3
ANS-Me (mm)	59.1	60.3
DENTAL		
U1-SN (degrees)	104.5	106.1
L1-GoMe (degrees)	104.0	104.8
U1-APo (mm)	6.0	4.0
L1-APo (mm)	0.0	0.0
SOFT TISSUE		
LS-PnPo′ (mm)	0.0	–1.0
LI-PnPo′ (mm)	2.0	1.5

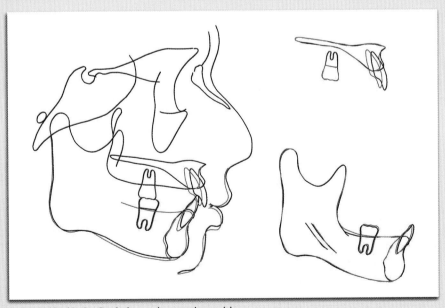

Fig. MPI 12-8. Cephalometric superimposition.

CR-MPI

13

Extrusion of a Deeply Impacted Lower First Molar Using an Upper MiniPlate Implant

Junji Sugawara, Takamasa Sannohe

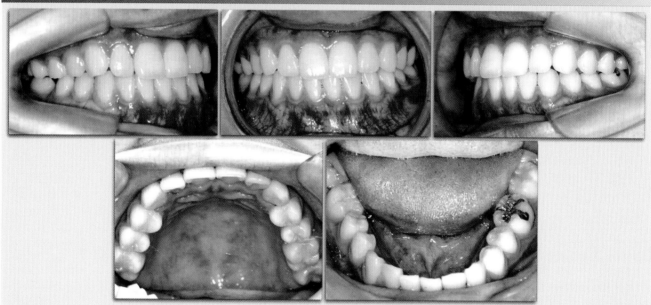

Fig. MPI 13-1. Pretreatment photographs.

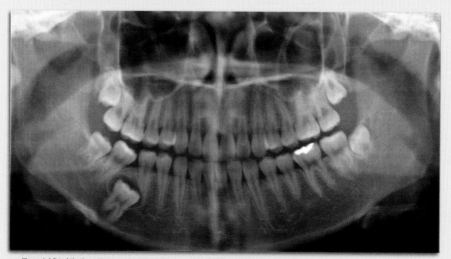

Fig. MPI 13-2. Pretreatment panoramic radiograph.

The treatment plan was to upright and distalize the lower right second molar to make space for the impacted first molar. After uprighting, the Skeletal Anchorage System (SAS) was to be placed in the upper right zygomatic buttress to extrude the deeply impacted lower right first molar.

Table MPI 13-1. Diagnosis and Treatment Goals		
	Diagnosis	Treatment Goals
SKELETAL		
Anteroposterior	Class I	Class I
Vertical	Normal	Normal
Transverse	Normal	Normal
DENTAL		
Right molar	Impacted	Class I
Right canine	Class I	Class I
Left molar	Class III	Class I
Left canine	Class III	Class I
Upper right	0 mm crowding	None
Upper left	0 mm crowding	None
Lower right	2.5 mm spacing	None
Lower left	2.5 mm crowding	None
Missing teeth	None	No. 18, 28, 38, 48
Restore teeth	N/A	N/A
Overjet	2.5 mm	2.5 mm
Overbite	2.8 mm	3 mm
Upper ML	0 mm to facial ML	0 mm to facial ML
Lower ML	2.5 mm right of facial ML	0 mm to facial ML
SOFT TISSUE		
Profile	Straight	Straight
Lips	Competent	Competent
PERIODONTIUM		
Inadequate KT/TT	None	None
Gingival recession	None	None
Bone loss	None	None
OTHER	No. 46 impacted; No. 47 tipped mesially	

KT/TT, Keratinized tissue/thin tissue; *ML*, midline; *N/A*, not applicable.

Table MPI 13-2. Temporary Anchorage Device Summary	
Procedure	Data
Appliances placed	15 May 2002
TAD placed	18 Sep 2002
Location of TAD	Zygomatic buttress apical No. 16-17
Type of TAD	MPI
TAD loaded	20 Jan 2003
Healing duration	56 days
Force in grams	50-100
Mechanics used	Direct
TAD unloaded	26 Mar 2004
TAD loading duration	17 months
TAD removed	14 Jun 2004
Appliances removed	26 Mar 2004
Treatment duration	22 months

TAD, Temporary anchorage device; *MPI*, miniplate implant.

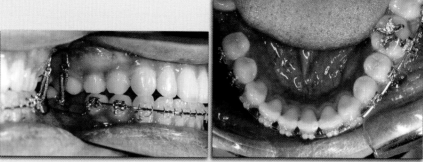

Fig. MPI 13-3. Initial temporary anchorage device (TAD) photographs.

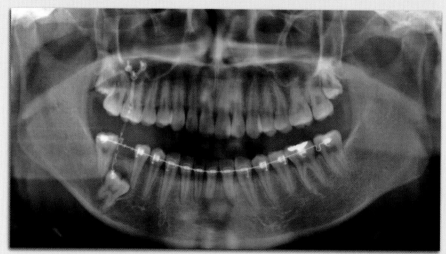

Fig. MPI 13-4. Initial TAD panoramic radiograph.

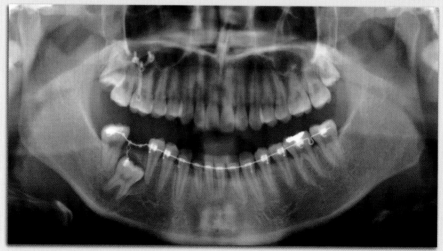

Fig. MPI 13-5. First progress TAD panoramic radiograph.

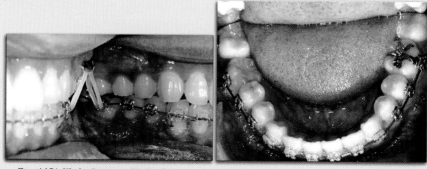

Fig. MPI 13-6. Progress TAD photographs.

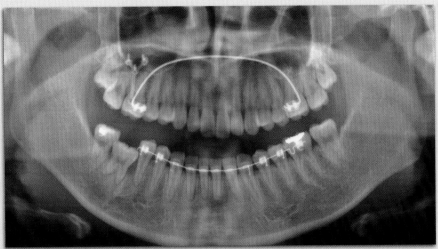

Fig. MPI 13-7. Second progress TAD panoramic radiograph.

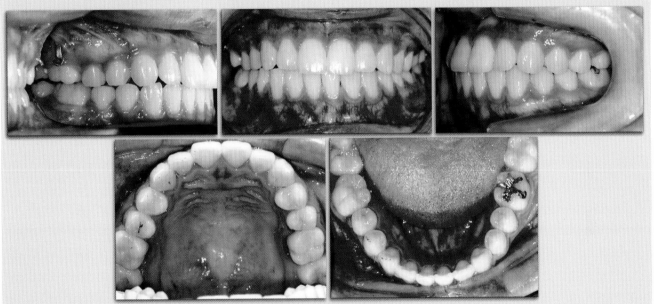

Fig. MPI 13-8.   Posttreatment photographs.

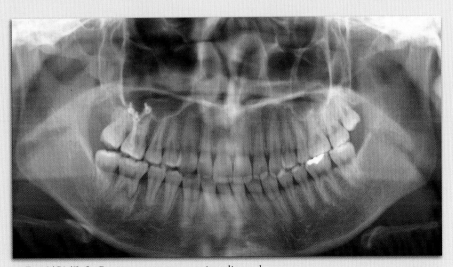

Fig. MPI 13-9. Posttreatment panoramic radiograph.

Table MPI 13–3.	Cephalometric Summary	
	Pretreatment	Posttreatment
SKELETAL		
SNA (degrees)	85.2	84.3
SNB (degrees)	81.9	81.2
ANB (degrees)	3.3	3.1
SN-ANS/PNS (degrees)	1.5	1.5
SN-GoMe (degrees)	30.7	31.8
N-ANS (mm)	56.5	56.9
ANS-Me (mm)	69.3	70.9
DENTAL		
U1-SN (degrees)	103.4	105.5
L1-GoMe (degrees)	90.8	95.1
U1-APo (mm)	4.0	6.5
L1-APo (mm)	1.5	2.5
SOFT TISSUE		
LS-PnPo′ (mm)	–2.0	–0.5
LI-PnPo′ (mm)	2.0	2.0

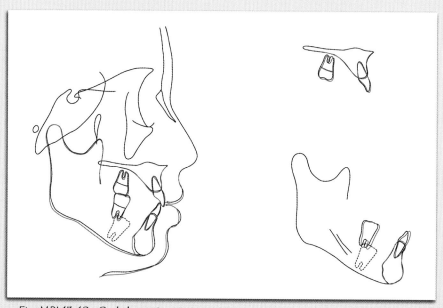

Fig. MPI 13–10. Cephalometric superimposition.

INDEX

Page numbers in bold type indicate case reports. Page numbers in italic type indicate illustrations.